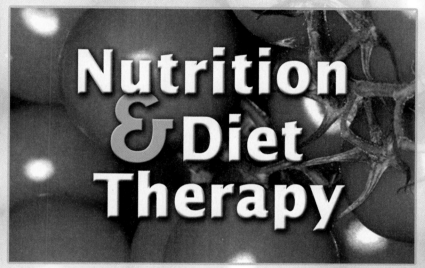

Nutrition & Diet Therapy

Nutrition & Diet Therapy

9th Edition

Ruth A. Roth, MS, RD

Park View Hospital, Fort Wayne, Indiana
and Indiana/Purdue University, Fort Wayne, Indiana

THOMSON

DELMAR LEARNING

Australia   Canada   Mexico   Singapore   Spain   United Kingdom   United States

THOMSON

DELMAR LEARNING

Nutrition & Diet Therapy, Ninth Edition
by Ruth A. Roth

Vice President,
Health Care Business Unit:
William Brottmiller

Director of Learning Solutions:
Matthew Kane

Acquisitions Editor:
Tamara Caruso

Senior Product Manager:
Elisabeth F. Williams

Editorial Assistant:
Tiffiny Adams

Marketing Director:
Jennifer McAvey

Marketing Channel Manager:
Michelle McTighe

Marketing Coordinator:
Danielle Pacella

Technology Director:
Laurie K. Davis

Technology Project Managers:
Mary Colleen Liburdi
Carolyn Fox

Production Director:
Carolyn Miller

Content Project Manager:
David Buddle

Library of Congress Cataloging-in-Publication Data

Roth, Ruth A.
  Nutrition & diet therapy / Ruth A. Roth—9th ed.
    p. cm.
  Includes bibliographical references and index.
    ISBN 1-4180-1826-0
    1. Diet therapy. 2. Nutrition. I. Title: Nutrition and diet therapy. II. Nutrition & diet therapy. III. Title

RM216.T738 2007
615.8/54 22

                              2006047296

ISBN-10: 1-4108-1826-0
ISBN-13: 978-1-4180-1826-9

NOTICE TO THE READER

*To my family and friends who love
and support me.*

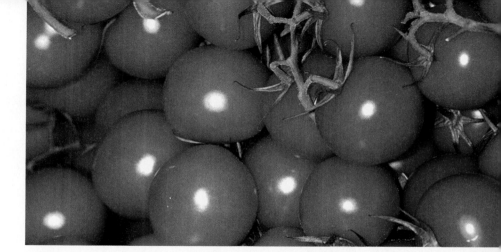

CONTENTS

vii

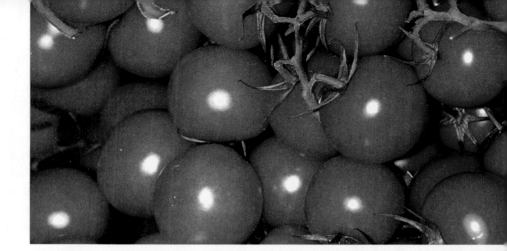

PREFACE

In our health-conscious society, the link between good nutrition and good health is seen everywhere, from magazine and newspaper headlines to television shows and web sites. Recipes for low-fat, heart healthy meals, fad diets, and stories about foods that claim to prevent certain diseases and health ailments abound. This presents a challenge to nurses working with clients to help them focus on improving both their nutrition and their overall health. *Nutrition & Diet Therapy,* 9th edition, provides sound nutritional information based upon fact. It is important that nurses have a solid foundation in the basic principles and concepts of good nutrition; then they can help clients debunk the myths and help them move toward better health through nutritional awareness.

Section 1, **Fundamentals of Nutrition,** includes chapters on the relationship of nutrition and health; planning a healthy diet; digestion, absorption, and metabolism; and chapters on each of the six nutrient groups (carbohydrates, lipids, proteins, vitamins, minerals, and water). Content has been thoroughly revised to embrace the MyPyramid guidelines.

Section 2, **Maintenance of Health Through Good Nutrition,** includes chapters on food related illnesses and allergies, diet planning during the various stages of life from pregnancy and lactation through infancy, childhood, adolescence, young and middle adulthood, and the senior years. This information provides sound knowledge of the changes in nutritional requirements across the lifespan.

Section 3, **Medical Nutrition Therapy,** includes discussion and research for many nutrition related disorders. It covers the effects of disease and surgery on nutrition, and the appropriate uses of diet therapy in restoring and

xiii

maintaining health. It includes chapters with specific nutritional information for clients requiring help with weight control, diabetes, cardiovascular disease, renal disease, gastrointestinal problems, and cancer. It also discusses the nutritional needs of surgical clients, clients suffering burns and infections including HIV, and clients requiring enteral and parenteral nutrition. There is also a chapter on the general nutritional care of clients.

Chapters follow a consistent format to help facilitate and enhance learning:

- **Objectives**—learning goals to be achieved upon completion of the chapter
- **Key Terms**—a list of terms used in text and defined in the margin, these are also included in the master glossary
- **In the Media**—new boxes highlight current trends, events, and fads, and the potential impact on clients' health
- **Exploring the Web**—directions to internet resources and web sites
- **Summary**—a brief narrative overview of the most important chapter highlights
- **Discussion Topics**—critical thinking activities which encourage synthesis and application of new concepts
- **Suggested Activities**—creative suggestions on how to implement the knowledge presented in the chapter
- **Review**—study questions to test understanding of content and to help prepare for examinations

NEW TO THIS EDITION

- The new **MyPyramid** guidelines and recommendations are embraced throughout the text.
- Many new and revised reality-based **Case in Points** have been incorporated; all case studies now include a new **Rate this Plate** challenge asking for evaluation of a proposed meal plan for a client.
- The national obesity epidemic is highlighted in a new feature box entitled **Supersize USA.**
- Expanded life span coverage is addressed with a new **Nutrition through the Life Cycle** feature, which outlines nutritional concerns at each stage of life.
- A **CD icon** is included with the key terms list, Case in Point, and Review Question features, to encourage use of this valuable electronic resource to further learning.
- A new **student tutorial CD** packaged with the text includes StudyWare activities, study questions, and responses to the Case in Point questions, Rate this Plate challenges, and review questions.
- A new appendix offers the updated **Dietary Guidelines for Americans.**

StudyWare™ CD-ROM

A free StudyWare CD-ROM is packaged with each text. It is a computerized flashcard question-and-answer program designed to help users learn and retain large amounts of information quickly and easily. This CD-ROM contains terms and definitions in a question-and-answer format to aid in overall understanding of the complexity of nutritional concepts. This unique program provides a fun, self-paced environment for anyone learning or brushing up on nutrition.

Minimum System Requirements

Operating System: Microsoft Windows 98 SE, Windows 2000, or Windows XP

Processor: Pentium PC 500 MHz or higher (750 Mhz recommended)

Memory: 64 MB of RAM (128 MB recommended)

Screen Resolution: 800 × 600 pixels

Color Depth: 16-bit color (thousands of colors)

Macromedia Flash Player V7.x. The Macromedia Flash Player is free, and can be downloaded from http://www.macromedia.com

SUPPLEMENTAL MATERIALS
Electronic Classroom Manager

This provides a complete customizable resource for the instructor. *The Electronic Classroom Manager* contains a customizable version of the Instructor's Manual that contains teaching strategies, answers to text questions, listings of additional resources, critical thinking exercises that can be done in small groups or as a whole class; a PowerPoint presentation correlating to each chapter of the text; and a computerized testbank with a variety of questions such as multiple choice, short answer, true and false, and matching to customize exams and quizzes.

ISBN 1-4180-1827-9

Web Tutor

WebTutor™ is an exciting online ancillary that takes your course beyond the classroom boundaries. WebTutor provides a content-rich, web-based teaching and learning environment that reinforces and helps clarify complex concepts. Elements include advance preparation, objectives, overview, class notes, discussion, glossary, multiple choice questions, and web links. Rich communication tools for instructors and students include a course calendar, chat, e-mail, threaded discussions, and a white board. WebTutor is available in both the WebCT and Blackboard platforms.

WebTutor on Blackboard
ISBN 1-4180-6239-1
WebTutor on WebCT
ISBN 1-4180-6240-5

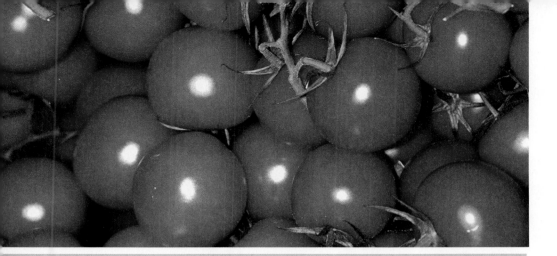

ACKNOWLEDGMENTS

The author wishes to express her appreciation to the following people:

Tom Donaldson
Rebecca Leichty, LPN
Beth Williams
Tiffiny Adams

Contributor to Case in Point Features
Margie Read, RN, BS, CNN
Clinical Educator
Renal Care Group
Fort Wayne, Indiana

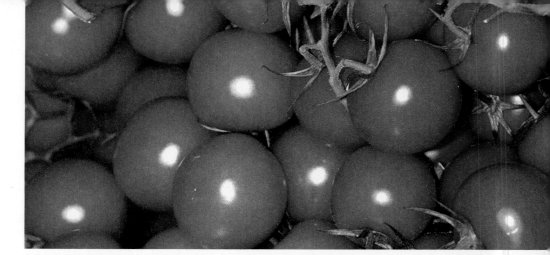

REVIEWERS

Jamie Erskine, RD, PhD
Associate Professor, Community Health & Nutrition
University of Northern Colorado
Greeley, Colorado

Paula Gribble, RN, BSN, MSAS
Chair, Nursing and Allied Health
Coastal Carolina Community College
Jacksonville, North Carolina

Teresa Grooms, RN, MSN
Nursing Instructor
Southern State Community College
Hillsboro, Ohio

Donna Headrick, RN, MSN, FNP
Professor
Bakersfield College
Bakersfield, California

Sandy Killam-Hall, MS, RD, LD
Adjunct Instructor of Culinary Arts
Art Institute of Atlanta
Atlanta, Georgia

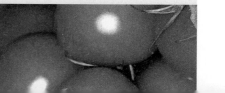

Susan Lamanna, RN, MA, MSN, ANP
Associate Professor
Onondaga Community College
Syracuse, New York

Patricia Lisk, RN, BSN
Instructor
Augusta Technical College
Augusta, Georgia

Marie Loisy, RN, MSN, FNP
Associate Professor of Nursing
Chattanooga State Technical Community College
Chattanooga, Tennessee

Pamela Y. Mahon, RN, PhD
Associate Professor of Nursing
Kingsborough Community College
Brooklyn, New York

Myrtle McCullock, RD, EdD
Clinical Assistant Professor
Georgetown University Schools of Medicine
Nursing and Health Studies
Washington, DC

Michael Meir, MD
Director
Technical Career Institute
New York, New York

Deborah Ochsner, MS, CMT
Dean of Allied Health Programs
Institute of Business and Medical Careers
Fort Collins, Colorado

Dr. Linda Parker, RD, LD, DSc
Assistant Professor in Nutrition
University of Miami
Miami, Florida

Patricia Terry, RD, PhD, LD
Chair, Department of Nutrition and Dietetics
Samford University
Birmingham, Alabama

Patricia Weaver Thompson, RN, BA
Program Director, Practical Nursing
West Central Technical College
Waco, Georgia

Karen Ward, RN, PhD
Professor
Middle Tennessee State University
School of Nursing
Murfreesboro, Tennessee

HOW TO USE THIS TEXT

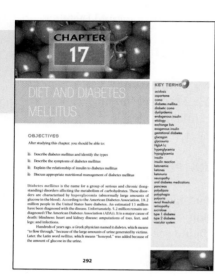

OBJECTIVES

Read the chapter Objectives before reading the chapter content to set the stage for learning. Return to the Objectives when the chapter study is complete to see which entries you can respond to with, "Yes, I can do that."

KEY TERMS

Glance over this list of terms before you tackle the chapter. Flip through the pages to check the definitions in the margins, and make a list of those terms which are unfamiliar. As you study, use the StudyWARE™ activities to test your learning; then when you complete the chapter, verify that you have mastered the meanings of the terms.

SUPERSIZE USA

Obesity has become a national health concern. Read over these boxes to find out why, and also for suggestions on what you, as a consumer and as a nurse, can do to help curb this trend.

SPOTLIGHT ON LIFE CYCLE

Nutritional concerns and needs will change at each stage of life. Test your knowledge of the needs of children, adolescents, pregnant women, and the elderly.

IN THE MEDIA

Which of these "hot topics" do you already know something about? Check here for current trends, events, and fads, and understand the potential impact on clients' health.

EXPLORING THE WEB

Be sure to visit these web sites for more depth on chapter topics. These are also excellent sources for information to make care plans and teaching guides.

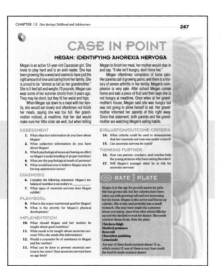

CASE IN POINTS

Two case studies conclude each chapter. Read these real-life stories, then look at the sample diet and **Rate this Plate.** Visit the StudyWARE™ disk to see how your answers match up to those of the experts.

SUMMARY

This brief narrative overview of the most important chapter highlights is ideal for testing your grasp of the chapter material. Always start your study sessions with a quick glance at the Summary to refresh your memory on the basics of the chapter.

DISCUSSION TOPICS

Critical thinking is key to your success as a nurse. Use these activities to synthesize and apply what you have read and learned.

SUGGESTED ACTIVITIES

Put your knowledge to the test; see how many of these activities you can successfully complete once you finish studying the chapter. Make a list of any areas needing additional attention.

REVIEW

These study questions are in multiple choice format, perfect for preparing for your nursing examinations.

ONLINE RESOURCES

A key study tool is available on the internet. Visit the **WebTutor** course for valuable course content, exercises, class notes, web links, and more.

HOW TO USE STUDYWARE™

The StudyWARE™ software helps you learn terms and concepts in *Nutrition & Diet Therapy*, 9th edition. As you study each chapter in the text, be sure to explore the activities in the corresponding chapter in the software. Use StudyWARE™ as your own private tutor to help you learn the material in your *Nutrition & Diet Therapy*, 9th edition, textbook.

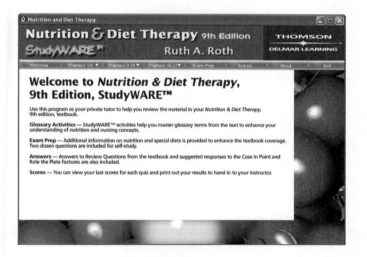

Getting started is easy. Install the software by inserting the CD-ROM into your computer's CD-ROM drive and following the on-screen instructions. When you open the software, enter your first and last name so the software can store your quiz results. Then choose a chapter from the menu to take a quiz or explore one of the activities.

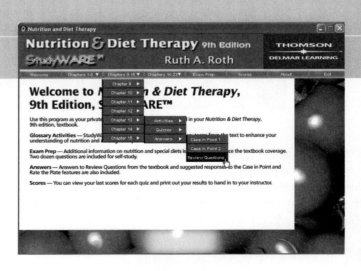

Menus

You can access the menus from wherever you are in the program. The menus include Chapter Activities, Exam Prep, and Scores.

Each chapter corresponds to a chapter in the *Nutrition & Diet Therapy*, 9th edition, textbook. You can start with glossary activities, which may include crossword puzzles and a concentration game. You can take quizzes to test your knowledge and verify your understanding of the content. Then proceed to check your responses to the Case in Point and Rate This Plate features from the text. Answers to the text Review Questions are also included.

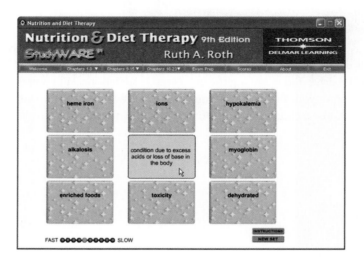

Have fun while increasing your knowledge!

Section One

FUNDAMENTALS

OF

NUTRITION

THE RELATIONSHIP OF NUTRITION AND HEALTH

OBJECTIVES

After studying this chapter, you should be able to:

- Name the six classes of nutrients and their primary functions
- Recognize common characteristics of well-nourished people
- Recognize symptoms of malnutrition
- Describe ways in which nutrition and health are related
- List the four basic steps in nutrition assessment

The United States was historically referred to as the "melting pot" because it represented people of many nationalities who immigrated to this country in hopes of finding a better life. The individuals in this country bring all their cultural diversities with them, including their cuisine. Many choose to assimilate immediately by learning the language and trying the foods of their new country; others may favor the foods and customs of their country of origin. The diet that individuals follow will determine, to a large extent, their health, growth, and development. It has never been more imperative that active measures be taken to make our social, cultural, political, and economic environment in relation to diet a health-promoting one.

Taking care of one's health is all about prevention. In the past, the focus was on treatment of diseases, with little, if any, attention to prevention. Prevention, however, can often be less costly than treatment and offer a better quality of life for an individual as well as the community. Nutrition and diet choice form a logical starting point for preventive health care measures and education to improve quality of life.

wellness
a way of life that integrates body, mind, and spirit

Achieving **wellness** that integrates body, mind, and spirit should be the main goal in life. This can be accomplished through lifestyle changes such as focusing on healthy food choices, not smoking, participating in regular physical activity, and maintaining a healthy weight. Expanding one's mind through continued education, in both nutrition and other areas, and finding a source of inner strength to deal with life changes will all contribute to one's sense of wellness.

Living a long life without major health problems is possible. The younger one is when positive changes are made, the healthier one is throughout the life span.

NUTRIENTS AND THEIR FUNCTIONS

nutrients
chemical substances found in food that are necessary for good health

To maintain health and function properly, the body must be provided with **nutrients.** Nutrients are chemical substances that are necessary for life. They are divided into six classes:

- Carbohydrates (CHO)
- Fats (lipids)
- Proteins
- Vitamins
- Minerals
- Water

essential nutrients
nutrients found only in food

The body can make small amounts of some nutrients, but most must be obtained from food in order to meet the body's needs. Those available only in food are called **essential nutrients.** There are about 40 of them, and they are found in all six nutrient classes.

The six nutrient classes are chemically divided into two categories: organic and inorganic (Table 1-1). Organic nutrients contain hydrogen, oxygen, and carbon. (Carbon is an element found in all living things.) Before the body can use organic nutrients, it must break them down into their smallest components. Inorganic nutrients are already in their simplest forms when the body ingests them, except for water.

Table 1-1 *The Six Essential Nutrients and Their Functions*

ORGANIC NUTRIENTS	FUNCTION
Carbohydrates	Provide energy
Fats	Provide energy
Proteins	Build and repair body tissues
	Provide energy
Vitamins	Regulate body processes
INORGANIC NUTRIENTS	**FUNCTION**
Minerals	Regulate body processes
Water	Regulates body processes

Each nutrient participates in at least one of the following functions:

- Providing the body with energy
- Building and repairing body tissue
- Regulating body processes

Carbohydrates (CHO), proteins, and **fats (lipids)** furnish energy. Proteins are also used to build and repair body tissues with the help of vitamins and minerals. **Vitamins, minerals,** and **water** help regulate the various body processes such as **circulation, respiration, digestion,** and **elimination.**

Each nutrient is important, but none works alone. For example, carbohydrates, proteins, and fats are necessary for energy, but to provide it, they need the help of vitamins, minerals, and water. Proteins are essential for building and repairing body tissue, but without vitamins, minerals, and water, they are ineffective. Foods that contain substantial amounts of nutrients are described as **nutritious** or **nourishing.** Nutrients are discussed in detail in Chapters 4 through 9.

CHARACTERISTICS OF GOOD NUTRITION

Most people find pleasure in eating. Eating allows one to connect with family and friends in pleasant surroundings. This connection creates pleasant memories. Unfortunately, in social situations it is easy for one to make food choices that may not be conducive to good health.

What determines when one needs to eat? Does one wait until the body signals hunger or eat when one sees food or when the clock says it is time? Hunger is the physiological need for food. Appetite is a psychological desire for food based on pleasant memories. When the body signals hunger, that is the indication that there is a decrease in blood glucose that supplies the body with energy. If one ignores the signal and hunger becomes intense, it is possible to make poor food choices. The choices one makes will determine one's nutrition status. A person who habitually chooses to eat, or not to eat, as a way of coping with life's emotional struggles may be suffering from an eating disorder. The various eating disorders will be discussed in Chapter 16.

Once foods have been eaten, the body must process it before it can be used. **Nutrition** is the result of the processes whereby the body takes in and uses food for growth, development, and the maintenance of health. These processes include digestion, absorption, and metabolism. (They are discussed in Chapter 3.) One's physical condition as determined by the diet is called **nutritional status.**

Nutrition helps determine the height and weight of an individual. Nutrition also can affect the body's ability to resist disease, the length of one's life, and the state of one's physical and mental well-being (Figure 1-1).

Good nutrition enhances appearance and is commonly exemplified by shiny hair, clear skin, clear eyes, erect posture, alert expressions, and firm flesh on well-developed bone structures. Good nutrition aids emotional adjustments, provides stamina, and promotes a healthy appetite. It also helps establish regular sleep and elimination habits (Table 1-2).

---

carbohydrates (CHO)
the nutrient class providing the major source of energy in the average diet

proteins
the only one of the six essential nutrient classes containing nitrogen

fats (lipids)
highest calorie-value nutrient class

vitamins
organic substances necessary for life although they do not, independently, provide energy

minerals
one of many inorganic substances essential to life and classified generally as minerals

water
major constituent of all living cells; composed of hydrogen and oxygen

circulation
the body process whereby the blood is moved throughout the body

respiration
breathing

digestion
breakdown of food in the body in preparation for absorption

elimination
evacuation of wastes

nutritious
foods or beverages containing substantial amounts of essential nutrients

nourishing
foods or beverages that provide substantial amounts of essential nutrients

nutrition
the result of those processes whereby the body takes in and uses food for growth, development, and the maintenance of health

nutritional status
one's physical condition as determined by diet

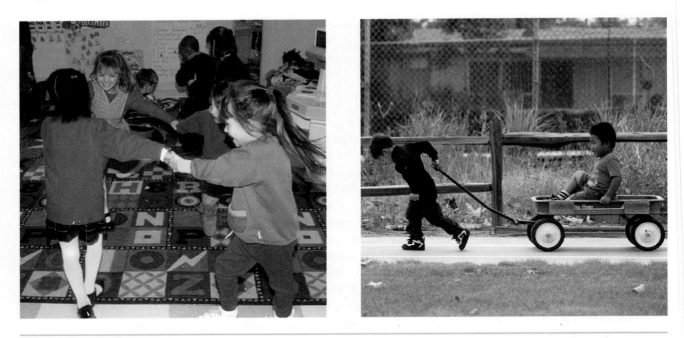

Figure 1-1 *Good nutrition shows in the happy faces of these children.*

Table 1-2 *Characteristics of Nutritional Status*

GOOD	POOR
Alert expression	Apathy
Shiny hair	Dull, lifeless hair
Clear complexion with good color	Greasy, blemished complexion with poor color
Bright, clear eyes	Dull, red-rimmed eyes
Pink, firm gums and well-developed teeth	Red, puffy, receding gums and missing or cavity-prone teeth
Firm abdomen	Swollen abdomen
Firm, well-developed muscles	Underdeveloped, flabby muscles
Well-developed bone structure	Bowed legs, "pigeon" breast
Normal weight for height	Overweight or underweight
Erect posture	Slumped posture
Emotional stability	Easily irritated; depressed; poor attention span
Good stamina; seldom ill	Easily fatigued; frequently ill
Healthy appetite	Excessive or poor appetite
Healthy, normal sleep habits	Insomnia at night; fatigued during day
Normal elimination	Constipation or diarrhea

MALNUTRITION

⟳ **malnutrition**
poor nutrition

Malnutrition can be caused by overnutrition (excess energy or nutrient intake) or undernutrition (deficient energy or nutrient intake). We usually think of malnutrition as a condition that results when the cells do not receive an ad-

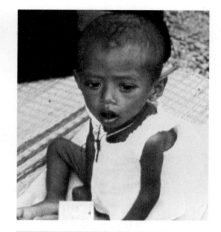

SUPERSIZE USA

Supersizing in the fast-food industry and large quantities served in restaurants lead to portion distortion. Those growing up in the supersized world may have no concept of what constitutes a normal portion. Children who are encouraged to, or have been made to, eat everything on their plates may feel compelled to finish their supersized meals, easily contributing to obesity and type 2 diabetes.

Figure 1-2 *The poor-quality hair, mottled complexion, dull expression, spindly arms and legs, and bloated abdomen of this baby girl exemplify many signs of malnutrition. (Courtesy of the Centers for Disease Control and Prevention, Public Health Image Library)*

equate supply of the essential nutrients because of poor diet or poor utilization of food (Figure 1-2). Sometimes it occurs because people do not or cannot eat enough of the foods that provide the essential nutrients to satisfy body needs. At other times people may eat well-balanced diets but suffer from diseases that prevent normal usage of the nutrients.

Overnutrition has become a larger problem in the United States than undernutrition. Overeating and the ingestion of megadoses of various vitamins and minerals (without prescription) are two major causes of overnutrition in the United States.

Nutrient Deficiency

A nutrient deficiency occurs when a person lacks one or more nutrients over a period of time. Nutrient deficiencies are classified as primary or secondary. Primary deficiencies are caused by inadequate dietary intake. Secondary deficiencies are caused by something other than diet, such as a disease condition that may cause malabsorption, accelerated excretion, or destruction of the nutrients. Nutrient deficiencies can result in malnutrition.

INDIVIDUALS AT RISK FROM POOR NUTRITIONAL INTAKE

Teenagers may eat often but at unusual hours. They may miss regularly scheduled meals, become hungry, and satisfy their hunger with foods that have low nutrient density such as potato chips, cakes, soda, and candy. Foods with low **nutrient density** provide an abundance of calories, but the nutrients are primarily carbohydrates and fats and, except for sodium, very limited amounts of proteins, vitamins, and minerals. Teenagers are subject to **peer pressure**; that is, they are easily influenced by the opinions of their friends. If friends favor foods with low nutrient density, it is difficult for a teenager to differ with them. Crash diets, which unfortunately are common among teens, sometimes result in a form of malnutrition. This condition occurs because some nutrients are eliminated from the diet when the types of foods eaten are severely restricted.

Pregnancy increases a woman's hunger and the need for certain nutrients, especially proteins, minerals, and vitamins. Pregnancy during adolescence requires extreme care in food selection. The young mother-to-be requires a diet that provides sufficient nutrients for the developing fetus as well as for her own still-growing body.

nutrient density
nutrient value of foods compared with number of calories

peer pressure
pressure of one's friends and colleagues of the same age

EXPLORING THE WEB

Search the Web to find information on iron deficiency and iron deficiency anemia. Is low iron intake the only cause? Who is at most risk? What mental and physical consequences of inadequate iron intake can occur?

SPOTLIGHT on Life Cycle

Infants, toddlers, adolescents (teenagers), the elderly, and pregnant women (especially teenagers) are at greater risk for malnutrition than the rest of the population. Infants and toddlers whose parents lack knowledge of proper nutrition and portion sizes will suffer the consequences of poor or inadequate nutrition choices. It may be difficult for toddlers who are "picky" eaters to obtain all their needed nutrients from food.

Many factors influence nutrition in the elderly. Depression, loneliness, lack of income, inability to shop, inability to prepare meals, and the state of overall health can all lead to malnutrition. Chapter 15 is another source of information on the elderly.

CUMULATIVE EFFECTS OF NUTRITION

There is an increasing concern among health professionals regarding the **cumulative effects** of nutrition. Cumulative effects are the results of something that is done repeatedly over many years. For example, eating excessive amounts of saturated fats (saturated fats are discussed in Chapter 5) for many years contributes to **atherosclerosis,** which leads to heart attacks. Years of overeating can cause **obesity** and may also contribute to hypertension, type 2 (non-insulin-dependent) diabetes, gallbladder disease, foot problems, certain cancers, and even personality disorders.

Deficiency Diseases

When nutrients are seriously lacking in the diet for an extended period, **deficiency diseases** can occur. The most common form of deficiency disease in the United States is **iron deficiency,** which is caused by a lack of the mineral iron and can cause iron deficiency anemia, which is discussed further in Chapter 8. Iron deficiency is particularly common among children and women. Iron is a necessary component of the blood and is lost during each menstrual period. In addition, the amount of iron needed during childhood and pregnancy is greater than normal because of the growth of the child or the fetus.

Rickets is another example of a deficiency disease. It causes poor bone formation in children and is due to insufficient calcium and vitamin D. These same deficiencies cause **osteomalacia** in young adults and **osteoporosis** in older adults. Osteomalacia is sometimes called "adult rickets." It causes the bones to soften and may cause the spine to bend and the legs to become bowed. Osteoporosis is a condition that causes bones to become porous and excessively

cumulative effects
results of something done repeatedly over many years

atherosclerosis
a form of arteriosclerosis affecting the intima (inner lining) of the artery walls

obesity
excessive body fat, 20% above average

deficiency diseases
disease caused by the lack of one or more specific nutrients

iron deficiency
intake of iron is adequate, but the body has no extra iron stored

rickets
deficiency disease caused by the lack of vitamin D; causes malformed bones and pain in infants and children

osteomalacia
a condition in which bones become soft, usually in adults because of calcium loss and vitamin D deficiency

osteoporosis
condition in which bones become brittle because there have been insufficient mineral deposits, especially calcium

Table 1-3 *Nutritional Deficiency Diseases and Possible Causes*

DEFICIENCY DISEASE	NUTRIENT(S) LACKING
Iron deficiency	Iron
Iron deficiency anemia	Iron
Beriberi	Thiamin
Night blindness	Vitamin A
Goiter	Iodine
Kwashiorkor	Protein
Marasmus	All nutrients
Osteomalacia	Calcium and vitamin D
Osteoporosis	Calcium and vitamin D, phosphorus, magnesium, and fluoride
Pellagra	Niacin
Rickets	Calcium and vitamin D
Scurvy	Vitamin C
Xerophthalmia (blindness)	Vitamin A

brittle. Too little iodine may cause **goiter,** and a severe shortage of vitamin A can lead to blindness.

Examples of other deficiency diseases (and their causes) are included in Table 1-3. Information concerning these conditions can be found in the chapters devoted to the given nutrients.

NUTRITION ASSESSMENT

That old saying, "You are what you eat," is true, indeed; but one could change it a bit to read, "You are *and will be* what you eat." Good nutrition is essential for the attainment and maintenance of good health. Determining whether a person is at risk requires completion of a **nutrition assessment,** which should, in fact, become part of a routine exam done by a registered **dietitian** or other health care professional specifically trained in the diagnosis of at-risk individuals. A proper nutrition assessment includes **anthropometric measurements, clinical examination, biochemical tests,** and **dietary-social history.**

Anthropometric measurements include height and weight and measurements of the head (for children), upper arm, and skinfold (Figure 1-3). The skinfold measurements are done with a **caliper.** They are used to determine the percentage of adipose and muscle tissue in the body. Measurements out of line with expectations may reveal failure to thrive in children, wasting (catabolism), edema, or obesity, all of which reflect nutrient deficiencies or excesses.

During the clinical examination, signs of nutrient deficiencies are noted. Some nutrient deficiency diseases, such as scurvy, rickets, iron deficiency, and

goiter
enlarged tissue of the thyroid gland due to a deficiency of iodine

nutrition assessment
evaluation of one's nutritional condition

dietitian
professional trained to assess nutrition status and recommend appropriate diet therapy

anthropometric measurements
of height, weight, head, chest, skinfold

clinical examination
physical observation

biochemical tests
laboratory analysis of blood, urine, and feces

dietary-social history
evaluation of food habits, including client's ability to buy and prepare food

caliper
mechanical device used to measure percentage of body fat by skinfold measurement

((⊶ In The Media

EATING BREAKFAST MAY BE GOOD FOR YOUR HEART

Breakfast really is the most important meal of the day. A small study in the United Kingdom found that women who skip breakfast eat more calories during the rest of the day. This could be a contributing factor to weight gain. Also, studies indicated that LDL, "bad cholesterol," was high and insulin sensitivity was poorer for those not consuming breakfast

(Source: *American Journal of Clinical Nutrition,* 2005).

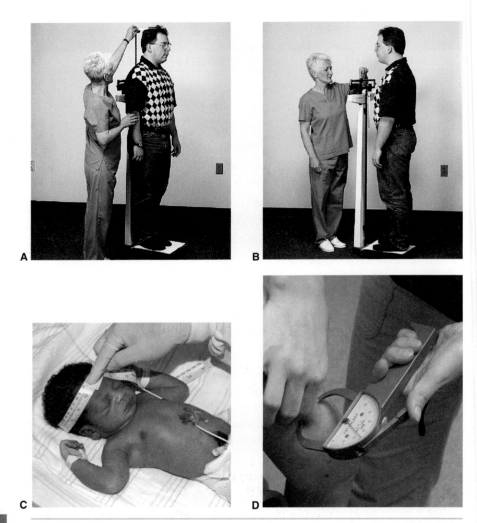

Figure 1-3 *(A) Height is one anthropometric measurement used in the nutrition assessment. (B) Weight is an anthropometric measurement used in the nutrition assessment. (C) Head circumference is an anthropometric measurement used to assess brain development during the first year of life. (D) Skinfold is an anthropometric measurement used to assess lean muscle mass versus fat.*

kwashiorkor, are obvious; other forms of nutrient deficiency can be far more subtle. Table 1-4 lists some clinical signs and probable causes of nutrient deficiencies.

Biochemical tests include various blood, urine, and stool tests. A deficiency or toxicity can be determined by laboratory analysis of the samples. The tests allow detection of malnutrition before signs appear. The following are some of the most commonly used tests for nutritional evaluation.

<u>**Serum albumin level**</u> measures the main protein in the blood and is used to determine protein status.

<u>**Serum transferrin level**</u> indicates iron-carrying protein in the blood. The level will be above normal if iron stores are low and below normal if the body lacks protein.

Table 1-4 *Clinical Signs of Nutrient Deficiencies*

CLINICAL SIGNS	POSSIBLE DEFICIENCIES
(Pale) Pallor; blue half circles beneath eyes	Iron, copper, zinc, B_{12}, B_6, biotin
Edema	Protein
Bumpy "gooseflesh"	Vitamin A
Lesions at corners of mouth	Riboflavin
Glossitis	Folic acid
Numerous "black-and-blue" spots and tiny, red "pinprick" hemorrhages under skin	Vitamin C
Emaciation	Carbohydrates, proteins; calories
Poorly shaped bones or teeth or delayed appearance of teeth in children	Vitamin D or calcium
Slow clotting time of blood	Vitamin K
Unusual nervousness, dermatitis, diarrhea in same client	Niacin
Tetany	Calcium, potassium, sodium
Goiter	Iodine
Eczema	Fat (linoleic acid)

Blood urea nitrogen (BUN) may indicate renal failure, insufficient renal blood supply, or blockage of the urinary tract.

Creatinine excretion indicates the amount of creatinine excreted in the urine over a 24-hour period and can be used in estimating body muscle mass. If the muscle mass has been depleted, as in malnutrition, the level will be low.

Serum creatinine indicates the amount of creatinine in the blood and is used for evaluating renal function.

Examples of other blood tests are hemoglobin (Hgb), hematocrit (Hct), red blood cells (RBCs), and white blood cells (WBCs). A low Hgb and Hct can indicate anemia. Not a routine test, but ordered on many clients with heart conditions, is the lipid profile, which includes total serum cholesterol, high-density lipoprotein (HDL), low-density lipoprotein (LDL), and serum triglycerides. Urinalysis also can detect protein and sugar in the urine, which can indicate kidney disease and diabetes.

The dietary-social history involves evaluation of food habits and is very important in the nutritional assessment of any client. It can be difficult to obtain an accurate dietary assessment. The most common method is the **24-hour recall**. In this method, the client is usually interviewed by the dietitian and is asked to give the types of, amounts of, and preparation used for all food eaten in the 24 hours prior to admission (PTA). Another method is the **food diary**. The client is asked to

⌒ **24-hour recall**
listing the types, amounts, and preparation of all foods eaten in past 24 hours

⌒ **food diary**
written record of all food and drink ingested in a specified period

EXPLORING THE WEB

Search the Web for nutritional assessment tools. What resources are available for the health care professional in making nutritional assessments of clients? Assess the advantages and disadvantages of each tool you find.

list all food eaten in a 3- or 4-day period. Neither method is totally accurate because clients forget or are not always totally truthful. They are sometimes inclined to say they have eaten certain foods because they know they should have done so. Computer analysis of the diet is the best way to determine if nutrient intake is appropriate. It will reveal any nutrient deficiencies or toxicities.

The dietary-social history is important to determine whether the client has the financial resources to obtain the needed food and the ability to properly store and cook food once home. After completing the dietary-social history, the dietitian can assess for risk of food-drug interactions that can lead to malnutrition (see Appendix E). Clients need to be instructed by a dietitian on possible interactions, if any.

When the preceding steps are evaluated together, and in the context of the client's medical condition, the dietitian has the best opportunity of making an accurate nutrition assessment of the client. This assessment can then be used by the entire health care team. The doctor will find it helpful in evaluating the client's condition and treatment. The dietitian can use the information to plan the client's dietary treatment and counseling, and other health care professionals will be able to use it in assisting and counseling the client.

CONSIDERATIONS FOR THE HEALTH CARE PROFESSIONAL

The practice of good nutrition habits would help eliminate many health problems caused by malnutrition (Figure 1-4). The health professional is obligated to have a sound knowledge of nutrition. One's personal health, as well as that of one's family, depends on it. Parents must have a good, basic knowledge of nutrition for the sake of their personal health and that of their children. Children learn by imitating their parents. Family members and friends who know that the health professional has studied nutrition will ask questions. Anyone, in fact, who plans and prepares meals should value, have knowledge of, and be able to apply the principles of sound nutrition practice.

Figure 1-4 *Hands-on experiences foster the development of positive feelings about food.*

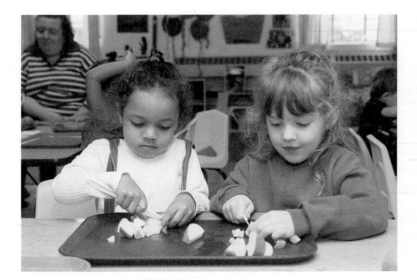

Clients will have questions and complaints about their diets. Their anxieties can be relieved by clear and simple explanations provided by the health professional. Sometimes clients must undergo diet therapy, prescribed by their physicians, which becomes part of their medical treatment in the hospital. The health professional must be able to check the client's tray quickly to see that it contains the correct foods for the diet prescribed. In many cases, diet therapy will have to be a lifelong practice for the client. In such cases, eating habits will have to be changed, and the client will need advice or instructions from a registered dietitian and support from other health professionals.

Nutrition is currently a popular subject. It is important to recognize that some books and articles concerning nutrition may not be scientifically correct. Also, food ads can be misleading. People with knowledge of sound nutrition practices will be less likely to be misled. They will recognize fad and distinguish it from fact.

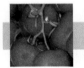

SUMMARY

Nutrition is directly related to health, and its effects are cumulative. Good nutrition is normally reflected by good health. Poor nutrition can result in poor health and even in disease. Poor nutrition habits contribute to atherosclerosis, osteoporosis, obesity, and some cancers.

To be well nourished, one must eat foods that contain the six essential nutrients: carbohydrates, fats, proteins, minerals, vitamins, and water. These nutrients provide the body with energy, build and repair body tissue, and regulate body processes. When there is a severe lack of specific nutrients, deficiency diseases may develop. The best way to determine deficiencies is to do a nutrition assessment.

With sound knowledge of nutrition, the health professional will be an effective health care provider and will also be helpful to family, friends, and self.

DISCUSSION TOPICS

1. Why is food commonly served at meetings and parties?
2. What relationship might nutrition and heredity have to each of the following?
   a. the development of physique
   b. the ability to resist disease
   c. the life span
3. What habits, in addition to good nutrition, contribute to making a person healthy?

4. What are the six classes of nutrients? What are their three basic functions?
5. Why are some foods called low-nutrient-density foods? Give some examples found in vending machines.
6. Ask anyone in the class who has been on a crash diet to discuss the diet's effects. Discuss possible reasons for those effects.
7. What is meant by the saying "You are what you eat"?
8. What is meant by the phrase "the cumulative effects of nutrition"? Describe some.
9. How could someone be overweight and at the same time suffer from malnutrition?
10. Discuss why health care professionals should be knowledgeable about nutrition.

SUGGESTED ACTIVITIES

1. List 10 signs of good nutrition and 10 signs of poor nutrition.
2. List the foods you have eaten in the past 24 hours. Underline those with low nutrient density.
3. Write a brief description of how you feel at the end of a day when you know you have not eaten wisely.
4. Name the laboratory tests used to determine nutritionally at-risk clients.

5. Write a brief paragraph discussing nutritional status.

6. Briefly describe rickets, osteomalacia, and osteoporosis. Include their causes.

7. Ask a registered dietitian to speak to your class about nutrition problems commonly seen in your area.

REVIEW

Multiple choice. Select the *letter* that precedes the best answer.

1. The result of those processes whereby the body takes in and uses food for growth, development, and maintenance of health is
   a. respiration
   b. diet therapy
   c. nutrition
   d. digestion

2. Nutritional status is determined by
   a. heredity
   b. employment
   c. personality
   d. diet

3. To nourish the body adequately, one must
   a. avoid all low-nutrient-density foods
   b. eat foods containing the six classes of nutrients
   c. include fats at every meal
   d. restrict proteins at breakfast

4. Nutrients used primarily to provide energy to the body are
   a. vitamins, water, and minerals
   b. carbohydrates, proteins, and fats
   c. proteins, vitamins, and fat
   d. vitamins, minerals, and carbohydrates

5. Nutrients used mainly to build and repair body tissues are
   a. proteins, vitamins, and minerals
   b. carbohydrates, fats, and minerals
   c. fats, water, and minerals
   d. fats, vitamins, and minerals

6. Foods such as potato chips, cakes, sodas, and candy are called
   a. dietetic foods
   b. essential nutrient foods
   c. low-nutrient-density foods
   d. nutritious foods

7. An inadequate intake of the six classes of nutrients in the diet may result in
   a. stamina
   b. malnutrition
   c. indigestion
   d. diabetes

8. The cumulative effect of a high-fat diet could be
   a. iron deficiency
   b. blindness
   c. heart disease
   d. diabetes mellitus

9. Malnutrition could be caused by
   a. poor posture
   b. constipation
   c. disease
   d. hypertension

10. A cumulative condition is one that develops
    a. within a very short period of time
    b. over several years
    c. only in women under 52
    d. in premature infants

11. Nutritional status
    a. is determined by heredity
    b. never changes
    c. is not reflected in one's appearance
    d. can affect the body's ability to resist disease

12. Infants, young children, adolescents, pregnant adolescents, and the elderly
    a. are commonly overweight
    b. are among those prone to malnutrition
    c. all commonly suffer from osteomalacia
    d. never suffer from primary nutrient deficiencies

13. Organic nutrients are
    a. only found in products grown without pesticides
    b. only sold at health food stores
    c. substances that cannot be broken down
    d. substances containing a carbon atom

14. Which of the following would be an organic nutrient?
    a. fat
    b. water
    c. calcium
    d. selenium

15. Hunger
    a. should be determined by the clock
    b. is a psychological response to food
    c. should be ignored
    d. is a physiological response by the body

CASE IN POINT

GARY: FENDING FOR HIMSELF

Gary, a 7-year-old Caucasian boy, was discovered searching a garbage can by a police officer. The officer noticed that Gary was <u>dirty</u>, unkempt, and <u>thin.</u> His skin was <u>pale.</u> Gary was taken to the police station, where he was turned over to social services. Gary told social services that his mother had been sick and was taken to the hospital; he had not seen her for many months. He did not know what hospital she was in, and he had been alone all this time. He told the social worker that he had run out of food immediately after she left; he had been able to survive by searching behind restaurants and in garbage bins. Social services brought Gary to the local hospital, and upon examination, it was found that Gary had a <u>distended abdomen, serosanguinous sores</u> on his body, and <u>swollen and painful lower limbs.</u> Gary limped and <u>found walking very tiring.</u>

[handwritten: Change in Gary Appearance]

ASSESSMENT

1. Identify three distinguishing signs of malnutrition.
2. What would you introduce first into Gary's diet? *[handwritten: Essential Nutrients]*
3. How frequently would you offer nutrition and how large a portion? *[handwritten: Sm. portions - Every couple Hrs.]*
4. What other signs of malnutrition would you expect to find? *[handwritten: Blood Work]*

DIAGNOSIS *[handwritten: Poor Inadequate Nutrition]*

5. Write a nursing diagnosis for Gary.

PLAN/GOAL *[handwritten: Bring Weight up Tolerate Food]*

6. What two changes can you predict will occur with the introduction of a good, nutritionally sound diet?
7. Whom can you refer to for assistance? *[handwritten: Social Services, possible Family members]*

IMPLEMENTATION

8. Name at least three methods that could be employed to improve Gary's nutrition.
9. Could a food diary be helpful? *[handwritten: Yes No His History would be]*
10. Would a home visit be beneficial for Gary and a caregiver? *[handwritten: Yes]*

EVALUATION/OUTCOME CRITERIA

11. What could the doctor measure at the next appointment to see if the plan is working?

[handwritten: His Blood levels, How his physical appearance looks]

12. What observations could the caregiver offer about the success of the plan?
13. What could be an important piece of information from Gary?

THINKING FURTHER *[handwritten: Research ways to help]*

14. How could the Internet be of benefit to the caregiver? *[handwritten: — Gary]*
15. Who would also benefit from this information?

RATE THIS PLATE

Gary has been through a lot of heartache for a child his age. Gary is placed in a foster home, and his foster mother asks him what he would like to eat for his first dinner with them. He thought and thought and finally decided on the following plate. Rate this plate. Take into consideration that Gary is malnourished, has not eaten much lately, and is lacking many nutrients.

[handwritten: Identify what he like to Eat.]

Fried chicken—leg and thigh

1/2 cup mashed potatoes and 2 Tbsp gravy

1/2 cup corn with butter

Biscuit with butter

2% milk—8 oz

Can Gary eat all of this, and should he? Does this plate need to be changed, and how would you change it?

CASE IN POINT

SHANNON: MAKING THAT PROM DRESS FIT

Shannon was a healthy 16-year-old Asian girl who was so happy to return to school this year. This is her junior year of high school, and she has been looking forward to attending the junior-senior prom with Mike.

Shannon is very active in cheerleading, Photo Club, gymnastics, and swimming. She has decided to join the Prom Committee this year so she can help plan the best prom that Wayne High has ever seen. Shannon has begun to look for prom dresses knowing that she will need to be saving every cent she can to afford the most perfect dress. Shannon has decided that she would like to lose a few extra pounds before the prom and decides to go on a strict diet.

Shannon's friends have noticed that the once perky, playful superstar of the swimming team has been losing her "shine." She has dull, limp hair, which is a total change from the full head of shiny, bouncy black hair. Shannon has developed a complexion problem and has started using all kinds of acne products. Her skin is very oily and feels dirty all the time. Shannon's friends also noticed that she is not as pleasant as before, and Shannon has started to lose lots of her friends. Shannon's friend Ruth contacted Shannon's mother and told her of her concerns. Shannon's mother agreed that she had also noticed the changes and would take Shannon to the doctor.

ASSESSMENT

— Less energenic
Attitud changes
Complexion

1. Identify three changes in Shannon to suggest that she was getting into trouble.

2. What information would be important to share with the physician?

3. In which category of nutritional assessment would you list Shannon's observations?

4. Which observation would you consider significant enough to cause concern?

5. Is there any other information that you could have that would help identify Shannon's problem?

DIAGNOSIS

6. Write a nursing diagnosis that most likely applies to Shannon's problem.

7. What contributed to the development of the problems?

PLAN/GOAL

8. Who can help with the plan?

9. What two changes are most significant for Shannon? *Attitude, Appearance.*

IMPLEMENTATION

Make meal times fun
Prepare meals she likes.

10. Name three methods that could be used to improve Shannon's nutrition.

11. How could friends and family help?

12. How could a food diary help?

EVALUATION/OUTCOME CRITERIA

13. What can the doctor measure at the next appointment to see if the plan is working?

14. What observations could Shannon's mother offer about the success of the plan?

15. What information from Shannon would benefit the success of the plan?

THINKING FURTHER

16. Who else could be at risk for the same or a similar problem?

17. How could information from the Internet be useful?

Social diet
diet diary
Her Complexion changes

Anthropometric & Biochemical Assessments

Lack of energy
Complexion changes
Attitude
Alteration in nutrition
psychological

Doctor Friends Family

RATE THIS PLATE

Read this case study about Shannon again. Rate this plate. For lunch Shannon has fixed herself:

one half peanut butter and jelly sandwich on white bread (1 Tbsp peanut butter and 1 Tbsp jelly)

Cup of tea with 1 tsp sugar

That was all she wanted. Answer the following questions about this plate:

1. Was the amount of peanut butter sufficient? If not, why not? How would you change the serving size?

2. Was the amount of jelly sufficient? If not, why not? How would you change the serving size?

3. Was the bread the best choice? Why or why not?

4. Is there any other food or foods that you would like to add to this lunch and why?

5. Why do you think Shannon is experiencing changes in appearance and demeanor?

I support Shannons efforts

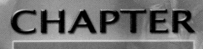

CHAPTER

2

PLANNING A
HEALTHY DIET

OBJECTIVES

After studying this chapter, you should be able to:

- Define a balanced diet
- List the U.S. government's Dietary Guidelines for Americans and explain the reasons for each
- Identify the food groups and their placement on the MyPyramid
- Describe information commonly found on food labels
- List some food customs of various cultural groups
- Describe the development of food customs

The statement "eat a balanced diet" has been repeated so often that its importance may be overlooked. The value of this statement is so great, however, that it deserves serious consideration by people of all ages. A **balanced diet** includes all six classes of nutrients and calories in amounts that preserve and promote good health.

Daily review of the **Dietary Reference Intakes (DRIs)** and the Recommended Dietary Allowances (RDAs) would provide enough information to plan balanced diets. However, ordinary meal planning would be cumbersome and time-consuming if that table had to be consulted each time a meal was planned. Fortunately, the U.S. Department of Agriculture (USDA) and the U.S. Department of Health and Human Services (USDHHS) developed a simple system to help with the selection of healthful diets. It is called the **Dietary Guidelines for Americans.** In addition, **MyPyramid** was released in 2005 by the USDA as an outline for daily food choices based on the Dietary Guidelines.

DIETARY GUIDELINES FOR AMERICANS, 2005

The Dietary Guidelines provide science-based advice to promote health and to reduce the risk for chronic diseases through diet and physical activity. The guidelines are targeted to the general public over 2 years of age in the United States. Below are the titles of the topics for each section; all of the following key recommendations are taken from www.health.gov/dietaryguidelines. The Dietary Guidelines themselves form an integrated set of key recommendations in each of the topic areas and will be discussed under the respective topics.

- Adequate nutrients within calorie needs
- Weight management
- Physical activity
- Food groups to encourage
- Fats
- Carbohydrates
- Sodium and potassium
- Alcoholic beverages
- Food safety

Adequate Nutrients within Calorie Needs

A basic premise of the Dietary Guidelines is that recommended diets will provide all the nutrients needed for growth and health and that the nutrients consumed should come primarily from foods. Foods contain not only the vitamins and minerals found in supplements, but also hundreds of naturally occurring substances, including carotenoids, flavonoids and isoflavones, and protease inhibitors that may protect against chronic health conditions.

not this

Key Recommendations.

- Consume a variety of nutrient-dense foods and beverages within and among the basic food groups while choosing foods that limit the intake of saturated and trans fats, cholesterol, added sugars, salt, and alcohol.
- Meet recommended intakes within energy needs by adopting a balanced eating pattern such as the USDA Food Guide or the Dietary Approaches to Stop Hypertension (DASH) Eating Plan (Appendix C-1).

○ **balanced diet**
one that includes all the essential nutrients in appropriate amounts

○ **Dietary Reference Intakes (DRIs)**
combines the Recommended Dietary Allowances, Adequate Intake, Estimated Average Requirements, and the Tolerable Upper Intake Levels for individuals into one value representative of the average daily nutrient intake of individuals over time

○ **Dietary Guidelines for Americans**
general goals for optimal nutrient intake

○ **MyPyramid**
outline for making food selections based on the Dietary Guidelines

EXPLORING THE WEB

The "Dietary Guidelines for Americans 2005," are science-based advice and suggestions for improving health through sound nutrition and physical activity. These guidelines serve as helpful reminders to many Americans, especially those who are overweight or obese, eat too much fat, and no longer think exercise is important. The Dietary Guidelines encourage a healthy diet, which means individuals should choose:
- Fruits, vegetables, whole grains, and fat-free or low-fat milk and milk products;
- Lean meats, poultry, fish, beans, eggs, and nuts; and beans
- Foods low in saturated fats, trans fats, cholesterol, salt (sodium), and added sugars. Read about the nine topic areas to see what you might need to change to ensure a healthy life: www.mypyramid. gov/guidelines

Key Recommendations for Specific Population Groups.

- *People over age 50.* Consume vitamin B_{12} in its crystalline form (e.g., fortified foods or supplements).
- *Women of childbearing age who may become pregnant.* Eat foods high in heme-iron and consume iron-rich plant foods or iron-fortified foods with an enhancer of iron absorption, such as vitamin C–rich foods.
- *Women of childbearing age who may become pregnant and those in the first trimester of pregnancy.* Consume adequate synthetic folic acid daily (from fortified foods or supplements) in addition to food forms of folate from a varied diet.
- *Older adults, people with dark skin, and people exposed to insufficient ultraviolet band-radiation (i.e., sunlight).* Consume extra vitamin D from vitamin D–fortified foods and supplements.

Weight Management

Over the last 20 years the prevalence of overweight in the general population, and especially among children and adolescents, has increased substantially; it is estimated that as many as 16% of children and adolescents are overweight. Overweight and obesity of both adults and children are of great public health concern because excess body fat leads to a higher risk of premature death, type 2 diabetes, hypertension, dyslipidemia, cardiovascular disease, stroke, gallbladder disease, and other chronic diseases.

High Cholesterol

Key Recommendations.

- To maintain body weight in a healthy range, balance calories from foods and beverages with calories expended.
- To prevent gradual weight gain over time, make small decreases in food and beverage calories and increase physical activity.

Key Recommendations for Specific Population Groups.

- *Those who need to lose weight.* Aim for a slow, steady weight loss by decreasing calorie intake while maintaining an adequate nutrient intake and increasing physical activity.
- *Overweight children.* Reduce the rate of body weight gain while allowing growth and development. Consult a health care provider before placing a child on a weight reduction diet.
- *Pregnant women.* Ensure appropriate weight gain as specified by a health care provider.
- *Breastfeeding women.* Moderate weight reduction is safe and does not compromise weight gain of the nursing infant.

Body Mass Index=BMI

⬐ *Overweight adults and overweight children with chronic disease and/or on medication.* Consult a health care provider about weight loss strategies before starting a weight reduction program to ensure appropriate management of other health conditions.

Physical Activity

Americans are relatively inactive. Regular physical activity and physical fitness make important contributions to one's health, sense of well-being, and maintenance of a healthy body weight. Physical activity is defined as any bodily movement produced by skeletal muscles resulting in energy expenditure. Regular physical activity has been shown to reduce the risk of certain chronic diseases, including high blood pressure, stroke, coronary artery disease, type 2 diabetes, colon cancer, and osteoporosis. Therefore, it is recommended that adults engage in at least 30 minutes of moderate-intensity physical activity on most days of the week. Regular physical activity is also a key factor in achieving and maintaining a healthy body weight for adults and children (Tables 2-1, 2-2, and 2-3). It is recommended that males over age 40 and females over age 50 check with their health care provider before beginning aerobic activities.

at least 30 minutes a day, 5 out of 7 DAYS a week

Key Recommendations.

⬐ Engage in regular physical activity and reduce sedentary activities to promote health, psychological well-being, and healthy body weight.

⬐ To reduce the risk of chronic disease in adulthood, engage in at least 30 minutes of moderate-intensity physical activity, above usual activity, at work or home on most days of the week. For most people, greater health benefits can be obtained by engaging in physical activity of more vigorous intensity or longer duration.

Table 2-1 *Health Benefits of Regular Physical Activity*

- Increases physical fitness
- Helps build and maintain healthy bones, muscles, and joints
- Builds endurance and muscular strength
- Helps manage weight
- Lowers risk factors for cardiovascular disease, colon cancer, and type 2 diabetes
- Helps control blood pressure
- Promotes psychological well-being and self-esteem
- Reduces feelings of depression and anxiety

Source: *Nutrition and Your Health: Dietary Guidelines for Americans* (6th ed.), 2005.

Table 2-2 *Examples of Physical Activities for Adults*

For at least 30 minutes most days of the week, preferably daily, do any one of the activities listed below—or combine activities. Look for additional opportunities among other activities that you enjoy.

AS PART OF YOUR ROUTINE ACTIVITIES:

- Walk, wheel, or bike-ride more; drive less.
- Walk up stairs instead of taking an elevator.
- Get off the bus a few stops early and walk or wheel the remaining distance.
- Mow the lawn with a push mower.
- Rake leaves.
- Garden.
- Push a stroller.
- Clean the house.
- Do exercises or pedal a stationary bike while watching television.
- Play actively with children.
- Take a brisk 10-minute walk or wheel in the morning, at lunch, and after dinner.

AS PART OF YOUR EXERCISE OR RECREATIONAL ROUTINE:

- Walk, wheel, or jog.
- Bicycle or use an arm pedal bicycle.
- Swim or do water aerobics.
- Play racket or wheelchair sports.
- Golf (pull cart or carry clubs).
- Canoe.
- Cross-country-ski.
- Play basketball.
- Dance.
- Take part in an exercise program at work, home, school, or gym.

Source: *Nutrition and Your Health: Dietary Guidelines for Americans* (6th ed), 2005.

➤ To help manage body weight and prevent gradual, unhealthy body weight gain in adulthood, engage in approximately 60 minutes of moderate- to vigorous-intensity activity on most days of the week while not exceeding caloric intake requirements.

➤ To sustain weight loss in adulthood, participate in at least 60 to 90 minutes of daily moderate-intensity physical activity while not exceeding caloric intake requirements. Some people may need to consult with a health care provider before participating in this level of activity.

As you get older =

Table 2-3 *Physical Activities for Children and Teens*

AIM FOR AT LEAST 60 MINUTES TOTAL PER DAY:

- Be spontaneously active.
- Play tag.
- Jump rope.
- Ride a bicycle or tricycle.
- Walk, wheel, skip, or run.
- Play actively during school recess.
- Roller-skate or in-line-skate.
- Take part in physical education activity classes during school.
- Join after-school or community physical activity programs.
- Dance.

Source: *Nutrition and Your Health: Dietary Guidelines for Americans* (6th ed.), 2005.

> Achieve physical fitness by including cardiovascular conditioning, stretching exercises for flexibility, and resistance exercises or calisthenics for muscle strength and endurance.

Key Recommendations for Specific Population Groups.

> *Children and adolescents.* Engage in at least 60 minutes of physical activity on most, preferably all, days of the week.

> *Pregnant women.* In the absence of medical or obstetric complications, incorporate 30 minutes or more of moderate-intensity physical activity on most, if not all, days of the week. Avoid activities with a high risk of falling or abdominal trauma.

> *Breastfeeding women.* Be aware that neither acute nor regular exercise adversely affects the mother's ability to successfully breastfeed.

> *Older adults.* Participate in regular physical activity to reduce functional declines associated with aging and to achieve the other benefits of physical activity identified for all adults.

Food Groups to Encourage

Increased intakes of fruits, vegetables, whole grains, and fat-free or low-fat milk products will have important health benefits. Those who eat more generous amounts of fruits and vegetables as part of a healthful diet may reduce the risk of chronic diseases, including stroke and other cardiovascular diseases, type 2 diabetes, and cancers in certain sites (oral cavity and pharynx, larynx, lung, esophagus, stomach, and colon-rectum). In addition to fruits and vegetables, whole grains are an important source of fiber and other nutrients. Consuming at least 3 or more ounce-equivalents of whole grains per day can reduce the

SPOTLIGHT on Life Cycle

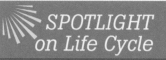

The most common nutrient deficiency in the world is lack of iron. This is particularly prevalent among infants, adolescents, and pregnant and menstruating women. It can result in iron-deficiency anemia. The health care provider can help by:
- Identifying those clients at risk (e.g., children under 2 years of age, adolescents, women with heavy menstrual flow, pregnant women, individuals with malabsorption syndromes, gastrointestinal bleedings, and gross dietary deficiencies).
- Performing complete nutritional assessments on high-risk clients.
- Encouraging clients to eat foods high in iron. These include lean meats, poultry, fish, enriched breads, legumes, leafy green vegetables, dried fruits, and nuts.

○ **legumes**

plant food that is grown in a pod; for example, beans and peas

Table 2-4 *Whole Grains That are Most Often Consumed in the United States*	
Whole wheat	Wild rice
Whole oats, oatmeal	Buckwheat
Whole-grain corn	Triticale
Popcorn	Bulgur (cracked wheat)
Brown rice	Millet
Whole rye	Quinoa
Whole-grain barley	Sorghum

Source: *Nutrition and Your Health: Dietary Guidelines for Americans*, 2005.

risk of several chronic diseases and may help with weight maintenance. Table 2-4 can help one recognize the names of whole grains.

Key Recommendations.

- Consume a sufficient amount of fruits and vegetables while staying within energy needs. For a 2,000-calorie intake, 2 cups of fruit and 2½ cups of vegetables per day are recommended, with higher or lower amounts depending on the calorie level.

- Choose a variety of fruits and vegetables each day. In particular, select from all five vegetable subgroups (dark green vegetables, orange vegetables, **legumes**, starchy vegetables, and other vegetables) several times a week.

- Consume 3 or more ounce-equivalents of whole-grain products per day, with the rest of the recommended grains coming from enriched or whole-grain products. In general, at least half the grains should come from whole grains.

- Consume 3 cups per day of fat-free or low-fat milk or equivalent milk products.

Key Recommendations for Specific Population Groups.

- *Children and adolescents.* Consume whole-grain products often; at least half the grains should be whole grains. Children 2 to 8 years should consume 2 cups per day of fat-free or low-fat milk or equivalent milk products. Children 9 years of age and older should consume 3 cups per day of fat-free or low-fat milk or equivalent milk products.

Fats

Fats and oils are part of a healthful diet, but the type of fat makes a difference to heart health, and the total amount of fat consumed is also important. High intake of saturated fats, trans fats, and cholesterol increases the risk of coronary heart disease due to high blood lipid levels. Fats supply energy and essential fatty acids and serve as a carrier for the absorption of the fat-soluble vitamins A, D, E, and K and carotenoids.

Key Recommendations.

- Consume less than 10% of calories from saturated fatty acids and less than 300 mg/day of cholesterol, and keep trans-fatty acid consumption as low as possible.

- Keep total fat intake between 20 and 35% of calories, with most fats coming from sources of polyunsaturated and monounsaturated fatty acids, such as fish, nuts, and vegetable oils.

- When selecting and preparing meat, poultry, dry beans, and milk or milk products, make choices that are lean, low fat, or fat-free.

- Limit intake of fats and oils high in saturated and trans-fatty acids, *that come from animal sources High in Cholesterol* and choose products low in such fats and oils.

Key Recommendations for Specific Population Groups.

- *Children and adolescents*. Keep total fat intake between 30 and 35% of calories for children 2 to 3 years of age and between 25 and 35% of calories for children and adolescents 4 to 18 years of age, with most fats coming from sources of polyunsaturated and monounsaturated fatty acids, such as fish, nuts, and vegetable oils.

Carbohydrates

Carbohydrates are part of a healthful diet. Foods in the basic food groups that provide carbohydrates—fruits, vegetables, grains, and milk—are important sources of many nutrients. Dietary fiber is composed of nondigestible carbohydrates. Sugars and starches supply energy to the body in the form of glucose. Sugars can be naturally present in foods or added to the food. The greater the consumption of foods containing large amounts of added sugars, the more difficult it is to consume enough nutrients without gaining weight. See Table 2-5 to help identify the names of added sugar on labels.

Table 2-5 *Names for Added Sugars That Appear on Food Labels*

A food is likely to be high in sugars if one of these names appears first or second in the ingredient list or if several names are listed.

Brown sugar	Glucose	Maltose
Corn sweetener	High-fructose corn syrup	Molasses
Corn syrup	Honey	Raw sugar
Dextrose	Invert sugar	Sucrose
Fructose	Lactose	Syrup
Fruit juice concentrate	Malt syrup	Table sugar

Source: *Nutrition and Your Health: Dietary Guidelines for Americans*, 2005.

Key Recommendations.

- Choose fiber-rich fruits, vegetables, and whole grains often.
- Choose and prepare foods and beverages with little added sugars or caloric sweeteners, such as the amounts suggested by the USDA MyPyramid and the DASH Eating Plan.
- Reduce the incidence of dental caries by practicing good oral hygiene and consuming foods and beverages containing sugar and starch less frequently. *promotes cavities.*

Key Recommendations for Specific Population Groups.

- *Older Adults.* Dietary fiber is important for laxation (the elimination of fecal waste through the anus). Since constipation may affect up to 20% of people over 65 years of age, older adults should choose to consume foods rich in dietary fiber.
- *Children.* Carbohydrate intakes of children need special considerations with regard to obtaining sufficient amounts of fiber, avoiding excessive amount of calories from added sugars, and prevention of dental caries. *make sure not too much from sugar.*

Sodium and Potassium

On average, the higher one's salt (sodium chloride) intake, the higher one's blood pressure. Keeping blood pressure in the normal range reduces one's risk of coronary heart disease, stroke, congestive heart failure, and kidney disease. When reading labels, look for the sodium content; foods that are low in sodium (less than 140 mg) are low in salt. Lifestyle changes including reducing salt intake, increasing potassium intake, losing excess body weight, increasing physical activity, and eating an overall healthful diet can prevent or delay the onset of high blood pressure and can lower elevated blood pressure.

Key Recommendations.

- Consume less than 2,300 mg of sodium (approximately 1 teaspoon of salt) per day.
- Choose and prepare foods with little salt. At the same time, consume potassium-rich foods, such as fruits and vegetables.

Key Recommendations for Specific Population Groups.

- *Individuals with hypertension, blacks, and middle-aged and older adults.* Aim to consume no more than 1,500 mg of sodium per day and meet the potassium recommendation (4,700 mg/day) with food.

Fruits & Veggies

Alcoholic Beverages

Alcoholic beverages supply calories but few essential nutrients. As a result, excessive alcohol consumption makes it difficult to eat sufficient nutrients within one's daily calories and to maintain a healthy weight. Alcoholic beverages are harmful when consumed in excess.

Key Recommendations.

- Those who choose to drink alcoholic beverages should do so sensibly and in moderation—defined as the consumption of up to one drink per day for women and up to two drinks per day for men.

- Alcoholic beverages should not be consumed by some individuals, including those who cannot restrict their alcohol intake, women of childbearing age who may become pregnant, pregnant and lactating women, children and adolescents, individuals taking medications that can interact with alcohol, and those with specific medical conditions.

- Alcoholic beverages should be avoided by individuals engaging in activities that require attention, skill, or coordination, such as driving or operating machinery.

Food Safety

Avoiding foods that are contaminated with harmful bacteria, viruses, parasites, toxins, and chemical and physical contaminants is vital for healthful eating. It is estimated that every year about 76 million people in the United States become ill from pathogens in food. Chapter 10 discusses this further.

Key Recommendations.

- Clean hands, food contact surfaces, and fruits and vegetables.
- Separate raw cooked and ready-to-eat foods while shopping, preparing, or storing foods.
- Cook foods to a safe temperature to kill microorganisms.
- Chill (refrigerate) perishable food promptly, and defrost foods properly.
- Avoid raw (unpasteurized) milk or any products made from unpasteurized milk, raw or partially cooked eggs or foods containing raw eggs, raw or undercooked meat and poultry, unpasteurized juices, and raw sprouts. *You can get Ecoli*

Key Recommendations for Specific Population Groups.

Should Not Eat Nothing

- *Infants and young children, pregnant women, older adults, and those who are immunocompromised.* Do not eat or drink raw (unpasteurized) milk or any products made from unpasteurized milk, raw or partially cooked eggs or foods containing raw eggs, raw or undercooked meat and poultry, and raw or undercooked fish or shellfish.

- *Pregnant women, older adults, and those who are immunocompromised.* Only eat certain deli meats and frankfurters that have been reheated to steaming hot.

*Salt 1 teaspoon
2300 mg.

Potassium 4700 mg.

Restricted salt under 500*

MYPYRAMID

Dietary Guidelines for Americans, 2005, serve as the U.S. federal nutrition policy (USDHHS and USDA, 2005). These guidelines form the basis for the MyPyramid Food guidance system unveiled in April 2005. MyPyramid is applicable to Americans over age 2. By introducing all Americans to MyPyramid and its slogan, "Steps to a Healthier you," the USDA hopes to help people make informed and healthier food choices. These choices can lead to a decrease in major nutrition-related chronic diseases, such as anemia, diabetes mellitus, coronary heart disease, hypertension, and alcoholic cirrhosis.

MyPyramid is the former Food Guide Pyramid tipped on its side. The color bands in MyPyramid represent the types of foods that should be consumed, and the width of the band denotes the approximate relative quantity of each food that should be consumed. In addition, MyPyramid incorporates the concept of physical activity into its design. A person climbing the stairs denotes the importance of physical activity in one's daily life, just as the food groups denote daily food intake. Personalization of one's diet is easier to accomplish by accessing the MyPyramid.gov Web site, where age, gender, and physical activity can be keyed in and more specific nutrition guidelines are provided. Twelve different pyramids are available on the Web site using these parameters. The 12 pyramids range from daily intake levels of 1,000 to 3,200 calories. By following the appropriate pyramid, the individual should be able to maintain a healthy body weight and decrease the risk of nutrition-related chronic diseases. Quantities are stated in household measures such as cups and ounces instead of the servings that were used in the Food Guide Pyramid.

MyPyramid has the following features:

- *MyPyramid Plan*. Provides a quick estimate of what and how much food you should eat from the different food groups by entering your age, gender, and activity level.

- *MyPyramid Tracker* (www.mypyramidtracker.gov). Provides more detailed information on your diet quality and physical activity status by comparing a day's work of foods eaten with current nutrition guidance.

- *Inside MyPyramid.* Provides in-depth information for every food group, including recommended daily amounts in commonly used measures, like cups and ounces, with examples and everyday tips. Included in this section are recommendations for choosing healthy oils, discretionary calories, and physical activity.

- *Start Today.* Offers tips and resources that include downloadable suggestions on all the food groups and physical activity and provides a downloadable worksheet to track what you are eating.

MyPyramid (Figure 2-1) has six color bands representing five food groups and oils. The bands are wider at the bottom, representing foods with little or no solid fats, added sugars, or caloric sweeteners, and become narrower at the top,

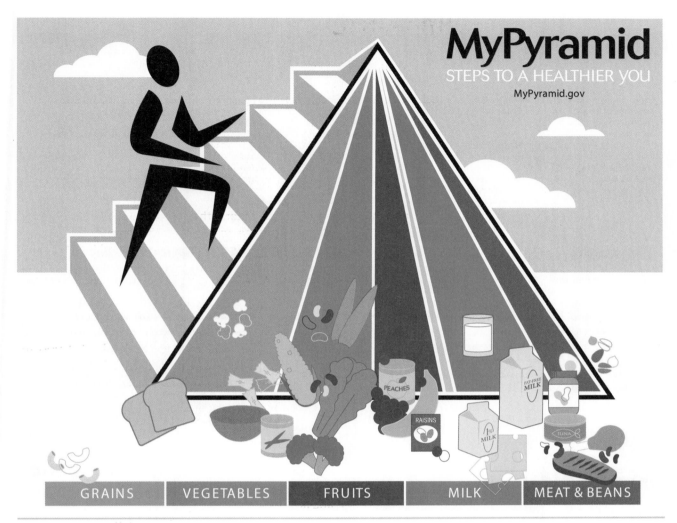

Figure 2-1 *MyPyramid Food Guidance System. (USDA and USHHS, 2005)*   *(continues)*

indicating that the foods that contain fats and sugars should be limited. The five food groups represented along with oils have not changed. They are:

- Grains—bread, cereal, rice, and pasta group
- Vegetable group
- Fruit group
- Milk, yogurt, and cheese group
- Meat, poultry, fish, dry beans, eggs, and nuts group
- Fats, oils, and sweets group

The emphasis of MyPyramid, which takes its guidance from the *Dietary Guidelines for Americans, 2005,* is not on a percentage of intake but on daily

GRAINS Make half your grains whole	VEGETABLES Vary your veggies	FRUITS Focus on fruits	MILK Get your calcium-rich foods	MEAT & BEANS Go lean with protein
Eat at least 3 oz. of whole-grain cereals, breads, crackers, rice, or pasta every day 1 oz. is about 1 slice of bread, about 1 cup of breakfast cereal, or ½ cup of cooked rice, cereal, or pasta	Eat more dark-green veggies like broccoli, spinach, and other dark leafy greens Eat more orange vegetables like carrots and sweetpotatoes Eat more dry beans and peas like pinto beans, kidney beans, and lentils	Eat a variety of fruit Choose fresh, frozen, canned, or dried fruit Go easy on fruit juices	Go low-fat or fat-free when you choose milk, yogurt, and other milk products If you don't or can't consume milk, choose lactose-free products or other calcium sources such as fortified foods and beverages	Choose low-fat or lean meats and poultry Bake it, broil it, or grill it Vary your protein routine — choose more fish, beans, peas, nuts, and seeds

For a 2,000-calorie diet, you need the amounts below from each food group. To find the amounts that are right for you, go to MyPyramid.gov.

Eat 6 oz. every day	Eat 2½ cups every day	Eat 2 cups every day	Get 3 cups every day; for kids aged 2 to 8, it's 2	Eat 5½ oz. every day

Find your balance between food and physical activity

- Be sure to stay within your daily calorie needs.
- Be physically active for at least 30 minutes most days of the week.
- About 60 minutes a day of physical activity may be needed to prevent weight gain.
- For sustaining weight loss, at least 60 to 90 minutes a day of physical activity may be required.
- Children and teenagers should be physically active for 60 minutes every day, or most days.

Know the limits on fats, sugars, and salt (sodium)

- Make most of your fat sources from fish, nuts, and vegetable oils.
- Limit solid fats like butter, stick margarine, shortening, and lard, as well as foods that contain these.
- Check the Nutrition Facts label to keep saturated fats, *trans* fats, and sodium low.
- Choose food and beverages low in added sugars. Added sugars contribute calories with few, if any, nutrients.

MyPyramid.gov
STEPS TO A HEALTHIER YOU

U.S. Department of Agriculture
Center for Nutrition Policy and Promotion
April 2005
CNPP-15

USDA

Figure 2-1 *(continued)*

servings. Depending on the information one enters into MyPyramid, a calorie level will be individually determined. See Table 2-6 for intake patterns for various caloric levels.

Bread, Cereal, Rice, and Pasta Group

The largest section of MyPyramid is made up of the grains—the bread, cereal, rice, and pasta group (Table 2-7). As the table shows, the number of servings from grains is established with the recommendation that at least half of the servings should be whole grains. Whole grains provide dietary fiber, B vitamins, iron, and magnesium. Enriched products also contain B vitamins and iron, but if they are not made from whole grains, they contain little dietary fiber.

Table 2-6 *MyPyramid Food Intake Patterns*

DAILY AMOUNT OF FOOD FROM EACH GROUP

The suggested amounts of food to consume from the basic food groups, subgroups, and oils to meet recommended nutrient intakes at 12 different calorie levels. Nutrient and energy contributions from each group are calculated according to the nutrient-dense forms of foods in each group (e.g., lean meats, and fat-free milk). The table also shows the discretionary calorie allowance that can be accommodated within each calorie level, in addition to the suggested amounts of nutrient-dense forms of foods in each group.

CALORIE LEVEL[1]

	1,000	1,200	1,400	1,600	1,800	2,000	2,200	2,400	2,600	2,800	3,000	3,200
Fruits	1 cup	1 cup	1.5 cups	1.5 cups	1.5 cups	2 cups	2 cups	2 cups	2 cups	2.5 cups	2.5 cups	2.5 cups
Vegetables	1 cup	1.5 cups	1.5 cups	2 cups	2.5 cups	2.5 cups	3 cups	3 cups	3.5 cups	3.5 cups	4 cups	4 cups
Grains	3 oz–eq	4 oz–eq	5 oz–eq	5 oz–eq	6 oz–eq	6 oz–eq	7 oz–eq	8 oz–eq	9 oz–eq	10 oz–eq	10 oz–eq	10 oz–eq
Meat and beans	2 oz–eq	3 oz–eq	4 oz–eq	5 oz–eq	5 oz–eq	5.5 oz–eq	6 oz–eq	6.5 oz–eq	6.5 oz–eq	7 oz–eq	7 oz–eq	7 oz–eq
Milk	2 cups	2 cups	2 cups	3 cups	3 cups	3 cups	3 cups	3 cups	3 cups	3 cups	3 cups	3 cups
Oils	3 tsp	4 tsp	4 tsp	5 tsp	5 tsp	6 tsp	6 tsp	7 tsp	8 tsp	8 tsp	10 tsp	11 tsp
Discretionary calorie allowance	165	171	171	132	195	267	290	362	410	426	512	648

[1] **Calorie levels** are set across a wide range to accommodate the needs of different individuals.

ESTIMATED DAILY CALORIE NEEDS

To determine which food intake pattern to use for an individual, the following chart gives an estimate of individual calorie needs. The calorie range for each age and gender is based on physical activity level, from sedentary to active. Sedentary means a lifestyle that includes only the light physical activity associated with typical day-to-day life. Active means a lifestyle that includes physical activity equivalent to walking more than 3 miles per day at 3 to 4 miles per hour, in addition to the light physical activity associated with typical day-to-day life.

	CALORIE RANGE				CALORIE RANGE		
	SEDENTARY	→	ACTIVE		SEDENTARY	→	ACTIVE
Children				**Males**			
2–3 years	1,000	→	1,400	4–8 years	1,400	→	2,000
Females				9–13	1,800	→	2,600
4–8 years	1,200	→	1,800	14–18	2,200	→	3,200
9–13	1,600	→	2,200	19–30	2,400	→	3,000
14–18	1,800	→	2,400	31–50	2,200	→	3,000
19–30	2,000	→	2,400	51+	2,000	→	2,800
31–50	1,800	→	2,200				
51+	1,600	→	2,200				

Note. *From MyPyramid Food Intake Patterns, by the U.S. Department of Agriculture, 2005, retrieved December 2, 2005, from http://www.mypyramid.gov/professionals/pdf_food_intake.html.*

Table 2-7 *Bread, Cereal, Rice, and Pasta Group*

BREADS

Whole wheat	Rolls or biscuits made with whole
Dark rye	wheat or enriched flour
Enriched	Flour, enriched
Oatmeal bread	whole wheat, other whole grain
Cornmeal, whole grain, or enriched	grits, enriched

CEREALS

Whole wheat	Other cereals, if whole grain or
Rolled oats	restored

RICE

Brown rice	Converted rice

PASTA

Noodles, spaghetti, macaroni

Table 2-8 *Vegetable Subgroup Amounts*

CALORIE LEVEL	1,000	1,200	1,400	1,600	1,800	2,000	2,200	2,400	2,600	2,800	3,000	3,200
Dark green veg.	1 c/wk	1.5 c/wk	1.5 c/wk	2 c/wk	3 c/wk	3 c/wk	3 c/wk	3 c/wk	3 c/wk	3 c/wk	3 c/wk	3 c/wk
Orange veg.	0.5 c/wk	1 c/wk	1 c/wk	1.5 c/wk	2 c/wk	2c/wk	2 c/wk	2 c/wk	2.5 c/wk	2.5 c/wk	2.5 c/wk	2.5 c/wk
Legumes	0.5 c/wk	1 c/wk	1 c/wk	2.5 c/wk	3 c/wk	3 c/wk	3 c/wk	3 c/wk	3.5 c/wk	3.5 c/wk	3.5 c/wk	3.5 c/wk
Starchy veg.	1.5 c/wk	2.5 c/wk	2.5 c/wk	2.5 c/wk	3 c/wk	3 c/wk	6 c/wk	6 c/wk	7 c/wk	7 c/wk	9 c/wk	9 c/wk
Other veg.	3.5 c/wk	4.5 c/wk	4.5 c/wk	5.5 c/wk	6.5 c/wk	6.5 c/wk	7 c/wk	7 c/wk	8.5 c/wk	8.5 c/wk	10 c/wk	10 c/wk

Note. *From* MyPyramid Food Intake Patterns, *by the U.S. Department of Agriculture, 2005, retrieved December 2, 2005, from* http://www.mypyramid.gov/professionals/pdf_food_intake.html.

Vegetable Group

The food intake patterns have established the number of daily servings per calorie level of vegetable. All vegetables are included in the vegetable group: green and leafy, yellow, starchy, and legumes (Table 2-8). Vegetables provide carbohydrates; dietary fiber; vitamins A, B-complex, C, E, and K; and iron, calcium, phosphorus, potassium, magnesium, copper, manganese, and sometimes, molybdenum.

This guideline, if followed, also guarantees that one will receive a variety of nutrients, phytochemicals, and **flavonoids.** One-half cup of cooked or chopped raw vegetables or two cups of uncooked, leafy vegetables is considered one serving.

⊙ **flavonoids**
naturally occurring water-soluble plant pigments that act as antioxidants

Table 2-9 *Fruit Group*		
SOURCES OF VITAMIN A	**SOURCES OF VITAMIN C**	
Bananas	Oranges	Cantaloupe
Cantaloupe	Lemons	Kiwi fruit
Avocados	Grapefruit	Honeydew melon
Apricots	Limes	Watermelon
Mangoes	Raspberries	Mangoes
	Strawberries	Papaya
	Pineapple	

Fruit Group

All fruits are included in the fruit group. They provide vitamins A and C, potassium, magnesium, iron, and carbohydrates, including dietary fiber (Table 2-9).

It is recommended that one eat a variety of fruit daily, following the food intake patterns for quantity, and go easy on the fruit juice. The calories in fruit juice add up quickly, especially if one is thirsty and drinks large amounts of juice. One serving is three-quarters cup of fruit juice; a half of a grapefruit; one whole raw medium apple, orange, peach, pear, or banana; a half cup of canned or cooked fruit; and a quarter cup of dried fruit.

Milk, Yogurt, and Cheese Group

Milk, yogurt, and cheese are excellent sources of carbohydrate (lactose); calcium, phosphorus, and magnesium; proteins; riboflavin, vitamins A, B_{12}, and, if the milk is fortified, vitamin D. Unfortunately, all contain sodium, and whole milk and whole-milk products also contain saturated fats and cholesterol. Fat-free milk has had the fats removed.

It is recommended that two to three servings of these foods be included in one's daily diet. The serving size is one 8-ounce glass of milk or the equivalent in terms of calcium content.

Children	2 servings
Adolescents	3 servings
Adults	3 servings
Pregnant or lactating women	3 servings
Pregnant or lactating teens	4 servings

The following dairy foods contain calcium equal to that found in one 8-ounce cup of milk. The best choices would be low fat.

- 1½ ounces cheddar cheese
- 2 cups cottage cheese
- 1¾ cups of ice cream
- 1 cup yogurt

Milk used in making cream sauces, gravies, or baked products fulfills part of the calcium requirement. A cheese sandwich would fulfill one of the serving requirements, and a serving of ice cream could fulfill half of one of the serving requirements. Obviously, drinking milk is not the only way to fulfill the calcium requirement.

Some clients suffer from lactose intolerance and cannot digest milk or milk products. If they eat or drink foods containing untreated lactose, they experience abdominal cramps and diarrhea. This condition is caused by a deficiency of lactase (see Chapter 4). In such cases, milk that has been treated with lactase can be used, or commercial lactase can be added to the milk or taken in tablet form before drinking milk or eating dairy products.

Meat and Beans Group

All meats, poultry, fish, eggs, soybeans, dry beans and peas, lentils, nuts, and seeds are included in this group (Table 2-10). These foods provide proteins, iron, copper, phosphorus, zinc, sodium, iodine, B vitamins, fats, and cholesterol.

Caution must be used so that the foods selected from this group are low in fat and cholesterol. Many meats contain large amounts of fats, and egg yolks and organ meats have very high cholesterol content.

Let the food intake patterns be the guide for the number of ounces one should eat daily. In general, 1 ounce of lean meat, poultry, or fish, 1 egg, 1 tablespoon of peanut butter, ¼ cup of cooked dry beans, or ½ ounce of nuts or seeds can be considered as a 1 ounce-equivalent from the meat and beans group.

Fats

This group contains butter, margarine, cooking oils, mayonnaise and other salad dressings, sugar, syrup, honey, jam, jelly, and sodas. All of these foods have a low nutrient density, meaning they have few nutrients other than fats and carbohydrates and have a high calorie content. One's limit for fat will be figured and listed as oils in accordance with the food intake patterns shown in Table 2-6. It is recommended that the fat sources be from fish, nuts, and vegetable oils.

Table 2-10 *Meats, Poultry, Fish, Dry Beans, Eggs, and Nuts*	
Beef	Dried beans
Lamb	Dried peas
Veal	Lentils
Pork, except bacon	Nuts
Organ meats, such as heart, liver, kidney, brain, tongue, sweetbread	Peanuts
	Peanut butter
Poultry, such as chicken, duck, goose, turkey	Soybean flour
	Soybeans
Fish, shellfish	

The Mediterranean diet has received attention because of the American Heart Association's recommendation to increase monounsaturated fats in the diet. The recommendations are outlined in Chapter 5. The following guidelines are recommended:

1. Eat the majority of food from plant sources, such as potatoes, grains and breads, beans, fruits, vegetables, nuts, and seeds.

2. Eat minimally processed foods, with an emphasis on fresh, locally grown foods.

3. Replace other fats and oils with olive oil.

4. Keep total fat in a range of less than 20–35% of energy. Saturated fat should be no more than 7–8% of energy.

5. Eat low to moderate amounts of cheese and yogurt (low fat and fat-free preferable).

6. Eat low to moderate amounts of fish and poultry and from zero to four eggs per week (those used in cooking need to be counted).

7. Eat fruit for dessert; desserts that contain a significant amount of sugar and saturated fat should be eaten only a few times per week.

8. Eat red meat a few times per month, not to exceed 12–16 ounces per month.

9. Engage in regular exercise to promote fitness, a healthy weight, and a feeling of physical well-being.

10. Drink wine in moderation (wine is optional). Wine with meals— one to two glasses per day for men and one glass per day for women.

FOOD LABELING

As a result of the passage by Congress of the Nutrition Labeling and Education Act (NLEA) in 1990, nutrition labeling regulations became mandatory in May 1994 for nearly all processed foods. The primary objective of the changes was to ensure that labels would be on most foods and would provide consistent nutrition information. The resulting food labels provide the consumer with more information on the nutrient contents of foods and how those nutrients affect health than former labels provided. Health claims allowed on labels are limited and set by the Food and Drug Administration (FDA). Serving sizes are determined by the FDA and not by the individual food processor. Descriptive terms used for foods are standardized. For example, "low fat" means that each serving contains 3 grams of fat or less.

Current Label

The nutrition label has a formatted space called Nutrition Facts (Figure 2-2) that includes required and optional information.

The items, with amounts per serving, that must be included on the food label are:

- Total calories
- Calories from fat

Nutrition Facts

Serving Size 1/2 cup (114g)
Servings Per Container 4

Amount Per Serving	
Calories 90	Calories from Fat 30

	% Daily Value
Total Fat 3g	5%
Saturated Fat 0g	0%
Cholesterol 0mg	0%
Sodium 300mg	13%
Total Carbohydrate 13g	4%
Dietary Fiber 3g	12%
Sugars 3g	
Protein 3g	

Vitamin A	80%	Vitamin C	60%
Calcium	4%	Iron	4%

* Percent Daily Values are based on a 2,000 calorie diet. Your daily values may be higher or lower depending on your calorie needs:

	Calories	2,000	2,500
Total Fat	Less than	65g	80g
Sat Fat	Less than	20g	25g
Cholesterol	Less than	300mg	300mg
Sodium	Less than	2,400mg	2,400mg
Total Carbohydrate		300g	375g
Fiber		25g	30g

Calories per gram:
Fat 9   •   Carbohydrate 4   •   Protein 4

Figure 2-2 *Food label. (Courtesy of the FDA)*

EXPLORING THE WEB

The Web site for the Center for Food Safety and Applied Nutrition, of the U.S. Food and Drug Administration, at www.cfsan.fda.gov, has an abundance of information on using the food label. Visit the Web site and create fact sheets on how to use the food label to lose weight, to lower salt intake, to control diabetes, and to prevent heart disease. These sheets can also be used to aid in the teaching of clients.

- Total fat
- Saturated fat
- Trans fat
- Cholesterol
- Sodium
- Total carbohydrates
- Dietary fiber
- Sugars
- Protein
- Vitamin A
- Vitamin C
- Calcium
- Iron

The food processor can voluntarily include additional information on food products. If a health claim is made about the food or if the food is enriched or fortified with an optional nutrient, then nutrition information about that nutrient becomes required. The standardized serving size is based on amounts of the specific food commonly eaten, and it is given in both English and metric measurements (Table 2-11).

daily values
represent percentage per serving of each nutritional item listed on food labels based on a daily intake of 2,000 calories

Daily values on the label give the consumer the percentage per serving of each nutritional item listed, based on a daily diet of 2,000 calories. For example, total fat on Figure 2-2 shows 3 grams, which represents 5% of the amount of fat someone on a 2,000-calorie diet should have. The label also shows the *maximum* amount of a nutrient that should be eaten (for example, fat) or the *minimum* requirement for specified nutrients (for example, carbohydrates) based on a daily diet of 2,000 calories and another based on 2,500 calo-

SUPERSIZE USA

The MyPyramid guidelines were developed in the atmosphere of the growing obesity epidemic in this country. One of the unique aspects of MyPyramid is that it recognizes that one size does not fit all. MyPyramid accounts for this by incorporating these concepts:

- *Activity.* The steps on the left side of the pyramid represent the daily need for physical activity to supplement the benefits of eating a healthy diet.
- *Moderation.* The pyramid's wide base and narrow tip highlight the concept of moderation. Foods with little or no solid fats or added sugars should be consumed often. As activity level increases, these foods can be eaten more. Also as activity level increases, added sugars, trans fatty acids, high-cholesterol foods, salt, and alcohol can be consumed, but they must be limited.
- *Proportionality.* The width of each food group band provides an approximate guide to suggest how much should be eaten from each food group.
- *Gradual improvement.* The "Steps to a Healthier You" slogan encourages small steps toward health benefits from observing the MyPyramid guidelines combined with physical activity.

Table 2-11 *Household and Metric Measures*

- 1 teaspoon (tsp) = 5 milliliters (ml)
- 1 tablespoon (Tbsp) = 15 ml
- 1 cup (C) = 240 ml
- 1 fluid ounce (fl oz) = 30 ml
- 1 ounce (oz) = 28 grams (g)

ries. The items included here are the amounts of total fat, saturated fat, cholesterol, sodium, total carbohydrate, and fiber. In addition, the label lists the calories per gram for fats, carbohydrates, and proteins.

Health Claims

Because diet has been implicated as a factor in heart disease, stroke, birth defects, and cancer, the following *health claims* linking a nutrient to a health-related condition are allowed on labels. They are intended to help consumers both choose foods that are the most healthful for them and avoid being deceived by false advertisements on the label. The allowed claims are for the relationship between:

- Calcium and *osteoporosis*
- Sodium and *hypertension*
- Diets low in saturated fat and cholesterol and high in fruits, vegetables, and grains containing dietary fiber and *coronary heart disease*
- Diets low in fat and high in fruits and vegetables containing dietary fiber and the antioxidants, vitamins A and C, and *cancer*
- Diets low in fat and high in fiber-containing grains, fruits, and vegetables and *cancer*
- Folic acid and *neural tube defects*
- Soy and reduced risk of cardiac heart disease

Two additional criteria must also be met:

1. A food whose label makes a health claim must be a naturally good source (containing at least 10% of the daily value) of at least one of the following nutrients: protein, vitamin A, vitamin C, iron, calcium, or fiber.
2. Health claims cannot be made for a food if a standard serving contains more than 20% of the daily value for total fat, saturated fat, cholesterol, or sodium.

Terminology

The FDA has also standardized **descriptors** (terms used by manufacturers to describe products) on food labels to help the consumer select the most appropriate and healthful foods. The following are examples:

- *Low calorie* means 40 calories or less per serving.
- *Calorie free* means less than 5 calories per serving.

descriptors
terms used to describe something

○ **food customs**
food habits

○ **dietary laws**
rules to be followed in meal planning in some religions

⚞ *Low fat* means a food has no more than 3 grams of fat per serving or per 100 grams of the food.

⚞ *Fat free* means a food contains less than 0.5 gram of fat per serving.

⚞ *Low saturated fat* means 1 gram or less of saturated fat per serving.

⚞ *Low cholesterol* means 20 mg or less of cholesterol per serving.

⚞ *Cholesterol free* means less than 2 mg of cholesterol per serving.

⚞ *No added sugar* means that no sugar or sweeteners of any kind have been added at any time during the preparation and packaging. When such a term is used, the package must also state that it is not low calorie or calorie reduced (unless it actually is).

⚞ *Low sodium* means less than 140 mg of sodium per serving.

⚞ *Very low sodium* means less than 35 mg of sodium per serving.

Obviously, the information on food labels is useful to all consumers and especially to those who must select foods for therapeutic diets. Health care professionals should become thoroughly knowledgeable about the labeling law. On request, many food manufacturers will provide the consumer with additional detailed information about their products.

FOOD CUSTOMS

MyPyramid and Nutrition Facts labels are useful in planning a nutritionally sound diet, but dietary and religious customs must also be taken into consideration. People from each country have favorite foods. Frequently, there are distinctive **food customs** originating in just a small section of a particular country. People of a particular area favor the foods that are produced in that area because they are available and economical. Some religions have **dietary laws** that require particular food practices. Because most people prefer the foods they were accustomed to while growing up, food habits are often based on nationality and religion.

One's economic status and social status also contribute to food habits. For example, the poor do not grow up with a taste for prime rib, whereas the wealthy may at least be accustomed to it—whether or not they like it. Those in a certain social class will be apt to consume the same foods as others in their class. And the foods they choose will probably depend on the work they do. For example, people doing hard, physical labor will require higher-calorie foods than will people in sedentary jobs.

When people move from one country to another, or from one area to another, their economic status may change. They will be introduced to new foods and new food customs. Although their original food customs may have been nutritionally adequate, their new environment may cause them to change their eating habits. For example, if milk was a staple (basic) food in their diet before moving and is unusually expensive in the new environment, milk may be replaced by a cheaper, nutritionally inferior beverage such as soda, coffee, or tea. Candy, possibly a luxury in their former environment, may be inexpensive and popular in their new environment. As a result, a family might increase consumption of soda or candy and reduce purchases of more nutritious foods.

Someone who is not familiar with the nutritive values of foods can easily make such mistakes in food selection.

The meal patterns of national and religious groups different from one's own may seem strange. However, the diet may well be nutritionally adequate. When a client's eating habits need to be corrected, such corrections are most easily made if the food customs of the client are known and understood. The health care professional can gain this knowledge by talking with the client and learning about her or his background. A dietitian can use that knowledge to plan nourishing menus consisting of foods that appeal to the client. The necessary adjustments in the diet can then be made gradually and effectively.

FOOD PATTERNS BASED ON CULTURE

American cuisine (cooking style) is a marvelous composite of countless national, regional, cultural, and religious food customs. Consequently, categorizing a client's food habits can be difficult. Nevertheless, it is sometimes helpful to be able to do so to a certain extent. People who are ill commonly have little interest in food. Sometimes comfort foods (foods that were familiar to them during their childhood) are more apt to tempt them than other types. The following section briefly discusses some food patterns typical of various cultures, regions, and countries. Of course, there can be and usually are enormous variations within any one classification.

Native American

It is thought that approximately half of the edible plants commonly eaten in the United States today originated with the Native Americans. Examples are corn, potatoes, squash, cranberries, pumpkins, peppers, beans, wild rice, and cocoa beans (Figure 2-3). In addition, wild fruits, game, and fish are also popular.

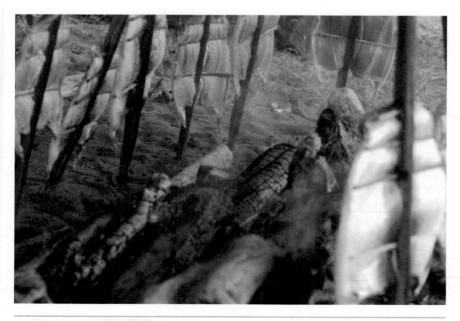

Figure 2-3 *Traditional Native American food.*

Foods are commonly prepared as soups and stews or are dried. The original Native American diets were probably more nutritionally adequate than are current diets, which frequently consist of too high a proportion of sweet and salty, snack-type low-nutrient-dense foods. Native American diets today may be deficient in calcium, vitamins A, C, and riboflavin.

U.S. Southern

Hot breads such as corn bread and baking powder biscuits are common in the U.S. South. Grits and rice are also popular carbohydrate foods. Favorite vegetables include sweet potatoes, squash, green beans, and lima beans. Green beans cooked with pork are commonly served. Watermelon, oranges, and peaches are popular fruits. Fried fish is served often, as are barbecued and stewed meats and poultry. These diets have a great deal of carbohydrate and fat and limited amounts of protein in some cases. Iron, calcium, and vitamins A and C may be deficient.

Mexican-Hispanic

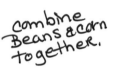

combine Beans & corn together.

Mexican food is a combination of Spanish and Native American foods. Beans, rice, chili peppers, tomatoes, and corn meal are favorites. Meat is often cooked with the vegetable. Corn meal or flour is used to make tortillas, which serve as bread. The combination of beans and corn makes a complete protein. Corn tortillas filled with cheese (called enchiladas) provide some calcium, but the use of milk should be encouraged. Additional green and yellow vegetables and vitamin C–rich foods would also improve these diets.

Puerto Rican

Rice is the basic carbohydrate food in Puerto Rican diets (Figure 2-4). Vegetables commonly used include beans, plantains, tomatoes, and peppers. Bananas, pineapple, mangoes, and papayas are popular fruits. Favorite meats are chicken, beef, and pork. Milk is not used as much as would be desirable from the nutritional point of view.

Italian

Pastas with various tomato or fish sauces and cheese are popular Italian foods. Fish and highly seasoned foods are common to southern Italian cuisine; meat and root vegetables are common to northern Italy. The eggs, cheese, tomatoes, green vegetables, and fruits common to Italian diets provide excellent sources of many nutrients, but additional fat-free milk and low-fat meat would improve the diet.

Northern and Western European

Northern and Western European diets are similar to those of the U.S. Midwest, but with a greater use of dark breads, potatoes, and fish and fewer green veg-

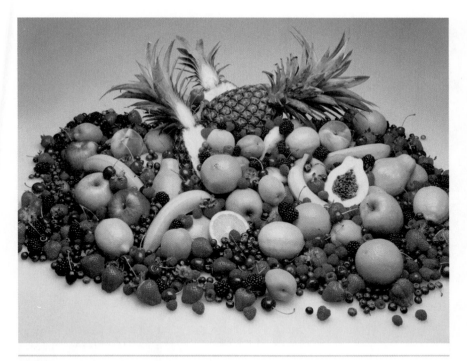

Figure 2-4 *Traditional Puerto Rican food.*

etable salads. Beef and pork are popular, as are various cooked vegetables, breads, cakes, and dairy products. The addition of fresh vegetables and fruits would add vitamins, minerals, and fiber to these diets.

Central European

Citizens of Central Europe obtain the greatest portion of their calories from potatoes and grain, especially rye and buckwheat. Pork is a popular meat. Cabbage cooked in many ways is a popular vegetable, as are carrots, onions, and turnips. Eggs and dairy products are used abundantly. Limiting the number of eggs consumed and using fat-free or low-fat dairy products would reduce the fat content in this diet. Adding fresh vegetables and fruits would increase vitamins, minerals, and fiber.

Middle Eastern

Grains, wheat, and rice provide energy in Middle Eastern diets. Chickpeas in the form of hummus are popular. Lamb and yogurt are commonly used, as are cabbage, grape leaves, eggplant, tomatoes, dates, olives, and figs (Figure 2-5). Black, very sweet coffee is a popular beverage. There may be insufficient protein and calcium in this diet, depending on the amounts of meat and calcium-rich foods eaten. Fresh fruits and vegetables should be added to the diet to increase vitamins, minerals, and fiber.

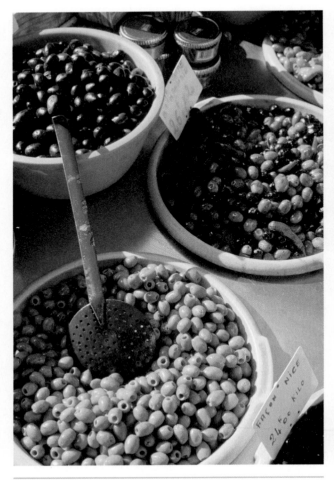

Figure 2-5 *Traditional Middle Eastern food.*

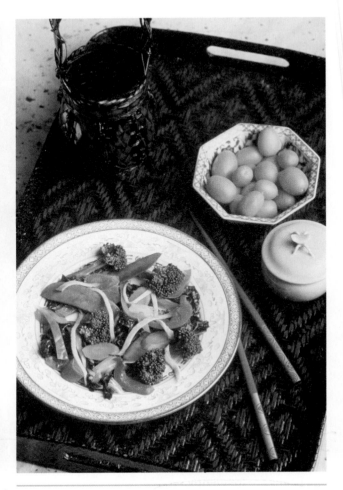

Figure 2-6 *Traditional Chinese food.*

Chinese

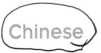

The Chinese diet is varied (Figure 2-6). Rice is the primary energy food and is used in place of bread. Foods are generally cut into small pieces. Vegetables are lightly cooked, and the cooking water is saved for future use. Soybeans are used in many ways, and eggs and pork are commonly served. Soy sauce is extensively used, but it is very salty and could present a problem for clients on low-salt diets. Tea is a common beverage, but milk is not. This diet may be low in fat.

Japanese

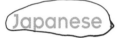

Japanese diets include rice, soybean paste and curd, vegetables, fruits, and fish. Food is frequently served tempura style, which means fried. Soy sauce (shoyu) and tea are commonly used. Current Japanese diets have been greatly influenced by Western culture. Japanese diets may be deficient in calcium, given the near total lack of milk in the diet. Although fish is eaten with bones, it may not supply sufficient calcium to meet needs. Japanese diets may contain excessive amounts of salt.

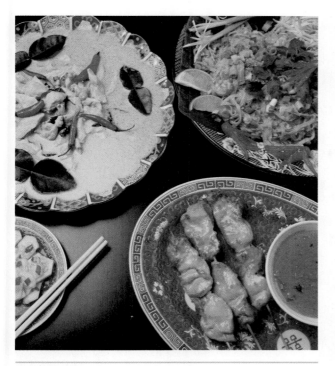

Figure 2-7 *Traditional Thai food.*

Indian

Many Indians are vegetarians who use eggs and dairy products. Rice, peas, and beans are frequently served. Spices, especially curry, are popular. Indian meals are not typically served in courses as Western meals are. They generally consist of one course with many dishes. Eating with one's fingers is considered acceptable.

Thai, Vietnamese, Laotian, and Cambodian

Rice, curries, vegetables, and fruit are popular in Thailand, Vietnam, Laos, and Cambodia (Figure 2-7). Meats and fish are used in small amounts. The wok (a deep, round fry pan) is used for sautéing many foods. A salty sauce made from fermented fish is commonly used. Thai, Vietnamese, Laotian, and Cambodian diets may contain inadequate amounts of protein and calcium.

FOOD PATTERNS BASED ON RELIGION OR PHILOSOPHY

Jewish

Interpretations of the Jewish dietary laws vary. Persons who adhere to the Orthodox view consider tradition important and always observe the dietary laws.

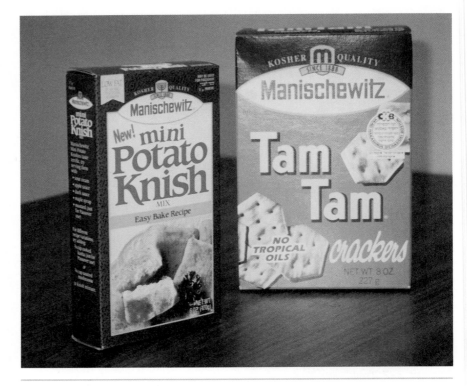

Figure 2-8 *Kosher food label.*

Foods prepared according to these laws are called *kosher* (Figure 2-8). Conservative Jews are inclined to observe the rules only at home. Reform Jews consider their dietary laws to be essentially ceremonial and so minimize their significance. Essentially the laws require the following:

- Slaughtering must be done by a qualified person in a prescribed manner. The meat or poultry must be drained of blood, first by severing the jugular vein and carotid artery, then by soaking in brine before cooking.
- Meat and meat products may not be prepared with milk or milk products.
- The dishes used in the preparation and serving of meat products must be kept separate from those used for dairy foods.
- Dairy products and meat may not be eaten together. At least 6 hours must elapse after eating meat before eating dairy products, and 30 minutes to 1 hour must elapse after eating dairy products before eating meat.
- The mouth must be rinsed after eating fish and before eating meat.
- There are prescribed fast days: Passover Week, Yom Kippur, and the Feast of Purim.
- No cooking is done on the Sabbath, from sundown Friday to sundown Saturday.

Jewish dietary laws forbid the eating of the following:

- The flesh of animals without cloven (split) hooves or that do not chew their cud
- Hindquarters of any animal
- Shellfish or fish without scales or fins
- Birds of prey
- Creeping things and insects
- Leavened (contains ingredients that cause it to rise) bread during the Passover

In general, the food served is rich. Chicken and fresh-smoked and salted fish are popular, as are noodles, eggs, and flour dishes. These diets can be deficient in fresh vegetables and milk.

Roman Catholic

Although the dietary restrictions of the Roman Catholic religion have been liberalized, meat is not allowed on Ash Wednesday and Good Friday, but the Pope requests adherents to abstain on the other Fridays during Lent.

Eastern Orthodox

The Eastern Orthodox religion includes Christians from the Middle East, Russia, and Greece. Although interpretations of the dietary laws vary, meat, poultry, fish, and dairy products are restricted on Wednesdays and Fridays and during Lent and Advent.

Seventh Day Adventist

In general, Seventh Day Adventists are **lacto-ovo vegetarians**, which means they use milk products and eggs, but no meat, fish, or poultry. They may also use nuts, legumes, and meat analogues (substitutes) and tofu (made from soybeans). They consider coffee, tea, and alcohol to be harmful.

lacto-ovo vegetarians
vegetarians who will eat dairy products and eggs, but no meat, poultry, or fish

Mormon (Latter Day Saints)

The only dietary restriction observed by the Mormons is the prohibition of coffee, tea, and alcoholic beverages.

Islamic

Adherents of Islam are called Muslims. Their dietary laws prohibit the use of pork and alcohol, and other meats must be slaughtered according to specific laws. During the month of Ramadan, Muslims do not eat or drink during daylight hours.

Hindu – Vegetarian

To the Hindus, all life is sacred, and animals contain the souls of ancestors. Consequently, most Hindus are vegetarians. They do not use eggs because eggs represent life.

OTHER FOOD PATTERNS
Vegetarians

There are several vegetarian diets. The common factor among them is that they do not include red meat. Some include eggs, some fish, some milk, and some even poultry. When carefully planned, these diets can be nutritious. They can even contribute to a reduction of obesity and a reduced risk of high blood pressure, heart disease, some cancers, and possibly diabetes. They must be carefully planned so that they include all the needed nutrients.

Lacto-ovo vegetarians use dairy products and eggs but no meat, poultry, or fish.

Lacto-vegetarians use dairy products but no meat, poultry, or eggs.

Vegans avoid all animal foods. They use soybeans, chickpeas, meat analogues, and tofu. It is important that their diets be carefully planned to include appropriate combinations of the essential amino acids. For example, beans served with corn or rice, or peanuts eaten with wheat, are better in such combinations than any of them would be if eaten alone. Vegans can show deficiencies of calcium; vitamins A, D, and B_{12}; and, of course, proteins.

lacto-vegetarians
vegetarians who eat dairy products

vegans
vegetarians who avoid all animal foods

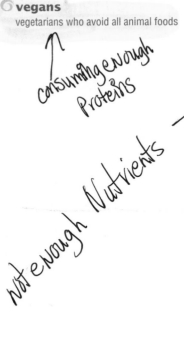

Zen-Macrobiotic Diets

The macrobiotic diet is a system of 10 diet plans, developed from Zen Buddhism. Adherents progress from the lower number diet to the higher, gradually giving up foods in the following order: desserts, salads, fruits, animal foods, soups, and ultimately vegetables, until only cereals—usually brown rice—are consumed. Beverages are kept to a minimum, and only organically grown foods are used. Foods are grouped as yang (male) or yin (female). A ratio of 5:1 yang to yin is considered important. Most macrobiotic diets are nutritionally inadequate. As the adherents give up foods according to plans, their diets become increasingly inadequate. These diets can be especially dangerous because avid adherents promise medical cures from the diets that cannot be attained, and so medical treatment may be delayed when needed.

CONSIDERATIONS FOR THE HEALTH CARE PROFESSIONAL

Learning and understanding the tools with which to plan a healthy diet are important for all health care professionals so that they can help their clients. All clients should be viewed as individuals whose food customs, which may be different from the health care professional's, must be respected. A registered dietitian will help with a specific diet plan for a hospitalized client. The dietitian will take into account the client's likes, dislikes, and food customs.

Bring Nutrition ATI Books

SUMMARY

MyPyramid emphasizes grains, fruits, and vegetables—all plant foods. It also includes milk, yogurt, and cheese; meat, poultry, fish, dry beans, eggs, and nuts; and fats, oils, and sweets. Each group has a recommended number of portions based on specific-calorie levels. The recommendations are useful in planning a nutritious diet. The Dietary Guidelines are important tools in the maintenance of good health through good nutrition. Their basic recommendation is to eat a balanced diet.

Food habits have many diverse origins. Nationality, religion, and economic and social status all affect their development. When food customs result in inadequate diets, corrections should be made gradually. Corrections are easier to make and are more effective when the reasons for the food habits are understood.

DISCUSSION TOPICS

1. Discuss the reasons why health care professionals should practice the rules of good nutrition themselves.

2. How do food habits originate?

3. What effects does environment have on particular food habits? When do the effects of a new environment improve diets, and when do they impair them?

4. From personal experience, explain why certain foods are enjoyed more than others that are commonly available in the local area.

5. Why might Scandinavians like fish more than Hungarians do?

6. Why are Zen-macrobiotic diets dangerous?

7. Discuss vegetarian diets. Are they safe? Explain.

8. Why is it difficult to convince someone to change her or his food habits? Discuss.

9. Define a balanced diet.

10. Describe MyPyramid, including number of servings or portion size recommended for each group.

11. How might one include milk in the diet of a 4-year-old who refuses to drink it?

12. Why would yogurt be a good snack or dessert for a pregnant woman?

13. Alcohol is not considered a food, so why is a Dietary Guideline devoted to it?

14. Why should "crash" or "fad" diets be avoided? What is a better alternative? Why?

15. Discuss the sale of foods with low nutrient density in school cafeterias. Is it a good practice? If so, why? If not, why not? What would your position be on this subject if you were principal of an elementary school? Of a junior or senior high school?

SUGGESTED ACTIVITIES

1. Give a series of short reports on food customs. Each student should select a different country or area within a country for study. After the reports have been presented, hold a class discussion on whether climate, availability of food, or economic or other factors determine the food customs of the countries studied. Include answers to the following questions: What is the climate of the country? What types of crops are grown there? Are modern methods of agriculture used? Does the country depend on imports for much of its food supply? If so, what foods are imported? Are the majority of the citizens poor? What types of foods are popular? What types are expensive? Which of these foods are produced in the country? Which are imported? What is the prevalent religion?

2. Plan a Good Friday menu for a client of the Roman Catholic faith.

3. Role-play a situation in which a diet counselor tries to persuade a client to use more milk.

4. Buy some fruits and vegetables that are new to you. Bring them to class and sample them. Share ideas about their potential uses. Perhaps these might be added to family menus.

5. Using a restaurant menu, choose breakfast, lunch, and dinner. Check the selection of foods

against MyPyramid. Are they balanced meals? Discuss the problems that people who eat all their meals in restaurants might have in maintaining a well-balanced diet.

6. Using the following table, fill in the "Menus" column with the foods eaten in the past two days. In the "Food Groups Used" column, list the group to which each food belongs. To evaluate personal dietary habits, fill in the "Food Groups Not Used" column. Compare the table with those of the rest of the class and discuss how your eating habits could be improved.

Menus	Food Groups Used	Food Groups Not Used
Breakfast		
Lunch		
Dinner		
Snacks		

7. Check labels on sour cream and yogurt containers. Which would be preferable for someone on a fat-restricted diet? Why? How does the calcium content compare?

8. Adapt the following menu for a person of the Orthodox Jewish faith.

Baked ham	Bread and butter
Scalloped potatoes	Fresh fruit
Buttered peas	Milk or coffee

REVIEW

Multiple choice. Select the *letter* that precedes the best answer.

1. Food customs mean one's
   a. food nutrients
   b. food habits
   c. food requirements
   d. all of the above

2. Food customs
   a. may be based on religion or nationality
   b. are always nutritious
   c. are easily changed
   d. are not affected by one's social status

3. Moving to a new environment or experiencing a change in salary
   a. rarely changes established food habits
   b. usually influences established food habits
   c. always reduces the amount of food eaten
   d. never reduces the quality of food eaten

4. Hot breads are common to diets of people from
   a. Mexico
   b. the U.S. Midwest
   c. China
   d. the U.S. South

5. Rice is a popular carbohydrate food in
   a. Puerto Rico
   b. Central Europe
   c. Northern Europe
   d. all of the above

6. In general, the diets of U.S. Southerners, Mexicans, Puerto Ricans, and Italians would be improved by the addition of more
   a. rice
   b. corn
   c. milk
   d. pasta

7. A diet of dried beans, corn, and chili peppers would most likely be used by a(n)
   a. Mexican family
   b. Italian family
   c. Armenian family
   d. Orthodox Jewish family

8. A balanced diet is one that includes
   a. equal amounts of carbohydrates and fats
   b. no animal products
   c. all six classes of nutrients
   d. more vegetables than fruits

9. Fruits and vegetables are rich sources of
   a. vitamins
   b. fats
   c. proteins
   d. all of the above

10. Teenagers should have a serving of milk (or its substitute)
    a. not more than twice a day
    b. three times a day
    c. not more than four times a week
    d. not at all if they are overweight

11. Milk products are made from milk and include
    a. butter and margarine
    b. yogurt and cottage cheese
    c. bean curd and coconut milk
    d. all of the above

12. Milk and its products are the best dietary source of
    a. proteins and fats
    b. calcium
    c. carbohydrates
    d. all of the above

13. Breads, cereals, rice, and pasta are rich sources of
    a. vitamin D
    b. fats
    c. carbohydrates
    d. all of the above

14. Daily intake from the meat group should be:
    a. 2 oz
    b. 5½ oz
    c. 8 oz
    d. 11 oz

15. Foods from the meat group are rich sources of
    a. proteins
    b. carbohydrates
    c. vitamin C
    d. all of the above

16. An example of a breakfast with high nutrient density is
    a. pancakes and cocoa
    b. melon, bran muffin, and cocoa made with fat-free milk
    c. fruit-flavored beverage, cinnamon bun, and coffee
    d. fried eggs, bacon, and coffee

17. Excessive amounts of salt in the diet
    a. raise cholesterol levels substantially
    b. are thought to contribute to hypertension
    c. cause cirrhosis of the liver
    d. have no relevance to one's nutritional status

18. MyPyramid
    a. food groups are nutritionally interchangeable
    b. is an outline for meal planning for adults only
    c. advises that fruits and vegetables be eaten in moderation
    d. recommends portion ranges of bread, cereal, rice, and pasta each day

19. The Nutrition Labeling and Education Act of 1990
    a. requires that descriptive words used for foods be standardized
    b. sets maximum amounts of cholesterol allowed for each food serving
    c. permits no health claims on food containers
    d. does not require the food manufacturer or processor to list the total amounts in each serving of calories, sodium, or dietary fiber

20. Foods rich in complex carbohydrates, such as breads and cereals, are also excellent sources of
    a. calcium and phosphorus
    b. vitamins C and D
    c. dietary fiber and B vitamins
    d. proteins and fats

21. When choosing foods from the meats, poultry, and fish food group, one should be careful to select foods that
    a. are rich in calcium and phosphorus
    b. provide at least one-half of one's daily need for carbohydrates
    c. have limited amounts of protein and iron
    d. are low in saturated fats and cholesterol

22. The two vitamins that the Nutrition Labeling and Education Act of 1990 requires be included as amounts per serving on food labels are
    a. vitamin A and thiamine
    b. niacin and folic acid
    c. vitamins A and C
    d. vitamins D and K

23. Immoderate use of alcoholic beverages
    a. by pregnant women can cause birth defects
    b. can cause cirrhosis of the liver only in men
    c. has little or no effect on one's nutritional status
    d. has no effect on one's appetite

CASE IN POINT

JEFFREY: PLANNING A HEALTHY DIET

Jeffrey, a Native American, has lived on his reservation in Idaho all his life. He and his family have enjoyed fresh home-grown vegetables, and fish has been a staple in his diet. Jeff attended the local reservation high school and earned a scholarship to move from Idaho to attend Arizona University in Scottsdale. Jeff's mother is concerned about his health. She knows that Jeff will experience some foods that may not be very good for him. She wants him to be aware of the consequences of alcohol, fast foods, and drugs. Upon freshmen orientation, she sets up a meeting for Jeff in the Student Health Clinic. He will be seeing a nurse practitioner and a dietitian.

ASSESSMENT

1. What factors will be influencing Jeff as he attends college?
2. List the subjective information that can be obtained from Jeff and his mother about his eating habits
3. What can you caution Jeff regarding his introduction into the college world of nutrition?
4. How significant are these problems?

DIAGNOSIS

5. Write a nursing diagnosis for Jeff.

PLAN/GOAL

6. What changes will Jeff expect to see if he decides to eat less healthily?
7. What situations will be most stressful to Jeff?

IMPLEMENTATION

8. List some strategies Jeff can use to help keep himself healthy.
9. What substitutes would Jeff be able to make to be able to fit in with the crowd and still be eating well?
10. What would you caution Jeff about in regard to stressful situations?

EVALUATION/OUTCOME CRITERIA

11. How will Jeff be able to determine his success for healthy eating?
12. How well will Jeff be able to associate body changes with poor food choices?

THINKING FURTHER

13. Who else will benefit from Jeff's food choices?
14. What information on the Internet could benefit Jeff?

◎ RATE THIS PLATE

Jeff met with the dietitian to better understand what types of food would be served in the dining hall and what would be the best choices for him to eat since he didn't want to gain the "freshman 15." The dietitian gave Jeff a copy of MyPyramid and figured his caloric needs to be 2,400 calories daily. The dietitian accessed www.mypyramid.gov, and the two of them went through the entire program together, with the dietitian showing Jeff how to input his foods to determine his caloric intake. The dietitian had Jeff plan a meal that he would eat, and then they analyzed it. Rate this plate.

1 1/2 cups beef and noodles
1/2 cup mashed potatoes
1/2 cup green beans
Tossed salad
2 Tbsp regular ranch dressing
2 whole-grain rolls with 2 tsp butter
1 cup mixed fruit
Ice cream cone with ½ cup ice cream

How did Jeff do with his planning? Does this meal follow the serving sizes on MyPyramid? Analyze Jeff's meal plan using the MyPyramid Web site and then determine how many servings in each food group he has left for the rest of the day? Would you change any portion sizes, and if so, which ones?

CASE IN POINT

TARA: LIVING WITH MIGRAINES

Tara, a native of Puerto Rico, has suffered from migraine headaches since she was 13. Tara does not like to take medicine and feels that the drugs and pharmacopeias of the Western world inhibit the body and cause more problems. At 25, Tara decides that she will follow the Zen Buddhism diet to rid herself of the migraines. For a long time she has felt that by following the Zen Buddhism way of life, she will be brought to a higher level of completeness. Tara has adopted the Zen diet.

ASSESSMENT

1. What subjective data do you have?
2. What objective data does the nurse need about Tara to assess her current state of health?
3. What information would be obtained from a food diary and food history?
4. What potential problems need to be addressed with Tara?

DIAGNOSIS

5. Write a nursing diagnosis for Tara.

PLAN/GOAL

6. What changes will there be in Tara's diet, and how can Tara measure changes in her health?

IMPLEMENTATION

7. Which dietary guidelines will be controversial for Tara's health?
8. What foods would be of benefit to Tara to give up?
9. How would you, as a dietition, advise Tara regarding her choice of diets?

EVALUATION/OUTCOME CRITERIA

10. If Tara does decide to follow a Zen diet, what criteria should be used to monitor Tara's health?
11. Which indicators would be present if the diet was harmful to Tara?

THINKING FURTHER

12. How would the Internet be helpful to Tara?
13. How could you use this lesson in other situations?

RATE THIS PLATE

Tara has decided to eliminate everything she can in her diet that would cause a migraine headache. This is the lunch she chose to eat. Rate this plate.

Black bean chili
    Black beans
    Jalapenos
    Bulgur
    Canned diced tomatoes
    Onion
    Green pepper
    Garlic
    Vegetable bouillon
    Chili powder, cayenne pepper, cumin
Sliced avocados
Tortilla chips
Decaf tea with aspartame (Equal)

Tara is new at being a vegan vegetarian. How did she do? Everything looks vegan, but will just being a vegan eliminate her migraine headaches? Is there an amino acid that may be triggering her headaches? Check out the Internet for a migraine diet to see if she has eliminated everything she needs to. What did you find?

CHAPTER 3

DIGESTION, ABSORPTION, AND METABOLISM

OBJECTIVES

After studying this chapter, you should be able to:

- Describe the processes of digestion, absorption, and metabolism
- Name the organs in the digestive system and describe their functions
- Name the enzymes or digestive juices secreted by each organ and gland in the digestive system
- Calculate your basal metabolic rate (BMR)

Although the body is infinitely more complex than the automobile engine, it may be compared to the engine because both require fuel to run. The body's fuel is, of course, food. For the body to use its fuel, it must first prepare the food and then distribute it appropriately. It does this through the processes of digestion and absorption. The actual use of the food as fuel, resulting in energy, is called **metabolism.**

DIGESTION

Digestion is the process whereby food is broken down into smaller parts, chemically changed, and moved through the gastrointestinal system. The **gastrointestinal (GI) tract** consists of the body structures that participate in digestion. Digestion begins in the mouth and ends at the anus. Along the entire GI tract secretions of mucus lubricate and protect the mucosal tissues. As the process of digestion is discussed, refer to Figure 3-1 and note the locations of the structures that perform the functions of digestion.

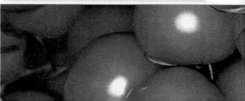

Digestion occurs through two types of action—mechanical and chemical. During **mechanical digestion,** food is broken into smaller pieces by the teeth. It is then moved along the gastrointestinal tract through the esophagus, stomach, and intestines. This movement is caused by a rhythmic contraction of the muscular walls of the tract called **peristalsis.** Mechanical digestion helps to prepare food for chemical digestion by breaking it into smaller pieces. Several small pieces collectively have more surface area than fewer large ones and thus are more readily broken down by digestive juices.

metabolism
the use of the food by the body after digestion which results in energy

digestion
breakdown of food in the body in preparation for absorption

gastrointestinal (GI) tract
pertaining to the digestive system

mechanical digestion
the part of digestion that requires certain mechanical movements such as chewing, swallowing, and peristalsis

peristalsis
rhythmical movement of the intestinal tract; moves the chyme along

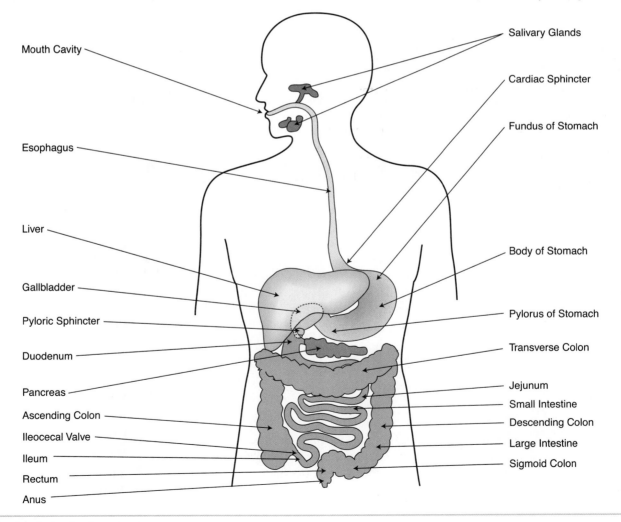

Figure 3-1 *The digestive system.*

◌ chemical digestion
chemical changes in foods during
digestion caused by hydrolysis

◌ hydrolysis
the addition of water resulting in the
breakdown of the molecule

◌ enzyme
organic substance that causes changes in
other substances

◌ catalyst
a substance that causes another
substance to react

◌ pancreas
gland that secretes enzymes essential for
digestion and insulin, which is essential
for glucose metabolism

◌ bolus
food in the mouth that is ready to be
swallowed

◌ saliva
secretion of the salivary glands

◌ salivary amylase
also called ptyalin; the enzyme secreted
by the salivary glands to act on starch

During **chemical digestion,** the composition of carbohydrates, proteins, and fats is changed. Chemical changes occur through the addition of water and the resulting splitting, or breaking down, of the food molecules. This process is called **hydrolysis.** Food is broken down into nutrients that the tissues can absorb and use. Hydrolysis also involves digestive **enzymes** that act on food substances, causing them to break down into simple compounds. An enzyme can also act as a **catalyst,** which speeds up the chemical reactions without itself being changed in the process. Digestive enzymes are secreted by the mouth, stomach, **pancreas,** and small intestine (Table 3-1). An enzyme is often named for the substance on which it acts. For example, the enzyme sucrase acts on sucrose, the enzyme maltase acts on maltose, and lactase acts on lactose.

Digestion in the Mouth

Digestion begins in the mouth, where the food is broken into smaller pieces by the teeth and mixed with saliva (Figure 3-2). At this point, each mouthful of food that is ready to be swallowed is called a **bolus. Saliva** is a secretion of the salivary glands that contains water, salts, and a digestive enzyme called **salivary amylase** (also called ptyalin), which acts on complex carbohydrates (starch). Food is normally held in the mouth for such a short time that only small amounts of carbohydrates are chemically changed there. The salivary glands also secrete a mucous material that lubricates and binds food particles to help in swallowing the bolus. The final chemical digestion of carbohydrates occurs in the small intestine.

Table 3-1 *Enzymes and Foods Acted Upon*

SOURCE	ENZYME	FOOD ACTED UPON
Mouth	Salivary amylase	Starch
Stomach	Pepsin	Proteins
	Rennin	Proteins in milk
	Gastric lipase	Emulsified fat
Small intestine	Pancreatic amylase	Starch
	Pancreatic proteases (trypsin) (chymotrypsin) (carboxypeptidases)	Proteins
	Pancreatic lipase (steapsin)	Fats
	Lactase	Lactose
	Maltase	Maltose
	Sucrase	Sucrose
	Peptidases	Proteins

1. Mouth: Teeth and tongue begin mechanical digestion by breaking food into smaller pieces.

2. Salivary Glands: Begin chemical digestion as salivary amylase begins to change starch to maltose.

3. Esophagus: Peristalsis and gravity move food along.

4. Stomach: Hydrochloric acid prepares the gastric area for enzyme action. Pepsin breaks down proteins. In children, rennin breaks down milk proteins. Lipase acts on emulsified fats.

5. Liver: Produces bile.

8. Small Intestine: Produces enzymes, prepares foods for absorption. Lactase converts lactose, maltase converts maltose, sucrase converts sucrose to simple sugars. Peptidases reduce proteins to amino acids.

6. Gallbladder: Stores bile and releases it into small intestine to emulsify fats.

7. Pancreas: Enzymes are released into the small intestine. Pancreatic amylase breaks down starch. Pancreatic lipase breaks down fats. Pancreatic proteases break down proteins.

9. Large Intestine: Absorbs water and some other nutrients, and collects food residue for excretion.

Figure 3-2 *Basic functions of the digestive system.*

The Esophagus

The **esophagus** is a 10-inch muscular tube through which food travels from the mouth to the stomach. When swallowed, the bolus of food is moved down the esophagus by peristalsis and gravity. At the lower end of the esophagus, the **cardiac sphincter** opens to allow passage of the bolus into the stomach. The cardiac sphincter prevents the acidic content of the stomach from flowing back into the esophagus. When this sphincter malfunctions, it causes acid reflux disease.

Digestion in the Stomach

The stomach consists of an upper portion known as the **fundus,** a middle area known as the body of the stomach, and the end nearest the small intestine called the **pylorus.** Food enters the fundus and moves to the body of the stomach, where the muscles in the stomach wall gradually knead the food, tear it, and mix it with gastric juices, and with the intrinsic factor necessary for the absorption of vitamin B_{12}, before it can be propelled forward in slow, controlled movements. The food becomes a semiliquid mass called **chyme** (pronounced "kime"). When the chyme enters the pylorus, it causes distention and the release of the hormone **gastrin,** which increases the release of gastric juices.

⊙ **esophagus**
tube leading from the mouth to the stomach; part of the gastrointestinal system

⊙ **cardiac sphincter**
the muscle at the base of the esophagus that prevents gastric reflux from moving into the esophagus

⊙ **fundus (of the stomach)**
upper part of the stomach

⊙ **pylorus**
the end of the stomach nearest the intestine

⊙ **chyme**
the food mass as it has been mixed with gastric juices

⊙ **gastrin**
hormone released by the stomach

gastric juices
the digestive secretions of the stomach

pepsin
an enzyme secreted by the stomach that is essential for the digestion of proteins

duodenum
first (and smallest) section of the small intestine

jejunum
middle section comprising about two-fifths of the small intestine

ileum
last part of the small intestine

secretin
hormone causing the pancreas to release sodium bicarbonate to neutralize acidity of the chyme

cholecystokinin
hormone that triggers the gallbladder to release bile

bile
secretion of the liver, stored in the gallbladder, essential for the digestion of fats

pancreatic protease
the enzyme secreted by the pancreas that is essential for the digestion of protein

pancreatic amylase
the enzyme secreted by the pancreas that is essential for the digestion of starch

pancreatic lipase
enzyme secreted by the pancreas that is essential for the digestion of fat

lactase
enzyme secreted by the small intestine for the digestion of lactose

maltase
enzyme secreted by the small intestine essential for the digestion of maltose

sucrase
enzyme secreted by the small intestine to aid in digestion of sucrose

peptidases
enzymes secreted by the small intestine that are essential for the digestion of protein

colon
large intestine

Gastric juices are digestive secretions of the stomach. They contain hydrochloric acid, **pepsin,** and mucus. Hydrochloric acid activates the enzyme pepsin, prepares protein molecules for partial digestion by pepsin, destroys most bacteria in the food ingested, and makes iron and calcium more soluble. As the hydrochloric acid is released, a thick mucus is also secreted to protect the stomach from this harsh acid. In children, there are two additional enzymes: rennin, which acts on milk protein and casein, and gastric lipase, which breaks the butterfat molecules of milk into smaller molecules.

In summary, the functions of the stomach include:

- Temporary storage of food
- Mixing of food with gastric juices
- Regulation of a slow, controlled emptying of food into the intestine
- Secretion of the intrinsic factor for vitamin B_{12} (to be discussed in Chapter 7)
- Destruction of most bacteria inadvertently consumed

Digestion in the Small Intestine

Chyme moves through the pyloric sphincter into the **duodenum,** the first section of the small intestine. Chyme subsequently passes through the **jejunum,** the midsection of the small intestine, and the **ileum,** the last section of the small intestine.

When food reaches the small intestine, the hormone **secretin** causes the pancreas to release sodium bicarbonate to neutralize the acidity of the chyme. The gallbladder is triggered by the hormone **cholecystokinin (CCK),** which is produced by intestinal mucosal glands when fat enters, to release **bile.** Bile is produced in the liver but stored in the gallbladder. Bile emulsifies fat after it is secreted into the small intestine. This action enables the enzymes to digest the fats more easily.

Chyme also triggers the pancreas to secrete its juice into the small intestine. Pancreatic juice contains the following enzymes:

- Trypsin, chymotrypsin, and carboxypeptidases split proteins into smaller substances. These are called **pancreatic proteases** because they are protein-splitting enzymes produced by the pancreas.
- **Pancreatic amylase** converts starches (polysaccharides) to simple sugars.
- **Pancreatic lipase** reduces fats to fatty acids and glycerol.

The small intestine itself produces an intestinal juice that contains the enzymes **lactase, maltase,** and **sucrase.** These enzymes split lactose, maltose, and sucrose, respectively, into simple sugars. The small intestine also produces enzymes called **peptidases** that break down proteins into amino acids.

The Large Intestine

The large intestine, or **colon,** consists of the cecum, colon, and rectum. The cecum is a blind pouchlike beginning of the colon in the right lower quadrant of the abdomen. The appendix is a diverticulum that extends off the cecum. The cecum is separated from the ileum by the ileocecal valve and is considered to be the beginning of the large intestine (colon). Its primary function is to absorb water and salts from undigested food. It has a muscular wall that can knead the contents to enhance absorption. One of the end products of fermentation in the cecum is volatile fatty acids. The major volatile fatty acids are acetate, propionate, and butyrate. These are absorbed from the large intestine and used as sources of energy. The digested food then enters the ascending colon and moves through the transverse colon and on to the descending colon, the sigmoid colon, the rectum, and, finally, the anal canal.

ABSORPTION

After digestion, the next major step in the body's use of its food is absorption (Figure 3-3). **Absorption** is the passage of nutrients into the blood or

absorption
passage of nutrients into the blood or lymphatic system

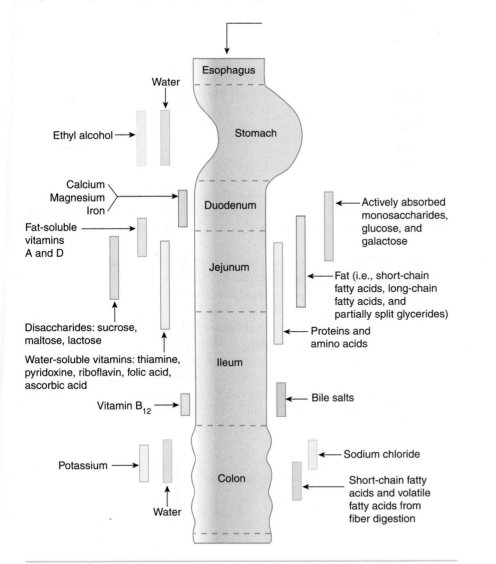

Figure 3-3 *Absorption in the gastrointestinal tract.*

⊙ lymphatic system
transports fat-soluble substances from the small intestine to the vascular system

⊙ villi
tiny, hairlike structures in the small intestines through which nutrients are absorbed

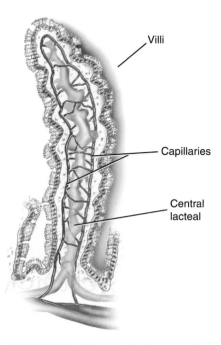

Figure 3-4 *Wall of the small intestine.*

⊙ capillaries
tiny blood vessels connecting veins and arteries

⊙ lacteals
lymphatic vessels in the small intestine that absorb fatty acids and glycerol

⊙ feces
solid waste from the large intestine

lymphatic system (the lymphatic vessels carry fat-soluble particles and molecules that are too large to pass through the capillaries into the bloodstream).

To be absorbed, nutrients must be in their simplest forms. Carbohydrates must be broken down to the simple sugars (glucose, fructose, and galactose), proteins to amino acids, and fats to fatty acids and glycerol. Most absorption of nutrients occurs in the small intestine, although some occurs in the large intestine. Water is absorbed in the stomach, small intestine, and large intestine.

Absorption in the Small Intestine

The small intestine is approximately 22 feet long. Its inner surface has mucosal folds, villi, and microvilli to increase the surface area for maximum absorption. The fingerlike projections called **villi** have hundreds of microscopic, hairlike projections called microvilli. The microvilli are very sensitive to the nutrient needs of our bodies (Figure 3-4). Each villus contains numerous blood **capillaries** (tiny blood vessels) and **lacteals** (lymphatic vessels). The villi absorb nutrients from the chyme by way of these blood capillaries and lacteals, which eventually transfer them to the bloodstream. Glucose, fructose, galactose, amino acids, minerals, and water-soluble vitamins are absorbed by the capillaries. Fructose and galactose are subsequently carried to the liver, where they are converted to glucose. Lacteals absorb glycerol and fatty acids (end products of fat digestion), in addition to the fat-soluble vitamins.

Absorption in the Large Intestine

When the chyme reaches the large intestine, most digestion and absorption have already occurred. The colon walls secrete mucus as a protection from the acidic digestive juices in the chyme, which is coming from the small intestine through the ileocecal valve.

The major tasks of the large intestine are to absorb water, to synthesize some B vitamins and vitamin K (essential for blood clotting), and to collect food residue. Food residue is the part of food that the body's enzyme action cannot digest and consequently the body cannot absorb. Such residue is commonly called dietary fiber. Examples include the outer hulls of corn kernels and grains of wheat, celery strings, and apple skins. It is important that the diet contain adequate fiber because it promotes the health of the large intestine by helping to produce softer stools and more frequent bowel movements (see Chapter 4).

Undigested food is excreted as **feces** by way of the rectum. In healthy people, 99% of carbohydrates, 95% of fat, and 92% of proteins are absorbed.

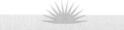

EXPLORING THE WEB

For a fun animation showing the process of digestion and absorption, visit www.kitses.com. Under animation, click on the BBC/Digestion sequence. This will take a short time to download. Geared toward children, this animation demonstrates the process of digestion and absorption. Create a Web link to this page to use as a teaching aid for pediatric clients.

METABOLISM

After digestion and absorption, nutrients are carried by the blood to the cells of the body. Within the cells, nutrients are changed into energy through a complex process called metabolism. During **aerobic metabolism,** nutrients are combined with oxygen within each cell. This process is known as oxidation. Oxidation ultimately reduces carbohydrates to carbon dioxide and water; proteins are reduced to carbon dioxide, water, and nitrogen. **Anaerobic metabolism** reduces fats without the use of oxygen. The complete oxidation of carbohydrates, proteins, and fats is commonly called the **Krebs cycle.**

As nutrients are oxidized, energy is released. When this released energy is used to build new substances from simpler ones, the process is called **anabolism.** An example of anabolism is the formation of new body tissues. When released energy is used to reduce substances to simpler ones, the process is called **catabolism.** This building up (anabolism) and breaking down (catabolism) of substances is a continuous process (metabolism) within the body and requires a continuous supply of nutrients.

Metabolism and the Thyroid Gland

Metabolism is governed primarily by the **hormones** secreted by the thyroid gland. These secretions are *triiodothyronine* (T_3) and *thyroxine* (T_4). When the thyroid gland secretes too much of these hormones, a condition known as hyperthyroidism may result. In such a case, the body metabolizes its food too quickly, and weight is lost. When too little T_4 and T_3 are secreted, the condition called hypothyroidism may occur. In this case, the body metabolizes food too slowly and the patient tends to become sluggish and accumulates fat.

ENERGY

Energy is constantly needed for the maintenance of body tissue and temperature and for growth (involuntary activity), as well as for voluntary activity. Examples of voluntary activity include walking, running, swimming, gardening, and so on. The three groups of nutrients that provide energy to the body are carbohydrates, proteins, and fats. Carbohydrates are and should be the primary energy source (see Chapter 4).

Energy Measurement

The unit used to measure the energy value of foods is the **kilocalorie,** or **kcal,** commonly known as the large calorie, or **calorie.** In the metric system it is known as the kilojoule. One kilocalorie is equal to 4.184 kilojoules, but this may be rounded off to 4.2 kilojoules. A calorie is the amount of heat needed to raise the temperature of 1 kilogram of water 1 degree Celsius (C).

The number of calories in a food is its energy value, or caloric density. Energy values of foods vary a great deal because they are determined by the types and amounts of nutrients each food contains.

---

aerobic metabolism
combining nutrients with oxygen within the cell; also called oxidation

anaerobic metabolism
reduces fats without use of oxygen

Krebs cycle
a series of enzymatic reactions that serve as the main source of cellular energy

anabolism
the creation of new compounds during metabolism

catabolism
the breakdown of compounds during metabolism

((• In The Media

CHEMICALS IN GRILLED MEAT INCREASE RISK OF CANCER

The Department of Health and Human Services has added heterocyclic amines to its list of carcinogens. These compounds are formed in red meat, poultry, and fish during grilling. In 1999 research conducted by the National Cancer Institute found that the odds of developing colorectal cancer was highly linked to the consumption of red meat, especially when grilled or well done. An outcome of this study indicates that these chemicals are primarily found in meat cooked at high temperatures or exposed to flames. A positive note is that marinating can have a protective effect on meat.

(Adapted from *The New York Times,* April 2005.)

hormone
substance secreted by the endocrine glands

kilocalorie (kcal)
the unit used to measure the fuel value of foods

calorie
represents the amount of heat needed to raise the temperature of one kilogram of water one degree Celsius (C)

One gram of carbohydrate yields 4 calories; 1 gram of protein yields 4 calories; and 1 gram of fat yields 9 calories. One gram of alcohol yields 7 calories.

The energy values of foods are determined by a device known as a **bomb calorimeter.** The inner part of a calorimeter holds a measured amount of food, and the outer part holds water. The food is burned, and its caloric value is determined by the increase in the temperature of the surrounding water. The number of calories in average servings of common foods is listed in Table A-D of the appendix.

Basal Metabolic Rate

One's basal metabolism is the energy necessary to carry on all involuntary vital processes while the body is at rest. These processes are respiration, circulation, regulation of body temperature, and cell activity and maintenance. The rate at which energy is needed only for body maintenance is called the **basal metabolism rate (BMR).** The BMR may be referred to as the **resting energy expenditure (REE).**

Medical tests can determine one's BMR (or REE). When such a test is given, the body is at rest and performing only the essential, involuntary functions. Voluntary activity is not measured in a BMR test. Factors that affect one's BMR are lean body mass, body size, sex, age, heredity, physical condition, and climate.

Lean body mass is muscle as opposed to fat tissue. Because there is more metabolic activity in muscle tissue than in fat or bone tissue, muscle tissue requires more calories than does fat or bone tissue. People with large body frames require more calories than do people with small frames because the former have more body mass to maintain and move than do those with small frames.

Men usually require more energy than women. They tend to be larger and to have more lean body mass than women do.

Children require more calories per pound of body weight than adults because they are growing. As people age, the lean body mass declines, and the basal metabolic rate declines accordingly. Heredity is also a determining factor. One's BMR may resemble one's parents', just as one's appearance may. One's physical condition also affects the BMR. For example, women require more calories during pregnancy and lactation than at other times. The basal metabolic rate increases during fever and decreases during periods of starvation or severely reduced calorie intake. People living and working in extremely cold or warm climates require more calories to maintain normal body temperature than they would in a more temperate climate.

Thermic Effect of Food

The body requires energy to process food (digestion, absorption, transportation, metabolism, and storage); this requirement represents 10% of daily energy (calorie) intake. Multiply BMR by 0.10 and add to the BMR (REE) before an activity factor is calculated.

Estimating BMR. Dietitians commonly use the Harris-Benedict equation to determine the BMR (REE) of persons over the age of 18. This equation uses

---

bomb calorimeter
device used to scientifically determine the kcal value of foods

basal metabolism rate (BMR)
the rate at which energy is needed for body maintenance

resting energy expenditure (REE)
same as BMR

lean body mass
percentage of muscle tissue

(handwritten margin notes) 2.2 lbs, 74
2.2 · 166 0
154
80

◉ SUPERSIZE **USA**

When you drive through the fast-food restaurant, keep in mind the following worst fast-food choices:

Order	Calories	Fat	Carbs	Protein	Sodium
Burger King Enormous					
Omelet Sandwich	730	47 g	43 g	32 g	1,860 mg
Carl's Jr. Breakfast Burger	830	46 g	65 g	38 g	N/A
Denny's Fabulous					
French Toast Platter	1,261	79 g	110 g	44 g	2,495 mg
Denny's French Slam	1,196	83 g	74 g	48 g	2,302 mg
Hardee's Monster					
Thickburger	1,417	107 g	49 g	64 g	2,651 mg
Burger King Double					
Whopper with Cheese	1,060	69 g	53 g	56 g	1,540 mg
Wendy's Big Bacon Classic	580	29 g	45 g	33 g	1,430 mg
McDonald's Double Quarter					
Pounder with Cheese	770	47 g	39 g	46 g	1,440 mg

Source: Nutrition information from each restaurant on the Internet.

height, weight, and age as factors and results in a more individualized estimate of the REE than some other methods (Figure 3-5).

Another method used to estimate one's BMR, or REE, is the following:

1. Convert body weight from pounds to kilograms (kg) by dividing pounds by 2.2 (2.2 pounds equal 1 kilogram).

2. Multiply the kilograms by 24 (hours per day).

3. Multiply the answer obtained in step 2 above by 0.9 for a woman and by 1.0 for a man.

For example, assume that a woman weighs 110 pounds. Divide 110 by 2.2 for an answer of 50 kg. Multiply 50 kg by 24 hours in a day for an answer of 1,200 calories. Then multiply 1,200 calories by 0.9 for an answer of 1,080 calories. This is the estimated basal metabolic energy requirement for that particular woman.

Female: **REE = 655 + (9.6 × weight in kg) + (1.8 × height in cm) − (4.7 × age)**

Male: **REE = 66 + (13.7 × weight in kg) + (5 × height in cm) − (6.8 × age)**

W = weight in kilograms (kg) (weight in pounds ÷ 2.2 = kg)
H = height in centimenters (cm) (height in inches × 2.54 = cm)
A = age in years

Figure 3-5 *Harris-Benedict equation.*

Table 3-2 *MyPyramid Food Intake Patterns*

ESTIMATED DAILY CALORIE NEEDS

To determine which food intake pattern to use for an individual, the following chart gives an estimate of individual calorie needs. The calorie range for each age and gender is based on physical activity level, from sedentary to active. Sedentary means a lifestyle that includes only the light physical activity associated with typical day-to-day life. Active means a lifestyle that includes physical activity equivalent to walking more than 3 miles per day at 3 to 4 miles per hour, in addition to the light physical activity associated with typical day-to-day life.

	CALORIE RANGE				CALORIE RANGE		
	SEDENTARY	→	ACTIVE		SEDENTARY	→	ACTIVE
Children				**Males**			
2–3 years	1,000	→	1,400	4–8 years	1,400	→	2,000
Females				9–13	1,800	→	2,600
4–8 years	1,200	→	1,800	14–18	2,200	→	3,200
9–13	1,600	→	2,200	19–30	2,400	→	3,000
14–18	1,800	→	2,400	31–50	2,200	→	3,000
19–30	2,000	→	2,400	51+	2,000	→	2,800
31–50	1,800	→	2,200				
51+	1,600	→	2,200				

Note: *From* MyPyramid Food Intake Patterns, *by the U.S. Department of Agriculture, 2005, retrieved April 26, 2005, from* http://www.mypyramid.gov/professionals/pdf_food_intake.html.

Calculating Total Energy Requirements

An individual's average daily **energy requirement** is the total number of calories needed in a 24-hour period. Energy requirements of people differ, depending on BMR (REE) and activities. More energy is burned playing soccer than playing the piano. Refer to Table 3-2 for calorie guidelines according to MyPyramid.

Table 3-3 shows suggested weights for adults according to height.

energy requirement
number of calories required by the body each day

adipose tissue
fatty tissue

energy balance
occurs when the caloric value of food ingested equals the calories expended

SPOTLIGHT on Life Cycle

Part of the latest research by the Food and Nutrition Board of the National Institute of Medicine focused on the energy requirements needed by individuals. The Estimated Energy Requirement (EER) is the dietary energy intake that will maintain energy balance in a healthy adult. A defined age, gender, weight, height (use the Harris-Benedict equation), thermic effect of food, and level of physical activity (Table 3-2) that would be consistent with good health were the parameters used. There is no Recommended Dietary Allowance for energy since energy intakes above the EER would most likely result in weight gain.

Energy Balance

A person who takes in fewer calories than she or he burns usually loses weight. If someone takes in more calories than she or he burns, the body stores them as **adipose tissue** (fat). Some adipose tissue is necessary to protect the body and support its organs. Adipose tissue also helps regulate body temperature, just as insulation helps regulate the temperature of a building. An excess of adipose tissue, however, leads to obesity, which can endanger health because it puts extra burdens on body organs and systems. For the healthy person, the goal is **energy balance.** This means that the number of calories consumed matches the number of calories required for one's BMR (REE) and activity.

CONSIDERATIONS FOR THE HEALTH CARE PROFESSIONAL

The health care professional will find that clients may make broad statements concerning the way their bodies work. An example would be: "Milk doesn't agree with me." This is when the appropriate questions need to be asked, such as "Does it cause flatulence (gas)?" or "Do you have to go to the bathroom immediately?" The first is a classic symptom of lactose intolerance, whereas the latter could indicate an allergy or other serious problems that would require further workup. Clients needing education about metabolism and energy requirements may tell you that they don't eat anything but keep gaining weight, or they exercise all the time but don't lose an ounce. Clients deserve current and correct health information; therefore health care professionals must continually educate themselves in order to provide the most accurate information to their clients.

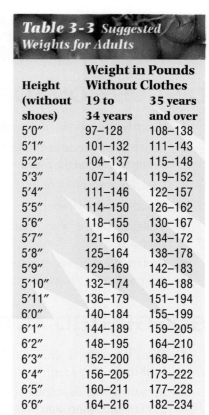

Table 3-3 *Suggested Weights for Adults*

Height (without shoes)	Weight in Pounds Without Clothes	
	19 to 34 years	35 years and over
5'0"	97–128	108–138
5'1"	101–132	111–143
5'2"	104–137	115–148
5'3"	107–141	119–152
5'4"	111–146	122–157
5'5"	114–150	126–162
5'6"	118–155	130–167
5'7"	121–160	134–172
5'8"	125–164	138–178
5'9"	129–169	142–183
5'10"	132–174	146–188
5'11"	136–179	151–194
6'0"	140–184	155–199
6'1"	144–189	159–205
6'2"	148–195	164–210
6'3"	152–200	168–216
6'4"	156–205	173–222
6'5"	160–211	177–228
6'6"	164–216	182–234

Note: *The higher weights in the ranges generally apply to men, who tend to have more muscle and bone; the lower weights more often apply to women, who have less muscle and bone.*

Source: *Reprinted from* Dietary Guidelines for Americans, *3rd ed., by U.S. Departments of Agriculture and Health and Human Services, 1990. Retrieved May 5, 2005, from http:// www.nal.usda.gov/fnic/dga/weight.htm.*

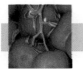

SUMMARY

The body is comparable to an automobile engine because both require fuel. Food acts as fuel, but to be usable, it must undergo a series of processes that includes digestion, absorption, and metabolism. Digestion is the process whereby food is broken down into smaller parts, chemically changed, and moved along the gastrointestinal tract. Mechanical digestion refers to that part of the process performed by the teeth and muscles of the digestive system. Chemical digestion refers to that part of the process wherein food is broken down to molecules that the blood can absorb. Enzymes are essential for chemical digestion. After digestion, nutrients are transported by the blood and lymphatic system, primarily in the small intestine, and then carried to all body tissues. After absorption, food is metabolized. During metabolism, carbohydrates and proteins are combined with oxygen in a process called oxidation. Energy released during oxidation is measured by the calorie.

Caloric values of foods vary, as do people's energy requirements. Requirements depend on age, body size, sex, lean body mass, physical condition, climate, and activity.

DISCUSSION TOPICS

1. Describe the process of digestion.
2. Of what value are enzymes to digestion? Name five enzymes and the nutrients on which they act.
3. Describe absorption of nutrients.
4. Describe metabolism.
5. Explain why the body requires fuel even during sleep.
6. Explain the differences between the terms *energy value* and *energy requirement*.

SUGGESTED ACTIVITIES

1. Using the method given in this chapter, calculate your total energy requirement.
2. Prepare a brief description of the processes of digestion and absorption that could be presented to a fourth grade class.
3. Role-play a situation where the client asks the health care provider to explain *metabolism*.

REVIEW

Multiple choice. Select the *letter* that precedes the best answer.

1. Digestion begins in the
   a. mouth
   b. stomach
   c. liver
   d. small intestine
2. Most of the digestive processes occur in the
   a. mouth
   b. stomach
   c. small intestine
   d. colon
3. The small intestine is divided into three segments. They are, in descending order,
   a. ileum, jejunum, duodenum
   b. jejunum, ileum, duodenum
   c. duodenum, ileum, jejunum
   d. duodenum, jejunum, ileum
4. The fluid mixture that moves from the stomach through the pyloric sphincter is called
   a. bolus
   b. chyme
   c. food
   d. gastrin
5. A muscular movement that moves food down the GI tract is called
   a. a pump
   b. peristalsis
   c. lymphatic circulation
   d. circular propulsion
6. The pyloric sphincter is between the
   a. ileum and colon
   b. stomach and duodenum
   c. small intestine and colon
   d. colon and rectum
7. A word ending in *ase* usually indicates that a substance is
   a. a hormone
   b. a bacterium
   c. an enzyme
   d. an acid
8. Maltase, sucrase, and lactase are produced in the
   a. stomach
   b. small intestine
   c. colon
   d. pancreas
9. Bile is needed to digest
   a. carbohydrates
   b. fiber
   c. proteins
   d. fats
10. When energy intake is greater than energy output, the body weight will
   a. remain the same
   b. decrease
   c. increase and then decrease
   d. increase

CASE IN POINT

JANESSA, AN OVERACHIEVER

Janessa is a 32-year-old African American factory worker who has been hyperactive all her life. She is 5 feet 2 inches tall and weighs 201 pounds. Janessa will admit that prior to her divorce 15 years ago, she was the smallest she had ever been, 123 pounds. After her divorce she was still an overachiever, but she began putting weight on. Since she has not stopped being active, she now believes she has a glandular problem. Janessa has always eaten very fast; in fact, some of her friends say she inhales food. She finds that she has frequent bouts of nausea and oftentimes is in the bathroom while others are out having a good time. She believes she has a nervous stomach. Janessa comes to the Employee Health Service for assistance. She is referred to a dietitian.

ASSESSMENT

1. Identify the significant data in this case study.
2. What metabolic problem do the data indicate?
3. Figure Janessa's REE using the Harris-Benedict, the thermic effect of food (TEF), and her calorie guidelines using Table 3-2.
4. What testing would you consider helpful in estimating Janessa's resting energy expenditure? How would you calculate her resting energy expenditure?

DIAGNOSIS

5. Write a nursing diagnosis for Janessa.

PLAN/GOAL

6. What changes can Janessa implement to help reduce her weight?
7. Set two measurable realistic goals for Janessa during this process to prevent further weight gain.
8. How could information on digestion be helpful to Janessa?

IMPLEMENTATION

9. What strategies can be used to help Janessa become aware of her food consumption and the time it takes her to eat?
10. What actions would help Janessa carry out these goals?
11. Who can help her?

EVALUATION/OUTCOME CRITERIA

12. What will Janessa be able to identify if the plan is successful?
13. What will she be able to measure as evidence of her success?

THINKING FURTHER

14. How could you help Janessa slow down when eating?

RATE THIS PLATE

Janessa continues to be active in spite of a weight gain of 78 pounds in the last 15 years. This is what Janessa packed for lunch. Lunch is 30 minutes, and she enjoys the time with her friends. Rate her plate.

2 bologna sandwiches with 2 Tbsp mayonnaise per sandwich

2.5-oz bag of potato chips

Chocolate pudding

Very large orange

6 sandwich cookies with double the filling

Will this plate help Janessa lose weight? Why or why not? Why would she become nauseated? Do you believe she has a glandular problem? Why or why not? What would you change on this plate, if anything? Why?

CASE IN POINT

CARL: LIVING WITH CROHN'S DISEASE

Carl is a 30-year-old Caucasian male with Crohn's disease, primarily of the large intestine and colon. He is 5 feet 9 inches tall and weighs 200 pounds. He knows he is prone to flare-ups of malabsorption of carbohydrate, protein, fats, and folate. He has been having diarrhea on and off for 3 weeks. It has been very bad this last 2 weeks. He has lost 10 pounds. He would like to get his weight down even more. His physician ordered blood for CBC, albumin, folic acid, and B$_{12}$. She has written for a dietary referral for a low-lactose, low-fat, high-fiber, high-protein diet.

ASSESSMENT

1. What are the pertinent objective and subjective data related to Carl's problem?

2. Calculate Carl's target caloric intake and weight according to Tables 3-2 and 3-3.

3. Calculate Carl's REE using the Harris-Benedict equation.

DIAGNOSIS

4. Write a nursing diagnosis for Carl.

5. What is the cause of Carl's problem with elimination?

PLAN/GOAL

6. Write a measurable goal for controlling Carl's diarrhea.

7. Write a goal to help Carl adapt to his new diet. Incorporate Carl's desire to lose weight.

8. Where could the dietitian direct Carl to obtain information to increase his understanding of his disease and the related nutrition issues?

IMPLEMENTATION

9. List at least one action to help Carl meet each goal.

10. List two foods Carl should avoid.

11. List three foods Carl needs to include.

12. How could the Web site http://qurlyjoe.bu.edu for Crohn's and ulcerative colitis be helpful to Carl?

EVALUATION/OUTCOME CRITERIA

13. What will Carl report when your plan for his diarrhea is effective?

14. How will Carl know his new diet is successful?

15. What can the doctor measure when all the goals are successful?

16. If the plan were not successful, what would Carl be experiencing?

17. What could be an unplanned, undesirable outcome of this diet change?

THINKING FURTHER

18. What challenges does Carl face with chronic progressive disease?

◎ RATE THIS PLATE

Carl has seen the dietitian and has written materials to help him plan his diet. Carl takes his lunch to work. Rate the plate.

Sandwich made from:

2 slices 100% whole wheat bread

4 oz roast beef

1 oz Colby cheese

2 Tbsp mayonnaise

2 slices tomato

2 large-leaf lettuce leaves

2 oz potato chips

Carrots and celery with dip of buttermilk ranch dressing

1 cup bread pudding

CARBOHYDRATES

KEY TERMS

adipose (fatty) tissue
bran
carbohydrates
cellulose
dietary fiber
disaccharides
endosperm
flatulence
fructose
galactose
germ
glucagon
glucose (dextrose)
glycogen
hemicellulose
hyperglycemia
hypoglycemia
insulin
islets of Langerhans
ketones
ketoacidosis
lactose
lactose intolerance
lignins
maltose
monosaccharides
mucilage
pectin
polysaccharides
starch
sucrose
whey

OBJECTIVES

After studying this chapter, you should be able to:

- Identify the functions of carbohydrates
- Name the primary sources of carbohydrates
- Describe the classification of carbohydrates

Energy foods are those that can be rapidly oxidized by the body to release energy and its by-product, heat. Carbohydrates, fats, and proteins provide energy for the human body, but carbohydrates are the primary source. They are the least expensive and most abundant of the energy nutrients. Foods rich in carbohydrates grow easily in most climates. They keep well and are generally easy to digest.

Carbohydrates provide the major source of energy for people all over the world (Figure 4-1). They provide approximately half the calories for people living in the United States. In some areas of the world, where fats and proteins are scarce and expensive, carbohydrates provide as much as 80 to 100% of calories. Carbohydrates are named for the chemical elements they are composed of—carbon, hydrogen, and oxygen.

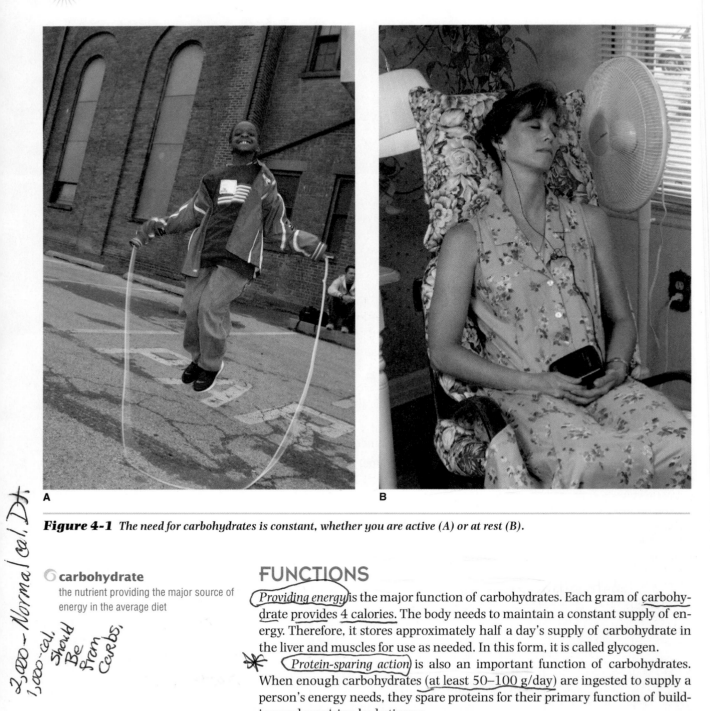

A   **B**

Figure 4-1 *The need for carbohydrates is constant, whether you are active (A) or at rest (B).*

(handwritten margin note, left side:) 2,000~Normal cal. Dt. 1,000~cal. Should Be from Carbs,

⊙ **carbohydrate**
the nutrient providing the major source of energy in the average diet

⊙ **ketones**
substances to which fatty acids are broken down in the liver

⊙ **ketoacidosis**
condition in which ketones collect in the blood; caused by insufficient glucose available for energy

FUNCTIONS

Providing energy is the major function of carbohydrates. Each gram of carbohydrate provides 4 calories. The body needs to maintain a constant supply of energy. Therefore, it stores approximately half a day's supply of carbohydrate in the liver and muscles for use as needed. In this form, it is called glycogen.

Protein-sparing action is also an important function of carbohydrates. When enough carbohydrates (at least 50–100 g/day) are ingested to supply a person's energy needs, they spare proteins for their primary function of building and repairing body tissues.

Normal fat metabolism requires an adequate supply of carbohydrates. If there is too little carbohydrate to fulfill the energy requirement, an abnormally large amount of fat is metabolized to help meet it. During such an emergency need for energy, fat oxidization in the cells is not complete and substances called ketones are produced. **Ketones** are acids that accumulate in the blood and urine, upsetting the acid-base balance. Such a condition is called **ketoacidosis**. It can result from IDDM (insulin-dependent diabetes

under 40 sugar cont

mellitus), also known as type 1 diabetes (see Chapter 17), from starvation, or from extreme low-carbohydrate diets. It can lead to coma and even death.

When sufficient carbohydrates are eaten, the body is protected against ketones. This is sometimes called the antiketogenic effect of carbohydrates.

Providing fiber in the diet is another important function of carbohydrates. Dietary fiber is found in grains, vegetables, and fruits. Fiber creates a soft, bulky stool that moves quickly through the large intestine.

20-35g/Day

FOOD SOURCES (Fiber Oatmeal) works as a sponge

The principal sources of carbohydrates are plant foods: cereal grains, vegetables, fruits, and sugars (Figure 4-2). The only substantial animal source of carbohydrates is milk.

Cereal grains and their products are dietary staples in nearly every part of the world. Rice is the basic food in Latin America, Africa, Asia, and many sections of the United States. Wheat and the various breads, pastas, and breakfast cereals made from it are basic to American and European diets. Rye and oats are commonly used in breads and cereals in the United States and Europe. Cereals also contain vitamins, minerals, and some proteins. During processing, some of these nutrients are lost. To compensate for this loss, food producers in the

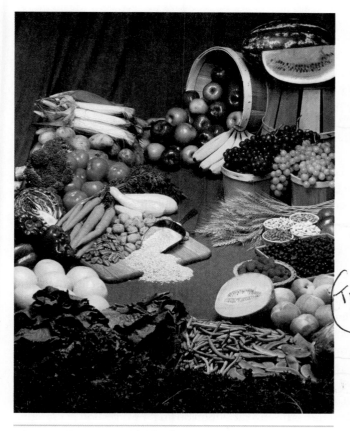

Figure 4-2 *Fruits, vegetables, grains, and some dairy products are good sources of carbohydrates. (Courtesy of Agricultural Research Service, USDA)*

7.35 - 7.45

6.9 or 7.0 acidotic-Diabetic

3,500 calories = 1 lb.

4 Kcal. of energy = 1 gram = carbs.

1 gram = protein

1 gram = fat

(Type I Diabetic Very thin)

Body Doesn't have enough carbs.
↓ Turns to
Stores Fats, protein - store
↓
Ketones (Acid products)
↳ Ketoneacidosis

Handwritten margin notes:
Diag 10% Dextrose — Ch, Blood Sugars
D25 25% Dextrose — everyshift
Babies every hour

(Fiber)
Only From Animal
as milk.

Brain will die if it doesn't have glucose.
Confusion — 1st indicator of Diabetic

United States commonly add the B vitamins—thiamine, riboflavin, and niacin—plus the mineral iron to the final product. The product is then called *enriched.* When a nutrient that has never been part of a grain is added, the grain is said to be fortified. An example of fortification is the addition of folic acid to cereal grains to prevent neural tube defects (see Chapter 7).

Vegetables such as potatoes, beets, peas, lima beans, and corn provide substantial amounts of carbohydrates (in the form of starch). Green leafy vegetables provide dietary fiber. All of them also provide vitamins and minerals.

Fruits provide sugar, fiber, vitamins, and minerals.

Sugars such as table sugar, syrup, and honey and sugar-rich foods such as desserts and candy provide carbohydrates in the form of sugar with few other nutrients except for fats. Therefore, the foods in which they predominate are commonly called low-nutrient-dense foods.

CLASSIFICATION

Carbohydrates are divided into three groups: monosaccharides, disaccharides, and polysaccharides (Table 4-1).

Monosaccharides

Monosaccharides are the simplest form of carbohydrates. They are sweet, require no digestion, and can be absorbed directly into the bloodstream from the small intestine. They include glucose, fructose, and galactose.

Glucose, also called dextrose, is the form of carbohydrate to which all other forms are converted for eventual metabolism. It is found naturally in corn syrup and some fruits and vegetables. The central nervous system, the red blood cells, and the brain use only glucose as fuel; therefore, a continuous source is needed.

Dextrose →

Fructose, also called levulose or fruit sugar, is found with glucose in many fruits and in honey. It is the sweetest of all the monosaccharides.

Galactose is a product of the digestion of milk. It is not found naturally.

Milk sugar → Lactoses gets digested.

Disaccharides

Disaccharides are pairs of the three sugars just discussed. They are sweet and must be changed to simple sugars by hydrolysis before they can be absorbed. Disaccharides include sucrose, maltose, and lactose.

Sucrose is composed of glucose and fructose. It is the form of carbohydrate present in granulated, powdered, and brown sugar and in molasses. It is one of the sweetest and least expensive sugars. Its sources are sugar cane, sugar beets, and the sap from maple trees.

Maltose is a disaccharide that is an intermediary product in the hydrolysis of starch. It is produced by enzyme action during the digestion of starch in the body. It also is created during the fermentation process that produces alcohol. It can be found in some infant formulas, malt beverage products, and beer. It is considerably less sweet than glucose or sucrose.

Not as sweet as glucose or sucrose

Glossary (margin)

○ **monosaccharides**
simplest carbohydrates; sugars that cannot be further reduced by hydrolysis; examples are glucose, fructose, and galactose

○ **glucose**
the simple sugar to which carbohydrate must be broken down for absorption; also known as *dextrose*

○ **fructose**
the simple sugar (monosaccharide) found in fruit and honey

○ **galactose**
the simple sugar (monosaccharide) to which lactose is broken down during digestion

○ **disaccharides**
double sugars that are reduced by hydrolysis to monosaccharides; examples are sucrose, maltose, and lactose

○ **sucrose**
a double sugar or disaccharide; examples are granulated, powdered, and brown sugar

○ **maltose**
the double sugar (disaccharide) occurring as a result of the digestion of grain

Table 4-1 *Carbohydrates*

TYPE	SOURCE		FUNCTIONS	DEFICIENCY SYMPTOMS
Monosaccharides (Simple Sugars)				
Glucose	Berries	Grapes	Furnish energy	Fatigue
	Sweet corn	Corn syrup	Spare proteins	Weight loss
			Prevent ketoacidosis	
Fructose	Ripe fruits	Soft drinks	Fruits and vegetables provide	
	Honey		vitamins, minerals, and fiber	
Galactose	Lactose			
Disaccharides				
Sucrose	Sugar cane		Furnish energy	Fatigue
	Sugar beets		Spare proteins	Weight loss
	Granulated sugar		Prevent ketoacidosis	
	Confectioner's sugar			
	Brown sugar			
	Molasses			
	Maple syrup			
	Candy			
	Jams and jellies			
Maltose	Digestion of starch			
Lactose	Milk			
Polysaccharides (Complex Carbohydrates)				
Starch	Cereal grains and their products:		Furnish energy	Fatigue
	cereals, breads, rice, flour,		Prevent ketoacidosis	Weight loss
	pasta, crackers		Fruits and vegetables provide	
	Potatoes	Corn	vitamins, minerals, and fiber	
	Lima beans	Yams		
	Navy beans	Green bananas		
	Sweet potatoes			
Dextrins	Starch hydrolysis			
Glycogen	Glucose stored in liver and muscles			
Cellulose	Wheat bran, whole-grain cereals,		Provide fiber	Constipation
	green and leafy vegetables,			Colon cancer
	fruits, especially apples, pears,			Diverticulosis
	oranges, grapefruit, grapes			

[handwritten notes: "Milk → Disaccharides"; "Your client complain of Bloating, abdominal cramps, & diarrhea milk or consuming a milk-based food such as processed cheese? A"; "Lact(ase) — Enzyme"]

Lactose is the sugar found in milk. It is distinct from most other sugars because it is not found in plants. It helps the body absorb calcium. Lactose is less sweet than monosaccharides or other disaccharides.

Many adults are unable to digest lactose and suffer from bloating, abdominal cramps, and diarrhea after drinking milk or consuming a milk-based

lactose
the sugar in milk; a disaccharide

galactose (handwritten)

lactose intolerance
inability to digest lactose because of a lack of the enzyme lactase; causes abdominal cramps and diarrhea

whey
liquid part of milk that separates from the curd (solid part) during the making of hard cheese

polysaccharides
complex carbohydrates containing combinations of monosaccharides; examples include starch, dextrin, cellulose, and glycogen

starch
polysaccharide found in grains and vegetables

endosperm
the inner part of the kernel of grain; contains the carbohydrate

bran
outer covering of grain kernels

germ
embryo or tiny life center of each kernel of grain

glycogen — *Important* (handwritten)
glucose as stored in the liver and muscles

glucagon — *Important* (handwritten)
hormone from alpha cells of the pancreas; helps cells release energy

dietary fiber
indigestible parts of plants; absorbs water in large intestine, helping to create soft, bulky stool; some is believed to bind cholesterol in the colon, helping to rid cholesterol from the body; some is believed to lower blood glucose levels

food such as process cheese. This reaction is called <u>lactose intolerance.</u> It is caused by insufficient lactase, the enzyme required for digestion of lactose. There are special low-lactose milk products that can be used instead of regular milk. Lactase-containing products are also available.

During the process of making hard cheese, milk separates into curd (solid part from which hard cheese is made) and **whey** (liquid part). Lactose becomes part of the whey and not the curd. Therefore, lactose is not a component of natural cheese. However, manufacturers can add milk or milk solids to process cheese, so it is important that persons who are lactose intolerant check the labels on cheese products.

There is no test for lactose intolerance. If eating dairy products consistently produces symptoms of flatulence, diarrhea, and abdominal pain, the doctor may recommend eliminating dairy products from the diet and adding them back after a period of time to ascertain the client's reaction. If the symptoms persist, the client is lactose intolerant.

Polysaccharides

Polysaccharides are commonly called *complex carbohydrates* because they are compounds of many monosaccharides (simple sugars). Three polysaccharides are important in nutrition: starch, glycogen, and fiber.

Starch is a polysaccharide found in grains and vegetables. It is the storage form of glucose in plants. Vegetables contain less starch than grains because vegetables have a higher moisture content. Legumes (dried beans and peas) are another important source of starch, as well as of dietary fiber and protein. Starches are more complex than monosaccharides or disaccharides, and it takes the body longer to digest them. Thus, they supply energy over a longer period of time. The starch in grain is found mainly in the **endosperm** (center part of the grain). This is the part from which white flour is made. The tough outer covering of grain kernels is called the **bran** (Figure 4-3). The bran is used in coarse cereals and whole wheat flour. The **germ** is the smallest part of the grain and is a rich source of B vitamins, vitamin E, minerals, and protein. Wheat germ is included in products made of whole wheat. It also can be purchased and used in baked products or as an addition to breakfast cereals.

Before the starch in grain can be used for food, the bran must be broken down. The heat and moisture of cooking break this outer covering, making the food more flavorful and more easily digested. Although bran itself is indigestible, it is important that some be included in the diet because of the fiber it provides.

Glycogen is sometimes called *animal starch* because it is the storage form of glucose in the body. In the healthy adult, approximately one-half day's supply of energy is stored as glycogen in the liver and muscles. The hormone **glucagon** helps the liver convert glycogen to glucose as needed for energy. (See Chapter 13 for information on glycogen loading.)

The Fibers

Dietary fiber, also called <u>roughage</u>, is <u>indigestible because</u> it cannot be broken down by digestive enzymes. Some fiber is insoluble (it does not readily dissolve in water), and some is soluble (it partially dissolves in water) (Figure 4-4). <u>Insoluble fibers include cellulose, some hemicellulose, and lignins.</u> Soluble fibers are gums, pectins, some hemicellulose, and mucilages.

CORN today corn tomorrow. (handwritten)   *Pears, peaches* (handwritten)

Insulin - lowers your Bloodsugar

Enriched - adding back nutrients that were already there. That should

Fortified - iron or calcium

milk - Vitamin D in

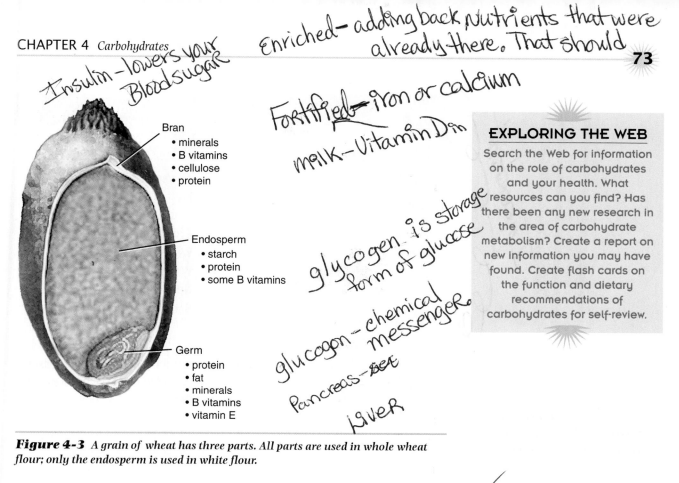

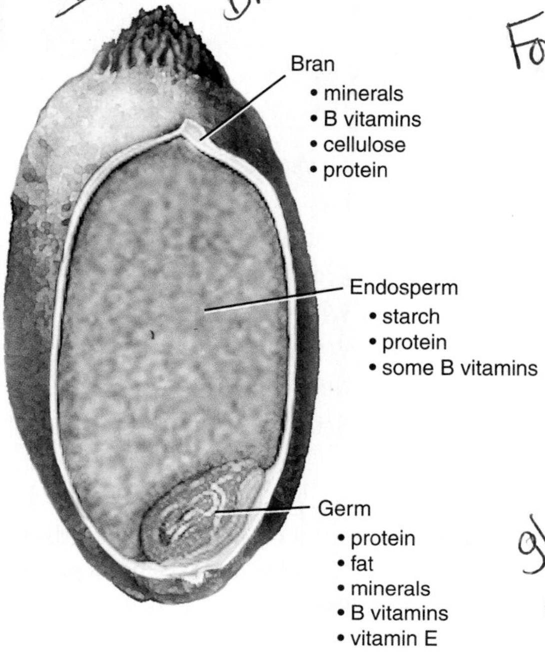
Bran
• minerals
• B vitamins
• cellulose
• protein
Endosperm
• starch
• protein
• some B vitamins
Germ
• protein
• fat
• minerals
• B vitamins
• vitamin E

glycogen is storage form of glucose

glucagon - chemical messenger.

Pancreas

Liver

Figure 4-3 ***A grain of wheat has three parts. All parts are used in whole wheat flour; only the endosperm is used in white flour.***

EXPLORING THE WEB

Search the Web for information on the role of carbohydrates and your health. What resources can you find? Has there been any new research in the area of carbohydrate metabolism? Create a report on new information you may have found. Create flash cards on the function and dietary recommendations of carbohydrates for self-review.

See Table 4-2 for food sources. **Cellulose** is a primary source of dietary fiber. It is found in the skins of fruits, the leaves and stems of vegetables, and legumes. Highly processed foods such as white bread, macaroni products, and pastries contain little if any cellulose because it is removed during processing. Because humans cannot digest cellulose, it has no energy value. It is useful because it provides bulk for the stool.

Hemicellulose is found mainly in whole-grain cereal. Some hemicellulose is soluble; some is not. **Lignins** are the woody part of vegetables such as carrots and asparagus or the small seeds of strawberries; they are not a carbohydrate.

Pectins, some hemicellulose, gums, and **mucilages** are soluble in water and form a gel that helps provide bulk for the intestines. They are useful also because they bind cholesterol, thus reducing the amount the blood can absorb.

Fiber is considered helpful to clients with diabetes mellitus because it lowers blood glucose levels. It may prevent some colon cancers by moving waste

cellulose
indigestible carbohydrate; provides fiber in the diet

hemicellulose
dietary fiber found in whole grains

lignins
dietary fiber found in the woody parts of vegetables

pectin
edible thickening agent

mucilage
gel-forming dietary fiber

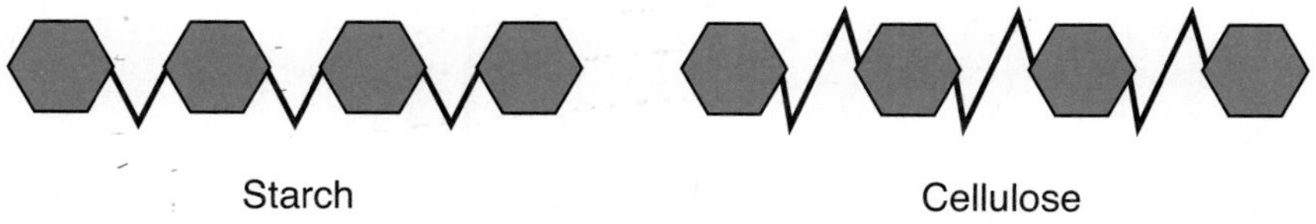
Starch
Cellulose

Figure 4-4 ***The alpha bonds that link glucose molecules together can be broken down during digestion. The beta bonds in cellulose cannot be broken by digestive enzymes and are eliminated without being digested (insoluble fiber).***

G.I. TRACT also natural soothing qualities for your throat

Table 4-2 *Sources of Fiber That Are Soluble in Water and Those That Are Insoluble in Water*

WATER-SOLUBLE FIBER		WATER-INSOLUBLE FIBER
Fruit (pectin)	**Grains**	All vegetables
Apples	Oats	Fruit
Peaches	Barley	Whole grains
Plums and prunes	**Legumes**	Brown rice
Bananas	Dried peas	Wild rice
	Beans	Wheat bran
	Lentils	Nuts
		Seeds

materials through the colon faster than would normally be the case, thereby reducing the colon's exposure time to potential carcinogens. Fiber helps prevent constipation, hemorrhoids, and diverticular disease by softening and increasing the size of the stool.

The optimal recommendation for fiber intake is 20–35 g/day. The normal U.S. diet is thought to contain approximately 11 grams. In general, Amer-

⊙ SUPERSIZE USA

Portion distortion is an enormous contribution to overweight and obesity. Having a realistic visual image of portion size is helpful when preparing meals and choosing foods. Did you know . . .

Portion	Visualization of Size or Amount
3 oz meat, poultry, or fish	Deck of playing cards, cassette tape, or the palm of a woman's hand
1 oz meat, poultry, or fish	Matchbook
1 pat butter or margarine (1 serving)	A scrabble tile
2 Tbsp peanut butter	Golf ball
1 oz cheese	1-in. cube
1 oz salad dressing	1 small restaurant ladle
1 cup fresh greens	Tennis ball
1 lb uncooked spaghetti	Circle thumb and index finger
1 Tbsp mayonnaise	Woman's thumb
1 oz chips or pretzels	One handful—not heaping
1 medium potato	Computer mouse
1 standard bagel	Hockey puck
1 slice cheese	3.5-in. computer disk
1 cup mashed potatoes, rice, or pasta	Person's fist or tennis ball
1 medium orange or apple	Baseball
1/2 cup cooked vegetable	1/2 a baseball or 7 to 8 baby carrots, 1 ear corn, 3 spears of broccoli
1/2 cup frozen yogurt	Small fist
1 oz nuts, raisins, candy	Small handful, 2 Tbsp

Atkins dt. No Carbs Ketone Acidosis
will have to Burn Fat & proteins

icans do not consume sufficient amounts of fruits and vegetables. They should eat no fewer than five servings of fruits and vegetables each day. Fiber intake should be increased gradually and should be accompanied by an increased intake of water. Eating too much fiber in a short time can produce discomfort, **flatulence** (abdominal gas), and diarrhea. It also could obstruct the GI tract if intake exceeds 50 grams. Insoluble fiber has binders (phytic acid or phytate), which are found in the outer covering of grains and vegetables. These can prevent the absorption of minerals such as calcium, iron, zinc, and magnesium, so excess intake should be avoided. The type of fiber consumed should be from natural food sources rather than from commercially prepared fiber products because the foods contain vitamins, minerals, and phytochemicals as well as fiber. Table 4-3 lists the dietary fiber content of selected foods.

DIGESTION AND ABSORPTION

Monosaccharides—glucose, fructose, and galactose—are simple sugars that may be absorbed from the intestine directly into the bloodstream. They are subsequently carried to the liver, where fructose and galactose are changed to glucose. The blood then carries glucose to the cells.

Disaccharides—sucrose, maltose, and lactose—require an additional step of digestion. They must be converted to the simple sugar glucose before they can be absorbed into the bloodstream. This conversion is accomplished by the enzymes sucrase, maltase, and lactase, which were discussed in Chapter 3 (see Table 3-1).

Polysaccharides are more complex, and their digestibility varies. After the cellulose wall is broken down, starch is changed to the intermediate product dextrin; it is then changed to maltose and finally to glucose. Cooking can change starch to dextrin. For example, when bread is toasted, it turns golden brown and tastes sweeter because the starch has been changed to dextrin.

The digestion of starch begins in the mouth, where the enzyme salivary amylase begins to change starch to dextrin. The second step occurs in the stomach, where the food is mixed with gastric juices. The final step occurs in the small intestine, where the digestible carbohydrates are changed to simple sugars by the enzyme action of pancreatic amylase and are subsequently absorbed into the blood.

METABOLISM AND ELIMINATION

All carbohydrates are changed to the simple sugar glucose before metabolism can take place in the cells. After glucose has been carried by the blood to the cells, it can be oxidized. Frequently, the volume of glucose that reaches the cells exceeds the amount the cells can use. In these cases, glucose is converted to glycogen and is stored in the liver and muscles. (Glycogen is subsequently broken down only from the liver and released as glucose when needed for energy.) When more glucose is ingested than the body can either use immediately or store in the form of glycogen, it is converted to fat and stored as **adipose (fatty) tissue.**

The process of glucose metabolism is controlled mainly by the hormone **insulin,** which is secreted by the **islets of Langerhans** in the pancreas and which maintains normal blood glucose at 70–110 mg/dl. When the secretion of insulin is impaired or absent, the glucose level in the blood becomes excessively

○ **flatulence**
gas in the intestinal tract

Insulin
↓
Lowers
Blood sugar

Glucagon
↑
RAISES
BS

Hypoglycemia
If a Diabetic
gives themselves
too much insulin

Diabetic—Insulin
Deficient

Pancreas
Insulin
glucagon } Pg

Insulin lowers your
Blood sugar.

✓ **adipose (fatty) tissue**
fatty tissue

○ **insulin**
secretion of the islets of Langerhans in the pancreas gland; essential for the proper metabolism of glucose

○ **islets of Langerhans**
part of the pancreas from which insulin is secreted

<70 Hypoglycemia   —Hyperglycemia

Table 4-3 *Dietary Fiber Content of Selected Foods*

GRAMS PER SERVING*	0.5 OR LESS	0.5–1.0	1.1–2.0	2.1–3.0	3.0 OR GREATER‡
Fruit†	Banana	Apricots (raw or dried)	Apple skin	Blackberries	Blackberries (4)
	Cherries	Apple (peeled or dried)	Cranberries, raw (1 cup)	Boysenberries	Elderberries (5)
	Coconut (shredded)	Applesauce	Figs	Gooseberries	Guava (5)
	Currants (dried)	Blueberries	Papaya	Kumquats	Raspberries (4)
	Dates	Cantaloupe		Pears	
	Fruit juice	Coconut, raw, 1/2 cup			
	Plums (cooked)	Cranberries, relish, 1/2 cup			
	Pomegranate	Honeydew			
	Prunes	Kiwifruit			
	Raisins	Mango			
	Rhubarb (raw)	Nectarine			
	Watermelon	Orange			
		Peach (raw or dried)			
		Pear (dried)			
		Pineapple			
		Plums (raw)			
		Prunes			
		Rhubarb, raw (1 cup) and cooked			
		Strawberries			
		Tangerine			
		Watermelon			
Vegetables†	Bamboo shoots	Artichoke hearts	Artichoke, Jerusalem		
	Bean sprouts (cooked or canned)	Asparagus	Broccoli (cooked)		
	Cabbage (cooked)	Bean sprouts (raw)	Brussels sprouts		
	Celery	Beans (string)	Chicory		
	Eggplant	Beets	Mushrooms		
	Endive	Broccoli (raw)	Pumpkin		
	Lettuce	Cabbage (raw)	Rutabagas		
	Onions	Carrots	Sauerkraut		
	Radishes	Cauliflower	Soybean sprouts (raw)		
	Summer squash	Cucumber	Spaghetti sauce		
	Vegetable juice	Green pepper	Tomato paste		
	Water chestnuts	Greens:	Turnips (raw)		
	Watercress	Beet			

(continued)

Table 4-3 *(continued)*

GRAMS PER SERVING*	0.5 OR LESS	0.5–1.0	1.1–2.0	2.1–3.0	3.0 OR GREATER‡
Vegetables†		Greens (cont'd): Collard Dandelion Kale Mustard Spinach Swiss chard Turnip Kohlrabi Mushrooms Okra Parsley Soybean sprouts (cooked) Summer squash (raw) Tomato puree Turnips (cooked)			
Starches	Cornflakes Corn grits Cream of Wheat or Rice Farina Graham crackers Maltomeal Plantain Potato chips Potatoes Puffed cereals Rice, white Rice Krispies Saltines Spaghetti (refined)	Bread, white Cheerios Corn Flour, white Granola Oatmeal (cooked) Roll or bun, white Spaghetti and macaroni from whole wheat flour	Black-eyed peas Bread, whole wheat Flour, whole wheat Grapenuts Green peas Lima beans Popcorn Ralston (cooked cereal) Rice, brown or white Sesame seed kernels Soybeans Squash, winter Sweet potatoes	Beans (dried) 40% Branflakes Bulgur Lentils Parsnips Peas (dried) Pumpkin Raisin Bran Shredded Wheat Wheat germ	All-Bran (9) Bran Buds (8) 100% Bran (6) Bran muffin (3.5) Bulgur (3.5) RY KRISP Wheat bran (9)

Reprinted with permission of the Mayo Clinic, Rochester, Minnesota.
Note: Based on the content of one diabetic exchange for each item listed.
* Serving sizes per the Dietary Guidelines for Americans.
† Includes all forms (raw, dried, cooked) for fruits and vegetables except where noted.
‡ Actual dietary fiber content listed in parentheses.

hyperglycemia
excessive amounts of glucose in the blood

hypoglycemia
subnormal levels of blood glucose

high. This condition is called **hyperglycemia** (blood glucose more than 126 mg/dl) and is usually a symptom of diabetes mellitus. If control by diet is ineffective, an oral hypoglycemic or insulin injections must be used to control blood sugar. When insulin is given, the diabetic client's intake of carbohydrates must be carefully controlled to balance the prescribed dosage of insulin (see Chapter 17). When blood glucose levels are unusually low, the condition is called **hypoglycemia** (blood glucose less than 70 mg/dl). A mild form of hypoglycemia may occur if one waits too long between meals or if the pancreas secretes too much insulin. Symptoms include fatigue, shaking, sweating, and headache.

Oxidation of glucose results in energy. With the exception of cellulose, the only waste products of carbohydrate metabolism are carbon dioxide and water. It is a very efficient nutrient.

DIETARY REQUIREMENTS

Although there is no specific daily dietary requirement for carbohydrates, the Food and Nutrition Board of the National Research Council recommends that half of one's energy requirement come from carbohydrates, preferably complex carbohydrates. (The recommendation is 10% of energy to come from simple carbohydrates.) For example, assume that one's total energy requirement is 2,000 calories. One-half of this is 1,000. Divide 1,000 calories by 4 (the number of calories in each gram of carbohydrate) for an estimated carbohydrate requirement of 250 g/day.

A mild deficiency of carbohydrates can result in weight loss and fatigue. A diet seriously deficient in carbohydrates could cause ketoacidosis, a stage in metabolism occurring when the liver has been depleted of stored glycogen and switches to a fasting mode. At this point, energy from fat is mobilized to the liver and used to synthesize glucose. The by-products of fat breakdown are ketones that build up in the bloodstream and are then released through the kidneys. To prevent these effects, one needs a minimum of 50–100 grams of carbohydrates each day.

The overweight population constitutes a major health problem in the United States. Some believe eating excess carbohydrates to be the most common cause of obesity. Although surplus carbohydrates are changed to glycogen, the major part of any surplus becomes adipose tissue. Also, an excess of carbohydrate in the form of sugar can spoil an appetite for other nutrients that are more important. Too many carbohydrates may cause tooth decay, irritate the lining of the stomach, or cause flatulence.

CONSIDERATIONS FOR THE HEALTH CARE PROFESSIONAL

The role of the health care professional in teaching about carbohydrates may be complicated. Some will have to be taught the nutritional differences between a baked potato and potato chips, between whole wheat toast and Danish pastry, between a fresh peach and canned fruit cocktail. Many will need to learn what dietary fiber is, where it can be found, and why it is needed. Some will need to learn that sugar can be used in moderation; others that it cannot be used in excess. All will require acceptance, understanding, and patience on the part of the health care professional.

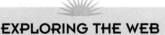

EXPLORING THE WEB

Search the Web for information on carbohydrate-reducing diets and products. Is the information provided at these sites accurate? If a client came to you with questions about a product such as these, how would you respond? Create a fact sheet that lists myths surrounding carbohydrates and the facts that dispel the myths.

SUMMARY

Energy foods are those that can be rapidly oxidized by the body to release energy. Carbohydrates are and should be the major source of energy. They are composed of carbon, hydrogen, and oxygen. One gram of carbohydrate provides 4 calories. Carbohydrates are the least expensive and most abundant nutrient. The principal sources of carbohydrates are plant products such as grains and their products, vegetables, fruits, legumes, and sugars. In addition to providing energy, carbohydrates spare proteins, maintain normal fat metabolism, and provide fiber. Digestion of carbohydrates begins in the mouth, continues in the stomach, and is completed in the small intestine. Although they are obviously essential to the health and well-being of the body, eating an excess of carbohydrates can cause dental caries, digestive disturbances, and obesity.

DISCUSSION TOPICS

1. What are the three basic groups of carbohydrates? Name several foods in each group.

2. Discuss the effects of regularly eating an excess of carbohydrates.

3. Why should one's diet contain dietary fiber? Name three sources of dietary fiber.

4. Describe the digestion and metabolism of carbohydrates.

5. Discuss the following menus. Which foods contain simple sugars and/or complex carbohydrates?

Orange juice	Baked chicken	Cheese sandwich
Cereal	Baked potato	on whole wheat
Milk and sugar	Green beans	bread with
Toast	Coleslaw	lettuce and tomato
Butter and jelly	Bread and	Carrot and
Coffee	butter	celery sticks
	Raspberry	Fresh fruit
	sherbet	Cookies
	Milk	Milk

6. Why are complex carbohydrates preferable to simple sugars?

7. Discuss *enrichment*. What does it mean? Why is it done? Which foods are typically enriched in the United States? Would you recommend that one purchase enriched foods? Why or why not?

8. Is it true, as many people say, that "carbs are fattening"? Explain your answer.

SUGGESTED ACTIVITIES

1. Hold a soda cracker in your mouth until you notice the change in flavor as the starch changes to dextrin.

2. Make a list of the foods you have eaten in the past 24 hours. Circle the carbohydrate-rich foods and underline the complex carbohydrates. Approximately what percentage of your calories were in the form of carbohydrates? In the form of complex carbs? Could your diet be improved? If so, how?

3. Role-play a situation between a diet counselor and a teenage girl who has placed herself on an extremely low-calorie diet. She refuses to eat anything that she thinks contains carbohydrates. Explain to her the functions of carbohydrates in the human body.

REVIEW

Multiple choice. Select the *letter* that precedes the best answer.

1. The three main groups of carbohydrates are
   a. fats, proteins, and minerals
   b. glucose, fructose, and galactose
   c. monosaccharides, disaccharides, and polysaccharides
   d. sucrose, cellulose, and glycogen

2. Galactose is a product of the digestion of
   a. milk
   b. meat
   c. breads
   d. vegetables

3. The simple sugar to which all forms of carbohydrates are ultimately converted is
   a. sucrose
   b. glucose
   c. galactose
   d. maltose

4. A fibrous form of carbohydrate that cannot be digested is
   a. glucose
   b. glycogen
   c. cellulose
   d. fat

5. Glycogen is stored in the
   a. heart and lungs
   b. liver and muscles
   c. pancreas and gallbladder
   d. small and large intestines

6. Glucose, fructose, and galactose are
   a. polysaccharides
   b. disaccharides
   c. enzymes
   d. monosaccharides

7. Before carbohydrates can be metabolized by the cells, they must be converted to
   a. glycogen
   b. glucose
   c. polysaccharides
   d. sucrase

8. The only form of carbohydrate that the brain uses for energy is
   a. glycogen
   b. galactose
   c. glucose
   d. glucagon

9. The substance that helps the liver convert glycogen to glucose is
   a. galactose
   b. estrogen
   c. thyroxin
   d. glucagon

10. Starch is
    a. the form in which glucose is stored in plants
    b. a monosaccharide
    c. an insoluble form of dietary fiber
    d. found only in grains

11. Insoluble dietary fiber
    a. can increase blood glucose
    b. can decrease blood cholesterol
    c. commonly causes diverticular disease
    d. is preferably provided by commercially prepared fiber products

12. The enzyme in the mouth that begins the digestion of starch is
    a. salivary ptyalin
    b. salivary amylase
    c. sucrase
    d. lipase

13. Cellulose is
    a. not digestible by humans
    b. not to be included in the human diet
    c. a monosaccharide
    d. an excellent substitute for dextrose

14. Carbohydrates
    a. are rich in fat
    b. are generally expensive
    c. should provide approximately half of the calories in the U.S. diet
    d. frequently are an excellent substitute for proteins in the human diet

15. Glucose metabolism is
    a. controlled mainly by the hormone insulin
    b. not affected by any secretion of the islets of Langerhans in the pancreas
    c. managed entirely by glucagon
    d. not related to human energy levels

CASE IN POINT

MARGARITA: MANAGING STEROID-INDUCED DIABETES

Margarita is a 59-year-old Hispanic nurse who has been admitted to the hospital for a left total knee replacement. She is 5 feet 6 inches and weighs 210 pounds. She has been NPO (nothing by mouth) all night and arrives to the hospital at 7 in the morning to be prepared for surgery. Once the operation is over, the healing process begins, and the physician notices that the incision is not healing as fast as expected. Margarita tells her nurse that since the surgery, she has noticed bilateral temporal pain.

Her hemoglobin drops dramatically, and she has been newly diagnosed with giant cell arteritis. The cure is large doses of prednisone. Large doses of prednisone cause steroid-induced diabetes. The doctor prescribed a 1,200-calorie diabetic diet. Margarita is overwhelmed with all that has happened.

ASSESSMENT

1. The dietitian can help Margarita regulate her diet and in so doing lose weight. Calculate Margarita's ideal weight using Table 3-3, Harris-Benedict, and thermic effect of food (TEF).

2. What does the dietitian need to know about Margarita's meal choices?

3. What does the dietitian need to know about Margarita's way of life?

4. What information will be helpful once Margarita is discharged and at home?

5. What sources of carbohydrates would be most helpful in weight loss and maintenance of blood sugar levels?

DIAGNOSIS

6. Write a nursing diagnosis for Margarita.

PLAN/GOAL

7. Write a goal related to weight loss that Margarita should achieve at the end of diabetic classes.

8. State two goals for Margarita related to her diet and blood sugar.

IMPLEMENTATION

9. List the topics that you would teach Margarita to achieve her goals.

10. What agencies or community resources can you provide to help Margarita achieve her goals?

EVALUATION/OUTCOME CRITERIA

11. What can you expect from Margarita to show she understands what you have taught?

12. What should Margarita's fasting blood sugar read?

13. How long do you think it would take Margarita to learn a new diet plan, check her blood sugar, learn a new exercise plan, and demonstrate integration into her everyday life?

THINKING FURTHER

14. What blood test could the doctor order to see if Margarita had maintained her blood sugar at a normal level?

15. What are some of the serious health consequences if Margarita does not manage her diabetes well?

◎ RATE THIS PLATE

Margarita was put on a 1,200-calorie ADA diet by her doctor. She is trying hard to adhere to her diet, but she is hungry all the time. Rate her plate.

6 oz broiled salmon
4 medium oven-roasted red potatoes
10 stalks of asparagus
2-oz hard roll with butter
1/2 cup peppermint stick ice cream
Iced tea with lemon

Is 1,200 calories realistic for Margarita? What is her BMR as figured by the Harris-Benedict equation? How was her planning? Is the plate correct? Would you change anything; what would you change and why? How many carbohydrates are allowed, each meal, on a 1,200-calorie ADA diet? How many carbohydrates are on this plate?

CASE IN POINT

JAMAL: ADJUSTING TO CORPORATE LIFE

Jamal is a 36-year-old African American accountant. He is 6 feet tall and weighs 305 pounds. In high school Jamal was a three-sports-a-year athlete. He was a trim 180 pounds. During college he was on the baseball team. His coach had the team in excellent condition, running sprints and drills. After college, Jamal stayed active with softball, but as the years progressed, he became more of a corporate man than an athlete. Jamal has been very upset with his weight and has tried Atkins and Weight Watchers. Because of the stress of owning two businesses, Jamal finds himself eating at all hours of the night and not even watching what he is eating; he is also occasionally constipated. Jamal seeks out his doctor for some helpful advice. Jamal's doctor advises him to go on a high-fiber diet and drink 13 glasses of water each day.

ASSESSMENT

1. What objective and subjective data do you have about Jamal?

2. What other issues could be influencing his weight?

3. What important information do you have regarding Jamal's eating habits?

4. What food consumption would be helpful to identify Jamal's present habits?

DIAGNOSIS

5. Write a nursing diagnosis for Jamal.

PLAN/GOAL

6. What changes do you want to see for Jamal?

7. What does Jamal need to learn about the relationship of carbohydrates and fiber?

IMPLEMENTATION

8. Name two dietary changes that will benefit Jamal.

9. What commercially available fiber will help Jamal?

10. How would increasing his exercise help Jamal?

11. How would adding raw fruits and vegetables help?

EVALUATION/OUTCOME CRITERIA

12. After adding more fiber and water and increasing his activity for 2 weeks, what might Jamal report about his bowel function?

13. What might Jamal relate about his new diet and exercise regime?

THINKING FURTHER

14. How is this lesson useful to a new corporate-type person?

RATE THIS PLATE

Jamal has a hectic schedule, but that shouldn't keep him from packing a cooler for those late-night snacks or meals. Jamal packed the following items in the cooler for one meal and snacks when he gets the munchies. Rate what has been packed for this evening and into the night.

Sandwich
   2 slices 100% whole wheat bread
   3 oz roasted turkey
   2 slices tomato
   2 large leaves of leaf lettuce
   1 tsp low-fat mayonnaise
   1 tsp tangy mustard
   1 cup diet gelatin
   1 large apple

Munchies
   1 bag pretzels
   1 large orange, peeled and separated into sections
   20 mini carrots
   2 celery sticks with peanut butter in the hollow (about 2 Tbsp of peanut butter)
   2 Rice Krispies squares (2 in. by 2 in.)
   1/2 cup diet applesauce
   1 bag baked potato chips

LIPIDS OR FATS

OBJECTIVES

After studying this chapter, you should be able to:

- State the functions of fats in the body
- Identify sources of dietary fats
- Explain common classifications of fats
- Describe disease conditions with which excessive use of fats is associated

Fats belong to a group of organic compounds called **lipids.** The word *lipid* is derived from *lipos,* a Greek word for fat. Forms of this word are found in several fat-related health terms such as blood *lipids* (fats in the blood), hyper*lipid*emia (high levels of fat in the blood), and *lipo*proteins (carriers of fat in human blood).

Fats are greasy substances that are not soluble in water. They are soluble in some solvents such as ether, benzene, and chloroform. They provide a more concentrated source of energy than carbohydrates; each gram of fat contains 9 calories. This is slightly more than twice the calorie content of carbohydrates. Fat-rich foods are generally more expensive than carbohydrate-rich foods. Like carbohydrates, fats are composed of carbon, hydrogen, and oxygen but with a substantially lower proportion of oxygen.

Cell membrane needs Fat

1yr - 2yr. Whole milk — for brain development.
Infants

○ **lipid**
fat

○ **adipose tissue**
fatty tissue

○ **satiety**
feeling of satisfaction; fullness

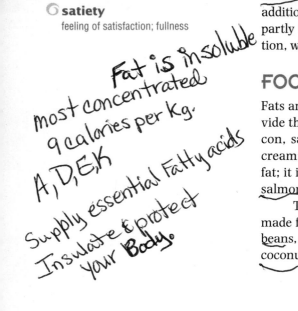

Fat is insoluble
most concentrated
9 calories per kg.
A, D, E, K
Supply essential Fatty acids
Insulate & protect
your Body.

FUNCTIONS

In addition to providing energy, fats are essential for the functioning and structure of body tissues (Table 5-1). Fats are a necessary part of cell membranes (cell walls). They contain essential fatty acids and act as carriers for fat-soluble vitamins A, D, E, and K. The fat stored in body tissues provides energy when one cannot eat, as may occur during some illness and after abdominal surgery. **Adipose** (fatty) **tissue** protects organs and bones from injury by serving as protective padding and support. Body fat also serves as insulation from cold. In addition, fats provide a feeling of **satiety** (satisfaction) after meals. This is due partly to the flavor fats give other foods and partly to their slow rate of digestion, which delays hunger.

FOOD SOURCES

Fats are present in both animal and plant foods. The animal foods that provide the richest sources of fats are meats, especially fatty meats such as bacon, sausage, and luncheon meats; whole, low-fat, and reduced-fat milk; cream; butter; cheeses made with cream; egg yolks (egg white contains no fat; it is almost entirely protein and water); and fatty fish such as tuna and salmon.

The plant foods containing the richest sources of fats are cooking oils made from sunflower, safflower, or sesame seeds, or from corn, peanuts, soybeans, or olives; margarine (which is made from vegetable oils); nuts; avocados; coconut; and cocoa butter.

Table 5-1 *Fats*

FUNCTIONS	DEFICIENCY SIGNS	SOURCES
Provide energy	Eczema	Animal
Carry fat-soluble vitamins	Weight loss	Fatty meats
Supply essential fatty acids	Retarded growth	Lard
Protect and support organs and bones		Butter
Insulate from cold		Cheese
Provide satiety to meals		Cream
		Whole milk
		Egg yolk
		Plant
		Vegetable oils
		Nuts
		Chocolate
		Avocados
		Olives
		Margarine

Production of the **85** *Food.*

Visible and Invisible Fats in Food

Sometimes fats are referred to as visible or invisible, depending on their food sources. Fats that are purchased and used as fats such as butter, margarine, lard, and cooking oils are called **visible fats**. Hidden or **invisible fats** are those found in other foods such as meats, cream, whole milk, cheese, egg yolk, fried foods, pastries, avocados, and nuts.

It is often the invisible fats that can make it difficult for clients on limited-fat diets to regulate their fat intake. For example, one 3-inch doughnut may contain 12 grams of fat, whereas one 3-inch bagel contains only 2 grams of fat. One fried chicken drumstick may contain 11 grams of fat, whereas one roasted drumstick may contain only 2 grams of fat.

It is essential that the health care professional confirm that clients on limited-fat diets are carefully educated about sources of hidden fats.

body makes cholesterol also consumes it

CLASSIFICATION

Triglycerides, phospholipids, and *sterols* are all lipids found in food and the human body. Most lipids in the body (95%) are triglycerides. They are in body cells, and they circulate in the blood.

Triglycerides are composed of three (tri) fatty acids attached to a framework of **glycerol**, thus their name (Figure 5-1). Glycerol is derived from a water-soluble carbohydrate. **Fatty acids** are organic compounds of carbon atoms to which hydrogen atoms are attached. They are classified in two ways: essential or nonessential. *Essential fatty acids (EFAs)* are necessary fats that humans cannot synthesize; EFAs must be obtained through diet. EFAs are long-chain polyunsaturated fatty acids derived from **linoleic, linolenic,** and oleic acids. There are two families of EFAs: omega-3 and omega-6. Necessary, but nonessential, are the omega-9 fatty acids because the body can manufacture a modest amount, provided EFAs are present. (Also see the later section on polyunsaturated fats.)

The other method of classification of fatty acids is by their degree of saturation with hydrogen atoms. In this method, they are described as *saturated, monounsaturated,* or *polyunsaturated,* depending on their hydrogen content (Figure 5-2).

Saturated Fats

When a fatty acid is **saturated,** each of its carbon atoms carries all the hydrogen atoms possible. In general, animal foods contain more saturated fatty acids than unsaturated. Examples include meat, poultry, egg yolks, whole milk, whole milk cheeses, cream, ice cream, and butter. Although plant foods generally contain more polyunsaturated fatty acids than saturated fatty acids, chocolate, coconut, palm oil, and palm kernel oils are exceptions. They contain substantial amounts of saturated fatty acids. Foods containing a high proportion of saturated fats are usually solid at room temperature. It is recommended that one consume no more than 7% of total daily calories as saturated fats.

visible fats
fats in foods that are purchased and used as fats, such as butter or margarine

invisible fats
fats that are not immediately noticeable such as those in egg yolk, cheese, cream, and salad dressings

triglyceride
three fatty acids attached to a framework of glycerol

glycerol
a component of fat; derived from a water-soluble carbohydrate

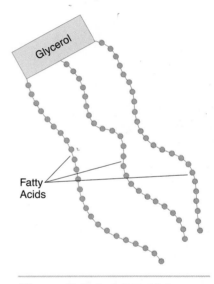

Figure 5-1 *A triglyceride is composed of three fatty acids attached to a framework of glycerol.*

fatty acids
a component of fats that determines the classification of the fat

linoleic acid
fatty acid essential for humans; cannot be synthesized by the body

linolenic acid
one of three fatty acids needed by the body; cannot be synthesized by the body

saturated fats
fats whose carbon atoms contain all of the hydrogen atoms they can; considered a contributory factor in atherosclerosis

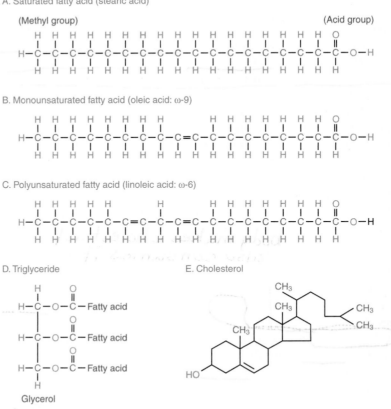

Figure 5-2 *Chemical formula for (A) saturated fatty acid, (B) monounsaturated fatty acid, (C) polyunsaturated fatty acid, (D) triglyceride, (E) cholesterol.*

Monounsaturated Fats

If a fat is **monounsaturated**, there is one place among the carbon atoms of its fatty acids where there are fewer hydrogen atoms attached than in saturated fats. Examples of foods containing monounsaturated fats are olive oil, peanut oil, canola oil, avocados, and cashew nuts. Research indicates that monounsaturated fats lower the amount of low-density lipoprotein (LDL) ("bad cholesterol") in the blood, but only when they replace saturated fats in one's diet. They have no effect on high-density lipoproteins (HDLs) ("good cholesterol"). It is recommended that one consume 15% of total daily calories as monounsaturated fats (Table 5-2).

Polyunsaturated Fats

If a fat is **polyunsaturated,** there are two or more places among the carbon atoms of its fatty acids where there are fewer hydrogen atoms attached than in saturated fats. The point at which carbon-carbon double bonds occur in a polyunsaturated fatty acid is the determining factor in how the body metabolizes it. The two major fatty acids denoted by the placement of their double bonds are the omega-3 and omega-6 fatty acids. **Omega-3 fatty acids** have been reported to help lower the risk of heart disease. Because omega-3 fatty acids are found in fish

◌ monounsaturated fats
fats that are neither saturated nor polyunsaturated and are thought to play little part in atherosclerosis

◌ polyunsaturated fats
fats whose carbon atoms contain only limited amounts of hydrogen

◌ omega-3 fatty acids
help lower the risk of heart disease

Table 5-2 *Sources of Saturated, Monounsaturated, and Polyunsaturated Fatty Acids*

SATURATED	MONOUNSATURATED	POLYUNSATURATED
Meats	Canola oil	Safflower oil
Coconut	Olive oil	Soybean oil
Palm oil, palm kernel oil	Peanut oil	Sunflower oil
Butter	Nuts	Soybeans
Egg yolks	Avocados	Tofu
Milk and milk products (except fat-free)	Sardines	

oils, an increased intake of fatty fish is recommended. Omega-6 (linoleic acid) has a cholesterol-lowering effect. The use of supplements of either of these fatty acids is not recommended. Examples of foods containing polyunsaturated fats include cooking oils made from sunflower, safflower, or sesame seeds or from corn or soybeans; soft margarines whose major ingredient is *liquid* vegetable oil; and fish. Foods containing high proportions of polyunsaturated fats are usually soft or oily. Polyunsaturated fats should not exceed 8% of total daily calories.

Trans-Fatty Acid

Trans-fatty acids (TFAs) are produced when hydrogen atoms are added to monounsaturated or polyunsaturated fats to produce a semisolid product like margarine and shortening. A product is likely to contain a significant amount of TFAs if partially hydrogenated vegetable oil is listed in the first three ingredients on the label. The major source of TFAs in the diet is from baked goods and foods eaten in restaurants. TFAs raise low-density lipoproteins (LDLs) and total cholesterol.

trans-fatty acids
produced by adding hydrogen atoms to a liquid fat making it solid

Hydrogenated Fats. Hydrogenated fats are polyunsaturated vegetable oils to which hydrogen has been added commercially to make them solid at room temperature. This process, called **hydrogenation**, turns polyunsaturated vegetable oils into saturated fats. Margarine is made in this way. (Soft margarine contains less saturated fat than firm margarine.)

hydrogenation
the combining of fat with hydrogen, thereby making it a saturated fat and solid at room temperature

CHOLESTEROL

Cholesterol is a sterol (Figure 5-2). It is not a true fat but a fatlike substance that exists in animal foods and body cells. It does not exist in plant foods. Cholesterol is essential for the synthesis of bile, sex hormones, cortisone, and vitamin D and is needed by every cell in the body. The body manufactures 800–1,000 mg of cholesterol a day in the liver.

cholesterol
fatlike substance that is a constituent of body cells; is synthesized in the liver; also available in animal foods

Cholesterol is a common constituent (part) of one's daily diet because it is found so abundantly in egg yolk, fatty meats, shellfish, butter, cream, cheese, whole milk, and organ meats (liver, kidneys, brains, sweetbreads) (Table 5-3).

Cholesterol is thought to be a contributing factor in heart disease because high serum cholesterol, also called **hypercholesterolemia,** is common in

hypercholesterolemia
unusually high levels of cholesterol in blood; also known as high serum cholesterol

SUPERSIZE USA

Twists and Turns of Fad Diets

Fad diets have been around for years. Look at these. Do you want to try any of them?

1960

Robert Cameron introduces the Drinking Man's Diet, which claims people can lose weight by eating steak and drinking red wine. Cameron subsequently undergoes coronary bypass surgery.

1967

Dr. Irwin Stillman publishes the *Quick Weight Loss Diet,* describing how he overcame middle-age obesity and a heart attack by cutting carbohydrates and consuming large quantities of water.

1972

Dr. Atkins' Diet Revolution, a high-protein, low-carbohydrate diet, promotes ketoacidosis, in which a semi-starving body burns fat for fuel.

1973

At age 25, Richard Simmons begins his career as fitness guru, video master and author by opening a Beverly Hills restaurant and exercise studio.

1978

The Complete Scarsdale Medical Diet, by Dr. Herman Tarnower, is the latest of the popular high-protein, low-carbohydrate diets.

1979

The restrictive Pritikin Program recommends a high-fiber diet with less than 10 percent of calories from fat, no added salt or sugar and regular aerobic exercise.

1980

Diarrhea is a common side effect of the six-week Beverly Hills Diet, which starts dieters off with 10 days of nothing but fruit and water.

1988

The liquid diet Optifast, made famous by Oprah Winfrey's 67-pound weight loss, becomes infamous when Winfrey gains all the weight back and then some.

1991

Robert Pritikin, following in his father Nathan's footsteps, publishes *The Pritikin Weight Loss Breakthrough* as part of the new Pritikin Program.

1995

High-protein diets make a comeback. In *Enter the Zone,* Barry Sears recommends eating lots of protein, fruits and vegetables, while greatly reducing carbohydrates, such as pastas, breads, rice and potatoes.

1996

Protein Power, by Michael and Mary Eades, claims the amount of carbohydrates required by humans for health is zero.

1997

Dr. Bob Arnot's *Revolutionary Weight Control Program* hits the stands, calling refined carbohydrates the dietary equivalent of "crack" because "you need them all day in order to feel good."

SugarBusters!, by H. Leighton Steward, Morrison C. Berthea, Sam S. Andrews and Luis A. Balart, claims all sugar is toxic and that potatoes, corn, white rice, white bread, sodas and beer must be completely eliminated from the diet.

Dr. Atkins *New Diet Revolution* is a slightly modified version of his 1972 book, referring to insulin as the "fat-producing hormone." Atkins' recipes call for heavy cream, butter and cheese and recommend bacon and eggs for breakfast every day. The newest craze, *Eat for Your Type,* by Dr. Peter D'Adamo, argues that blood type is an evolutionary marker of which foods each person will process well and which will be useless calories.

(Source: The Wheat Foods Council, 2005. The Wheat Foods Council is a national nonprofit organization formed to help increase awareness of dietary grains as an essential component to a healthy diet. Information or graphics included in this Web site may be used for educational purposes as long as the information is not altered. The information cannot be used for advertising.)

Table 5-3 *Fat and Cholesterol Content of Some Common Foods*

FOOD	AMOUNT	SATURATED FAT (g)	CHOLESTEROL (mg)	TOTAL FAT (g)	TOTAL KCAL
Dairy					
Creamed cottage cheese (4% fat)	1 cup	6.4	34	10	235
Uncreamed cottage cheese (0.5% fat)	1 cup	0.4	10	1	125
Cream cheese	1 oz	6.2	31	10	100
Swiss cheese	1 oz	5.0	26	8	105
American processed cheese	1 oz	5.6	27	9	105
Half and half	1 Tbsp	1.1	6	2	20
Heavy cream	1 Tbsp	3.5	21	6	54
Nondairy creamer	1 Tbsp	1.4	0	1	20
Whole milk	1 cup	5.1	33	8	150
Reduced-fat milk	1 cup	2.9	18	5	120
Low-fat milk	1 cup	1.6	10	3	100
Fat-free milk	1 cup	0.3	4	Trace	85
Chocolate milk shake	10 oz	4.8	30	8	335
Ice cream (11% fat)	1/2 cup	8.9	59	14	270
Egg	1	1.7	274	6	80
Oils					
Butter	1 Tbsp	7.1	31	11	100
Margarine	1 Tbsp	2.2	0	11	100
Corn oil	1 Tbsp	1.8	0	14	125
Seafood					
Crabmeat (canned)	1 cup	0.5	135	3	135
Salmon (canned)	3 oz	0.9	34	5	120
Shrimp (canned)	3 oz	0.2	128	1	100
Tuna					
Water-packed	3 oz	0.3	48	1	135
Oil-packed	3 oz	1.4	55	7	165
Vegetable					
Avocado	1/2	2.2	0	15	150
Bread					
Bagel	1	0.3	0	2	200
Doughnut	1	2.8	20	12	210
English muffin	1	0.3	0	1	140
Nuts					
Peanuts (dry roasted)	1 oz	2.0	0	15	170
Meat					
Ground beef (lean)	3 oz	6.2	74	16	230
Roast beef (lean)	4.4 oz	7.2	100	18	300
Leg lamb (lean)	5.2 oz	4.8	130	12	280
Leg lamb (lean and fat)	6 oz	11.2	156	26	410
Bacon	3 slices	3.3	16	9	110
Pork chop (lean)	5 oz	5.2	142	16	330
Frankfurter	1.5 oz	4.8	23	13	145
Chicken leg, fried (meat and skin)	5 oz	6.0	124	22	390
Chicken leg, roasted (meat only)	3.2 oz	1.4	82	4	150

Source: *Adapted from* Nutritive Value of Foods, *USDA Home and Garden Bulletin No. 72, 1981.*

atherosclerosis
a form of arteriosclerosis affecting the intima (inner lining) of the artery walls

 plaque
fatty deposit on interior of artery walls

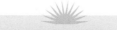

EXPLORING THE WEB

Search the Web for cholesterol-lowering products. What claims do these products make? Are food-drug interactions mentioned? Are the claims based on scientific research and facts? What advice would you give a client who is inquiring about such products? Create a fact sheet that lists the myths regarding fats and cholesterol and present the facts that dispel these myths.

clients with **atherosclerosis.** Atherosclerosis is a cardiovascular disease in which **plaque** (fatty deposits containing cholesterol and other substances) forms on the inside of artery walls, reducing the space for blood flow. When the blood cannot flow through an artery near the heart, a heart attack occurs. When this is the case near the brain, stroke occurs. (See Chapter 18.)

It is considered advisable that blood cholesterol levels not exceed 200 mg/dl (200 milligrams of cholesterol per 1 deciliter of blood). A reduction in the amount of total fat, saturated fats, and cholesterol and an increase in the amounts of monounsaturated fats in the diet, weight loss, and exercise all help to lower serum cholesterol levels. Soluble dietary fiber also is considered helpful in lowering blood cholesterol because the cholesterol binds to the fiber and is eliminated via the feces, thus preventing it from being absorbed in the small intestine. In some cases, medication may be prescribed if diet, weight loss, and exercise do not sufficiently lower serum cholesterol.

Because the development of plaque is cumulative, the preferred means of avoiding or at least limiting its development is to limit cholesterol and fat intake throughout life. If children are not fed high-cholesterol foods on a regular basis, their chances of overusing them as adults are reduced. Thus, their risk of heart attack and stroke is also reduced.

DIGESTION AND ABSORPTION

Although 95% of ingested fats are digested, it is a complex process. The chemical digestion of fats occurs mainly in the small intestine. Fats are not digested in the mouth. They are digested only slightly in the stomach, where gastric lipase acts on emulsified fats such as those found in cream and egg yolk. Fats must be mixed well with the gastric juices before entering the small intestine. In the small intestine, bile emulsifies the fats, and the enzyme pancreatic lipase reduces them to fatty acids and glycerol, which the body subsequently absorbs through villi (Figure 5-3).

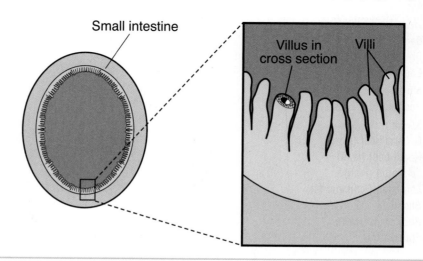

Small intestine

Villus in cross section   Villi

Figure 5-3 *The body absorbs fatty acids and glycerol through the villi of the small intestine.*

Lipoproteins

Fats are insoluble in water, which is the main component of blood. Therefore, special carriers must be provided for the fats to be absorbed and transported by the blood to body cells. In the initial stages of absorption, bile joins with the products of fat digestion to carry fat. Later, protein combines with the final products of fat digestion to form special carriers called **lipoproteins.** The lipoproteins subsequently carry the fats to the body cells by way of the blood.

Lipoproteins are classified as **chylomicrons, very-low-density lipoproteins (VLDLs), low-density lipoproteins (LDLs),** and **high-density lipoproteins (HDLs),** according to their mobility and density. Chylomicrons are the first lipoprotein identified after eating. They are the largest lipoproteins and the lightest in weight. They are composed of 80 to 90% triglycerides. Lipoprotein lipase acts to break down the triglycerides into free fatty acids and glycerol. Without this enzyme, fat could not get into the cells.

Very-low-density lipoproteins are made primarily by the liver cells and are composed of 55 to 65% triglycerides. They carry triglycerides and other lipids to all cells. As the VLDLs lose triglycerides, they pick up cholesterol from other lipoproteins in the blood and they then become LDLs. Low-density lipoproteins are approximately 45% cholesterol with few triglycerides. They carry most of the blood cholesterol from the liver to the cells. Elevated blood levels greater than 130 mg/dL of LDL are thought to be contributing factors in atherosclerosis. Low-density lipoprotein is sometimes termed *bad cholesterol.*

High-density lipoproteins carry cholesterol from the cells to the liver for eventual excretion. The level at which low HDL becomes a major risk factor for heart disease has been set at 40 mg/dL. Research indicates that an HDL level of 60 mg/dL or more is considered protective against heart disease. High-density lipoproteins are sometimes called *good cholesterol.* Exercising, maintaining a desirable weight, and giving up smoking are all ways to increase one's HDL.

lipoproteins
carriers of fat in the blood

chylomicron
largest lipoprotein; transports lipids after digestion into the body

very-low-density lipoproteins (VLDLs)
lipoproteins made by the liver to transport lipids throughout the body

low-density lipoproteins (LDLs)
carry blood cholesterol to the cells

high-density lipoproteins (HDLs)
lipoproteins that carry cholesterol from cells to the liver for eventual excretion

METABOLISM AND ELIMINATION

The liver controls fat metabolism. It hydrolyzes triglycerides and forms new ones from this hydrolysis as needed. Ultimately, the metabolism of fats occurs in the cells, where fatty acids are broken down to carbon dioxide and water, releasing energy. The portion of fat that is not needed for immediate use is stored as adipose tissue. Carbon dioxide and water are byproducts that are used or removed from the body by the circulatory, respiratory, and excretory systems.

FATS AND THE CONSUMER

Fats continue to be of particular interest to the consumer. Most people know that fats are high-calorie foods and that they are related to heart disease. But people who are not in the health field may not know *how* fats affect health. Consequently, they may be easily duped by clever ads for or salespersons of nutritional supplements or new "health food" products.

It is important that the health care professional carefully evaluate any new dietary "supplement" for which a nutrition claim is made. If the item is not included in the RDA, DRI, or AI, it is safe to assume that medical research has not determined that it is essential. Ingestion of dietary supplements of unknown value could, ironically, be damaging to one's health.

Lecithin

⚪ lecithin
fatty substance found in plant and animal foods; a natural emulsifier that helps transport fats in the bloodstream; used commercially to make food products smooth

Lecithin is a fatty substance classified as a phospholipid. It is found in both plant and animal foods and is synthesized in the liver. It is a natural emulsifier that helps transport fat in the bloodstream. It is used commercially to make food products smooth.

Lecithin supplements have been promoted by some health food salespersons as being able to prevent cardiovascular disease. To date, this has not been scientifically proven.

Fat Alternatives

Research into fat alternatives has been in progress for decades. Olestra, the newest product on the market, is made from carbohydrates and fat. The FDA has approved olestra for use only in snack foods such as potato chips, tortilla chips, and crackers. The government requires that food labels indicate that olestra "inhibits the absorption of some vitamins and other nutrients." Therefore, the fat-soluble vitamins A, D, E, and K have been added to foods containing olestra. Olestra contains no calories, but it can cause cramps and diarrhea. The products manufactured with olestra should be used in moderation.

Simplesse is made from either egg white or milk protein and contains 1.3 kcal/g. Simplesse can be used only in cold foods such as ice cream because it becomes thick or gels when heated. Simplesse is not available for home use.

Oatrim is carbohydrate-based and is derived from oat fiber. Oatrim is heat-stable and can be used in baking but not in frying. Manufacturers have used carbohydrate-based compounds for years as thickeners. Oatrim does provide calories, but significantly less than fat.

The long-term effects these products may have on human health and nutrition are unknown. If they are used in the way the U.S. population uses artificial sweeteners, they probably will not reduce the actual fat content in the diet. They may simply be additions to it. One concern among nutritionists is that they will be used in place of nutritious food that, in addition to fat, also provides vitamins, minerals, proteins, and carbohydrates.

DIETARY REQUIREMENTS

Although no specific dietary requirement for fats is included in the RDA and DRIs, deficiency symptoms do occur when fats provide less than 10% of the total daily calorie requirement. When gross deficiency occurs, eczema (inflamed and scaly skin condition) can develop. This has been observed in infants who were fed formulas lacking the essential fatty acid linoleic acid and in clients maintained for long periods on intravenous feedings that lack linoleic acid.

SPOTLIGHT on Life Cycle

Are you a TV watcher? Have you always been a TV watcher? One-fourth of U.S. children spend 4 hours or more a day watching television, and only 27% of high school students engage in moderate physical activity at least 30 minutes a day for 5 or more days of the week. Children who watch 4 or more hours of TV daily are shown to have significantly greater body mass indexes compared with those who watch less than 2 hours a day. Having a TV in the bedroom is a strong predictor of being overweight. The absence of family meals is associated with lower fruit and vegetable consumption and increased consumption of more fried foods and carbonated beverages.
(Source: The News Sentinel, November 2003.)

Also, growth may be retarded, and weight loss can occur when diets are seriously deficient in fats.

On the other hand, excessive fat in the diet can lead to obesity or heart disease. In addition, studies point to an association between high-fat diets and cancers of the colon, breast, uterus, and prostate.

The Food and Nutrition Board's Committee on Diet and Health recommends that people reduce their fat intake to 30% of total calories. The American Heart Association's newest recommendation is to consume less or no more than 7% of saturated fats, 8% polyunsaturated fats, and 15% monounsaturated fats. At present, 36% of calories in U.S. diets is derived from fats.

CONSIDERATIONS FOR THE HEALTH CARE PROFESSIONAL

To accomplish dietary change, the health care professional should review clients' usual diets *with* them. Changes then can be introduced clearly and sensitively and with the clients' active participation. Unless clients understand *why* dietary changes are needed and want to make them, they are unlikely to change their diets.

> ### ((In The Media
>
> **FAT IN THE DIET**
>
> The media keep their readers informed about the positives and negatives of fat in the diet. If you listen to the American Heart Association, and you should, you will follow its recommendations of only 30% of daily calories from fat, with the emphasis on "good fats." But if you listen to the spokesperson for Dr. Atkins Diet Revolution, you will believe that there is no "bad fat." This diet recommends as much meat and fat as you want! It is imperative that the health care professional have up-to-date knowledge of the various types of fat and the positives and negatives of overconsumption and underconsumption.

SUMMARY

In addition to providing an important source of energy, fats carry essential fatty acids and fat-soluble vitamins, protect organs and bones, insulate from cold, and provide satiety to meals. They are composed of carbon, hydrogen, and oxygen and are found in both animal and plant foods. Each gram of fat provides 9 calories. Digestion of fats occurs mainly in the small intestine, where they are reduced to fatty acids and glycerol. An excess of fat in the diet can result in obesity and possibly heart disease or cancer.

DISCUSSION TOPICS

1. Why are fats considered a more concentrated source of energy than carbohydrates?

2. Of what value are fats to the body? List some foods rich in fats.

3. Discuss adipose tissue. Is it good? Is it bad? Explain.

4. Describe atherosclerosis. It is said that its effects are cumulative. Explain.

5. Describe the digestion and metabolism of fats. What are the end products of fat digestion?

6. Why might a client on a low-fat diet complain? How might the health care professional be helpful in such a case?

7. What are hydrogenated fats? Are they polyunsaturated? Explain.

8. Why is there a greater danger of excess fat in the U.S. diet than a deficiency of fat?

9. Discuss invisible fats and their potential impact on low-fat diets.

10. What are the probable reasons that omega-3 fatty acid capsules and lecithin have become so popular with the general public?

SUGGESTED ACTIVITIES

1. List the foods you ate yesterday. Circle those containing visible fats. Underline those containing invisible fats. Explain why some foods are both

circled and underlined. Revise your list, making it appropriate for someone on a limited-fat diet.

2. Using a cookbook, review recipes for baked products and answer the following questions about them.
   a. Why do bagels contain no cholesterol?
   b. Why does angel cake contain no cholesterol?
   c. Why does a doughnut contain cholesterol when an English muffin does not?
   d. Why does French toast contain cholesterol when the white bread it is made from may not?
   e. Why does lemon meringue pie filling contain cholesterol when apple pie filling does not?
   f. Why does a cheeseburger contain more cholesterol than a ham- burger?

3. Write down five typical meals in your family's diet—one breakfast, one lunch, one dinner, and two snacks. How could you modify them to reduce the fat content?

4. Visit a fast-food restaurant and review the menu. How many items are high in fat? How many are not? Is there any invisible fat in the more "healthy" items? Share your findings with the class.

REVIEW

Multiple choice. Select the *letter* that precedes the best answer.

1. Fats provide the most concentrated form of
   a. carbon   c. lipase
   b. oxygen   d. energy

2. Adipose tissue is useful because it
   a. can synthesize triglycerides
   b. prevents eczema
   c. provides satiety
   d. protects and insulates

3. Atherosclerosis is thought to increase the risk of
   a. cancer   c. heart attacks
   b. plaque   d. hypercholesterolemia

4. A diet grossly deficient in fats may be deficient in
   a. lipase   c. cholesterol
   b. linoleic acid   d. triglycerides

5. Invisible fats can be found in
   a. cake and cookies
   b. orange and tomato juice
   c. egg white and skim milk
   d. lettuce and tomatoes

6. Plant foods that contain saturated fats are
   a. olives and avocados   c. corn and soybeans
   b. coconut and chocolate   d. cashew nuts and canola oil

7. When a polyunsaturated vegetable oil is changed to a saturated fat, the process is called
   a. hydrolysis   c. hydrogenation
   b. hypercholesterolemia   d. hyperlipidemia

8. Linoleic acid is one of the fatty acids that is known to be
   a. a triglyceride   c. monounsaturated
   b. saturated   d. essential to the human diet

9. Cholesterol is
   a. not essential to the human diet
   b. thought to contribute to atherosclerosis
   c. not found in animal foods
   d. classified as a mineral

10. Another name for fats is
    a. lipase   c. lipoproteins
    b. lipidemia   d. lipids

11. Three groups of lipids found naturally in the human body and in food are triglycerides, phospholipids, and
    a. cortisone   c. sterols
    b. steroids   d. hydrogenated fats

12. Fatty acids are organic compounds of carbon atoms and
    a. hydrogen atoms   c. triglycerides
    b. arachidonic acids   d. glycerol

13. Cholesterol
    a. is found in both plants and animals
    b. is found only in plants
    c. does not contribute in any way to heart disease
    d. is a sterol

14. HDL (high-density lipoprotein)
    a. is sometimes called good cholesterol
    b. carries lipids to the cells
    c. is the same as lipase
    d. levels should be less than 40 mg/dl of human blood

15. For digestion, fats require the help of gastric lipase,
    a. bile, and fatty acids
    b. bile, and pancreatic lipase
    c. pancreatic lipase, and glycerol
    d. cholesterol, and bile

CASE IN POINT

AFZOL: GETTING CHOLESTEROL UNDER CONTROL

Afzol is a 61-year-old Indian man who has a family history of high cholesterol. His father and brother (respectively) died at the ages of 49 and 45 of heart attacks. Afzol's wife, Anyra, had been very careful in what she prepared for Afzol when they were first married. Afzol's cholesterol was well within the high normal limits. He was feeling good and did not need his medications. Years later, Afzol is in the midst of buying out a competitor's plastics company. He is wining and dining many people and taking them to the best restaurants. He is not paying attention to his diet. This has been going on for many months, and now that the buyout has been successful, Afzol finds himself in a larger role and busier than ever. He seldom eats right and is smoking more than ever. Even though he is busier, he is less active. Anyra convinces Afzol to see his physician. Tests reveal that Afzol has a cholesterol level of 450 mg/dl, an LDL of 250 mg/dl, and an HDL of 30 mg/dl. His physician refers him to the cardiac education classes for diet education and fitness assessment. The physician is seriously considering increasing Afzol's cholesterol lowering medication but would like to wait until his assessment is completed.

ASSESSMENT

1. What data do you have about Afzol?
2. What conclusion can you draw from Afzol's lab results?
3. What do you need to know about his current eating habits? Could foods with invisible fat have a bearing on his current diet? How could a 24-hour food diary help?
4. What about his health habits like smoking and alcohol use?
5. What is Afzol doing that is healthy for his heart?

DIAGNOSIS

6. What is the cause of Afzol's imbalanced nutrition, more than body requirements?
7. Complete this statement: Afzol's change of lifestyle is related to _____ ?

PLAN/GOAL

8. What two goals do you have for Afzol?

IMPLEMENTATION

9. What topics do you need to cover related to dietary fats?

10. Name three things Afzol can do to help him recognize hidden fats in fast-food restaurants.
11. Who else should be in class with Afzol?
12. What agencies or resources could you provide to support Afzol at home?
13. How could the information on the American Heart Association Web site, at www.americanheart.org, be helpful to Afzol?

EVALUATION/OUTCOME CRITERIA

14. What can the physician measure to determine the effectiveness of the plan?
15. What can Afzol provide to demonstrate his compliance with the plan?

THINKING FURTHER

16. What is the worst consequence if Afzol does not reduce his cholesterol?
17. What does family history have to do with Afzol's results?
18. What are the challenges of maintaining a diet and exercise plan for the rest of your life?

RATE THIS PLATE

Afzol met with the dietitian at the cardiac education class and indicated that he would like to learn to make better choices when eating out. Below is what Afzol usually ordered. Is this alright for his new low-cholesterol diet? Rate the plate.

12 oz prime rib

Baked potato with butter and sour cream

Steamed vegetables with butter

House salad with bacon bits, hard-cooked egg, tomato, cucumber, and croutons

Honey mustard salad dressing—about 1/4 cup

Cheesecake with cherries

Coffee with cream

CASE IN POINT

FRANCESCA: LOSING WEIGHT

Francesca is a 40-year-old Italian schoolteacher who has been heavy most of her life. She is active and loves playing handball and racquetball. She was always active during school and does not know why she cannot lose her weight. She has about 100 pounds to lose. She has an Italian mother who loves to cook, and she brings Francesca a lot of traditional

Italian meals. Francesca loves her mom and does not want to offend her by not eating the food. Francesca wants to lose weight and is now ready to forge ahead. She knows that the diet programs offered on TV, "lose weight fast and drop a dress size in a week," are not for her. Francesca asked her doctor for a referral to a dietitian to discuss the best way to lose weight.

ASSESSMENT

1. What data do you currently have about Francesca?
2. What has contributed to her current problem?
3. Is this an unusual problem for a woman of 40?
4. What do you know about Francesca's personality?
5. What do you know about her knowledge of weight reduction strategies?

DIAGNOSIS

6. What is the cause of Francesca's weight?
7. What can you tell Francesca about eating carbohydrates and fats?

PLAN/GOAL

8. What are two reasonable, measurable goals for Francesca and her weight loss program?

IMPLEMENTATION

9. What is the recommended rate of weight loss?

10. What is the recommended percentage of fat in the diet during weight loss?
11. What else can Francesca do besides modify her diet?
12. Given your assessment data, would you recommend Francesca diet alone or in a group? Why?
13. What other resources could be helpful to Francesca?
14. How could the Shape Up America! web site at www.shapeup.org be helpful to Francesca?

EVALUATION/OUTCOME CRITERIA

15. How often should Francesca weigh herself?
16. What other signs will indicate that Francesca is losing weight?

THINKING FURTHER

17. Who else could benefit from Francesca's change in diet and activity? How?
18. For whom else could this lesson be useful?

◎ RATE THIS PLATE

Francesca doesn't want to hurt her mother's feelings, so she continues to eat more than her body needs. What can she do? Let's see if you can take a dinner her mother brought and make the portion sizes right for weight loss. Let's say she is on 1,600 calories per day. Create the plate. Then rate your plate.

3 cups spaghetti with 1 cup sauce

4 2-oz meatballs

Tossed salad with cucumbers, tomatoes, black olive slices, grated cheddar cheese, and red onion slices

Homemade Italian dressing (oil, vinegar, and herbs)

2 slices garlic bread (1 1/2 oz per slice of Italian bread)

Crème brûlée

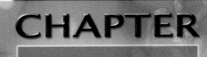

CHAPTER

6

PROTEINS

OBJECTIVES

After studying this chapter, you should be able to:

- State the functions of proteins in the body
- Identify the elements of which proteins are composed
- Describe the effects of protein deficiency
- State the energy yield of proteins
- Identify at least six food sources of complete proteins and six food sources of incomplete proteins

Proteins are the basic material of every body cell. By the age of 4 years, body protein content reaches the adult level of about 18% of body weight. An adequate supply of proteins in the daily diet is essential for normal growth and development and for the maintenance of health. Proteins are appropriately named. The word **protein** is of Greek derivation and means "of first importance."

FUNCTIONS

Proteins build and repair body tissue, play major roles in regulating various body functions, and provide energy if there is insufficient carbohydrate and fat in the diet.

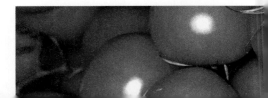

Ꮞ **protein**
the only one of six essential nutrients containing nitrogen

SPOTLIGHT on Life Cycle

Did you realize that from conception to death, proteins are either building, as in babies that are developing, or repairing, as in body cells that are constantly wearing out? When an injury happens and the skin is broken, what repairs the skin? Proteins, of course. Of the six nutrient groups, only proteins can make new cells and rebuild tissue; proteins are essential throughout the entire life span, from birth through advanced age.

Building and Repairing Body Tissue

The primary function of proteins is to build and repair body tissues. This is made possible by the provision of the correct type and number of amino acids in the diet. Also, as cells are broken down during metabolism (catabolism), some amino acids released into the blood are recycled to build new and repair other tissue (anabolism). The body uses the recycled amino acids as efficiently as those obtained from the diet.

Regulating Body Functions

Proteins are important components of hormones and enzymes that are essential for the regulation of metabolism and digestion. Proteins help maintain fluid and electrolyte balances in the body and thus prevent edema (abnormal retention of body fluids). Proteins also are essential for the development of antibodies and, consequently, for a healthy immune system.

Providing Energy

Proteins can provide energy if and when the supply of carbohydrates and fats in the diet is insufficient. Each gram of protein provides 4 calories. This is not a good use of proteins, however. In general, they are more expensive than carbohydrates, and most of the complete proteins also contain saturated fats and cholesterol.

FOOD SOURCES

Proteins are found in both animal and plant foods (Table 6-1). The animal food sources provide the highest quality, of complete, proteins. They include meats, fish, poultry, eggs, milk, and cheese.

Despite the high biologic value of proteins from animal food sources, they also provide saturated fats and cholesterol. Consequently, complete proteins

Table 6-1 *Rich Sources of Proteins*			
COMPLETE PROTEINS		**INCOMPLETE PROTEINS**	
Meats	Eggs	Corn	Grains
Fish	Milk	Peanuts	Nuts
Poultry	Cheese	Peas	Sunflower seeds
		Navy beans	Sesame seeds
		Soybeans	

should be carefully selected from low-fat animal foods such as fish, lean meats, and low-fat dairy products. Whole eggs should be limited to two or three a week if hyperlipidemia is a problem.

Proteins found in plant foods are incomplete proteins and are of a lower biologic quality than those found in animal foods. Even so, plant foods are important sources of protein. Examples of plant foods containing protein are corn, grains, nuts, sunflower seeds, sesame seeds, and legumes such as soybeans, navy beans, pinto beans, split peas, chickpeas, and peanuts.

Plant proteins can be used to produce textured soy protein and tofu, also called analogues. Meat alternatives (analogues) made from soybeans contain soy protein and other ingredients mixed together to simulate various kinds of meat. Meat alternatives may be canned, dried, or frozen. Analogues are excellent sources of protein, iron, and B vitamins.

Tofu is a soft cheeselike food made from soy milk. Tofu is a bland product that easily absorbs the flavors of other ingredients with which it is cooked. Tofu is rich in high-quality proteins and B vitamins, and it is low in sodium. Textured soy protein and tofu are both economical and nutritious meat replacements.

Because of their inclusion of either dairy products and eggs or dairy products alone, most individuals who follow lacto-ovo vegetarian or lacto-vegetarian diets will be able to meet their protein requirements through a balanced diet that includes milk and milk products, enriched grains, nuts, and legumes. Strict vegetarians who consume no animal products will need to be more careful to include other protein-rich food sources such as soybeans, soy milk, and tofu.

CLASSIFICATION

The classification and quality of a protein depends on the number and types of amino acids it contains. There are 20 amino acids, but only 10 are considered essential to humans (Table 6-2). Two additional amino acids are sometimes incorporated into proteins during translation: selenocyteine and pyrrolysine. Essential amino acids are necessary for normal growth and development and must be provided in the diet. Proteins containing all the essential amino acids are of high biologic value; these proteins are called **complete proteins** and are extremely **bioavailable.** The nonessential amino acids can be produced in the body from the essential amino acids, vitamins, and minerals.

○ **complete proteins**
proteins that contain all the essential amino acids

○ **bioavailable**
means that a nutrient can be absorbed and used by the body

Table 6-2 *Amino Acids*			
ESSENTIAL		**NONESSENTIAL**	
Arginine*	Phenylalanine	Alanine	Glutamine
Histidine*	Threonine	Arginine*	Glycine
Isoleucine	Tryptophan	Asparagine	Histidine*
Leucine	Valine	Aspartic acid	Proline
Lysine		Cysteine	Serine
Methionine		Glutamic acid	Tyrosine

*Essential during childhood only.

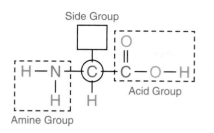

Figure 6-1 *Two different foods (e.g., grains and diary products) alone may not provide all the essential amino acids. Combined, however, they form a complete protein and therefore are considered complementary.*

Table 6-3 Examples of Complementary Protein Foods		
Corn	and	Beans
Rice	and	Beans
Bread	and	Peanut butter
Bread	and	Split pea soup
Bread	and	Cheese
Bread	and	Baked beans
Macaroni	and	Cheese
Cereal	and	Milk

Incomplete proteins are those that lack one or more of the essential amino acids. Consequently, incomplete proteins cannot build tissue without the help of other proteins. The value of each is increased when it is eaten in combination with another incomplete protein, not necessarily at the same meal, but during the same day. In this way, one incomplete protein food can provide the essential amino acids the other lacks. The combination may thereby provide all the essential amino acids (Figure 6-1). When this occurs, the proteins are called complementary proteins (Table 6-3). Gelatin is the only protein from an animal source that is an incomplete protein.

incomplete proteins
proteins that do not contain all of the essential amino acids

COMPOSITION

Like carbohydrates and fats, proteins contain carbon, hydrogen, and oxygen, but in different proportions. In addition, and most important, they are the only nutrient group that contains **nitrogen,** and some contain sulfur.

Proteins are composed of chemical compounds called **amino acids** (Figure 6-2). Amino acids are sometimes called the building blocks of protein because they are combined to form the thousands of proteins in the human body. Heredity determines the specific types of proteins within each person.

nitrogen
chemical element found in protein; essential to life

amino acids
nitrogen-containing chemical compounds of which protein is composed

DIGESTION AND ABSORPTION

The mechanical digestion of protein begins in the mouth, where the teeth grind the food into small pieces. Chemical digestion begins in the stomach.

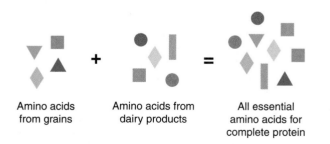

Amino acids from grains   +   Amino acids from dairy products   =   All essential amino acids for complete protein

Figure 6-2 *All amino acids have a chemical backbone of a carbon atom; an amine group, which contains nitrogen; an acid group; and a side group. It is the chemical structure of the side group that gives each amino acid its unique identity.*

○ **pepsin**
an enzyme secreted by the stomach that is essential for the digestion of proteins

○ **polypeptides**
ten or more amino acids bonded together

○ **trypsin**
pancreatic enzyme; helps digest proteins

○ **chymotrypsin**
pancreatic enzyme necessary for the digestion of proteins

○ **carboxypeptidase**
pancreatic enzyme necessary for protein digestion

Hydrochloric acid prepares the stomach so that the enzyme **pepsin** can begin its task of reducing proteins to **polypeptides.**

After the polypeptides reach the small intestine, three pancreatic enzymes (**trypsin, chymotrypsin,** and **carboxypeptidase**) continue chemical digestion. Intestinal peptidases finally reduce the proteins to amino acids.

After digestion, the amino acids in the small intestine are absorbed by the villi and are carried by the blood to all body tissues. There, they are used to form needed proteins.

METABOLISM AND ELIMINATION

All essential amino acids must be present to build and repair the cells as needed. When amino acids are broken down, the nitrogen-containing amine group is stripped off. This process is called deamination. Deamination produces ammonia, which is released into the bloodstream by the cells. The liver picks up the ammonia, converts it to urea, and returns it to the bloodstream for the kidneys to filter out and excrete. The remaining parts are used for energy or are converted to carbohydrate or fat and stored as glycogen or adipose tissue.

DIETARY REQUIREMENTS

One's protein requirement is determined by size, age, sex, and physical and emotional conditions. A large person has more body cells to maintain than a small person. A growing child, a pregnant woman, or a woman who is breast-feeding needs more protein for each pound of body weight than the average adult. When digestion is inefficient, fewer amino acids are absorbed by the body; consequently the protein requirement is higher. This is sometimes thought to be the case with the elderly. Extra proteins are usually required after surgery, severe burns, or during infections in order to replace lost tissue and to manufacture antibodies. In addition, emotional trauma can cause the body to excrete more nitrogen than it normally does, thus increasing the need for protein foods.

◉ SUPERSIZE USA

Smaller portions are an important solution to the obesity epidemic. Research indicates that young adults are more apt to overeat when served larger portions of food. The study's findings suggest that the growing obesity problems in the United States are due in large part to expanding portion sizes. The study found that when participants were served 125 to 150% of their normal amounts of food, they consumed an average of 273 extra calories per person (*Journal of Nutrition* 134: 2546–2549, October 2004). This can be especially troublesome with protein overconsumption, as may be seen in double burger patties and breakfast sandwiches that include eggs, meat, and sausage. Excessive protein consumption means higher fat and cholesterol intake, potential inadequate intake of calcium, nuts, and vegetables, and increased risk of certain diseases.

The National Research Council of the National Academy of Sciences considers the average adult's daily requirement to be 0.8 gram of protein for each kilogram of body weight. To determine your requirement:

1. Divide body weight by 2.2 (the number of pounds per kilogram).
2. Multiply the answer obtained in step 1 by 0.8 (gram of protein per kilogram of body weight).

In 2002 the Dietary Reference Intakes (DRIs) for protein were published by the National Academy of Science (see Table 6-4). An Adequate Intake (AI) was established for infants 0 to 6 months, with all other recommendations

Table 6-4 *Dietary Reference Intakes (DRIs): Protein*

LIFE STAGE GROUP	AGE	PROTEIN (GRAMS/DAY)
Infants		
	0–6 mo	9.1
	7–12 mo	11.0
Children		
	1–3 y	13
	4–8 y	19
Males		
	9–13 y	34
	14–18 y	52
	19–30 y	56
	31–50 y	56
	51–70 y	56
	> 70 y	56
Females		
	9–13 y	34
	14–18 y	46
	19–30 y	46
	31–50 y	46
	51–70 y	46
	> 70 y	46
Pregnancy		
	14–18 y	71
	19–30 y	71
	31–50 y	71
Lactation		
	14–18 y	71
	19–30 y	71
	31–50 y	71

Source: Adapted from Food and Nutrition Board, Institute of Medicine, National Academies of Sciences *Dietary Reference Intakes for Energy, Carbohydrate, Fiber, Fat, Fatty Acids, Cholesterol, Protein, and Amino Acids* (2002).

Table 6-5 *Protein in an Average Diet for One Day*

	SERVING SIZE	PROTEIN (g)	CALORIE
Breakfast			
Orange juice	1/2 cup	1	45
Cornflakes	3/4 cup	1	75
with sugar	2 tsp		30
Toast	2 slices	4	140
Butter	1 Tbsp		65
Jelly	1 Tbsp		60
Fat-free milk	1/2 cup	4	50
Lunch			
Grapefruit juice	1/2 cup	1	50
Tuna salad sandwich	2/3 cup tuna salad	20	220
on bread with	2 slices bread	4	140
lettuce			
Carrot sticks	1 carrot	1	25
Canned pears	1/2 cup	1	100
Oatmeal cookies	2	1	160
Fat-free milk	1 cup	8	100
Dinner			
Chicken breast	3 oz	26	160
Baked potato	1	4	145
Asparagus	1/2 cup		25
Sliced tomato salad	1 tomato	1	25
Roll	1	2	100
with butter	1 Tbsp		65
Ice cream	2/3 cup	3	200
Fat-free milk	1 cup	8	100
		90	2,080

based on 0.8 g/kg of body weight. Table 6-5 provides an idea of the amount of protein in an average day's diet. (For specific amounts of protein in other foods, refer to Appendix D.)

Protein Excess

It is easy for people living in the developed parts of the world to ingest more protein than the body requires. There are a number of reasons why this should be avoided. The saturated fats and cholesterol common to complete protein foods may contribute to heart disease and provide more calories than are desirable. Some studies seem to indicate a connection between long-term high-protein diets and colon cancer and high calcium excretion, which depletes the bones of calcium and may contribute to osteoporosis. People who eat excessive amounts of protein-rich foods may ignore the also essential fruits and vegetables, and excess protein intake may put more demands on the liver, (which converts nitrogen to urea) and the kidneys to excrete excess urea than they are prepared to handle. Therefore, the National Research Council recommends that protein intake represent no more than 15 to 20% of one's daily calorie intake and not exceed double the amount given in the table of DRIs (Table 6-4).

Protein and Amino Acid Supplements

Protein and amino acid supplements are taken for a number of reasons, such as "bulking up" by athletes, growing fingernails, and sparing body protein in weight loss. It is weight lifting, not protein bars or protein supplements, that builds muscles. Fingernails have never been affected by extra protein, and dieters need a balanced diet using the guidelines of MyPyramid.

High-quality protein foods are more bioavailable than expensive supplements. Single amino acids can be harmful to the body and never occur naturally in food. The body was designed to handle food, not supplements. If a single amino acid has been recommended, it is very important that a physician be consulted before the amino acid is used.

Nitrogen Balance

Protein requirements may be discussed in terms of **nitrogen balance**. This occurs when nitrogen intake equals the amount of nitrogen excreted. **Positive nitrogen balance** exists when nitrogen intake exceeds the amount excreted. This indicates that new tissue is being formed, and it occurs during pregnancy, during children's growing years, when athletes develop additional muscle tissue, and when tissues are rebuilt after **physical trauma** such as illness or injury. **Negative nitrogen balance** indicates that protein is being lost. It may be caused by fevers, injury, surgery, burns, starvation, or immobilization.

Protein Deficiency

When people are unable to obtain an adequate supply of protein for an extended period, muscle wasting will occur, and arms and legs become very thin. At the same time, **albumin** (protein in blood plasma) deficiency will cause edema, resulting in an extremely swollen appearance. The water is excreted when sufficient protein is eaten. People may lose appetite, strength, and weight, and wounds may heal very slowly. Patients suffering from edema become lethargic and depressed. These signs are seen in grossly neglected children or in the elderly, poor, or incapacitated. It is essential that people following vegetarian diets, especially vegans, carefully calculate the types and amount of protein in their diets so as to avoid protein deficiency.

EXPLORING THE WEB

Search the Web for information on protein supplements. What are some of the claims of these products? Are they based on solid research and fact? Create fact sheets on protein supplements citing common myths and providing the truth behind the myths. How would you approach a client inquiring about the use of protein supplements?

nitrogen balance
when nitrogen intake equals nitrogen excreted

positive nitrogen balance
nitrogen intake exceeds outgo

physical trauma
extreme physical stress

negative nitrogen balance
more nitrogen lost than taken in

albumin
protein that occurs in blood plasma

○ **protein energy
   malnutrition (PEM)**
   protein energy malnutrition; marasmus

○ **marasmus**
   severe wasting caused by lack of protein
   and all nutrients or faulty absorption; PEM

○ **kwashiorkor**
   deficiency disease caused by extreme
   lack of protein

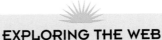

EXPLORING THE WEB

Search the Web for information
on protein deficiency disorders.
Are there any types of these
disorders found commonly in
the United States? In your area
of the country? For each
disorder you find, create a fact
sheet stating signs and
symptoms of the disorder and
dietary changes that can be
made to correct the deficiency.

○ **mental retardation**
   below-normal intellectual capacity

Protein Energy Malnutrition (PEM)

People suffering from **protein energy malnutrition (PEM)** lack both protein and energy-rich foods. Such a condition is not uncommon in developing countries where there are long-term shortages of both protein and energy foods. Children who lack sufficient protein do not grow to their potential size. Infants born to mothers eating insufficient protein during pregnancy can have permanently impaired mental capacities.

Two deficiency diseases that affect children are caused by a grossly inadequate supply of protein or energy, or both. **Marasmus,** a condition resulting from severe malnutrition, afflicts very young children who lack both energy and protein foods as well as vitamins and minerals. The infant with marasmus appears emaciated, but does not have edema. Hair is dull and dry, and the skin is thin and wrinkled (Figure 6-3). The other protein deficiency disease that affects children as well as adults is kwashiorkor (Figure 6-4). **Kwashiorkor** appears when there is a sudden or recent lack of protein-containing food (such as during a famine). This disease causes fat to accumulate in the liver, and the lack of protein and hormones results in edema, painful skin lesions, and changes in the pigmentation of skin and hair. The mortality rate for kwashiorkor patients is high.

Those who survive these deficiency diseases may suffer from permanent **mental retardation.** The ultimate cost of food deprivation among young children is high, indeed.

Table 6-6 lists some signs that help distinguish marasmus from kwashiorkor.

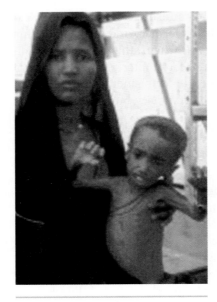

Figure 6-3 *Visible signs of marasmus include extreme wasting, wrinkled skin, and irritability. (Courtesy of the World Health Organization)*

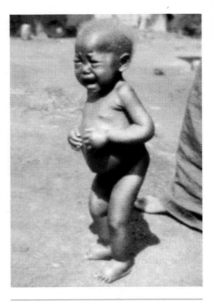

Figure 6-4 *Edema, skin lesions, and hair changes are common signs of kwashiorkor. (Courtesy of the UNHCR, The UN Refugee Agency)*

Table 6-6 *Differentiating Marasmus and Kwashiorkor*

MARASMUS	KWASHIORKOR
Total surface fat (TSF)* and midarm circumference (MAC) decreased	TSF and MAC within normal limits
Weight decreased	Weight possibly within normal limits
Visceral proteins (albumin) within normal limits or decreased	Visceral proteins decreased
Immune function within normal limits	Immune function decreased
Dull, dry hair	Reddish-color hair
Emaciated, wrinkled appearance	Puffy appearance
Lack of protein and total energy	Edema

*TSF and MAC can be determined by anthropometric measurements (see Chapter 1), which are done by a dietitian. The results are then compared with standard values obtained from measurement of a large number of people.

CONSIDERATIONS FOR THE HEALTH CARE PROFESSIONAL

Proteins have acquired an unfairly high value among the general public in the United States. Also, many people think that proteins are found only in animal food sources. As a result, complete proteins tend to be overused in most diets.

Research about the cumulative effects of the overuse of proteins in the diet is beginning to suggest that excessive use of protein could damage kidneys, possibly contribute to osteoporosis and cancer, and cause overweight and heart disease.

The health care professional may find that reeducating patients about the need to reduce their protein intake to 15% to 20% of total calories is a challenging task.

SUMMARY

Proteins contain nitrogen, an element that is necessary for growth and the maintenance of health. In addition to building and repairing body tissues, proteins regulate body processes and can supply energy. Each gram of protein provides 4 calories. Proteins are composed of amino acids, ten of which are essential for growth and repair of body tissues.

Complete proteins contain all of the essential amino acids and can build tissues. The best sources of complete proteins are animal foods such as meat, fish, poultry, eggs, milk, and cheese. Incomplete proteins do not contain all of the essential amino acids, and two or more of these proteins must be combined in order to build tissues. The best sources of incomplete proteins are legumes, corn, grains, and nuts. The nutritional value of incomplete protein foods can be increased by eating two or more incomplete protein foods during the day. Chemical digestion of proteins occurs in the stomach and small intestine. Proteins are reduced to amino acids and ultimately are absorbed into the blood through the villi in the small intestine.

A severe deficiency of protein in the diet can cause kwashiorkor and can contribute to marasmus in children. Both conditions can result in impaired physical and mental development.

DISCUSSION TOPICS

1. Why are proteins especially important to children, pregnant women, and people who are ill?
2. Of which elements are proteins composed?
3. What functions do proteins perform in the body?
4. Discuss why it may be unwise to use protein foods as energy foods.
5. Discuss the effects of protein deficiency.
6. Describe the digestion of proteins.
7. Describe the metabolism of proteins.
8. Tell what amino acids are and explain their importance. Tell where they are found.
9. Describe complete and incomplete protein foods and name several of each type.
10. How does one determine protein requirements?
11. Why might someone with a broken hip develop negative nitrogen balance in the hospital?

SUGGESTED ACTIVITIES

1. Keep a record of the foods you eat in a 24-hour period. Using Appendix D or the diet analysis software at MyPyramid, compute the grams of protein consumed. Did your diet provide the recommended amount of protein as indicated in Table 6-4?
2. Plan a day's menu for yourself. Include foods especially rich in complete proteins.
   a. Alter your planned menu by replacing some of the complete protein foods with those containing incomplete proteins.
   b. Visit a local supermarket and compute the cost of the menu that contains complete proteins. Compute the cost of the menu that contains incomplete proteins. Which is less expensive? Why?

REVIEW

Multiple choice. Select the *letter* that precedes the best answer.

1. The building blocks of proteins are
   a. ascorbic acids
   b. amino acids
   c. nitrogen and sulfur only
   d. meat and fish

2. Proteins are essential because they are the only nutrient that contains
   a. nitrogen
   b. niacin
   c. hydrochloric acid
   d. carbon

3. Corn, peas, and beans
   a. are complete protein foods
   b. are incomplete protein foods
   c. contain no protein
   d. lose proteins during cooking

4. Protein deficiency may result in
   a. beriberi
   b. goiter
   c. edema
   d. leukemia

5. Good sources of complete protein foods are
   a. eggs and ground beef
   b. breads and cereals
   c. butter and margarine
   d. legumes and nuts

6. One gram of protein provides
   a. 4 calories
   b. 9 calories
   c. 7 calories
   d. 19 calories

7. Complete proteins contain all the essential
   a. nutrients
   b. ascorbic acids
   c. amino acids
   d. calories

8. The *primary* function of protein is to
   a. build and repair body cells
   b. provide energy
   c. digest minerals and vitamins
   d. none of the above

9. Once proteins reach the small intestine, chemical digestion continues through the action of
   a. rennin
   b. pancreatic enzymes
   c. bile
   d. hydrochloric acid

10. It is unwise to regularly ingest excessive amounts of protein because
    a. it can cause positive nitrogen balance
    b. it can contribute to heart disease
    c. it may reduce the work of the kidneys
    d. it may cause uremic poisoning

Arrange the following foods into two lists, one containing those that are the best sources of complete proteins and one containing those that are the best sources of incomplete proteins.

Scrambled eggs	Refried beans
Corn on the cob	Hot chocolate milk
Chickpeas and rice	Fat-free milk
Beefburgers	Baked navy beans
Filet of sole	Fried chicken
Peanuts	Swiss cheese

CASE IN POINT

ANIKA: FOLLOWING A PROTEIN DIET

Anika, a college student from Germany, has been on the Atkins diet for 6 months and finds that she misses eating fruit and vegetables. She has seen a weight reduction with Atkins but is tired of all the meat and fats. Anika has been investigating the new rage—the South Beach diet. Because this diet allows for more vegetables and fruits, Anika thinks this is the way to go to lose the weight she wants, keep it off, and have fruits and vegetables.

ASSESSMENT

1. What data do you have about Anika's eating habits? *Atkins Dt. missing Fruits & veggies*
2. What do you know about her ability to develop habits?
3. What is the cause of the current dissatisfaction?

DIAGNOSIS

4. Complete the following diagnostic statement: Imbalanced nutrition, more than body requirements, as evidenced by _Fatigue_ .
5. Complete the following diagnostic statement: Deficient knowledge related to a lack of information about _Nutrition_ .

PLAN/GOAL

6. What are two measurable, reasonable goals for Anika?

IMPLEMENTATION

7. What factors need to be altered in Anika's diet?
8. What does Anika need to add to her diet?
9. Using preferences, suggest some alternative menus that would help Anika lose weight.

EVALUATION/OUTCOME CRITERIA

10. What criterion would a dietitian use to measure Anika's success?
11. What diseases would Anika avoid by reducing her long-term protein intake?

THINKING FURTHER

12. Which protein sources are most economical and are low in calories? How could this information be useful in other situations?

RATE THIS PLATE

Anika wants more fruits and vegetables in her diet. Good for her! Unfortunately, for the first 2 weeks on the South Beach diet there will be no carbohydrates. Anika didn't know that, but she thinks she can do it for two long weeks. Anika has chosen to eat the following for one of her meals. Rate this plate.

3-egg cheese omelet made with butter in the skillet

4 slices crisp bacon

3 sausage links

Kale and an orange wedge

CASE IN POINT

EDNA: RECOVERING FROM A SERIOUS ACCIDENT

Edna is a 78-year-old Caucasian female who was the driver in a very serious car accident with her husband, Tom. The emergency medical team had to cut open the car to get them out. Miraculously, Tom had only scrapes and bruises. But Edna suffered bilateral leg fractures, head injury, and internal abdominal injuries. Edna required numerous life-saving surgeries. Although Edna had been seriously injured, the doctors were confident that she would survive.

Initially, Edna was on intravenous feedings of hyperalimentation (see Chapter 22). The hospital dietitian monitored her nutritional status closely. Finally, Edna made the transition to oral nutrition. Edna was going to be hospitalized for at least three more weeks, followed by six to eight weeks of bed rest for her fractures. She was eating between 40% and 50% of her meals and at times forced herself to eat. The most recent note by the physician read, "Her wounds are healing, but slower than expected." The physical therapist documented, "She can tolerate only 15 minutes of range-of-motion exercises and complains about being too tired to continue." The dietitian ordered another 48-hour calorie count.

ASSESSMENT

1. What information do you have about Edna and her nutrition?
2. What deficit does the dietitian suspect?
3. What does the physician suspect?
4. How significant is the problem?
5. If Edna were 5 feet 2 inches tall and weighed 110 pounds before the accident, what would her daily protein requirements be?
6. What two benefits of protein is Edna missing?

DIAGNOSIS

7. What is the cause of Edna's nutritional problem? *No Carbs,*
8. Complete the following nursing diagnosis statement: Edna's imbalanced nutrition less than body requirements, related to *Hospital Stay* resulting in *Slowed Healing & fatigued disoriented without proper diet.*

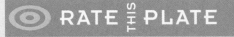

PLAN/GOAL

9. What is your goal for Edna?

IMPLEMENTATION

10. What will the calorie count reveal?
11. What do you need to know about Edna's food preferences?
12. What could Tom do to help during meals?
13. What should be the size and frequency of Edna's meals?
14. Should appetite stimulants be used?
15. Should liquid nutritional supplements be used?
16. Which proteins could provide the highest quality per bite?

EVALUATION/OUTCOME CRITERIA

17. What criteria would the doctor, physical therapist, and dietitian use to evaluate the effectiveness of the plan?
18. Would weight gain be an effective criterion? If not, why not?

THINKING FURTHER

19. How could the lessons from this case be used in other situations?

◎ RATE ᴛʜɪs PLATE

Edna needs protein for healing and carbohydrates for energy. Without carbohydrates Edna's body will pull protein from her lean muscle mass. Edna is still in the hospital, and so the dietitian can give her supplements with extra calories and protein. The calorie count will determine if the dietitian will recommend that Edna be given tube feeding along with oral intake. For patients who are not eating, it is advantageous to give them six small meals per day so as to not overwhelm them with so much food at one time.

Lunch
1/2 slice meatloaf
1/4 cup mashed potatoes and 1 Tbsp gravy
1/4 cup green beans

1/2 cup egg custard
1/2 cup apple juice
1/2 scoop protein powder mixed with food and drinks
2:00 p.m.
High-protein milkshake
  4 oz whole milk
  1 cup ice cream
  1 scoop protein powder (5 grams protein and 28 calories)

Using MyPyramid or Diet Analysis Plus, determine how many calories and how much protein Edna got from this meal and snack. You will have to add the protein powder by hand.

CHAPTER 7

VITAMINS

OBJECTIVES

After studying this chapter, you should be able to:

- State one or more functions of each of the 13 vitamins discussed
- Identify at least two food sources of each of the vitamins discussed
- Identify some symptoms of, or diseases caused by, deficiencies of the vitamins discussed

Vitamins are organic (carbon-containing) compounds that are essential in small amounts for body processes. Vitamins themselves do not provide energy. They enable the body to use the energy provided by fats, carbohydrates, and proteins. The name **vitamin** implies their importance. *Vita* in Latin, means life. They do not, however, represent a panacea (universal remedy) for physical or mental illness or a way to alleviate the stressors in life. They should not be over-used—more is not necessarily better. In fact, **megadoses** can be toxic (poisonous). In the past it was believed that a healthy person eating a balanced diet would obtain all the nutrients—including vitamins—needed. That was in the past. Today's reality is such that with after-school sports, dance lessons, music practice or lessons, both parents working, and more, people are in a time and energy crunch. So in many homes, home-cooked family meals have been replaced by fast food, home delivery, vending machines, and processed foods. Most of these choices are not found in the fruit and vegetable recommendation from MyPyramid.

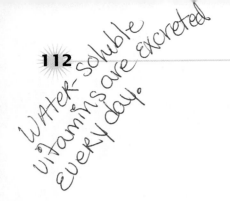

Water-Soluble Vitamins are excreted every day.

Table 7-1 *Vitamins*

FAT-SOLUBLE (4)	WATER-SOLUBLE (9)	
Vitamin A	Vitamin B complex includes:	
Vitamin D	Thiamine (B_1)	Vitamin B_{12} (cobalamin)
Vitamin E	Riboflavin (B_2)	Folate
Vitamin K	Niacin	Biotin
	Vitamin B_6	Pantothenic acid
	Vitamin C (ascorbic acid)	

⊙ **vitamins**
organic substances necessary for life although they do not, independently, provide energy

⊙ **megadose**
extraordinarily large amount

The existence of vitamins has been known since early in the twentieth century. It was discovered that animals fed diets of pure proteins, carbohydrates, fats, and minerals did not thrive as did those fed normal diets that included vitamins.

Vitamins were originally named by letter. Subsequent research has shown that many of the vitamins that were originally thought to be a single substance are actually groups of substances doing similar work in the body. Vitamin B proved to be more than one compound—B_1, B_6, B_{12}, and so on—and consequently is now known as B complex. Many of the 13 known vitamins are currently named according to their chemical composition or function in the body (Table 7-1).

Vitamins are found in minute amounts in foods. The specific amounts and types of vitamins in foods vary.

DIETARY REQUIREMENTS

Since 1997, the Food and Nutrition Board of the Institute of Medicine has been establishing Dietary Reference Intakes (DRIs) to replace the Recommended Dietary Allowances (RDAs) as outlined in Table 7-2. Tolerable Upper Limits (ULs) have also been set for some vitamins and minerals. The UL is the maximum

Table 7-2 *Adequate Intakes for Biotin and Pantothenic Acid*

CATEGORY	AGE (YEARS)	BIOTIN (mg)	PANTOTHENIC ACID (mg)
Infants	0–0.5	10	2
	0.5–1.0	15	3
Children and adolescents	1–3	20	3
	4–6	25	3–4
	7–10	30	4–5
	11+	30–100	4–7
Adults		30–100	4–7

Reprinted with permission of the National Academy of Science. (Table taken from the DRI report. See *www.nap.edu*.)

SPOTLIGHT on Life Cycle

Hypervitaminosis can be very dangerous. Several years ago, I received a letter from my sister informing me that she had been diagnosed with Alzheimer's and she had approximately 3 years until she would no longer recognize me. I was devastated. My sister is a very intelligent person who keeps up with the latest nutrition information about diabetes (she has type 2), nutrition in general, and supplements. Over the years, we had many discussions about what supplements would be beneficial for her age, which is currently 79.

What I didn't know was that she and my brother-in-law, who live in Florida, had been going to a health food store and had been talked into taking a multitude, I mean handfuls, of vitamins, minerals, and herbal supplements. During my next visit, I discovered one entire dresser drawer full of bottles of vitamins, minerals, and herbal supplements that they had been taking for about 2 years. My brother, who visited more often than I, knew that there had been a change in my sister's cognition. She would stop talking in mid-sentence, lose her train of thought, and even slur her speech. That explained why, when I would call, she would not want to talk very long. My brother and I found it hard to believe she really had Alzheimer's, given her symptoms.

During my next visit, my brother and I got rid of all the supplements, and we helped my sister apply and thankfully be accepted into the assisted-living section of a retirement community. We did this so that my sister's medication and approved supplements would be given at designated times. Since then, 2 years have gone by, and my sister does not have Alzheimer's. Her cognition is fine, no more slurred speech or low blood pressure (caused by excessive potassium), and just a little forgetfulness. I almost lost my sister because of overconsumption of vitamins, minerals, and herbal supplements, and now I have her back. I am so grateful!

level of daily intake unlikely to cause adverse effects and is not a recommended level of intake. Vitamin allowances are given by weight—milligrams (mg) or micrograms (µg or mcg).

Vitamin deficiencies can occur and can result in disease. Persons inclined to vitamin deficiencies because they do not eat balanced diets include alcoholics, the poor and incapacitated elderly, patients with serious diseases that affect appetite, mentally retarded persons, and young children who receive inadequate care. Also, deficiencies of fat-soluble vitamins occur in patients with chronic malabsorption diseases such as cystic fibrosis, celiac disease, and Crohn's disease.

The term **avitaminosis** means "without vitamins." This word followed by the name of a specific vitamin is used to indicate a serious lack of that particular vitamin. **Hypervitaminosis** is the excess of one or more vitamins. Either a lack or excess of vitamins can be detrimental to a person's health.

Vitamins taken in addition to those received in the diet are called **vitamin supplements.** These are available in concentrated forms in tablets, capsules, and drops. Vitamin concentrates are sometimes termed natural or synthetic (manufactured). Some people believe that a meaningful difference exists between the two types and that the natural are far superior in quality to the synthetic. However, according to the U.S. Food and Drug Administration (FDA), the body cannot distinguish between a vitamin of plant or animal origin and one manufactured in a laboratory, because once they have been dismantled by the digestive system, the two types of the same vitamin are chemically identical.

Synthetic vitamins are frequently added to foods during processing. When this is done, the foods are described as enriched or fortified. Examples of these foods are enriched breads and cereals to which thiamine, niacin, riboflavin, folate, and the mineral iron have been added. Vitamins A and D are added to milk and fortified margarine.

avitaminosis
without vitamins

hypervitaminosis
condition caused by excessive ingestion of one or more vitamins

vitamin supplements
concentrated forms of vitamins; may be in tablet or liquid form

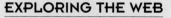

EXPLORING THE WEB

Search the Web for vitamin supplements. Choose a supplement to report on. What claims are made by this product? What are they based on? Prepare a fact sheet that highlights the health benefits of this product and the adverse effects this product may have. What should consumers be aware of if they are taking this product?

Preserving Vitamin Content in Food

Occasionally, vitamins are lost during food processing. In most cases, food producers can replace these vitamins with synthetic vitamins, making the processed food nutritionally equal to the unprocessed food. Foods in which vitamins have been replaced are called restored foods.

Because some vitamins are easily destroyed by light, air, heat, and water, it is important to know how to preserve the vitamin content of food during its preparation and cooking. Vitamin loss can be avoided by:

- Buying the freshest, unbruised vegetables and fruits and using them raw whenever possible
- Preparing fresh vegetables and fruits just before serving
- Heating canned vegetables quickly and in their own liquid
- Following package directions when using frozen vegetables or fruit
- Using as little water as possible when cooking and having it boiling before adding vegetables, or, preferably, steaming them
- Covering the pan (except for the first few minutes when cooking strongly flavored vegetables such as broccoli and cauliflower) and cooking as short a time as possible
- Saving the cooking liquid for later use in soups, stews, and gravies
- Storing fresh vegetables and most fruits in a cool, dark place

CLASSIFICATION

Vitamins are commonly grouped according to solubility. A, D, E, and K are **fat-soluble,** and B complex and C are **water-soluble** (Table 7-3). In addition, vitamin D is sometimes classified as a **hormone,** and the B-complex group may be classified as **catalysts** or **coenzymes.** When a vitamin has different chemical forms but serves the same purpose in the body, these forms are sometimes called vitamers. Vitamin E is an example. Sometimes a **precursor,** or **provitamin,** is found in foods. This is a substance from which the body can synthesize (manufacture) a specific vitamin. **Carotenoids** are examples of precursors of vitamin A, and are referred to as provitamin A.

FAT-SOLUBLE VITAMINS

The fat-soluble vitamins A, D, E, and K are chemically similar. They are not lost easily in cooking, but are lost when mineral oil is ingested. Mineral oil is not absorbed by humans. Consequently, it may be used in salad dressings to avoid the calories of vegetable oils. It is sometimes used as a laxative by the elderly. Its use should be discouraged because it picks up and carries with it fat-soluble vitamins that are then lost to the body. After absorption, fat-soluble vitamins are transported through the blood by lipoproteins because they are not soluble in water. Excess amounts can be stored in the liver. Therefore, deficiencies of fat-soluble vitamins are slower to appear than are those caused by a lack of water-soluble vitamins. Because of the body's ability to store them, megadoses of fat-soluble vitamins should be avoided as they can reach toxic levels.

fat-soluble
can be dissolved in fat

water-soluble
can be dissolved in water

hormone
chemical messengers secreted by a variety of glands

catalyst
a substance that causes another substance to react

coenzyme
an active part of an enzyme

precursor
something that comes before something else; in vitamins it is also called a provitamin, something from which the body can synthesize the specific vitamin

provitamin
see precursor

carotenoids
plant pigments, some of which yield vitamin A

Table 7-3 *Fat-Soluble Vitamins and Water-Soluble Vitamins*

NAME	FOOD SOURCES	FUNCTIONS	DEFICIENCY/TOXICITY
Fat-soluble vitamins			

Vitamin A (retinol)	Animal
	  Liver
	  Whole milk
	  Butter
	  Cream
	  Cod liver oil
	Plants
	  Dark green leafy vegetables
	  Deep yellow or orange fruit
	  Fortified margarine
		Maintenance of vision in dim light
		Maintenance of mucous membranes and healthy skin
		Growth and development of bones
		Reproduction
		Healthy immune system
			Deficiency
			  Night blindness
			  Xerophthalmia
			  Respiratory infections
			  Bone growth ceases
			Toxicity
			  Birth defects
			  Bone pain
			  Anorexia
			  Enlargement of liver

Vitamin D (calciferol)	Animal
	  Eggs
	  Liver
	  Fortified milk
	  Fortified margarine
	  Oily fish
	Plants
	  None
	Sunlight
		Regulation of absorption of calcium and phosphorus
		Building and maintenance of normal bones and teeth
		Prevention of tetany
			Deficiency
			  Rickets
			  Osteomalacia
			  Osteoporosis
			  Poorly developed teeth and bones
			  Muscle spasms
			Toxicity
			  Kidney stones
			  Calcification of soft tissues

Vitamin E (tocopherol)	Animal
	  None
	Plants
	  Green and leafy vegetables
	  Margarines
	  Salad dressing
	  Wheat germ and wheat germ oils
	  Vegetable oils
	  Nuts
		Antioxidant
		Considered essential for protection of cell structure, especially of red blood cells
			Deficiency
			  Destruction of red blood cells
			Toxicity

(continued)

Table 7-3 *Continued*

NAME	FOOD SOURCES	FUNCTIONS	DEFICIENCY/TOXICITY

Vitamin K	Animal
	  Liver
	  Milk
	Plants
	  Green leafy vegetables
	  Cabbage, broccoli
		Blood clotting	Deficiency
			  Prolonged blood clotting
			  or hemorrhaging
			Toxicity
			  Hemolytic anemia
			  Interferes with anticlotting medications

Water-soluble vitamins			

Thiamine (vitamin B$_1$)	Animal
	  Lean pork
	  Beef
	  Liver
	  Eggs
	  Fish
	Plants
	  Whole and enriched grains
	  Legumes
	  Brewer's yeast
		Metabolism of carbohydrates and some amino acids
		Maintains normal appetite and functioning of nervous system
			Deficiency
			  Gastrointestinal tract, nervous system, and cardiovascular system problems
			  Beriberi
			Toxicity
			  None

Riboflavin (vitamin B$_2$)	Animal
	  Liver, kidney, heart
	  Milk
	  Cheese
	Plants
	  Green, leafy vegetables
	  Cereals
	  Enriched bread
		Aids release of energy from food
		Health of the mouth tissue
		Healthy eyes
			Deficiency
			  Cheilosis
			  Eye sensitivity
			  Dermatitis
			  Glossitis
			  Photophobia
			Toxicity
			  None

Niacin (nicotinic acid)	Animal
	  Milk
	  Eggs
	  Fish
	  Poultry
	Plants
	  Enriched breads and cereals
		Energy metabolism
		Healthy skin and nervous and digestive systems
			Deficiency
			  Pellagra—dermatitis, dementia, diarrhea
			Toxicity
			  Vasodilation of blood vessels

(continued)

Table 7-3 *Continued*

NAME	FOOD SOURCES	FUNCTIONS	DEFICIENCY/TOXICITY

Pyridoxine (vitamin B_6)	Animal
	  Pork
	  Fish
	  Poultry
	  Liver, kidney
	  Milk
	  Eggs
	Plants
	  Whole-grain cereals
	  Legumes
		Conversion of tryptophan to niacin
		Release of glucose from glycogen
		Protein metabolism and synthesis of nonessential amino acids
			Deficiency
			  Cheilosis
			  Glossitis
			  Dermatitis
			  Confusion
			  Depression
			  Irritability
			Toxicity
			  Depression
			  Nerve damage

Vitamin B_{12} (cobalamin)	Animal
	  Seafood
	  Poultry
	  Liver, kidney
	  Muscle meats
	  Eggs
	  Milk
	  Cheese
	Plants
	  None
		Synthesis of red blood cells
		Maintenance of myelin sheaths
		Treatment of pernicious anemia
		Folate metabolism
			Deficiency
			  Degeneration of myelin sheaths
			  Pernicious anemia
			  Sore mouth and tongue
			  Anorexia
			  Neurological disorders
			Toxicity
			  None

Folate (folic acid)	Animal
	  Liver
	Plants
	  Leafy green vegetables
	  Spinach
	  Legumes
	  Seeds
	  Broccoli
	  Cereal fortified with folate
	  Fruit
		Synthesis of RBCs
		Synthesis of DNA
			Deficiency
			  Anemia
			  Glossitis
			  Neural tube defects such as anencephaly and spina bifida
			Toxicity
			  Could mask a B_{12} deficiency

(continued)

Table 7-3 *Continued*

NAME	FOOD SOURCES	FUNCTIONS	DEFICIENCY/TOXICITY

Biotin	Animal
	  Milk
	  Liver and kidney
	  Egg yolks
	Plants
	  Legumes
	  Brewer's yeast
	  Soy flour
	  Cereals
	  Fruit
		Coenzyme in carbohydrate and amino acid metabolism
		Niacin synthesis from tryptophan
			Deficiency
			  Dermatitis
			  Nausea
			  Anorexia
			  Depression
			  Hair loss
			Toxicity
			  None

Pantothenic acid	Animal
	  Eggs
	  Liver
	  Salmon
	  Poultry
	Plants
	  Mushrooms
	  Cauliflower
	  Peanuts
	  Brewer's yeast
		Metabolism of carbohydrates, lipids, and proteins
		Synthesis of fatty acids, cholesterol, steroid hormones
			Deficiency
			  Rare: burning feet syndrome; vomiting; fatigue
			Toxicity
			  None

Vitamin C (ascorbic acid)	Animal
	  None
	Plants
	  All citrus fruits
	  Broccoli
	  Melons
	  Strawberries
	  Tomatoes
	  Brussels sprouts
	  Potatoes
	  Cabbage
	  Green peppers
		Prevention of scurvy
		Formation of collagen
		Healing of wounds
		Release of stress hormones
		Absorption of iron
		Antioxidant
		Resistance to infection
			Deficiency
			  Scurvy
			  Muscle cramps
			  Ulcerated gums
			  Tendency to bruise easily
			Toxicity
			  Raised uric acid level
			  Hemolytic anemia
			  Kidney stones
			  Rebound scurvy

Vitamin A

Vitamin A consists of two basic dietary forms: preformed vitamin A, also called **retinol,** which is the active form of vitamin A; and carotenoids, the inactive form of vitamin A, which are found in plants.

Functions. Vitamin A is a family of fat-soluble compounds that play an important role in vision, bone growth, reproduction, and cell division. Vitamin A helps regulate the immune system, which helps fight infections. Vitamin A has been labeled as an **antioxidant** when, in fact, provitamin A (carotenoids) is the part of the family that functions as an antioxidant. Antioxidants protect cells from **free radicals.** Free radicals are atoms or groups of atoms with an odd (unpaired) number of electrons and can be formed when oxygen interacts with certain molecules. Once formed, these highly reactive radicals can start a chain reaction. When they react with important cellular components such as DNA or cell membranes, the most damage occurs. Antioxidants have the capability of safely interacting with free radicals and stopping the chain reaction before vital cells are damaged.

The first organic free radical was discovered in 1900 by Moses Gomberg. In the 1950s, Denman Harman, M.D., was the first to propose the free radical theory of aging.

Sources. There are two forms of vitamin A: preformed vitamin A and provitamin A. Retinol is a preformed vitamin A and is one of the most active and usable forms of vitamin A. Retinol can be converted to retinal and retinoic acid, other active forms of vitamin A.

Provitamin A carotenoids can be converted to vitamin A from darkly colored pigments, both green and orange, in fruits and vegetables. Common carotenoids are beta-carotene, lutein, lycopene, and zeaxanthin. Beta-carotene is most efficiently converted to retinol. Eating "five-a-day" of fruits and vegetables is highly recommended. The best sources of beta-carotene are carrots, sweet potatoes, spinach, broccoli, pumpkin, squash (butternut), mango, and cantaloupe.

Research has shown that regular consumption of foods rich in carotenoids decreases the risk of some cancers because of its antioxidant effect. Taking a beta-carotene supplement has not shown the same results.

Preformed vitamin A (retinol) is found in fat-containing animal foods such as liver, butter, cream, whole milk, whole milk cheeses, and egg yolk. It is also found in low-fat milk products and in cereals that have been fortified with vitamin A, but these are not the best sources.

Requirements. A well-balanced diet is the preferred way to obtain the required amounts of vitamin A. Vitamin A values are commonly listed as **retinol equivalents (RE).** A retinol equivalent is 1 µg retinol or 6 µg beta carotene. Refer to the inside back cover of this text for the dietary reference intakes of vitamin A as prescribed by the Food and Nutrition Board of the Institute of Medicine.

Hypervitaminosis. The use of vitamin supplements should be discouraged because an excess of vitamin A can have serious consequences. Signs of hypervitaminosis A may include birth defects, hair loss, dry skin, headaches, nausea, dryness of mucous membranes, liver damage, and bone and joint pain. In general, these symptoms tend to disappear when excessive intake is discontinued.

retinol
the preformed vitamin A

antioxidant
a substance preventing damage from oxygen

free radical
are atoms or groups of atoms with an odd (unpaired) number of electrons and can be formed when oxygen interacts with certain molecules

retinol equivalent (RE)
the equivalent of 3.33 international units of vitamin A

xerophthalmia

serious eye disease characterized by dry mucous membranes of the eye, caused by a deficiency of vitamin A

Deficiency. Signs of a deficiency of vitamin A include night blindness; dry, rough skin; and increased susceptibility to infections. Avitaminosis A can result in blindness or **xerophthalmia,** a condition characterized by dry, lusterless, mucous membranes of the eye. Lack of vitamin A is the leading cause of blindness in the world (discounting accidents).

Vitamin D

Vitamin D exists in two forms—D_2 (ergocalciferol) and D_3 (cholecalciferol). Each is formed from a provitamin when irradiated with (exposed to) ultraviolet light. They are equally effective in human nutrition, but D_3 is the one that is formed in humans from cholesterol in the skin. D_2 is formed in plants. Vitamin D is considered a **prohormone** because it is converted to a hormone in the human body.

prohormone

substance that precedes the hormone and from which the body can synthesize the hormone

Vitamin D is heat-stable and not easily oxidized, so it is not harmed by storage, food processing, or cooking.

Functions. The major function of vitamin D is the promotion of calcium and phosphorus absorption in the body. By contributing to the absorption of these minerals, it helps to raise their concentration in the blood so that normal bone and tooth mineralization can occur and tetany (involuntary muscle movement) can be prevented. (Tetany can occur when there is too little calcium in the blood. This condition is called hypocalcemia.)

Vitamin D is absorbed in the intestines and is chemically changed in the liver and kidneys. Excess amounts of vitamin D are stored in the liver and in adipose tissue.

Sources. The best source of vitamin D is sunlight, which changes a provitamin to vitamin D_3 in humans. It is sometimes referred to as the sunshine vitamin. The amount of vitamin D that is formed depends on the individual's pigmentation (coloring matter in the skin) and the amount of sunlight available. The best food sources of vitamin D are milk, fish liver oils, egg yolk, butter, and fortified margarine. Because of the rather limited number of food sources of vitamin D and the unpredictability of sunshine, health authorities decided that the vitamin should be added to a common food. Milk was selected. Conse-

Table 7-4 *Adequate Intakes for Vitamin D*	
Newborns through 51 years	5.0 µg (200 international units)
51–70 years	10.0 µg (400 international units)
70+ years	15.0 µg (600 international units)
Pregnant and lactating women	5.0 µg (200 international units)

Source: Dietary Reference Intakes, Food and Nutrition Board, National Academy of Sciences–Institute of Medicine, 1997.

quently, most milk available in the United States today has had 10 µg of vitamin D concentrate added per quart.

Requirements. Under the DRIs, there are several reference values included. Vitamin D levels are given as Adequate Intake levels, or AI (Table 7-4).

People who are seldom outdoors, those who use sunscreens, and those who live in areas where there is little sunlight for 3 to 4 months a year should be especially careful that their diets provide their Adequate Intake levels of vitamin D. Drinking 2 cups of vitamin D–fortified fat-free milk each day will provide sufficient vitamin D to those between birth and 50 years of age. Between the ages of 51 and 70, 1 quart of such milk will be needed each day to fulfill the AI. After 70, 1½ quarts will be needed daily. In this last age group, a vitamin D supplement may be needed.

Vitamin D or, specifically, cholecalciferol values are given in micrograms (mg or mcg.) or in **international units;** 5 mg equals 200 international units.

Hypervitaminosis. Hypervitaminosis D must be avoided because it can cause deposits of calcium and phosphorus in soft tissues, kidney and heart damage, and bone fragility.

Deficiency. The deficiency of vitamin D inhibits the absorption of calcium and phosphorus in the small intestine and results in poor bone and tooth formation. Young children suffering vitamin D deficiency may develop **rickets,** which causes malformed bones and pain, and their teeth may be poorly formed, late in appearing, and particularly subject to decay. Adults lacking sufficient vitamin D may develop **osteomalacia,** softening of bones. It is thought that a deficiency of vitamin D may contribute to **osteoporosis** (brittle, porous bones).

Vitamin E

Vitamin E consists of two groups of chemical compounds. They are the **tocopherols** and the **tocotrienols.** There are four types of tocopherols: alpha, beta, delta, and gamma. The most biologically active of these is alpha-tocopherol.

Functions. Vitamin E is an antioxidant. It is aided in this process by vitamin C and the mineral selenium. It is carried in the blood by lipoproteins. When the amount of vitamin E in the blood is low, the red blood cells become vulnerable to a higher than normal rate of **hemolysis.** Vitamin E has been found

international units
units of measurement of some vitamins; 5 µg = 200 international units

rickets
deficiency disease caused by the lack of vitamin D; causes malformed bones and pain in infants

osteomalacia
a condition in which bones become soft, usually in adult women, because of calcium loss

osteoporosis
a condition in which bones become brittle and porous

tocopherols
vitamers of vitamin E

tocotrienols
a form of vitamin E

hemolysis
the destruction of red blood cells

helpful in the prevention of hemolytic anemia among premature infants. It also may enhance the immune system. Because of its antioxidant properties, it is commonly used in commercial food products to retard spoilage.

Sources. Vegetable oils made from corn, soybean, safflower, and cottonseed, and products made from them, such as margarine, are the best sources of vitamin E. Wheat germ, nuts, and green leafy vegetables also are good sources. Animal foods, fruits, and most vegetables are poor sources.

Requirements. Research indicates that the vitamin E requirement increases if the amount of polyunsaturated fatty acids in the diet increases. In general, however, the U.S. diet is thought to contain sufficient vitamin E.

Hypervitaminosis. Although vitamin E appears to be relatively nontoxic, it is a fat-soluble vitamin, and the excess is stored in adipose tissue. Consequently, it would seem advisable to avoid long-term megadoses of vitamin E.

Deficiency. A deficiency of vitamin E has been detected in premature, low-birthweight infants and in patients who are unable to absorb fat normally. Malabsorption can cause serious neurological defects in children, but in adults, it takes 5 to 10 years before deficiency symptoms occur.

Vitamin K

Vitamin K is made up of several compounds that are essential to blood clotting. Vitamin K_1, commonly called phylloquinone, is found in dietary sources, especially green leafy vegetables such as broccoli and in animal tissue. Vitamin K_2, called menaquinone, is synthesized in the intestine by bacteria and is also found in animal tissue. In addition, there is a synthetic vitamin K, called menadione. Vitamin K is destroyed by light and alkalies.

Vitamin K is absorbed like fats, mainly from the small intestine and slightly from the colon. Its absorption requires a normal flow of bile from the liver, and it is improved when there is fat in the diet.

Functions. Vitamin K is essential for the formation of prothrombin, which permits the proper clotting of the blood. It may be given to newborns immediately after birth because human milk contains little vitamin K and the intestines of newborns contain few bacteria. With insufficient vitamin K, newborns may be in danger of intracranial hemorrhage (bleeding within the head).

Vitamin K may be given to patients who suffer from faulty fat absorption; to patients after extensive antibiotic therapy (ingestion of antibiotic drugs to combat infection) because these drugs destroy the bacteria in the intestines; as an antidote for an overdose of anticoagulant (blood thinner such as warfarin—sometimes sold as Coumadin or Warnerin); or to treat cases of **hemorrhage.**

Sources. The best dietary sources of vitamin K are green leafy vegetables such as broccoli, cabbage, spinach, and kale. Dairy products, eggs, meats, fruits, and cereals also contain some vitamin K. Cow's milk is a much better source of vitamin K than human milk. The synthesis of vitamin K by bacteria

⊙ hemorrhage
unusually heavy bleeding

in the small intestine does not provide a sufficient supply by itself. It must be supplemented by dietary sources.

Requirements. Vitamin K is measured in micrograms. The Adequate Intake for vitamin K is 120 μg for men and 90 μg for women. This is not increased during pregnancy or lactation. Infants up to 6 months should have 2.0 μg a day. Those between 6 months and 1 year should receive 2.5 μg a day.

Hypervitaminosis. Ingestion of excessive amounts of synthetic vitamin K can be toxic and can cause a form of anemia.

Deficiency. The only major sign of a deficiency of vitamin K is defective blood **coagulation.** This increases clotting time, making the client more prone to hemorrhage. Human deficiency may be caused by faulty fat metabolism, antibiotic therapy, inadequate diet, or anticoagulants.

coagulate
to thicken

WATER-SOLUBLE VITAMINS

Water-soluble vitamins include B complex and C. These vitamins dissolve in water and are easily destroyed by air, light, and cooking. They are not stored in the body to the extent that fat-soluble vitamins are stored.

Vitamin B Complex

Beriberi is a disease that affects the nervous, cardiovascular, and gastrointestinal systems. The legs feel heavy, the feet burn, and the muscles degenerate. The patient is irritable and suffers from headaches, depression, anorexia, constipation, tachycardia (rapid heart rate), edema, and heart failure.

Toward the end of the nineteenth century, a doctor in Indonesia discovered that chickens that were fed table scraps of polished rice developed symptoms much like those of his patients suffering from beriberi. When these same chickens were later fed brown (unpolished) rice, they recovered.

Some years later, this mysterious component of unpolished rice was recognized as an essential food substance and was named vitamin B. Subsequently, it was named vitamin *B complex* because the vitamin was found to be composed of several compounds. The B-complex vitamins are listed in Table 7-1.

beriberi
deficiency disease caused by a lack of vitamin B_1 (thiamine)

Thiamine

Thiamine, a coenzyme, was originally named vitamin B_1. It is partially destroyed by heat and alkalies, and it is lost in cooking water.

thiamine
vitamin B_1

Functions. Thiamine is essential for the metabolism of carbohydrates and some amino acids. It is also essential to nerve and muscle action. It is absorbed in the small intestine.

Sources. Thiamine is found in many foods, but generally in small quantities. (See Appendix D.) Some of the best natural food sources of thiamine are unrefined and enriched cereals, yeast, wheat germ, lean pork, organ meats, and legumes.

Requirements. Thiamine is measured in milligrams. The daily thiamine requirement for the average adult female is 1.1 mg a day, and for the average adult male it is 1.2 mg a day. The requirement is not thought to increase with age. In general, however, an increase in calories increases the need for thiamine.

Most breads and cereals in the United States are enriched with thiamine, so that the majority of people can and do easily fulfill their recommended intake.

Deficiency. Symptoms of thiamine deficiency include loss of appetite, fatigue, nervous irritability, and constipation. An extreme deficiency causes beriberi. Its deficiency is rare, however, occurring mainly among alcoholics whose diets include reduced amounts of thiamine while their requirements of it are increased and their absorption of it is decreased. Others at risk include renal clients undergoing long-term dialysis, clients fed intravenously for long periods, and clients with chronic fevers.

Because some raw fish contain thiaminase, an enzyme that inhibits the normal action of thiamine, frequent consumption of large amounts of raw fish could cause thiamine deficiency. Eating raw fish is not recommended. Cooking inactivates this enzyme.

There are no known ill effects from excessive oral intake of thiamine, but it may be toxic if excessive amounts are given intravenously.

Riboflavin

⊙ **riboflavin**
vitamin B$_2$

Riboflavin is sometimes called B$_2$. It is destroyed by light and irradiation and is unstable in alkalies.

Functions. Riboflavin is essential for carbohydrate, fat, and protein metabolism. It is also necessary for tissue maintenance, especially the skin around the mouth, and for healthy eyes. Riboflavin is absorbed in the small intestine.

Sources. Riboflavin is widely distributed in animal and plant foods but in small amounts. Milk, meats, poultry, fish, and enriched breads and cereals are some of its richest sources. Some green vegetables such as broccoli, spinach, and asparagus are also good sources.

Requirement. Riboflavin is measured in milligrams. The average adult female daily requirement is thought to be 1.1 mg, and the adult male requirement is 1.3 mg. The riboflavin requirement appears to increase with increased energy expenditure. The requirement does not diminish with age.

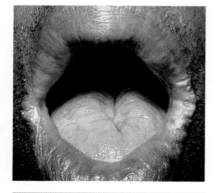

Figure 7-1 *Cheilosis at the corners of the mouth is an indication of a riboflavin deficiency. (Courtesy of Dr. Joseph Konzelman, School of Dentistry, Medical College of Georgia)*

Deficiency. Because of the small quantities of riboflavin in foods and its limited storage in the body, deficiencies of riboflavin can develop. The generous use of fat-free milk in the diet is a good way to prevent deficiency of this vitamin. It is important, however, that milk be stored in opaque containers because riboflavin can be destroyed by light. It appears that fiber laxatives can reduce riboflavin absorption, and their use over long periods should be discouraged.

A deficiency of riboflavin can result in cheilosis, a condition characterized by sores on the lips and cracks at the corners of the mouth (Figure 7-1);

glossitis (inflammation of the tongue); dermatitis; and eye strain in the form of itching, burning, and eye fatigue. Its toxicity is unknown.

Niacin

Niacin is the generic name for nicotinic acid and nicotinamide. Niacin is fairly stable in foods. It can withstand reasonable amounts of heat and acid and is not destroyed during food storage.

Functions. Niacin serves as a coenzyme in energy metabolism and consequently is essential to every body cell. In addition, niacin is essential for the prevention of **pellagra.** Pellagra is a disease characterized by sores on the skin and by diarrhea, anxiety, confusion, irritability, poor memory, dizziness, and untimely death if left untreated. Niacin, when used as a cholesterol-lowering agent, must be closely supervised by a physician because of possible adverse side effects such as liver damage and peptic ulcers.

Sources. The best sources of niacin are meats, poultry, and fish. Peanuts and other legumes are also good sources. Enriched breads and cereals also contain some. Milk and eggs do not provide niacin per se, but they are good sources of its precursor, tryptophan (an amino acid). Vegetables and fruits contain little niacin.

Requirements. Niacin is measured in **niacin equivalents (NE)**. One NE equals 1 mg of niacin or 60 mg of tryptophan. The general recommendation is a daily intake of 14 mg/NE for adult women and 16 mg/NE for adult men. Because excessive amounts of niacin have caused flushing due to vascular dilation (expansion of blood vessels), self-prescribed doses of niacin concentrate should be discouraged. Other symptoms include gastrointestinal problems and itching. If excessive amounts of niacin are ingested, liver damage may result.

Deficiency. A deficiency of niacin is apt to appear if there is a deficiency of riboflavin. Symptoms of niacin deficiency include weakness, anorexia, indigestion, anxiety, and irritability. In extreme cases, pellagra may occur.

Vitamin B$_6$

Vitamin B$_6$ is composed of three related forms: pyridoxine, pyridoxal, and pyridoxamine. It is stable to heat but sensitive to light and alkalies.

Functions. Vitamin B$_6$ is essential for protein metabolism and absorption, and it aids in the release of glucose from glycogen. With the help of vitamin B$_6$, amino acids present in excessive amounts can be converted to those in which the body is temporarily deficient. It also serves as a catalyst in the conversion of tryptophan to niacin, and it is helpful in the formation of other substances from amino acids. An example is the synthesis of neurotransmitters such as serotonin and dopamine.

Sources. Some of the nutrient-dense sources of vitamin B$_6$ are poultry, fish, liver, kidney, potatoes, bananas, and spinach. Whole grains, especially oats

niacin
B vitamin

pellagra
deficiency disease caused by a lack of niacin

niacin equivalent (NE)
unit of measuring niacin; 1 NE equals 1 mg niacin or 60 mg tryptophan

and wheat, are good sources of vitamin B_6, but because this vitamin is lost during milling and is not replaced during the enrichment process, refined grains are not a good source.

Requirements. Vitamin B_6 is measured in milligrams, and the need increases as the protein intake increases. For adult females, the daily requirement is 1.3–1.5 mg and for males, 1.3–1.7 mg. Oral contraceptives interfere with the metabolism of vitamin B_6 and can result in a deficiency.

Deficiency. A deficiency of vitamin B_6 is usually found in combination with deficiencies of other B vitamins. Symptoms include irritability, depression, and dermatitis. In infants, its deficiency can cause various neurological symptoms and abdominal problems. Although its toxicity is rare, it can cause temporary neurological problems.

Vitamin B_{12}

○ **cobalamin**
organic compound known as vitamin B_{12}

○ **myelin**
lipoprotein essential for the protection of nerves

○ **intrinsic factor**
secretion of stomach mucosa essential for B_{12} absorption

○ **pernicious anemia**
severe, chronic anemia caused by a deficiency of vitamin B_{12}; usually due to the body's inability to absorb B_{12}

Vitamin B_{12} **(cobalamin)** is a compound that contains the mineral cobalt. It is slightly soluble in water and fairly stable to heat, but it is damaged by strong acids or alkalies and by light. It can be stored in the human body for 3 to 5 years.

Functions. Vitamin B_{12} is involved in folate metabolism, maintenance of the **myelin** sheath, and healthy red blood cells. In order for vitamin B_{12} to be absorbed, it must bind with a glycoprotein **(intrinsic factor)** present in gastric secretions in the stomach and travel to the small intestine, where it combines with pancreatic proteases, then travels to the ileum, where it attaches to special receptor cells to complete the absorption process. A patient who has lost the ability to produce the gastric secretions, pancreatic proteases, intrinsic factor, or the special receptor cells because of disease or surgery will develop **pernicious anemia**.

Sources. The best food sources of B_{12} are animal foods, especially organ meats, lean meat, seafood, eggs, and dairy products.

Requirements. Vitamin B_{12} is measured in micrograms. The DRI for adults is 2–4 μg a day, but it increases during pregnancy and lactation. The amount absorbed will depend on current needs.

Deficiency. Fortunately, a vitamin B_{12} deficiency is rare and is thought to be caused by congenital problems of absorption, which inhibit the body's ability to absorb or synthesize sufficient amounts of vitamin B_{12}. It may also be due to years of a strict vegetarian diet that contains no animal foods.

When the amount of B_{12} is insufficient, megaloblastic anemia may result. If the intrinsic factor is missing, pernicious anemia develops. Intrinsic factor could be missing because of surgical removal of the stomach, or a large portion of it, or because of disease or surgery affecting the ileum. Dietary treatment will be ineffective; the patient must be given intramuscular injections of B_{12}, usually on a monthly basis.

Vitamin B_{12} deficiency may also result in inadequate myelin synthesis. This deficiency causes damage to the nervous system. Signs of vitamin B_{12} deficiency include anorexia, glossitis, sore mouth and tongue, pallor, neurological upsets such as depression and dizziness, and weight loss.

Folate

Folate, *folacin*, and **folic acid** are chemically similar compounds. Their names are often used interchangeably.

Functions. Folate is needed for DNA synthesis, protein metabolism, and the formation of hemoglobin.

Sources. Folate is found in many foods, but the best sources are cereals fortified with folate, green leafy vegetables, legumes, sunflower seeds, and fruits such as orange juice and strawberries. Heat, oxidation, and ultraviolet light all destroy folate, and it is estimated that 50% to 90% of folate may be destroyed during food processing and preparation. Consequently, it is advisable that fruits and vegetables be eaten uncooked or lightly cooked whenever possible.

Requirements. Folate is measured in micrograms. The average daily requirement for the adult female is 400 µg, and for the adult male it is also 400 µg. There is an increased need for folate during pregnancy and periods of growth because of the increased rate of cell division and the DNA synthesis in the body of the mother and of the fetus. Consequently, it is extremely important that women of childbearing age maintain good folate intake. The recommended amount for a woman 1 month before conception and through the first 6 weeks of pregnancy is 600 µg a day.

Deficiency. Folate deficiency has been linked to **neural tube defects (NTDs)** in the fetus, such as **spina bifida** (spinal cord or spinal fluid bulge through the back) and **anencephaly** (absence of a brain). Other signs of deficiency are inflammation of the mouth and tongue, poor growth, depression and mental confusion, problems with nerve functions, and **megaloblastic anemia**. Megaloblastic anemia is a condition wherein red blood cells are large and immature and cannot carry oxygen properly.

Hypervitaminosis. The FDA limits the amount of folate in over-the-counter (OTC) supplements to 100 µg for infants, 300 µg for children, and 400 µg for adults because consuming excessive amounts of folate can mask a vitamin B_{12} deficiency and inactivate phenytoin, an anticonvulsant drug used by epileptics.

⌕ **folate/folic acid**
a form of vitamin B, also called folacin; essential for metabolism

⌕ **neural tube defects (NTDs)**
congenital malformation of brain and/or spinal column due to failure of neural tube to close during embryonic development

⌕ **spina bifida**
spinal cord or spinal fluid bulge through the back

⌕ **anencephaly**
absence of brain

⌕ **megaloblastic anemia**
anemia in which the red blood cells are unusually large and are not completely mature

Biotin

Function and Sources.

Biotin participates as a coenzyme in the synthesis of fatty acids and amino acids. Some of its best dietary sources are liver, egg yolk, soy flour, cereals, and yeast. Biotin is also synthesized in the intestine by microorganisms, but the amount that is available for absorption is unknown.

Requirements.

Biotin is measured in micrograms. The Food and Nutrition Board of the Institute of Medicine has established an AI of 30 μg for adults (see Table 7-2).

Deficiency.

Deficiency symptoms include nausea, anorexia, depression, pallor (paleness of complexion), dermatitis (inflammation of skin), and an increase in serum cholesterol. Toxicity from excessive intake is unknown.

⊙ **biotin**
　a B vitamin; necessary for metabolism

Pantothenic Acid

Pantothenic acid is appropriately named, because the Greek word *pantothen* means "from many places." It is fairly stable, but it can be damaged by acids and alkalies.

Functions.

Pantothenic acid is involved in metabolism of carbohydrates, fats, and proteins. It is also essential for the synthesis of the neurotransmitter acetylcholine and of steroid hormones.

Sources.

Pantothenic acid is found extensively in foods, especially animal foods such as meats, poultry, fish, and eggs. It is also found in whole-grain cereals and legumes. In addition, it is thought to be synthesized by the body.

Requirements.

There is no DRI for pantothenic acid, but the Food and Nutrition Board has provided an estimated intake of 4–7 mg a day for normal adults (see Table 7-2).

Deficiency.

Natural deficiencies are unknown. However, deficiencies have been produced experimentally. Signs include weakness, fatigue, and a burning sensation in the feet. Toxicity from excessive intake has not been confirmed.

⊙ **pantothenic acid**
　a B vitamin

Vitamin C

Vitamin C is also known as **ascorbic acid.** It has antioxidant properties and protects foods from oxidation, and it is required for all cell metabolism. It is readily destroyed by heat, air, and alkalies, and it is easily lost in cooking water.

Functions.

Vitamin C is known to prevent **scurvy.** This is a disease characterized by gingivitis (soft, bleeding gums, and loose teeth); flesh that is easily bruised; tiny, pinpoint hemorrhages of the skin; poor wound healing; sore joints and muscles; and weight loss. In extreme cases, scurvy can result in death. Scurvy used to be common among sailors, who lived for months on

⊙ **ascorbic acid**
　vitamin C

⊙ **scurvy**
　a deficiency disease caused by a lack of
　vitamin C

bread, fish, and salted meat, with no fresh fruits or vegetables. During the middle of the eighteenth century, it was discovered that the addition of limes or lemons to their diets prevented this disease.

Vitamin C also has an important role in the formation of **collagen**, a protein substance that holds body cells together, making it necessary for wound healing. Therefore, the requirement for vitamin C is increased during trauma, fever, and periods of growth. Tiny, pinpoint hemorrhages are symptoms of the breakdown of collagen.

Vitamin C aids in the absorption of **nonheme iron** (from plant and animal sources and less easily absorbed than **heme iron**—see Chapter 8) in the small intestine when both nutrients are ingested at the same time. Because of this, it is called an iron enhancer.

Vitamin C also appears to have several other functions in the human body that are not well understood. For example, it may be involved with the formation or functioning of norepinephrine (a neurotransmitter and vasoconstrictor that helps the body cope with stressful conditions), some amino acids, folate, leukocytes (white blood cells), the immune system, and allergic reactions.

It is believed to reduce the severity of colds because it is a natural antihistamine, and it can reduce cancer risk in some cases by reducing nitrites in foods.

Vitamin C is absorbed in the small intestine.

Sources. The best sources of vitamin C are citrus fruits, melon, strawberries, tomatoes, potatoes, red and green peppers, cabbage, and broccoli.

Requirements. Vitamin C is measured in milligrams. Under normal circumstances, an average female adult in the United States requires 75 mg a day, and an average male 90 mg. In times of stress, the need is increased. Regular cigarette smokers are advised to ingest 35 mg or more a day.

It is generally considered nontoxic, but this has not been confirmed. An excess can cause diarrhea, nausea, cramps, an excessive absorption of food iron, rebound scurvy (when megadoses are stopped abruptly), and possibly oxalate kidney stones.

Deficiency. Deficiencies of vitamin C are indicated by bleeding gums, loose teeth, tendency to bruise easily, poor wound healing and, ultimately, scurvy.

SUPPLEMENTS

Healthy people who eat a variety of foods using the guidelines of MyPyramid should be able to obtain all the vitamins needed to maintain good health. However, some people take supplements because they believe that (1) food no longer contains the right nutrients in adequate quantities, (2) supplements can "bulk up" muscles and enhance athletic performance, (3) vitamins provide needed energy, and (4) vitamins and minerals can cure anything, including heart trouble, the common cold, and cancer.

The facts are as follows: (1) A balanced diet would provide for the nutritional needs of healthy people, but many do not follow a healthy eating plan, relying on fast food, processed foods, and heat, eat, and go foods. Therefore, the American Medical Association has recommended that everyone take one multiple vitamin a

collagen
protein substance that holds body cells together

nonheme iron
iron from animal foods that is not part of the hemoglobin molecule, and all iron from plant foods

heme iron
part of hemoglobin molecule in animal foods

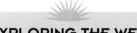

EXPLORING THE WEB

Search the Web for information on vitamin deficiency disorders. Choose a disorder and research the signs and symptoms related to it. Prepare a diet for a client suffering from the disorder that would provide the vitamin content that is lacking in the client's current diet. What other factors do you need to consider in regard to planning a therapeutic diet?

EXPLORING THE WEB

Search the Web for information on herbal dietary supplements. What claims are made by these products? Distinguish fact from fiction in the information that you uncover. Create a fact sheet for each of the herbal supplements you found and present the facts and the myths regarding use of the supplement. In addition, provide alternative food choices that would furnish the same benefits the supplement claims to make. What advice would you give a client inquiring about the use of these products?

day. (2) No amount of vitamins will build muscles; only weight lifting will do that. (3) Vitamins do not provide energy themselves. They help to release the energy within the carbohydrates, proteins, and fats that people ingest. (4) Only certain diseases caused by vitamin deficiencies (such as beriberi, scurvy, rickets) can be cured with the help of vitamin supplements. Heart disease, cancer, and the common cold cannot.

Almost everyone can take a daily multivitamin and mineral supplement without fear of toxicity, but a megadose (10 times the RDA/DRI) to correct a deficiency or to help prevent disease should be prescribed by a physician. If a multivitamin-mineral is taken as a supplement, it is best not to exceed 100% of the RDA/DRI for each vitamin and mineral. An excess of one vitamin or one mineral can negatively affect the absorption or utilization of other vitamins and minerals. If vitamin supplements are thought to be necessary, it is best to consult a physician or registered dietitian.

Herbal products also are included under the heading "dietary supplements." Some people are interested in herbs because they believe certain ones can improve their health, they require no prescription, and they are often less expensive than prescription drugs.

The U.S. Food and Drug Administration (FDA) requires that manufacturers of prescription and over-the-counter drugs run, monitor, and report results of clinical trials of their products before selling them. Doses are established and side effects and adverse reactions are reported in scientific journals. Also the FDA can inspect drug manufacturing facilities to confirm the purity of ingredients.

The *Dietary Supplement Health and Education Act of 1994 exempts dietary supplements from FDA evaluation unless the FDA has evidence that a product is harmful.* But before a suspect product can be removed from store shelves, the FDA must prove it is not safe. Manufacturers of supplements cannot claim their products can treat or prevent diseases, but they can make "structure-function" claims. For example, they cannot say vitamin A prevents cancer, but they can say vitamin A has antioxidant properties and antioxidants have been linked to reduced rates of cancer.

Misinformation concerning supplements is widely available. Health care professionals must stay well informed concerning supplements, provide accurate information to their clients, and urge clients to consult with their physicians or registered dietitians before using any supplement. Some herbal products may indeed be helpful, but some may be harmful.

CONSIDERATIONS FOR THE HEALTH CARE PROFESSIONAL

Vitamins are a popular subject about which many people have strong beliefs. Some beliefs are based on fact; many are incorrect. Today's magazines and newspapers frequently contain articles about vitamins, but they are not always factual. Clients who have no other source of nutrition information tend to believe the statements in those articles. It is important that the client have correct information about vitamins (Figure 7-2). Continuation of a poor diet or continued abuse of vitamin supplements is potentially dangerous to the client.

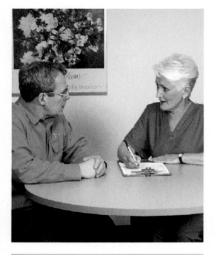

Figure 7-2 *Client education about vitamins is important.*

Health care professionals will need a solid knowledge of vitamins, a convincing manner, and enormous patience to reeducate patients as may be needed. Some will believe that vitamin E will prevent heart attack, that the only source of vitamin C is orange juice, or that megadoses of vitamin A will prevent cancer. Others will confuse milligrams with grams.

Client education about vitamins may be difficult until the health care professional gains the confidence of the client. Simple and clear written materials to reinforce the information will be helpful to the client.

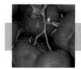

SUMMARY

Vitamins are organic compounds that regulate body functions and promote growth. Each vitamin has a specific function or functions within the body. Food sources of vitamins vary, but generally a well-balanced diet provides sufficient vitamins to fulfill body requirements. Vitamin deficiencies can result from inadequate diets or from the body's inability to utilize vitamins. Vitamins are available in concentrated forms, but their use should be carefully monitored because overdoses can be detrimental to health. Vitamins A, D, E, and K are fat-soluble. Vitamin B complex and vitamin C are water-soluble. Water-soluble vitamins can be destroyed during food preparation. It is important that care is taken during the preparation of food to preserve its vitamin content.

DISCUSSION TOPICS

1. How do vitamins help to provide energy to the body?

2. Discuss possible times when avitaminosis of one or more vitamins may occur.

3. Discuss any vitamin deficiencies that class members have observed. What treatments were prescribed?

4. Discuss why it may be unwise for anyone but a physician to prescribe vitamin supplements.

5. Discuss the terms *enriched* and *fortified.* What do they mean in relation to food products? Name foods that are enriched or fortified.

6. Discuss the proper storage and cooking of foods to retain their vitamin content.

7. If any member of the class has experienced night blindness, ask her or him to describe it. Discuss how this condition occurs and how it can be prevented.

8. Why is it advisable to use liquids left over from vegetable cooking? How might these be used?

9. Explain the role of vitamin C in collagen formation and wound healing.

10. If anyone in the class has taken concentrated vitamin C, ask why. If it was useful, ask how it helped.

11. Why are some vitamins called prohormones? Coenzymes? Give examples.

12. What is a precursor? Give an example.

13. Discuss appropriate nutritional advice for a young mother who is giving her 4-year-old 50 μg of vitamin D each day.

14. What is beriberi, and how can it be prevented?

15. Why should milk be sold in opaque containers?

SUGGESTED ACTIVITIES

1. Write a menu for one day that is especially rich in the B-complex vitamins. Underline the foods that are the best sources of these vitamins.

2. List the foods you have eaten in the past 24 hours. Write the names of the vitamins supplied

by each food. What percentage of your day's food did *not* contain vitamins? Could this diet be nutritionally improved? How?

3. Plan a day's menu for a person who has been instructed to eat an abundance of foods rich in vitamin A.

REVIEW

Multiple choice. Select the *letter* that precedes the best answer.

1. The daily vitamin requirement is best supplied by
    a. eating a well-balanced diet
    b. eating one serving of citrus fruit for breakfast
    c. taking one of the many forms of vitamin supplements
    d. eating at least one serving of meat each day

2. All of the following measures preserve the vitamin content of food except
    a. using vegetables and fruits raw
    b. preparing fresh vegetables and fruits just before serving
    c. adding raw, fresh vegetables to a small amount of cold water and heating to boiling
    d. storing fresh vegetables in a cool place

3. Fat-soluble vitamins
    a. cannot be stored in the body
    b. are lost easily during cooking
    c. are dissolved by water
    d. are slower than water-soluble vitamins to exhibit deficiencies

4. Night blindness is caused by a deficiency of
    a. vitamin A
    b. thiamine
    c. niacin
    d. vitamin C

5. Good sources of thiamine include
    a. citrus fruits and tomatoes
    b. wheat germ and liver
    c. carotene and fish liver oils
    d. nuts and milk

6. Water-soluble vitamins include
    a. A, D, E, and K
    b. A, B_6, and C
    c. thiamine, niacin, and retinol
    d. thiamine, riboflavin, niacin, B_6, B_{12}

7. Injections of B_{12} are given in the treatment of
    a. scurvy
    b. pernicious anemia
    c. pellagra
    d. beriberi

8. Blindness can result from a severe lack of
    a. vitamin K
    b. vitamin A
    c. thiamine
    d. vitamin E

9. Organ meats are good sources of the vitamins
    a. thiamine, riboflavin, B_{12}
    b. biotin, vitamin C
    c. vitamins E and K
    d. all of the above

10. Irradiated milk is a good source of
    a. vitamin E
    b. vitamin D
    c. vitamin K
    d. vitamin C

11. Good sources of vitamin C are
    a. meats
    b. milk and milk products
    c. breads and cereals
    d. citrus fruits

12. The vitamin that aids in the prevention of rickets is
    a. vitamin A
    b. thiamine
    c. vitamin C
    d. vitamin D

13. The vitamin that is necessary for the proper clotting of the blood is
    a. vitamin A
    b. vitamin K
    c. vitamin D
    d. niacin

14. Vitamins commonly added to breads and cereals are
    a. vitamins A, D, and K
    b. thiamine, riboflavin, niacin, and folate
    c. vitamins E, B_6, and B_{12}
    d. ascorbic acid, pantothenic acid, and folate

15. The vitamin known to prevent scurvy is
    a. vitamin A
    b. vitamin B complex
    c. vitamin C
    d. vitamin D

CASE IN POINT

KASIA: INCREASING VITAMIN AND MINERAL INTAKE

Kasia is a 13-year-old girl of Polish descent who has nine siblings and lives in the mountains of Kentucky with her family. She attended school for a short time but had to drop out because she was needed at home after her mother died. Her father works very hard in a local mine but does not make enough money to feed and clothe his family. Kasia worries all the time about her younger siblings and knows that they are not healthy. Kasia cannot remember when she had a glass of milk or enough to eat; she feels hungry all the time. She has not started her menses yet, and she is concerned about her recent loss of hair. Kasia was preparing breakfast, using a dulled knife to cut some bacon, when the knife slipped and she cut her thumb. She tried to stem the bleeding but could not get it to stop for hours. Kasia was frightened about the bleeding. Knowing that she needed to get help from someone, Kasia walked to the local school, 8 miles away, and asked to see the school nurse. Kasia spoke with the nurse and then agreed to see a dietitian.

ASSESSMENT

1. What data do you have about Kasia?
2. What might be lacking in Kasia's diet?
3. As the dietitian, what would you find helpful in Kasia's history?

DIAGNOSIS

4. Complete the following sentence: Kasia's delayed menses and growth and development problems are related to _____ .

PLAN/GOAL

5. What are two specific measurable goals for Kasia's diet?

IMPLEMENTATION

6. What food category is a priority for Kasia? What other food categories would be helpful to her health?
7. What else can be done to improve her health?

EVALUATION/OUTCOME CRITERIA

8. What criteria should Kasia use to evaluate the success of her actions?

THINKING FURTHER

9. Who else will benefit from Kasia's information?
10. Who else should be involved in discussions regarding diet and health?

RATE THIS PLATE

Kasia needs to learn how to prepare meals that are healthy but inexpensive. The dietitian learned that the family has a sow that it will butcher in the fall. The family also has a goat that is milked; and Kasia uses the milk for cooking and her brothers and sisters drink it. In the spring, it would be a good idea to plant a large garden and seek help if she doesn't know how to can the excess food. In the meantime, she has planned a dinner that she hopes will be good. Rate the plate.

Fried bacon

Boiled potatoes

Fried cabbage (using the bacon grease)

Bread and jelly

Apple pie

Did Kasia plan a healthy meal? What does this meal have too much of? What would you change to make it a better meal, but still inexpensive?

CASE IN POINT

KAYLA: LACKING PROTEIN

Kayla is a 6-year-old Hispanic girl who lives with her mom and dad and older sister. Her mother and father have full-time jobs away from the home. Kayla is a lively imp who has a great outlook on life. She loves to play and has a lot of energy. Her mother often refers to Kayla as a "bull in a china shop" because she is always running into things, especially at night, and she seems not to notice things in her way. Kayla is a lot smaller than kids her own age. She is always first in line when standing in line according to height.

During a routine physical, the nurse talks to Kayla about what she likes to eat. Kayla loves macaroni and spaghetti sauce, no added meat. She eats bread-and-jelly sandwiches and loves chocolate candy. The nurse asks her parents about meat and vegetables. Kayla doesn't eat vegetables and hates the texture of meat in her mouth. The nurse is somewhat concerned about the dietary habits, especially since Kayla's parents informed her of the complaints of bone pain that Kayla has. Her mom attributed the pain to growing pains. Since starting school this year, her parents told the nurse that Kayla has had a continuous runny nose and a cold. The nurse suggests that Kayla see a dietitian.

ASSESSMENT

1. What data do you have about Kayla?
2. What factors about Kayla would concern you about her eating habits?
3. After reviewing Kayla's history, what do you, as the nurse, suspect could be causing Kayla's bone pain?
4. What can you surmise about Kayla's family situation that could contribute to her lack of proper diet?

DIAGNOSIS

5. What could you attribute the "bull in a china shop" symptom to?
6. What would you caution Kayla's parents about her eating habits?

PLAN/GOAL

7. What is a reasonable, measurable goal for Kayla in regard to her eating habits?

IMPLEMENTATION

8. What three strategies can Kayla's parents institute that will help Kayla to begin a healthy eating regime?
9. What information would be helpful to give to Kayla's parents about vitamins?
10. Would you reward Kayla for improving her eating habits?

EVALUATION/OUTCOME CRITERIA

11. How will Kayla's parents be able to identify improvement in eating habits?
12. What impact of better eating will Kayla notice?

THINKING FURTHER

13. What questions might you want to ask Kayla's family about the older sister?

◎ RATE THIS PLATE

Kayla is lacking protein in her diet and is eating mostly carbohydrates. Kayla is too young to truly understand the importance of learning to eat a variety of food, so her parents will have to become inventive. On Kayla's plate is:

1/2 cup macaroni with a three-cheese sauce

1/2 cup applesauce

1/2 cup chocolate pudding

1 cup chocolate milk

How can Kayla's parents get vegetables into this meal? Is she getting enough protein? How about calcium? What else can you do to replace the nutrients Kayla would get from vegetables?

CHAPTER

8

MINERALS

OBJECTIVES

After studying this chapter, you should be able to:

- List at least two food sources of given minerals
- List one or more functions of given minerals
- Describe the recommended method of avoiding mineral deficiencies

Chemical analysis shows that the human body is made up of specific chemical elements. Four of these elements—oxygen, carbon, hydrogen, and nitrogen—make up 96% of body weight. All the remaining elements are *minerals*, which represent only 4% of body weight. Nevertheless, these minerals are essential for good health.

A mineral is an inorganic (non-carbon-containing) element that is necessary for the body to build tissues, regulate body fluids, or assist in various body functions. Minerals are found in all body tissues. Any abnormal concentration of minerals in the blood can help diagnose different disorders. Minerals cannot provide energy by themselves, but in their role as body regulators, they contribute to the production of energy within the body.

Minerals are found in water and in natural (unprocessed) foods, together with proteins, carbohydrates, fats, and vitamins. Minerals in the soil are absorbed by growing plants. Humans obtain minerals by eating plants grown in mineral-rich soil or by eating animals that have eaten such plants. The specific mineral content of food is determined by burning the food and then chemically analyzing the remaining ash.

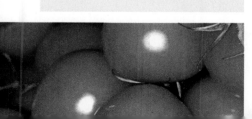

135

Highly processed or refined foods such as sugar and white flour contain almost no minerals. Iron, together with the vitamins thiamine, riboflavin, niacin, and folate, are commonly added to white flour and cereals, which are then labeled **enriched.**

Most minerals in food occur as salts, which are soluble in water. Therefore, the minerals leave the food and remain in the cooking water. Foods should be cooked in as little water as possible or, preferably, steamed, and any cooking liquid should be saved to be used in soups, gravies, and white sauces. Using this liquid improves the flavor as well as the nutrient content of foods to which it is added.

CLASSIFICATION

Minerals are divided into two groups. They are the major minerals, so named because each is required in amounts greater than 100 mg a day, and the trace minerals, which are needed in amounts smaller than 100 mg a day (Tables 8-1 and 8-2).

As mineral salts dissolve in water, they break into separate, electrically charged particles called **ions.** Ions, if positively charged, are called cations. When negatively charged, they are anions. The cations and anions must be balanced within the body fluids to maintain electroneutrality. For example, if body fluid contains 200 positive ($+$) charges, it must also contain 200 negative ($-$) charges. These ions are known as **electrolytes.**

enriched foods
foods to which nutrients, usually B vitamins and iron, have been added to improve their nutritional value

ions
electrically charged atoms resulting from chemical reactions

electrolyte
chemical compound that in water breaks up into electrically charged atoms called ions

Table 8-1 *Major Minerals*

NAME	FOOD SOURCES	FUNCTIONS	DEFICIENCY/TOXICITY
Calcium (Ca^{++})	Milk, cheese Sardines Salmon Some dark green, leafy vegetables	Development of bones and teeth Transmission of nerve impulses Blood clotting Normal heart action Normal muscle activity	Deficiency Osteoporosis Osteomalacia Rickets Tetany Retarded growth Poor tooth and bone formation
Phosphorus (P)	Milk, cheese Lean meat Poultry Fish Whole-grain cereals Legumes Nuts	Development of bones and teeth Maintenance of normal acid-base balance of the blood Constituent of all body cells Necessary for effectiveness of some vitamins Metabolism of carbohydrates, fats, and proteins	Deficiency Poor tooth and bone formation Weakness Anorexia General malaise

(continued)

Table 8-1 *Continued*

NAME	FOOD SOURCES	FUNCTIONS	DEFICIENCY/TOXICITY

Potassium (K^+)	Oranges, bananas
	Dried fruits
	Vegetables
	Legumes
	Milk
	Cereals
	Meat
		Contraction of muscles
		Maintenance of fluid balance
		Transmission of nerve impulses
		Osmosis
		Regular heart rhythm
		Cell metabolism
			Deficiency
			  Hypokalemia
			  Muscle weakness
			  Confusion
			  Abnormal heartbeat
			Toxicity
			  Hyperkalemia
			  Potentially life-threatening irregular heartbeats

Sodium (Na^+)	Table salt
	Beef, eggs
	Poultry
	Milk, cheese
		Maintenance of fluid balance
		Transmission of nerve impulses
		Osmosis
		Acid-base balance
		Regulation of muscle and nerve irritability
			Deficiency
			  Nausea
			  Exhaustion
			  Muscle cramps
			Toxicity
			  Increase in blood pressure
			  Edema

Chloride (Cl^-)	Table salt
	Eggs
	Seafood
	Milk
		Gastric acidity
		Regulation of osmotic pressure
		Osmosis
		Fluid balance
		Acid-base balance
		Formation of hydrochloric acid
			Deficiency
			  Imbalance in gastric acidity
			  Imbalance in blood pH
			  Nausea
			  Exhaustion

Magnesium (Mg^{++})	Green, leafy vegetables Whole grains Avocados Nuts Milk Legumes Bananas	Synthesis of ATP Transmission of nerve impulses Activation of metabolic enzymes Constituent of bones, muscles, and red blood cells Necessary for healthy muscles and nerves	Deficiency Normally unknown Mental, emotional, and muscle disorders
Sulfur (S)	Eggs Poultry Fish	Maintenance of protein structure For building hair, nails, and all body tissues Constituent of all body cells	Unknown

Table 8-2 *Trace Minerals*

NAME	FOOD SOURCES	FUNCTIONS	DEFICIENCY/TOXICITY

Iron (Fe^+)	Muscle meats
	Poultry
	Shellfish
	Liver
	Legumes
	Dried fruits
	Whole grain or enriched breads and cereals
	Dark green and leafy vegetables
	Molasses
		Transports oxygen and carbon dioxide
		Component of hemoglobin and myoglobin
		Component of cellular enzymes essential for energy production
			Deficiency
			  Iron deficiency anemia characterized by weakness, dizziness, loss of weight, and pallor
			Toxicity
			  Hemochromatosis (genetic)
			  Can be fatal to children
			  May contribute to heart disease
			  Injure liver

Iodine (I^-)	Iodized salt
	Seafood
		Regulation of basal metabolic rate	Deficiency
			  Goiter
			  Cretinism
			  Myxedema

Zinc (Zn^+)	Seafood, especially oysters
	Liver
	Eggs
	Milk
	Wheat bran
	Legumes
		Formation of collagen
		Component of insulin
		Component of many vital enzymes
		Wound healing
		Taste acuity
		Essential for growth
		Immune reactions
			Deficiency
			  Dwarfism, hypogonadism, anemia
			  Loss of appetite
			  Skin changes
			  Impaired wound healing
			  Decreased taste acuity

Selenium (Se^-)	Seafood
	Kidney
	Liver
	Muscle meats
	Grains
		Constituent of most body tissue
		Needed for fat metabolism
		Antioxidant functions
			Deficiency
			  Unclear, but related to Keshan disease
			  Muscle weakness
			Toxicity
			  Vomiting
			  Loss of hair and nails
			  Skin lesions

Copper (Cu^+)	Liver
	Shellfish, oysters
	Legumes
	Nuts
	Whole grains
		Essential for formation of hemoglobin and red blood cells
		Component of enzymes
		Wound healing
		Needed metabolically for the release of energy
			Deficiency
			  Anemia
			  Bone disease
			  Disturbed growth and metabolism
			Toxicity
			  Vomiting; diarrhea
			  Wilson's disease (genetic)

(continued)

Table 8-2 Continued			
NAME	**FOOD SOURCES**	**FUNCTIONS**	**DEFICIENCY/TOXICITY**
Manganese (Mn^+)	Whole grains Nuts Fruits Tea	Component of enzymes Bone formation Metabolic processes	Deficiency 　Unknown Toxicity 　Possible brain disease
Fluoride (F^-)	Fluoridated water Seafood	Increases resistance to tooth 　decay Component of bones and teeth	Deficiency 　Tooth decay 　Possibly osteoporosis Toxicity 　Discoloration of teeth 　(mottling)
Chromium (Cr)	Meat Vegetable oil Whole-grain cereal and nuts Yeast	Associated with glucose and 　lipid metabolism	Deficiency 　Possibly disturbances of 　glucose metabolism
Molybdenum (Mo)	Dark green, leafy vegetables Liver Cereal Legumes	Enzyme functioning Metabolism	Deficiency 　Unknown Toxicity 　Inhibition of copper 　absorption

Electrolytes are essential in maintaining the body's fluid balance, and they contribute to its electrical balance, assist in its transmission of nerve impulses and contraction of muscles, and help regulate its acid-base balance (see Chapter 9).

Normally, a balanced diet will maintain electrolyte balance. However, in cases of severe diarrhea, vomiting, high fever, or burns, electrolytes are lost and the electrolyte balance can be upset. Medical intervention will be necessary to replace the lost electrolytes.

Scientists lack exact information on some of the trace elements, although they do know that trace elements are essential to good health. The study of these elements continues to reveal their specific relationships to human nutrition. A balanced diet is the only safe way of including minerals in the amounts necessary to maintain health.

EXPLORING THE WEB

Search the Web for information on sports drinks or drinks containing electrolytes. What are the claims made by the makers of these drinks? What are the benefits, if any, that these drinks provide? Who is the target market for these drinks? What are some other dietary alternatives to these drinks? Are any warnings included for giving these drinks to babies?

Table 8-3 *Adequate Intakes for Selected Trace Minerals*

CATEGORY	AGE (YEARS)	COPPER (μg)	MANGANESE (Mg)	CHROMIUM (μg)	MOLYBDENUM (μg)
Infants	0–0.6	200	0.003	0.2	2
	0.6–1.0	220	0.6	5.5	3
Children and	1–3	340	1.2	11	17
adolescents	4–8	440	1.5	15	22
	9–13	700	1.9	25	34
	14–18	890	2.2	35	43
Adults		900	1.8–2.3	20–35	45

Reprinted with permission from the National Academy of Sciences. Copyright 2001 National Academy Press, Washington, D.C.

The Food and Nutrition Board of the National Academy of Sciences–National Research Council (hereafter NRC) has recommended dietary allowances for minerals where research indicates knowledge is adequate to do so.

For those minerals where there remains some uncertainty as to amounts of specific human requirements, the NRC has provided a table of Adequate Intakes of selected minerals (Table 8-3). The NRC recommends that the upper levels of listed amounts not be habitually exceeded. (Tables 8-1 and 8-2 list the best sources, functions, and deficiency symptoms of minerals.)

In addition, the Institute of Medicine has developed Daily Reference Intakes (DRIs) for calcium, fluoride, phosphorus, and magnesium. The DRI incorporates Estimated Average Requirements (EAR), the RDA, and Tolerable Upper Intake Levels.

TOXICITY

Because it is known that minerals are essential to good health, some would-be nutritionists will make claims that "more is better." Ironically, more can be hazardous to one's health when it comes to minerals. In a healthy individual eating a balanced diet, there will be some normal mineral loss through perspiration and saliva, and amounts in excess of body needs will be excreted in urine and feces. However, when concentrated forms of minerals are taken on a regular basis, over a period of time, they become more than the body can handle, and **toxicity** develops. An excessive amount of one mineral can sometimes cause a deficiency of another mineral. In addition, excessive amounts of minerals can cause hair loss and changes in the blood, hormones, bones, muscles, blood vessels, and nearly all tissues. Concentrated forms of minerals should be used only on the advice of a physician.

toxicity
state of being poisonous

MAJOR MINERALS
Calcium (Ca)

The human body contains more calcium than any other mineral. The body of a 154-pound person contains approximately 4 pounds of calcium. Ninety-nine percent of that calcium is found in the skeleton and teeth. The remaining 1% is found in the blood.

Functions. Calcium, in combination with phosphorus, is a component of bones and teeth, giving them strength and hardness. Bones, in turn, provide storage for calcium. Calcium is needed for normal nerve and muscle action, blood clotting, heart function, and cell metabolism.

Regulation of Blood Calcium. Each cell requires calcium. It is carried throughout the body by the blood, and its delivery to the cells is regulated by the hormonal system. Normal blood calcium levels are maintained even if intake is poor.

When blood calcium levels are low, the parathyroid glands release a hormone that tells the kidneys to retrieve calcium before it is excreted. In addition, this hormone, working with calcitriol (the active hormone form of vitamin D), causes increased release of calcium from the bones by stimulating the activity of the osteoclasts (cells that break down bones). Both of these actions increase blood calcium levels. If calcium intake is low for a period of years, the amount withdrawn from the bones will cause them to become increasingly fragile. Osteoporosis may result.

If the blood calcium level is high, osteoblasts (cells that make bones) will increase bone mass. During growth, osteoblasts will make more bone mass than will be broken down. Bone mass is acquired until one is approximately 30 years old. With adequate consumption of calcium, phosphorus, and vitamin D, bone mass will remain stable in women until menopause. After menopause, bones will begin to weaken owing to the lack of the hormone estrogen. A special X-ray, a DEXA scan, can be taken to determine bone density. If a person is at risk for injury due to decreased bone density, the physician will decide the best course of action. Drugs that help prevent further loss of bone mass are available.

Sources. The best sources of calcium are milk and milk products. They provide large quantities of calcium in small servings. For example, 1 cup of milk provides 300 mg of calcium (Figure 8-1). One ounce of cheddar cheese provides 250 mg of calcium.

Calcium is also found in some dark green, leafy vegetables. However, when the vegetable contains oxalic acid, as spinach and Swiss chard do, the calcium remains unavailable because the oxalic acid binds it and prevents it from being absorbed. When the intake of fiber exceeds 35 grams a day, calcium will also bind with phytates (phosphorus compounds found in some high-fiber cereal), which also limits its absorption.

Factors that are believed to enhance the absorption of calcium include adequate vitamin D, a calcium-to-phosphorus ratio that includes no more phosphorus than calcium, and the presence of lactose. A lack of weight-bearing exercise reduces the amount of calcium absorbed.

Requirements. The estimated requirement for calcium is now given as an Adequate Intake level (AI). Calcium is measured in milligrams (mg). The AIs

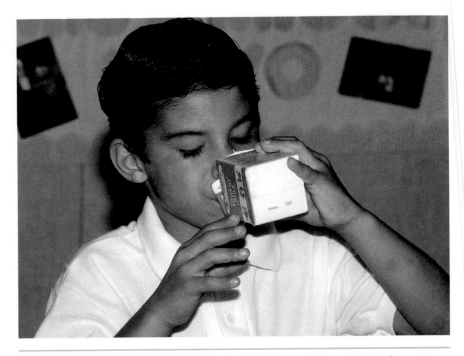

Figure 8-1 *Milk is an important source of calcium and phosphorus. These minerals are essential for the normal growth and development of bones and teeth.*

Table 8-4 *Adequate Intakes for Calcium*	
0–6 months	210 mg
6–12 months	270 mg
1–3 years	500 mg
4–8 years	800 mg
9–18 years	1,300 mg
19–50 years	1,000 mg
51–70+ years	1,200 mg
Pregnant women, 14–18 years	1,300 mg
Pregnant women, 19–50 years	1,000 mg
Lactating women	Same as for nonlactating women of same age

Source: *Dietary Reference Intakes*, Food and Nutrition Board, National Academy of Sciences–Institute of Medicine, 1997.

for calcium at different ages and conditions are shown in Table 8-4. The recommendations were made to achieve optimal bone health and to reduce the probability of fractures in later life.

Calcium supplements are recommended for persons who are lactose intolerant, those who dislike milk, and those who are unable to consume enough dairy products to meet their needs. Calcium carbonate, the form found in calcium-based antacid tablets, has the highest concentration of bioavailable calcium. Calcium supplements appear to be absorbed most efficiently when consumed in doses of 500 mg.

When purchasing calcium supplements, check for the USP (United States Pharmacopeia) seal of approval on the product you select (Figure 8-2). USP-approved products are unlikely to contain lead or other toxins. Avoid bone meal products, because they may contain lead.

Deficiency. Calcium deficiency may result in **rickets.** This is a disease that occurs in early childhood and results in poorly formed bone structure. It causes bowed legs, "pigeon breast," and enlarged wrists or ankles. Severe cases can result in stunted growth. Insufficient calcium can also cause "adult rickets" (osteomalacia), a condition in which bones become soft. And although the precise **etiology** of osteoporosis is not known, it is thought that long-term calcium deficiency is a contributing factor. Other factors contributing to osteoporosis include deficiency of vitamin D and certain hormones.

Insufficient calcium in the blood can cause a condition characterized by involuntary muscle movement, known as **tetany.** Excessive intake may cause constipation, or it may inhibit the absorption of iron and zinc.

Phosphorus (P)

Phosphorus, together with calcium, is necessary for the formation of strong, rigid bones and teeth. Phosphorus is also important in the metabolism of carbohydrates, fats, and proteins. Phosphorus is a constituent of all body cells. It is necessary for a proper acid-base balance of the blood and is essential for the effective action of several B vitamins. Like calcium, phosphorus is stored in bones, and its absorption is increased in the presence of vitamin D.

Sources. Although phosphorus is widely distributed in foods, its best sources are protein-rich foods such as milk, cheese, meats, poultry, and fish. Cereals, legumes, nuts, and soft drinks also contain substantial amounts of this mineral.

Requirements. The requirement for phosphorus is provided as AI (Adequate Intake) for the first 12 months and as EAR (Estimated Average Requirements) after that (Table 8-5). Phosphorus is measured in milligrams.

Deficiency. Because phosphorus is found in so many foods, its deficiency is rare. Excessive use of antacids can cause it, however, because they affect its absorption. Symptoms of phosphorus deficiency include bone **demineralization** (loss of minerals), fatigue, and anorexia.

Potassium (K)

Potassium is an electrolyte found primarily in **intracellular** fluid. Like sodium, it is essential for fluid balance and osmosis. Potassium maintains the fluid level *within* the cell, and sodium maintains the fluid level *outside* the cell. **Osmosis** moves the fluid into and out of cells as needed to maintain electrolyte (and

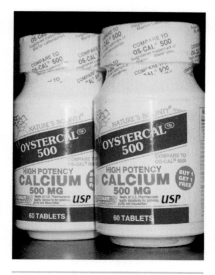

Figure 8-2 *Always look for the USP seal of approval when purchasing supplements.*

⚬ **rickets**
deficiency disease caused by the lack of calcium and vitamin D; causes malformed bones and pain in infants

⚬ **etiology**
cause

⚬ **tetany**
involuntary muscle movement

⚬ **demineralization**
loss of mineral or minerals

⚬ **intracellular**
within the cell

⚬ **osmosis**
movement of a substance through a semipermeable membrane

Table 8-5 *Adequate Intakes and Estimated Average Requirements for Phosphorus*

AI FOR PHOSPHORUS	
0–6 months	100 mg
6–12 months	275 mg
EAR FOR PHOSPHORUS	
1–3 years	380 mg
4–8 years	405 mg
9–18 years	1,055 mg
19–70+ years	580 mg
Pregnant and lactating women	Same as for nonpregnant and nonlactating women of same age

Source: *Dietary Reference Intakes*, Food and Nutrition Board, National Academy of Sciences–Institute of Medicine, 1997.

fluid) balance. There is normally more potassium than sodium inside the cell and more sodium than potassium outside the cell. If this balance is upset and the sodium inside the cell increases, the fluid within the cell also increases, swelling it and causing edema. If the sodium level outside the cell drops, fluid enters the cell to dilute the potassium level, thereby causing a reduction in **extracellular** fluid. With the loss of sodium and reduction of extracellular fluid, a decrease in blood pressure and dehydration can result.

Potassium is also necessary for transmission of nerve impulses and for muscle contractions.

Sources. Potassium is found in many foods. Fruits—especially melons, oranges, bananas, and peaches—and vegetables—notably mushrooms, Brussels sprouts, potatoes, tomatoes, winter squash, lima beans, and carrots—are particularly rich sources of it.

Deficiency or Excess. Potassium deficiency (**hypokalemia**) can be caused by diarrhea, vomiting, diabetic acidosis, severe malnutrition, or excessive use of laxatives or **diuretics.** Nausea, anorexia, fatigue, muscle weakness, and heart abnormalities (tachycardia) are symptoms of its deficiency. **Hyperkalemia** (high blood levels of potassium) can be caused by dehydration, renal failure, or excessive intake. Cardiac failure can result.

Sodium (Na)

Sodium is an electrolyte whose primary function is the control of fluid balance in the body. It controls the extracellular fluid and is essential for osmosis. Sodium is also necessary to maintain the acid-base balance in the body. In addition, it participates in the transmission of nerve impulses essential for normal muscle function.

extracellular
outside the cell

hypokalemia
low level of potassium in the blood

diuretics
substances used to increase the amount of urine excreted

hyperkalemia
excessive amounts of potassium in the blood

Sources. The primary dietary source of sodium is table salt (sodium chloride), which is 40% sodium. (One teaspoon of table salt contains 2,000 mg sodium.) It is also naturally available in animal foods. Salt is typically added to commercially prepared foods because it enhances flavor and helps to preserve some foods by controlling growth of microorganisms. Fruits and vegetables contain little or no sodium. Drinking water contains sodium but in varying amounts. "Softened" water has a much higher sodium content than "hard," or unsoftened, water.

Requirements. The DRI for sodium has been established at 1,500 mg, or 3,800 mg of salt. The UL for salt is 5,800 mg, with the majority of men and women exceeding that limit.

Deficiency or Excess. Either deficiency or excess of sodium can cause upsets in the body's fluid balance. Although rare, a deficiency of sodium can occur after severe vomiting, diarrhea, or heavy perspiration. In such cases, **dehydration** can result. A sodium deficiency also can upset the acid-base balance in the body. Cells function best in a neutral or slightly **alkaline** medium. If too much acid is lost (which can happen during severe vomiting), tetany due to **alkalosis** may develop. If the alkaline reserve is deficient as a result of starvation or faulty metabolism, as in the case of diabetes, **acidosis** (too much acid) may develop.

An excess of sodium is a more common problem and may cause **edema.** This edema adds pressure to artery walls that can cause **hypertension.** Thus, an excess of sodium is frequently associated with **cardiovascular** conditions such as hypertension and congestive heart failure. Certain groups have greater (or lesser) reduction in blood pressure in response to reduced sodium intake. Those with the greatest reductions in blood pressure have been termed *salt sensitive,* while those with little or no reduction in blood pressure have been termed *salt resistant.* Working with your cardiologist is the best way to determine which you are, sensitive or resistant. Depending on the diagnosis, the diet order may

dehydration
loss of water

alkaline
base; capable of neutralizing acids

alkalosis
condition in which excess base accumulates in, or acids are lost from, the body

acidosis
condition in which excess acids accumulate or there is a loss of base in the body

SPOTLIGHT on Life Cycle

Older individuals, African Americans, and those with chronic diseases including hypertension, diabetes, and kidney disease are especially sensitive to the blood pressure-raising effects of salt and should follow their physician's or dietitian's advice on the amount of salt to consume daily. Their UL may be lower. These groups also experience an especially high incidence of high blood pressure related to cardiac vascular disease.

edema
abnormal retention of fluid by the body

hypertension
higher than normal blood pressure

cardiovascular
pertaining to the heart and entire circulatory system

be either a 3- to 4-gram (also called no-added salt, or NAS) or a 1- to 2-gram sodium-restricted diet. A physician rarely prescribes a diet of 1 gram of sodium because compliance is difficult.

Chloride (Cl)

Chloride is an electrolyte that is essential for maintenance of fluid, electrolyte, and acid-base balance in the body. Like sodium, it is a constituent of extracellular fluid. It is also a component of gastric juices, where, in combination with hydrogen, it is found in hydrochloric acid, cerebrospinal (of the brain and spinal cord) fluid, and muscle and nerve tissue. It helps the blood carry carbon dioxide to the lungs and is necessary during immune responses when white blood cells attack foreign cells.

Sources. Chloride is found almost exclusively in table salt (sodium chloride) or in foods containing sodium chloride.

Requirements. The DRI for chloride for normal adults is 2,300 mg a day.

Deficiency. Because chloride is found in salt, deficiency is rare. It can occur, however, with severe vomiting, diarrhea, or excessive use of diuretics, and alkalosis can result. Also, it could occur in patients who must follow long-term sodium-restricted diets. In such cases, patients can be provided with an alternative source of chloride.

Magnesium (Mg)

Magnesium is vital to both hard and soft body tissues. It is essential for metabolism and regulates nerve and muscle function, including the heart, and plays a role in the blood-clotting process.

Sources. Like phosphorus, magnesium is widely distributed in foods, but it is found primarily in plant foods. The nutrient-dense foods are green leafy vegetables, legumes, nuts, whole grains, and some fruits such as avocados and bananas. Milk is also a good source if taken in sufficient quantity. For example, 2 cups of fat-free milk provide about 60 mg of magnesium.

Magnesium is lost during commercial food processing and in cooking water, so it is preferable to eat vegetables and fruits raw rather than cooked.

Requirements. The requirement for magnesium is provided as AIs (Table 8-6). Magnesium is measured in milligrams.

Deficiency. Because of the wide availability of magnesium, its deficiency among people on normal diets is unknown. When deficiency was experimentally induced, the symptoms included nausea and mental, emotional, and muscular disorders.

Sulfur (S)

Sulfur is necessary to all body tissue and is found in all body cells. It contributes to the characteristic odor of burning hair and tissue. It is necessary for metabolism.

Table 8-6 *Adequate Intakes for Magnesium*

AI FOR MAGNESIUM		
Boys and girls	0–6 months	30 mg
	6–12 months	75 mg
	1–3 years	80 mg
	4–8 years	130 mg
	9–13 years	240 mg
Boys	14–18 years	410 mg
Girls	14–18 years	360 mg
Men	19–30 years	400 mg
Women	19–30 years	310 mg
Men	31–70+ years	420 mg
Women	31–70+ years	320 mg
Pregnant women	14–18 years	400 mg
	19–30 years	350 mg
	31–50 years	360 mg
Lactating women	14–18 years	360 mg
	19–30 years	310 mg
	31–50 years	320 mg

Source: *Dietary Reference Intakes,* Food and Nutrition Board, National Academy of Sciences–Institute of Medicine, 2001.

Sources. Sulfur is a component of some amino acids and consequently is found in protein-rich foods.

Requirements or Deficiency. Neither the amount of sulfur required by the human body nor its deficiency is known.

TRACE MINERALS

Iron (Fe)

The principal role of iron is to deliver oxygen to body tissues. It is a component of hemoglobin, the coloring matter of red blood cells (erythrocytes). Hemoglobin allows red blood cells to combine with oxygen in the lungs and carry it to body tissues.

Iron is also a component of **myoglobin,** a protein compound in muscles that provides oxygen to cells, and it is a constituent of other body compounds involved in oxygen transport. Iron is utilized by enzymes that are involved in the making of amino acids, hormones, and neurotransmitters.

Sources. Meat, poultry, and fish are the best sources of iron because only the flesh of animals contains **heme iron.** Heme iron is absorbed more than

myoglobin
protein compound in muscle that provides oxygen to cells

heme iron
part of hemoglobin molecule in animal foods

Table 8-7 *Factors That Affect Iron Absorption*

INCREASE	DECREASE
Acid in the stomach	Phytic acid (in fiber)
Heme iron	Oxalic acid
High body demand for red blood cells (blood loss, pregnancy)	Polyphenols in tea and coffee
Low body stores of iron	Full body stores of iron
Meat protein factor (MPF)	Excess of other minerals (Zn, Mn, Ca) (especially when taken as supplements)
Vitamin C	Some antacids

⊙ **nonheme iron**
iron from animal foods that is not part of the hemoglobin molecule; and all iron from plant foods

twice as efficiently as nonheme iron. **Nonheme iron** is found in whole-grain cereals, enriched grain products, vegetables, fruit, eggs, meat, fish, and poultry. The rate of absorption of nonheme iron is strongly influenced by dietary factors and the body's iron stores. Factors affecting the absorption of both heme and nonheme iron are listed in Table 8-7.

For iron to be absorbed, it must be chemically changed from ferric to ferrous iron. This change is accomplished by the hydrochloric acid in the stomach. Absorption of nonheme iron can be enhanced by consuming a vitamin C–rich food and a nonheme iron–rich food at the same meal. Vitamin C holds onto and keeps the iron in its ferrous form, which facilitates absorption. Meat protein factor (MPF) is a substance in meat, poultry, and fish that aids in the absorption of nonheme iron.

Phytic acid and oxalic acid can bind iron and reduce the body's absorption of it. Polyphenols, such as tannins in tea and related substances in coffee, also reduce the absorption of iron. Antacids containing calcium and calcium supplements should be taken several hours before or after a meal high in iron because calcium also interferes with iron absorption.

Requirements. The NRC has determined that men lose approximately 1 mg of iron a day and that women lose 1.5 mg a day. On the assumption that only 10% of ingested iron is absorbed, the DRI for men has been set at 10 mg and for women from the age of 11 through the childbearing years at 15 mg. This is doubled during pregnancy and is difficult to meet by diet alone. Consequently, an iron supplement is commonly prescribed during pregnancy. Women should make a special effort to include iron-rich foods in their diets at all times. The rapid growth periods of infancy and adolescence also produce a heavy need for iron.

Deficiency or Toxicity. Iron deficiency continues to be a problem, especially for women. **Iron deficiency** can be caused by insufficient intake, malabsorption, lack of sufficient stomach acid, or excessive blood loss, any or all of which can deplete iron stores in the body. Decreased stores of iron prevent hemoglobin synthesis. The result is an insufficient number of red blood cells to carry needed oxygen. What begins as iron deficiency can be-

⊙ **iron deficiency**
intake of iron is adequate, but the body has no extra iron stored

come **iron deficiency anemia**. Iron deficiency anemia takes a long time to develop, but it is the most common nutrient deficiency worldwide. Symptoms include fatigue, weakness, irritability, and shortness of breath. Clinical signs include pale skin and spoon-shaped fingernails.

Some people suffer from *hemochromatosis*. This is a condition due to an inborn error of metabolism and causes excessive absorption of iron. The onset of this disorder can happen at any age. Unless treated, this condition can damage the liver, spleen, and heart. To control the buildup of iron, patients with this condition must give blood on a regular basis.

Iodine (I)

Iodine is a component of the thyroid hormones, thyroxine (T_4) and triiodothyronine (T_3). It is necessary for the normal functioning of the thyroid gland, which determines the rate of metabolism.

Sources. The primary sources of iodine are **iodized salt**, seafood, and some plant foods grown in soil bordering the sea. Iodized salt is common table salt to which iodine has been added in an amount that, if used in normal cooking, provides sufficient iodine.

Requirements. The DRI for adults is 150 mg a day. Additional amounts are needed during pregnancy and lactation.

Deficiency. When the thyroid gland lacks sufficient iodine, the manufacture of thyroxine and triiodothyronine is retarded. In its attempt to take up more iodine, the gland grows, forming a lump on the neck called a **goiter** (Figure 8-3). Goiter appears to be more common among women than among men. A thyroid gland that doesn't function properly causes myxedema (hypothyroidism) in adults. The children of mothers lacking sufficient iodine may suffer from cretinism (retarded physical and mental development).

Zinc (Zn)

Zinc is a cofactor for more than 300 enzymes. Consequently, it affects many body tissues. It appears to be essential for growth, wound healing, taste acuity, glucose tolerance, and the mobilization of vitamin A within the body.

Sources. The best sources of zinc are protein foods, especially meat, fish, eggs, and dairy products, and wheat germ and legumes.

Requirements. The DRI for zinc in normal adult males is 11 mg, and in adult females, it is 8 mg, with increased requirements during pregnancy and further increases during lactation.

Deficiency. Decreased appetite and taste acuity, delayed growth, dwarfism, hypogonadism (subnormal development of male sex organs), poor wound healing, anemia, acnelike rash, and impaired immune response are all symptoms of zinc deficiency.

iron deficiency anemia
condition resulting from inadequate amount of iron in the diet, reducing the amount of oxygen carried by the blood to the cells

iodized salt
salt that has had the mineral iodine added for the prevention of goiter

goiter
enlarged tissue of the thyroid gland due to a deficiency of iodine

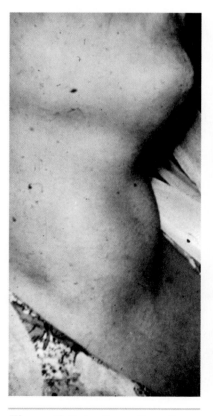

Figure 8-3 *A goiter on the neck, which results primarily from iodine deficiency, is an enlargement of the thyroid gland. (Courtesy of the Centers for Disease Control and Prevention, Public Health Image Library)*

Selenium (Se)

Selenium is a constituent of most body tissues, but the heaviest concentration of the mineral is in the liver, kidneys, and heart.

Functions. Selenium is a component of an enzyme that acts as an antioxidant. In this way, it protects cells against oxidation and spares vitamin E.

Sources. The best sources of selenium are seafood, kidney, liver, and muscle meats.

Requirements. The DRI for selenium for an adult male and female is 70 μg.

Deficiency or Toxicity. Symptoms of selenium deficiency are unclear, but selenium supplements appear to be effective in treating **Keshan disease.** High doses (1 mg or more daily) are toxic and can cause vomiting, loss of hair and nails, and skin lesions.

⊙ **Keshan disease**
condition causing abnormalities in the heart muscle

Copper (Cu)

Copper is found in all tissues, but its heaviest concentration is in the liver, kidneys, muscles, and brain. As an essential component of several enzymes, it helps in the formation of hemoglobin, aids in the transport of iron to bone marrow (soft tissue in bone center) for the formation of red blood cells, and participates in energy production.

Sources. Copper is available in many foods, but its best sources include organ meats, shellfish, legumes, nuts, cocoa, and whole-grain cereals. Human milk is a good source of copper, but cow's milk is not.

Requirements. The DRI for copper is 900 mg for adults.

Deficiency or Toxicity. Copper deficiency is extremely rare among adults, occurring only in people with malabsorption conditions and in cases of gross protein deficiency, such as kwashiorkor. It is apparent sometimes in premature infants and in people on long-term parenteral nutrition (feeding via a vein) programs lacking copper. A copper deficiency can be caused by taking excess zinc supplements. Anemia, bone demineralization, and impaired growth may result.

Excess copper can be highly toxic. A single dose of 10–15 mg can cause vomiting. Wilson's disease is an inherited condition resulting in accumulation of copper in the liver, brain, kidneys, and cornea. It can cause damage to liver cells and neurons. If the excess is detected early, copper-binding agents can be used to bind copper in the bloodstream and increase excretion.

Manganese (Mn)

Manganese is a constituent of several enzymes involved in metabolism. It is also important in bone formation.

Sources. The best sources of manganese are whole grains and tea. Vegetables and fruits also contain moderate amounts.

Requirements. The Adequate Intake for adults is 2.3 mg for men and 1.8 mg for women.

Deficiency and Toxicity. Its deficiency has not been documented. Toxicity from excessive ingestion of manganese is unknown. However, people who have inhaled high concentrations of manganese dust have developed neurological problems.

Fluoride (F)

Fluoride increases one's resistance to dental caries. It appears to strengthen bones and teeth by making the bone mineral less soluble and thus less inclined to being reabsorbed.

Sources. The principal source of fluoride is fluoridated water (water to which fluoride has been added). In addition, fish and tea contain fluoride. Commercially prepared foods in which fluoridated water has been used during the preparation process also contain fluoride.

Requirements. The requirement for fluoride is given as AI levels (Table 8-8). Fluoride is measured in milligrams.

Deficiency or Toxicity. The deficiency of fluoride can result in increased tooth decay. Excessive amounts of fluoride in drinking water have been known to cause permanent discoloration or mottling of children's teeth.

Chromium (Cr)

Chromium is associated with glucose and lipid metabolism. Chromium levels decrease with age except in the lungs, where chromium accumulates.

Sources. The best sources of chromium include meat, mushrooms, nuts, yeast, organ meats, and wheat germ.

Table 8-8 *Adequate Intakes for Fluoride*		
Boys and girls	0–6 months	0.01 mg
	6–12 months	0.5 mg
	1–3 years	0.7 mg
	4–8 years	1.0 mg
	9–13 years	2.0 mg
Boys	14–18 years	3.1 mg
Girls	14–18 years	3.0 mg
Males	19+ years	4.0 mg
Females	19+ years	3.0 mg
Pregnant and lactating women	Same as for nonpregnant and nonlactating women of same age	

Source: *Dietary Reference Intakes*, Food and Nutrition Board, National Academy of Sciences–Institute of Medicine, 1997.

Requirements. Although there is no DRI for chromium, there is AI for adults, which is 35 mg for men and 25 mg for women. There appears to be no difficulty fulfilling this requirement when one has a balanced diet.

Deficiency. Chromium deficiency appears to be related to disturbances in glucose metabolism.

Molybdenum (Mo)

Molybdenum is a constituent of enzymes and is thought to play a role in metabolism.

Sources. The best sources of molybdenum include milk, liver, legumes, and cereals.

Requirements. The estimated safe and adequate daily intake for adults is 45 µg. This is normally fulfilled with a balanced diet.

Deficiency or Toxicity. No deficiencies have been noted in people who consume a normal diet. Excessive intake can inhibit copper absorption.

CONSIDERATIONS FOR THE HEALTH CARE PROFESSIONAL

Second to vitamins, minerals are of great interest to the general public. They often are given mythic powers in current articles.

It is imperative that the health care professional be aware of the dangers of even small doses of minerals and be able to transmit this information in a meaningful way to the patients.

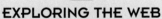

EXPLORING THE WEB

Search the Web for information on mineral supplements. What claims are made regarding the use of these substances? Make a teaching checklist for a client outlining the health benefits and risks related to the use of these minerals. State other sources of attaining these minerals without the use of supplements.

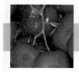

SUMMARY

Minerals are necessary to promote growth and regulate body processes. They originate in soil and water and are ingested via food and drink. Deficiencies can result in conditions such as anemia, rickets, and goiter. A well-balanced diet can prevent mineral deficiencies. Concentrated forms of minerals should be taken only on the advice of a physician. Excessive amounts of minerals can be toxic, causing hair loss and changes in nearly all body tissues.

DISCUSSION TOPICS

1. Discuss the special importance of calcium and phosphorus to children and to pregnant women.

2. List ways of supplying an adequate amount of calcium in the diet of an adult who dislikes milk. Plan a day's menu for this adult.

3. Ask if any member of the class has suffered from anemia. If anyone has, ask the class member to describe the symptoms and treatment. What kind of anemia was it? If it's preventable, what measures are being taken to prevent a recurrence of the condition?

4. If a person is to decrease sodium in her or his diet, should animal foods be increased or decreased?

5. Why does the FNB/NAS recommend that the upper limits of DRIs for minerals not be habitually exceeded?

6. If anyone in class knows someone with osteoporosis, ask for a description of the patient, including sex, age, physical appearance, physical complaints, lifelong dietary habits, and medical treatment.

7. Explain the relationship of sodium and edema.

8. Why is it recommended that patients on sodium-restricted diets have the mineral content of their local water supply evaluated?

9. Explain the relationship of sodium and potassium.

10. Why would a doctor prescribe potassium at the same time a diuretic is prescribed?

11. Although rare, why does chloride deficiency sometimes occur in patients on long-term sodium-restricted diets?

12. Discuss the differences between heme and nonheme iron.

13. Why is iron commonly prescribed for pregnant women?

14. Why is selenium said to spare vitamin E?

SUGGESTED ACTIVITIES

1. Using outside sources, prepare a report on how sodium and potassium regulate the body's fluid balance.

2. Using other sources, write a report on at least one of the following:

   Rickets
   Goiter
   Hypothyroidism and hyperthyroidism
   Edema
   Osteoporosis
   Osteomalacia

3. Check four or five varieties of bread at the local supermarket. Using the labels on the breads, evaluate their mineral content.

4. List five good sources of heme iron and five sources of nonheme iron.

5. Spend 5 or 10 minutes observing customers at a drugstore display of various vitamin and mineral compounds. Write a short report on which minerals were most frequently purchased. Include your opinion about why this was the case.

6. Write a short essay on why iodized salt is a better choice than plain salt.

REVIEW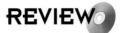

Multiple choice. Select the *letter* that precedes the best answer.

1. Minerals are inorganic elements that
   a. help to build and repair tissues
   b. are found only in bones
   c. provide energy when carbohydrates are lacking
   d. can substitute for proteins

2. The trace minerals in the human body are defined as
   a. those minerals that cannot be detected in laboratory tests
   b. those essential minerals found in very small amounts
   c. those minerals that are not essential to health
   d. only those minerals that are found in the blood

3. Calcium is necessary for
   a. healthy bones and teeth
   b. normal red blood cells
   c. preventing goiter
   d. energy

4. Phosphorus is found in
   a. poultry   c. vegetable oils
   b. common table salt   d. leafy vegetables

5. The coloring matter of the blood is
   a. hemoglobin   c. marrow
   b. lymph   d. plasma

6. Some of the common signs of iron deficiency anemia are
   a. muscle spasms and pain in the liver
   b. bowed legs and an enlarged thyroid gland
   c. edema and loss of vision
   d. fatigue and weakness

7. Iodine is essential to health because it
   a. is necessary for red blood cells
   b. strengthens bones and teeth
   c. helps the blood to carry oxygen to the cells
   d. affects the rate of metabolism

8. Sodium is often restricted in cardiovascular conditions because it
   a. causes the heart to beat slowly
   b. encourages the growth of the heart
   c. contributes to edema
   d. raises the blood sugar

9. Iron is known to be a necessary component of
   a. thyroxine
   b. adipose tissue
   c. hemoglobin
   d. amino acids

10. Liquid from cooking vegetables should be used in preparing other dishes because
    a. mineral salts are soluble in water
    b. the hydrogen and oxygen in water aid the digestion of minerals
    c. the amino acids are soluble in water
    d. none of the above

11. Goiter can result from a deficiency of
    a. manganese   c. copper
    b. magnesium   d. iodine

12. A deficiency of calcium can cause
    a. lactose intolerance   c. tetany
    b. severe nausea   d. hypertension

13. Sodium is especially important in
    a. the blood-clotting process
    b. curing osteoporosis
    c. the prevention of osteomalacia
    d. osmosis

14. Sulfur
    a. is found only in bones and teeth
    b. is richly supplied in carbohydrates
    c. is found in all body cells
    d. deficiency is very common

15. Hypokalemia is
    a. caused by an abnormal heartbeat
    b. caused by potassium deficiency
    c. often a precursor of hyperkalemia
    d. a common result of chronic overeating

CASE IN POINT

MI-LING: CONTROLLING EDEMA AND HIGH BLOOD PRESSURE

Mi-Ling is a 53-year-old Asian librarian who has been noticing that her hands and feet have been swelling. She is not a particularly active woman and is overweight by 70 pounds. She has been experiencing shortness of breath upon climbing stairs and walking more than 30 yards. She blames these symptoms on her physical lack of exercise. But the swelling is causing her some concern. She goes to her doctor for a checkup.

Her doctor tells her that her blood pressure is up, 186/92; her heart is working hard at 100 bpm. The doctor hears no anomalies with her heart, and her electrocardiogram looks within normal limits. Mi-Ling's doctor suggests following a no-added-salt diet, increasing her physical stamina, and losing weight, and she prescribes a diuretic. Mi-Ling is concerned about the no-added-salt diet; she is referred to a dietitian.

ASSESSMENT

1. How would you identify hidden sources of sodium in Mi-Ling's diet?
2. What contributing factors would cause her to have swelling?
3. What questions about thirst would be helpful to pinpoint?
4. What information from a 24-hour food diary could the doctor obtain?
5. What information about no added salt could be causing stress for Mi-Ling?

DIAGNOSIS

6. What information about Mi-Ling's lack of physical activity could benefit her in the future?
7. What prepared foods can Mi-Ling have when starting to diet that would not interfere with her sodium restriction?

PLAN/GOAL

8. What two goals would you set for Mi-Ling?

IMPLEMENTATION

9. What are the main topics you would have Mi-Ling understand about a no-added-salt, low-fat diet?
10. List three foods that have high sodium content that Mi-Ling should avoid or have in moderation.
11. Explain the importance of drinking lots of water even with edema.

EVALUATION/OUTCOME CRITERIA

12. How will Mi-Ling know if she is successful?

THINKING FURTHER

13. Look ahead to Chapter 18. What other factors could be influencing Mi-Ling's hypertension?
14. Why is it important for Mi-Ling to control her hypertension? What are some of the consequences of uncontrolled hypertension?

RATE THIS PLATE

Mi-Ling had her appointment with the dietitian and was given written and verbal information about her no-added-salt (NAS) diet. The dietitian also told her that it would take 2 to 4 months for her mouth to get used to lower salt. She had Mi-Ling write a sample dinner that she could prepare. This is Mi-Ling's plate:

4 oz roast prepared with onion soup and cream of mushroom soup
4 quarter pieces potatoes and 6 mini carrots cooked with the roast
2 tsp horseradish
3/4 cup Waldorf salad
1/2 cup ice cream

What food items are high in sodium? What would happen to the potatoes and carrots cooked in the gravy? Is there any appreciable salt in the salad, and if so, from where? Is the ice cream allowed on a weight loss diet? Why or why not? Is a diet of NAS adequate given Mi-Ling's symptoms? What other mineral should the doctor prescribe to go with the diuretic? Any idea?

CASE IN POINT

SHANESA: ADDRESSING PAINFUL MENSES THROUGH DIET

Shanesa is a 34-year-old African American woman and mother of two. She has had a history of difficult menses. When she was 12, she started her periods and had very irregular patterns to her cycles. Her cycle was and still is accompanied by heavy bleeding. Shanesa would be off school for days with each difficult cycle. Shanesa visited her family practice physician many times during her life to see if he could help with the fatigue. What she reported was that the family practice physician said she would have better cycles after her children were born. After that, Shanesa never thought anything more about it.

After the birth of her first daughter, she found that her periods were more regular but just as heavy. After her second daughter was born, Shanesa felt just as tired and did not find her periods improved. Shanesa is often short-tempered with her husband, and is finding that she is more irritated with "little things." She continues to complain of fatigue and takes naps on most days during her cycle. Shanesa asks her physician for a dietary consult in order to better understand her needs. Before her dietary visit, her physician draws blood and learns that Shanesa has low iron stores and a low iron count.

ASSESSMENT

1. Would a 48-hour diet diary be helpful to a dietitian?

2. What would you look for in the diet diary that would indicate a low iron store for Shanesa?

3. What blood tests do you expect to see the doctor order for Shanesa?

4. How much iron is lost by women, per day, according to the NRC (National Academy of Sciences–National Research Council)?

5. What is the daily requirement for iron for women?

DIAGNOSIS

6. Complete the following diagnostic statement: Deficient knowledge related to _____.

7. Complete the following diagnostic statement: Health-seeking behaviors related to lack of understanding of iron deficiency anemia _____ .

PLAN/GOAL

8. Name two reasonable goals for Shanesa.

IMPLEMENTATION

9. Which food categories are a priority to include in Shanesa's diet?

10. What can Shanesa include as part of daily living to assist in absorption of iron?

11. Would Shanesa benefit from taking an iron supplement?

EVALUATION/OUTCOME CRITERIA

12. In four months, when Shanesa sees her doctor again what could the doctor measure to evaluate the effectiveness of Rhonda's compliance.

THINKING FURTHER

13. What changes could Shanesa expect to see if she complies with her program?

RATE THIS PLATE

Shanesa has heavy bleeding monthly with her menses. With this excess bleeding comes iron loss. She needs to plan meals with the potential for high iron absorption. Rate her plate.

1 cup Total cereal

1 cup milk

Banana

Will she get enough iron from her breakfast? What type of iron is in cereal? Will her absorption be high quality? Does Shanesa have a deficiency or anemia? What is the difference?

WATER

OBJECTIVES

After studying this chapter, you should be able to:

- Describe the functions of water in the body
- Explain fluid balance and its maintenance
- Name causes and consequences of water depletion
- Give causes and consequences of positive fluid balance
- Describe the acid-base balance of the human body

Although humans can live about 30 to 45 days without food, it is possible to live only 10 to 14 days without water. Water is a component of all body cells and constitutes from 50% to 60% of the body weight of normal adults. The percentage is higher in males than females because men usually have more muscle tissue than women. The water content of muscle tissue is higher than that of fat tissue. The percentage of water content is highest in newborns (75%) and decreases with age.

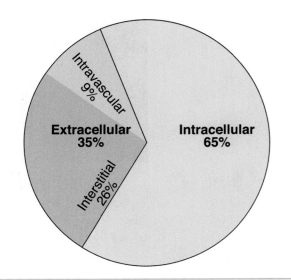

Figure 9-1 *Body fluid compartments as percentage of total body fluid. All fluid in the body can be classified as either intracellular or extracellular.*

intracellular fluid
water within cells; approximately 65% of total body fluid

extracellular fluid
water outside the cells; approximately 35% of total body fluid

interstitial fluid
fluid between cells

solvent
liquid part of a solution

Body water is divided into two basic compartments: intracellular and extracellular. **Intracellular fluid** (ICF) is water within the cells and accounts for about 65% of total body fluid (Figure 9-1). **Extracellular fluid** (ECF) is water outside the cells and accounts for about 35% of total body fluid. Extracellular fluid is found in the intravascular fluid (water in the bloodstream), **interstitial fluid,** and glandular secretions.

Although it is a component of all body tissues, water is the major component of blood plasma. It is a **solvent** for nutrients and waste products and helps transport both to and from body cells by way of the blood. It is necessary for the hydrolysis of nutrients in the cells, making it essential for metabolism. It functions as a lubricant in joints and in digestion. In addition, it cools the body through perspiration and may, depending on its source, provide some mineral elements (Table 9-1).

Table 9-1 *Functions of Water*
Component of all body tissues providing structure and form
Solvent for nutrients and body wastes and chemical reactions
Provides transport for nutrients and wastes via the blood and lymphatic system
Essential for hydrolysis and thus metabolism
Lubricant of joints and in digestion
Helps regulate body temperature by evaporation of perspiration
Serves as a shock absorber

Table 9-2 *Estimated Daily Fluid Intake for an Adult*	
Ingested liquids	1,500 ml
Water in foods	700 ml
Water from oxidation	200 ml
Total	2,400 ml

The best source of water is drinking water. Beverages of all types are the second-best source. A considerable amount is also found in foods, especially fruits, vegetables, soups, milk, and gelatin desserts. In addition, energy metabolism produces water. When carbohydrates, fats, and proteins are metabolized, their end products include carbon dioxide and water (Table 9-2). See Appendix D for water content of foods.

FLUID AND ELECTROLYTE BALANCE

For optimum health there must be **homeostasis**. For this to exist, the body must be in *fluid and electrolyte balance.* This means the water lost by healthy individuals through urination, feces, perspiration, and the respiratory tract must be replaced in terms of both volume and electrolyte content. Electrolytes are measured in **milliequivalents** (mEq/L). An illness causing vomiting and diarrhea can result in large losses of water and electrolytes and must be addressed quickly. Water lost through urine is known as sensible (noticeable) water loss. Insensible (unnoticed) water loss is in feces, perspiration, and respiration. The body must excrete 500 ml of water as urine each day in order to get rid of the waste products of metabolism (Table 9-3).

Water moves through cell walls by **osmosis** (Figure 9-2). Water flows from the side with the lesser amount of **solute** to the side with the greater solute concentration. The electrolytes sodium, chloride, and potassium are the

homeostasis
state of physical balance; stable condition

milliequivalent
the concentration of electrolytes in a solution

osmosis
movement of a substance through a semipermeable membrane

solute
the substance dissolved in a solution

((In The Media

RUNNERS: BEWARE TOO MUCH WATER

Drinking too much water during long-distance races, marathons, and other endurance exercises can cause hyponatremia, which can be fatal. Low sodium can cause headaches, confusion, seizures, and even death. Researchers found that the strongest indicator or hyponatremia was weight gain during a race. To prevent hyponatremia, runners should weigh themselves before practice and after practice to determine how much water weight was lost and to replace that much water during the actual race. Plain water is absorbed faster than sports drinks, but researchers stated it didn't matter which runners drank. The small amount of sodium in the sports drink did not make a difference.

(Source: Adapted from CBS News, April 2005. Retrieved from www.cbsnews.com.)

Table 9-3 *Factors That Lead to Fluid Imbalances*

	FLUID DEFICIT	FLUID EXCESS
Environmental factors	Exposure to sun or high atmospheric temperatures	
Personal behaviors	Fasting Fad diets Exercise without adequate fluid replacement	Excessive sodium or water intake Venous compression due to pregnancy

Psychological influences	Decreased motivation to drink due to:
	  Fatigue
	  Depression
	Excessive use of:
	  Laxatives
	  Enemas
	  Alcohol
	  Caffeine
		Low protein intake due to anorexia

Consequences of diseases	Fluid losses due to:
	  Fever
	  Wound drainage
	  Vomiting
	  Diarrhea
	  Heavy menstrual flow
	  Burns
	Difficulty swallowing due to:
	  Oral pain
	  Fatigue
	  Neuromuscular weakness
	Excessive urinary output due to uncontrolled:
	  Diabetes mellitus
	  Diabetes insipidus
		Fluid retention due to:
		  Renal failure
		  Cardiac conditions
		  Congestive heart failure
		  Valvular diseases
		  Left ventricular failure
		  Cirrhosis
		  Cancer
		  Impaired venous return

⚬ **osmolality**
number of particles per kilogram of solution; solutions with high osmolality exert more pressure than do those with fewer particles

⚬ **hypothalamus**
area at base of brain that regulates appetite and thirst

⚬ **dehydrated**
having lost large amounts of water

solutes that maintain the balance between intracellular and extracellular fluids. Potassium is the principal electrolyte in intracellular fluid. Sodium is the principal electrolyte in extracellular fluid. **Osmolality** is the measure of particles in a solution.

When the electrolytes in the extracellular fluid are *increased,* ICF moves to the ECF in an attempt to equalize the concentration of electrolytes on both sides of the membrane. This movement reduces the amount of water in the cells. The cells of the **hypothalamus** (regulates appetite and thirst) then become **dehydrated,** as do those in the mouth and tongue, and the body experiences thirst. The hypothalamus stimulates the pituitary gland to excrete ADH (antidiuretic

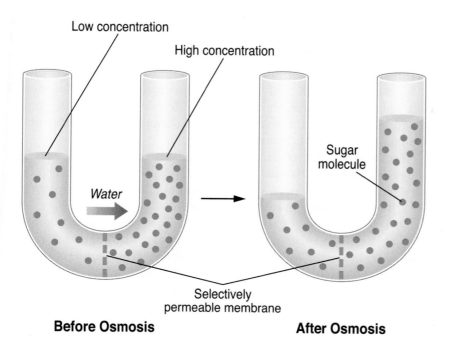

Before Osmosis **After Osmosis**

Figure 9-2 *In osmosis, water passes through the selectively permeable cell membrane from an area of low-solute concentration to an area of high-solute concentration.*

hormone) whenever the electrolytes become too concentrated in the blood or whenever blood volume or blood pressure is too low. (This measurement is called **vascular osmotic pressure**.) The ADH causes the kidneys to reabsorb water rather than excrete it. At such times, thirst causes the healthy person to drink fluids, which provide the water and electrolytes needed by the cells.

When the sodium in the ECF is reduced, water flows from the ECF into the cells, causing **cellular edema**. When this occurs, the adrenal glands secrete aldosterone, which triggers the kidneys to increase the amount of sodium reabsorbed. When the missing sodium is replaced in the ECF, the excess water that has been drawn from the ECF into the cells moves back to the ECF, and the edema is relieved.

The amount of water used and thus needed each day varies, depending on age, size, activity, environmental temperature, and physical condition. The average adult water requirement is 1 ml (milliliter) for every calorie in food consumed. For example, for every 1,800 kcal in food consumed, one needs to drink 7.5 glasses of fluid. For optimal health, it is recommended that adults drink at least thirteen 8-ounce glasses of fluid a day, preferably eight glasses of water but at least seven of water and five of other fluids. Youth, fever, diarrhea, unusual perspiration, and hyperthyroidism increase the requirement.

Dehydration

When the amount of water in the body is inadequate, **dehydration** can occur. It can be caused by inadequate intake or abnormal loss. Such loss can occur from severe diarrhea, vomiting, hemorrhage, burns, diabetes mellitus, excessive perspiration, excessive urination, or the use of certain medications such as diuretics. Symptoms of dehydration include low blood pressure, thirst, dry skin, fever, and mental disorientation.

vascular osmotic pressure
high concentration of electrolytes in the blood; low blood volume or blood pressure

cellular edema
swelling of body cells caused by inadequate amount of sodium in extracellular fluid

dehydration
loss of water

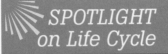
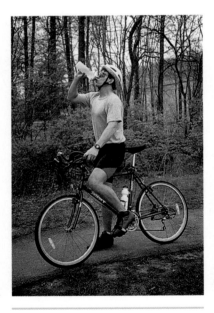

Figure 9-3 *Preventing dehydration is an important element of proper nutrition.*

As water is lost, electrolytes are also lost. Thus, treatment includes replacement of electrolytes and fluids. Electrolyte content must be checked and corrections made if necessary. A loss of 10% of body water can cause serious problems. Blood volume and nutrient absorption are reduced, and kidney function is upset. A loss of 20% of body water can cause circulatory failure and death. Infants, for example, are at high risk of dehydration when fever, vomiting, and diarrhea occur. Intravenous fluids are often necessary if sufficient fluids cannot be consumed by mouth.

The thirst sensation often lags behind the body's need for water, especially in the elderly, children, athletes, and the ill. Feeling thirsty is not a reliable indicator of when the body needs water. Fluids should be drunk throughout the day to prevent dehydration (Figure 9-3 and Table 9-4).

Dehydration can occur in hot weather when one perspires excessively but fails to drink sufficient water to replace the amount lost through perspiration. Failure to replace water lost through perspiration could lead to one of the four stages of heat illness or could progress through all four. The four stages of heat illness are: (1) *Heat fatigue*, which causes thirst, feelings of weakness, or fatigue. To combat this, one should go to a cool place, rest, and drink fluids. (2) *Heat cramp*, due to the loss of sodium and potassium, which causes leg cramps and thirst. One should go to a cool place, rest, and drink fluids. (3) *Heat exhaustion*, which causes thirst, dizziness, nausea, headache, and profuse sweating. Treatment includes sponge baths with cool water, a 2- to 3-day rest, and the ingestion of a great deal of water. (4) *Heat stroke*, which involves fever and could produce brain and kidney damage. Emergency medical service (911) should be called, and the patient should be put in chilled water and transported to the hospital. People can die from heat stroke. People who are unable to perspire are at high risk for any of the stages of heat illness.

Excess Water Accumulation

Some conditions cause an excessive accumulation of fluid in the body. This condition is called positive water balance. It occurs when more water is taken in than is used and excreted, and edema results. Hypothyroidism, congestive heart failure, hypoproteinemia (low amounts of protein), some infections, some cancers, and some renal conditions can cause such water retention be-

Table 9-4 *Signs of Dehydration*
Health history reveals inadequate intake of fluids.
Decrease in urine output.
Weight loss (% body weight): 3%–5% for mild, 6%–9% for moderate, and 10%–15% for severe dehydration.
Eyes appear sunken; tongue has increased furrows and fissures.
Oral mucous membranes are dry.
Decreased skin turgor (normal skin resiliency).
Changes in neurological status may occur with moderate to severe dehydration.

cause sodium is not being excreted normally. Fluids and sodium may then be restricted. Excess water drinking is a recognized characteristic of schizophrenia. Also it has been reported that acute psychological stress had led to excessive water drinking that resulted in brain damage (Mukherjee et al., 2005). Those without a medical or psychological condition are not prone to excess water intake.

ACID-BASE BALANCE

In addition to maintaining fluid and electrolyte balance, the body must also maintain **acid-base balance.** This is the regulation of hydrogen ions in body fluids (**pH** balance).

In a water solution, an acid gives off hydrogen ions and a base picks them up. Hydrochloric acid is an example of an acid found in the body. It is secreted by the stomach and is necessary for the digestion of proteins. Ammonia is a base produced in the kidneys from amino acids.

Acidic substances run from pH 1 to 7, with the lowest numbers representing the most acidic (which contain the most hydrogen ions). Alkaline substances run from pH 7 to 14, with the alkalinity increasing with the number (as the number of hydrogen ions decreases). A pH of 7 is considered neutral. Blood plasma runs from pH 7.35 to 7.45. Intracellular fluid has a pH of 6.8. The kidneys play the primary role in maintaining the acid-base balance by selecting which ions to retain and which to excrete. For the most part, what a person eats affects the acidity not of the body but of the urine.

Buffer Systems

The body has **buffer systems** that regulate hydrogen ion content in body fluids. Such a system is a mixture of a weak acid and a strong base that reacts to protect the nature of the solution in which it exists. In a normal buffer system, the ratio of base to acid is 20:1. For example, when a strong acid is added to a buffered solution, the base takes up the hydrogen ions of the strong acid, thereby weakening it. When a strong base is added to a solution, the acid of the buffer system combines with this base and weakens it.

A mixture of carbonic acid and sodium bicarbonate forms the body's main buffer system. Carbonic acid moves easily to buffer a strong alkali, and sodium bicarbonate moves easily to buffer a strong acid. Amounts are easily adjusted by the lungs and kidneys to suit needs. For example, the end products of metabolism are carbon dioxide and water, and together they can form carbonic acid. The hemoglobin in the blood carries carbon dioxide to the lungs, where the excess is excreted. If the amount of carbon dioxide is more concentrated than it should be, the medulla oblongata in the brain causes the breathing rate to increase. This increase, in turn, increases the rate at which the body rids itself of carbon dioxide. Excess sodium bicarbonate is excreted via the kidneys. The kidneys can excrete urine from pH 4.5 to pH 8. The pH of average urine is 6.

EXPLORING THE WEB

Search the Web for information related to the water needs of elderly and pediatric clients. How do the water needs differ in these two client populations? Why is there a difference? Why are these two populations at increased risk for dehydration? What tips can you provide to clients to maintain adequate water intake in these two client groups?

acid-base balance
the regulation of hydrogen ions in body fluids

pH
symbol for the degree of acidity or alkalinity of a solution

buffer systems
protective systems regulating amounts of hydrogen ions in body fluids

Acidosis and Alkalosis

⊙ **acidosis**
condition in which excess acids accumulate or there is a loss of base in the body

⊙ **alkalosis**
condition in which excess base accumulates in, or acids are lost from, the body

The healthy person eating a balanced diet does not normally have to think about acid-base balance. Upsets can occur in some disease conditions, however. Renal failure, uncontrolled diabetes mellitus, starvation, or severe diarrhea can cause **acidosis**. This is a condition in which the body is unable to balance the need for bases with the amount of acids it is retaining. **Alkalosis** can occur when the body has suffered a loss of hydrochloric acid from severe vomiting or has ingested too much alkali, such as too many antacid tablets.

CONSIDERATIONS FOR THE HEALTH CARE PROFESSIONAL

Clients who are required to limit both their salt and liquid intake will probably be unhappy with their diets. In such cases, it is helpful when the dietitian can discuss realistic ways of planning menus for them and *with* them. These menus should be based, of course, on good nutrition, but they also must be based on the client's normal habits and desires as much as is possible. The client's former diet should be reviewed with the client. The high-salt and high-liquid foods should be pointed out and alternative foods presented in a positive manner.

⊙ SUPERSIZE USA

Lance Armstrong is my idol. I too love cycling and have competed in some short races. Now I am ready for my first long race that will take at least 5 hours and maybe longer. The day of the race is hot and humid, but I have my water, and there will be stations for water along the way. I am racing well and have downed my first bottle of water (480 ml) and have been riding for about 1 hour. I am drinking my second bottle of water (480 ml) and am into my second hour of racing. The hot and humid weather is taking its toll on me, and I am feeling dehydrated, so I start my third bottle (480 ml) and a fourth bottle (480 ml)—I have been riding for 3 hours. I continue to drink, and after two more bottles of water I begin to feel nauseated, really tired; I feel like I can't remember how much water I have had or how much more I need—I'm confused. I have to stop racing. I learn from the physician that I have hyponatremia (low sodium concentrations) caused by overhydration. How did I end up drinking too much water? I thought I needed a lot of water because I was perspiring so much.

The physician recognized my symptoms. After he obtained my weight and discovered I had gained weight, he knew definitively that I was suffering from overhydration. I was told that fluid intake of 500 ml/hr would have been sufficient for this 5-hour race. I also learned that I should not limit my sodium intake before the race. I will be better prepared for the next race.

SUMMARY

Water is a component of all tissues. It is a solvent for nutrients and body wastes and provides transport for both. It is essential for hydrolysis, lubrication, and maintenance of normal temperature. Its best sources are water, beverages, fruits, vegetables, soups, and water-based desserts.

Fluid balance and electrolyte balance are dependent upon one another. An upset in one can cause an upset in the other. An inadequate supply of water can result in dehydration, which can be caused by severe diarrhea, vomiting, hemorrhage, burns, or excessive perspiration or urination. Symptoms include thirst, dry skin, fever, lowered blood pressure, and mental disorientation. Dehydration can result in death. Positive water balance is an excess accumulation of water in the body. It causes edema.

Acid-base balance is the regulation of hydrogen ions in the body. Excessive acids or inadequate amounts of base can cause acidosis. Excessive base or inadequate amounts of acids can cause alkalosis.

Healthy people eating a balanced diet need not be concerned about fluid, electrolyte, or acid-base balance, as the body has intricate maintenance systems for all.

DISCUSSION TOPICS

1. Why can people live longer without food than without water?

2. Why does water constitute a larger proportion of a man's body weight than of a woman's?

3. Describe homeostasis.

4. How do the lungs help to prevent excess acid from developing in the body?

5. What happens to the skin when it touches a red-hot pan? How might such developments on a large scale upset the body's fluid and electrolyte balance?

6. What is alkalosis? What causes it?

7. Explain how dehydration is dangerous in adults and in infants and children.

8. What does pH mean? How is it related to the homeostasis of the body?

SUGGESTED ACTIVITIES

1. Ask a nurse to describe what happens to body tissue when it is badly burned. Also ask about the treatment of burn clients, including diet.

2. Ask a nurse to describe a diabetic coma, explaining what causes it, why it can be life-threatening, and how it can be treated.

REVIEW

Multiple choice. Select the *letter* that precedes the best answer.

1. Fluid within the cells is called
   a. interstitial fluid
   b. extracellular fluid
   c. intracellular fluid
   d. none of the above

2. Intravascular fluid contains
   a. interstitial fluid
   b. extracellular fluid
   c. intracellular fluid
   d. none of the above

3. In a mixture of sugar and water, water is the
   a. solvent
   b. solute
   c. solution
   d. none of the above

4. Water
   a. is essential for hydrolysis
   b. causes hydrogenation
   c. reduces hypoproteinemia
   d. is produced by hypothyroidism

5. Good sources of water include
   a. oranges and melon
   b. seafood and meats
   c. baked desserts and rice
   d. all of the above

6. The solute in the extracellular fluid principally responsible for maintaining fluid balance is
   a. potassium
   b. phosphorus
   c. calcium
   d. sodium

7. The solute in the intracellular fluid principally responsible for maintaining fluid balance is
   a. potassium
   b. phosphorus
   c. calcium
   d. sodium

8. ADH causes the kidneys to
   a. conserve fluid
   b. reabsorb water
   c. release additional sodium
   d. excrete increased amounts of urine

9. The amount of water needed by individuals
   a. varies from day to day
   b. is not affected by one's activities
   c. decreases with fever
   d. all of the above

10. Positive water balance
    a. means one's intake is equal to output
    b. can cause hydrogenation
    c. may cause edema
    d. is a good thing

CASE IN POINT

UTE: REACTING TO DEHYDRATION

Ute is a nurse from South Africa who has just changed jobs and career paths. She no longer is working as an office nurse in a physician's office but has embarked into the field of nephrology. Ute has been in orientation and is learning about the kidney and its functions as well as about the dialysis equipment. Ute is impressed by all the precautions needed to prevent the spread of infection to the patients with catheters and prevent the possible cross-contamination of hidden diseases to the staff.

Ute will be initiating treatment for a dialysis patient. She finds it very exciting and very frightening as well. Ute has learned that she could kill a patient in a matter of 3 minutes if she is not careful and diligent regarding her practice.

Ute has been dialyzing patients for 3 weeks now. The hours are long, and the treatment schedules are close together. She has come to hate putting on the plastic cover-ups prior to initiating treatment. She says that she perspires so heavily in the plastic that she feels like a terrarium. Her scrub top is saturated by the time she takes off her plastic cover-ups. Besides the cover-ups, she must wear latex-free gloves, a mask, and eye protection. She knows that the patient changeover shifts are 2 hours in length, and she must comply with the policies to protect her patients and herself.

She has noticed that she has not been able to drink as much water as she would like because of her schedule. At night she has been awakened with grueling thigh and ankle cramps.

ASSESSMENT

1. What can you tell Ute that is happening to her?
2. What data support your conclusion?
3. What does Ute's increasing her physical exertion at work have to do with her condition?
4. What can be expected to occur if Ute ignores the leg cramps?

DIAGNOSIS

5. Complete the following nursing diagnosis statement: Ute's deficient fluid volume is related to _____ as evidenced by her behavior of _____.

PLAN/GOAL

6. What would be your immediate concern for Ute?
7. What is your concern for her nursing shift?

IMPLEMENTATION

8. What fluid is most helpful to Ute? Why?
9. How much fluid does she need to drink?
10. What else should Ute be aware of during her nursing shift?

EVALUATION/OUTCOME CRITERIA

11. What should Ute look for when her plan is effective?
12. Who else could benefit from this information?

THINKING FURTHER

13. At what point could Ute have avoided her cramping problem?

◎ RATE THIS PLATE

Ute is becoming dehydrated due to excessive perspiration and not drinking enough fluids. Can Ute's hydration be helped with food? Rate the plate.

4 oz broiled chicken on a bun with lettuce and tomato

1 oz corn chips

1 large carrot

1 stalk of celery

8-oz glass of fat-free milk

Which food has the most percentage of water and the least percentage? Look in Appendix D for percent of water content in foods. Were you surprised with any percentages you found? Would you change anything, and if so, what?

CASE IN POINT

MOSES: MANAGING DIARRHEA

Moses is a 72-year-old Egyptian gentleman who has been living in an assisted nursing home for the past 8 months, since his wife died. Moses's son could not relocate to Michigan to help his father after his mother's death, and he felt that his father needed assistance for daily living. Moses misses his wife very much and at first had difficulty accepting the need for a nursing home. After a few months, Moses has met some of his home mates and has become interested in playing bingo and bridge and singing in the choir. He likes being out with his friends now and is happy to have his days filled with activity. Two weeks ago Moses had a bout of what he called the stomach flu. He had persistent diarrhea for 9 days, along with a temperature of 102. His mental status, usually clear, is now classified as disorientated.

ASSESSMENT

1. What has happened to Moses?
2. What data do you have to support your findings?
3. What conditions will occur if Moses's diarrhea and temperature are not treated?
4. Because of his age, what do you know about Moses's total body water content?

DIAGNOSIS

5. Complete the following nursing diagnosis statement: Moses's deficient fluid volume is related to _____ as evidenced by his behavior of _____ .

PLAN/GOAL

6. What is your immediate concern for Moses?
7. What is your concern for the next 24 hours?

IMPLEMENTATION

8. What fluid would be most helpful to Moses and why?
9. How much fluid should he have?
10. What else should be done to treat Moses?
11. What should Moses do the next time he starts to have diarrhea?

EVALUATION/OUTCOME CRITERIA

12. What changes will you expect to see if your plan is effective?

THINKING FURTHER

13. At what point could Moses have avoided this problem?
14. How could you use this lesson in your future experiences?

◎ RATE ᴛʜɪꜱ PLATE

Moses has been ill for a long time and may be dehydrated. He is having diarrhea without vomiting. I don't believe food will cure his problem, but let's see if we can make eating pleasant and easy on his GI system. Rate this plate.

1 glass orange juice

2 poached eggs

1 to 2 slices 100% whole wheat toast with jelly

Tea with sugar and cream

Would you change any food? If so, what would you substitute in its place?

Section Two

MAINTENANCE

OF HEALTH

THROUGH

GOOD

NUTRITION

FOOD-RELATED ILLNESSES AND ALLERGIES

OBJECTIVES

After studying this chapter, you should be able to:

- Identify diseases caused by contaminated food, their signs, and the means by which they are spread

- List signs of food contamination

- State precautions for protecting food from contamination

- Describe allergies and elimination diets and their uses

The most nutritious food can cause illness if it is contaminated with **pathogens** (disease-causing agents) or certain chemicals. Some of the pathogens that can cause foodborne illness include certain bacteria, viruses, molds, worms, and protozoa. The chemicals may be a natural component of specific foods, intentionally added during production or processing or accidentally added through carelessness or pollution.

○ **pathogens**
disease-causing agents

○ **food poisoning**
foodborne illness

○ **enterotoxins**
toxins affecting mucous membranes

○ **neurotoxins**
toxins affecting the nervous system

There are always microorganisms in the environment. Some are useful, such as the bacteria used to make yogurt and certain cheeses. Others are pathogens. Pathogens may be in the air, on equipment, in food, on the skin, or in mucus and feces. Food is a particularly good breeding place for them because it provides nutrients, moisture, and often warmth. Although pathogens can be found in all food groups, they are most commonly found in foods from animal sources. Contaminated food seldom smells, looks, or tastes different from non-contaminated food.

Food poisoning is a general term for foodborne illness. When food poisoning develops as a result of a pathogen's infecting someone, it is a *foodborne infection*. When it is caused by toxins produced by the pathogen, it is called *food intoxication* and, in the case of botulism, can kill. Toxins can be produced by bacteria during food preparation or storage or by bacteria in one's digestive tract. **Enterotoxins** affect mucous membranes in the digestive tract, and **neurotoxins** affect the nervous system.

It is thought that as many as one-third of the population of the United States may experience food poisoning each year. Its typical symptoms include vomiting, diarrhea, headache, and abdominal cramps. Many never know they are suffering from food poisoning and assume they have the flu. Others, especially young children, the elderly, or those with compromised immune systems (such as people who are HIV positive) may become very ill, and some may die.

BACTERIA THAT CAUSE FOODBORNE ILLNESS

Campylobacter jejuni, Clostridium botulinum, Clostridium perfringens, Cyclospora Cayentanensis, Escherichia coli 0157:H7, Listeria monocytogenes, Salmonella, Shigella, and *Staphylococcus aureas* are examples of bacteria that can cause foodborne illness. Refer to Table 10-1.

Campylobacter jejuni

Campylobacter jejuni is believed to be one of the most prevalent causes of diarrhea. It is commonly found in the intestinal tracts of cattle, pigs, sheep, chickens, turkeys, dogs, and cats, and can contaminate meat during slaughter. It is caused by the ingestion of live bacteria.

It can take from 2 to 5 (or more) days to develop after infection, and may last up to 10 days. Symptoms include diarrhea (sometimes bloody), fever, headache, muscle and abdominal pain, and nausea. It can be transmitted to humans via unpasteurized milk, contaminated water, and raw or undercooked meats, poultry, and shellfish.

Clostridium botulinum

Clostridium botulinum is found in soil and water, on plants, and in the intestinal tracts of animals and fish. The spores of these bacteria can divide and produce toxin in the absence of oxygen. (Spores are single cells that are produced asexually, each of which is able to develop into a new organism. They have thick, protective walls that allow them to survive unfavorable conditions.) This means

Table 10-1 *Foodborne Illnesses*

BACTERIA	TRANSMISSION	SYMPTOMS	PREVENTION
Campylobacter jejuni	Unpasteurized milk, contaminated water, raw and undercooked meat and shellfish.	Diarrhea, fever, headache, abdominal pain, and nausea.	Avoid unpasteurized milk and questionable water. Cook meat and fish thoroughly.
Clostridium botulinum	Home-canned and, rarely, improperly prepared commercially canned food.	Double vision, speech difficulties, inability to swallow, respiratory paralysis.	Avoid bulging cans. Boil home-canned green beans for 10 minutes.
Clostridium perfringens	Sometimes referred to as the "cafeteria germ." Outbreaks occur when large quantities of food are served at room temperature or from a steam table. Meat, poultry, cooked dried beans, and gravies are the most common carriers.	Diarrhea and gas pains beginning between 6 and 24 hours after ingestion and lasting approximately 24 hours.	Keep hot food hot (at or above 140°F) and cold food cold (at or below 40°F). Leftovers should be heated to at least 165°F before serving. Wash all soil from vegetables.
Cyclospora cayentanensis	Feces-contaminated food or water.	Watery diarrhea, abdominal cramps, decreased appetite, and low-grade fever. Could last off and on for several weeks.	Thorough hand washing. Washing fruit before eating, using and drinking only clean water.
Escherichia coli (E. coli 0157:H7)	Eating contaminated foods such as undercooked hamburger, ground poultry, and unpasteurized milk and apple juice.	Abdominal cramps, watery diarrhea, nausea, and vomiting. Serious complications: bloody diarrhea and severe abdominal cramps. Onset within 3–9 days. Duration 2–9 days if no complications.	Cook ground meat to 160°F. Eat no raw ground meat. Wash all fruits and vegetables before eating.
Listeria monocytogenes	Unpasteurized milk, raw and cooked poultry, and meat, raw leafy vegetables.	Fever, chills, headache, backache, and occasional abdominal pain and diarrhea. Onset 12 hours to 8 days.	Avoid unpasteurized milk and dairy products. Cook ground meats to 160°F, ground poultry to 165°F. Hot foods should be kept hot and cold foods cold. Wash produce thoroughly.

(continued)

Table 10-1 *Continued*

BACTERIA	TRANSMISSION	SYMPTOMS	PREVENTION
Salmonella	Raw or undercooked food such as eggs, poultry, unpasteurized milk, or other dairy products and meats. Cross-contamination by uncooked foods.	Headache, abdominal pain, diarrhea, fever, and nausea. Onset: 6–48 hours. Duration: 1–8 days.	Avoid cross-contamination of raw and cooked foods. Do not eat raw eggs. Cook ground beef to 160°F. Keep hot foods hot and cold foods cold. Do not eat any unpasteurized raw or undercooked food of animal origin.
Shigella	Contamination of food by infected food handlers. Primarily transmitted in cold salads such as tuna, chicken, and potato.	Severe diarrhea, nausea, headaches, chills, and dehydration. Onset 1 day to a week.	Good hygiene of food handlers and sanitary food preparation. Keep hot foods hot and cold foods cold. Always wash hands in hot soapy water after going to the bathroom and before preparing or eating food.
Staphylococcus aureas	Transmitted by infected food handlers.	Vomiting, diarrhea, abdominal cramps. Onset: ½–8 hours. Duration: 1–2 days.	Good hygiene of food handlers. Always wash hands thoroughly in hot soapy water before preparing food. Keep hot food hot and cold food cold.

Source: Centers for Disease Control and Prevention. (2005). Retrieved from www.cdc.gov.

botulism

deadliest of food poisonings; caused by the bacteria *Clostridium botulinum*

that toxin can be produced in sealed containers such as cans, jars, and vacuum-packaged foods.

The spores are extremely heat resistant and must be boiled for 6 hours before they will be destroyed. Such a lengthy time will, of course, destroy the food they have infected. The toxin, however, can be destroyed by boiling for 20 minutes. This toxin causes **botulism**, which is perhaps the rarest but most deadly of all food poisonings. Symptoms usually appear within 4 to 36 hours after eating and include double vision, speech difficulties, inability to swallow, and respiratory paralysis. If botulism is not properly treated, death will result in 3 to 10 days. The fatality rate in the United States is about 65%.

Great care must be taken to prevent botulism when canning foods at home. The Centers for Disease Control and Prevention (CDC) reported that from 1950 through 1996, 289 botulism outbreaks have been traced to home-processed foods and 31 to commercially processed foods, including foods served in restaurants. The type of food processing was unknown for the remaining 124 outbreaks. Vegetables were the most important carrier for the botulism toxin in the United States during this time period. Raw honey has also been identified as a source. If a can bulges, *Clostridium botulinum* may be present and can be fatal. A good rule of thumb is: "If in doubt, throw it out" where children and animals cannot reach it.

Clostridium perfringens

Clostridium perfringens is often called the "cafeteria" or "buffet germ" because it tends to infect those who eat food that has been standing on buffets or steam tables for long periods. *Clostridium perfringens* is found in soil dust, sewage, and the intestinal tracts of animals. It is a spore-forming pathogen that needs little oxygen. The bacteria are destroyed by cooking, but the spores can survive it.

  Clostridium perfringens is transmitted by eating heavily contaminated food. Symptoms include nausea, diarrhea, and inflammation of the stomach and intestine. Symptoms may appear within 6 to 24 hours of ingestion and last approximately 24 hours.

  To best prevent it, hot foods should be kept at or above 140°F and cold foods below 40°F. Leftovers should be heated to 165°F before serving. Foods should be stored at temperatures of 40°F or lower. People with compromised immune systems should be very cautious concerning *Clostridium perfringens*.

Cyclospora cayentanensis

Cyclospora cayentanensis is a parasite that causes gastroenteritis. Until 1996 most cases were experienced by overseas travelers, but several domestic outbreaks have been reported in recent years. This bacteria is commonly found in the feces of an infected person and can be transmitted by poor hygiene. It has been found in unclean water.

  Symptoms are watery diarrhea, abdominal cramps, decreased appetite, and a low-grade fever. These symptoms could last off and on for several weeks. Those with compromised immune systems, children, and the elderly are at greatest risk of complications.

  Cyclospora has an incubation period of 1 week, is associated with invasion of the small intestine, and is manifested by the preceding symptoms. The parasite's natural ecology, infective dose, and host range are unknown. It is known that *Cyclospora* does not multiply outside the host.

  It is strongly recommended that clean water be used for drinking and the irrigation of produce. Thorough washing of fruits and vegetables and the practice of good hygiene by food handlers help to prevent the spread of this bacteria.

Escherichia coli (E. coli 0157:H7)

Escherichia coli, commonly called *E. coli*, is a group of bacteria that can cause illness in humans. E. coli 0157:H7 is a very infectious strain of this group. These bacteria can be found in the intestines of some mammals (including humans and animals used for food), in raw milk, and in water contaminated by animal or human feces.

E. coli are transmitted to humans through contaminated water, unpasteurized milk or apple juice, raw or rare ground beef products, unwashed fruits or vegetables, and directly from person to person. Plant foods can be contaminated by fertilization with raw manure or irrigation with contaminated water.

Symptoms include severe abdominal cramps, diarrhea that may be watery or bloody, and nausea. Sometimes, however, E. coli 0157:H7 can cause hemorrhagic colitis (inflammation of the colon). This in turn can result in *hemolytic uremic syndrome* (HUS) in children, which can damage the kidneys.

E. coli can be controlled by careful choice and cooking of foods. All meats and poultry should be cooked thoroughly. Ground beef, veal, and lamb should be cooked to 160°F and ground poultry to at least 165°F. Fruits and vegetables should be carefully washed, and unpasteurized milk and other dairy products and vegetable and fruit juices should be avoided. People with compromised immune systems should be especially vigilant.

Listeria monocytogenes

Listeria monocytogenes is a bacteria often found in human and animal intestines and in milk, leafy vegetables, and soil. It can grow in the refrigerator and can be transmitted to humans by unpasteurized dairy foods such as milk, soft cheeses, and ice creams and via raw leafy vegetables and processed meats.

Listeria monocytogenes can affect a person from 12 hours to 8 days after ingestion. Symptoms include fatigue, fever, chills, headache, backache, abdominal pain, and diarrhea. It can develop into more serious conditions and cause respiratory distress, spontaneous abortion, or meningitis.

To prevent infection by *Listeria monocytogenes*, meats and poultry should be thoroughly cooked and salad greens carefully washed. Attention must be paid to all dairy products—especially the unfamiliar from new sources—to be certain they have been pasteurized.

Salmonellosis

salmonella
an infection caused by the *Salmonella* bacteria

Salmonellosis (commonly called *salmonella*) is an infection caused by the *Salmonella* bacteria. **Salmonella** can be found in raw meats, poultry, fish, milk, and eggs. It is transmitted by eating contaminated food or by contact with a carrier. Salmonellosis is characterized by headache, vomiting, diarrhea, abdominal cramps, and fever. Symptoms generally begin from 6 to 48 hours after eating. In severe cases, it can result in death. One species of *Salmonella* causes typhoid fever. Those who suffer the most severe cases are typically the very young, the elderly, and the weak or incapacitated.

Refrigeration (40°F or lower) inhibits the growth of these bacteria, but they can remain alive in the freezer and in dried foods. *Salmonella* bacteria are destroyed by heating to at least 140°F for a minimum of 10 minutes.

To prevent contamination, thaw poultry and meats in the refrigerator or microwave and cook immediately. Avoid cross-contamination of raw and cooked foods by carefully cleaning utensils and counter surfaces that were in contact with raw food. Raw or undercooked eggs, or foods that contain them, should not be eaten. Even a taste of raw cookie dough or Caesar salad dressing made with raw egg yolk can cause contamination. People with compromised immune systems should be especially careful.

Shigella

Shigella bacteria are found in the intestinal tract and thus the feces of infected individuals. The disease they cause is called *shigellosis.* These bacteria are typically passed on by an infected food handler who did not wash his or her hands properly after using the toilet. They are also found on plants that were fertilized with untreated animal feces or given contaminated water. *Shigella* are destroyed by heat, but infected cold foods such as tuna, chicken, or egg salads are common carriers.

Shigellosis can occur from 1 day to a week following infection. Symptoms include diarrhea (sometimes with blood and mucus), fever, chills, headache, nausea, and abdominal cramps, and can lead to dehydration. Some people, however, experience no symptoms.

Staphylococcus aureus

Staphylococcus aureas bacteria are found on human skin, in infected cuts and pimples, and in noses and throats. Staphylococcal poisoning is commonly called **staph.** These bacteria grow in meats; poultry; fish; egg dishes; salads such as potato, egg, macaroni, and tuna; and cream-filled pastries. This poisoning is transmitted by carriers and by eating foods that contain the toxin these bacteria create.

staph
staphylococcal poisoning

Symptoms, which include vomiting, diarrhea, and abdominal cramps, begin within 1/2 to 8 hours after ingestion of the toxin and last from 24 to 48 hours. Staph is considered a mild illness.

The growth of these bacteria is inhibited if foods are kept at temperatures above 140°F or below 40°F. Their toxin can be destroyed by boiling the food for several hours or by heating it in a pressure cooker at 240°F for 30 minutes. Both of these methods would destroy both the appeal and nutrient content of the infected foods. It is more practical to safely discard foods suspected of being contaminated.

OTHER SUBSTANCES THAT CAUSE FOOD POISONING

Mold is a type of fungus. Its roots go down, into the food, and it grows a stalk upward on which spores form. The green "fuzzy" part that can be seen by the naked eye is where the spores are found. Some spores cause respiratory problems and allergic reactions for some people. For this reason, moldy food should never be smelled.

mold
a type of fungus

Some molds produce a dangerous mycotoxin called aflatoxin that can cause cancer. It can develop in spoiled peanuts and peanut butter, soybeans, grains, nuts, and spices. Symptoms of such an infection include abdominal pain, vomiting, and diarrhea, and may occur from 1 day to several months after ingestion. It can cause liver and skin damage and, ultimately, cancer.

The Food and Drug Administration observes the aflatoxin content of foods closely, and although this toxin cannot as yet be totally eradicated, foods containing more than a very minute amount of it cannot be sold by one state to another.

Neither cooking nor refrigeration destroys this toxin. Cheese may develop mold, and that part should be cut away to a depth of at least an inch. (Cheeses such as bleu or Roquefort that were intentionally ripened by harmless molds are safe to eat.) Fruits and vegetables showing signs of mold should not be purchased.

Trichinella spiralis is a parasitic worm that causes **trichinosis.** This disease is transmitted by eating inadequately cooked pork from pigs that are infected with the *Trichinella spiralis* parasite. Symptoms include abdominal pain, vomiting, fever, chills, and muscle pain. Symptoms occur about 24 hours after ingesting infected pork. Cooking all pork to an internal temperature of at least 170°F kills the organism and prevents this disease. It can also be destroyed by freezing.

Dysentery is a disease caused by protozoa (tiny, one-celled animal). The protozoa are introduced to food by carriers or contaminated water. They cause severe diarrhea that can occur intermittently until the patient is treated appropriately.

PREVENTION OF FOODBORNE ILLNESSES

Strict federal, state, and local laws regulate the commercial production of food in the United States, and dairies, canneries, bakeries, and meat-packing plants are all subject to government inspection. Nevertheless, errors and accidents can and do occur, and illness can result. *Most foodborne illnesses occur because of the ignorance or carelessness of people who handle food.* People can introduce pathogens to food, prevent them from reaching it, or kill them with appropriate cooking temperatures.

Cleanliness is especially important in preventing foodborne illness. When kitchen equipment such as a cutting board, meat grinder, or countertop is used for preparing pathogen-infected foods and not cleaned properly afterward, noninfected food that is subsequently prepared with this equipment can become infected by the same pathogen(s). This is called cross-contamination. Dishes used to hold uncooked meat, poultry, fish, or eggs must always be washed before cooked foods are placed on them.

⊙ trichinosis

disease caused by the parasitic roundworm *Trichinella spiralis;* can be transmitted through undercooked pork

⊙ dysentery

disease caused by microorganism; characterized by diarrhea

EXPLORING THE WEB

Choose one of the pathogens in the text that causes foodborne illness. Research this pathogen using the Web. What sources can you find on the pathogen? Create a fact sheet listing the signs and symptoms of the illness, the foods commonly infected with the pathogen, assessment of the client for the presence of the illness, and treatment. Also include tips on prevention of the illness.

((In The Media

FOOD SAFETY MADE EASY: FOOD SAFETY TIPS OFFERED IN NEW ONLINE BROCHURE

Responding to consumer research that revealed that consumers needed more food safety information, the Partnership for Food Safety Education released a new brochure available at fightbac.org. The brochure details how to properly *clean, separate, cook,* and *chill* to reduce the risk of foodborne illness. Their research showed that consumers are familiar with clean, separate, cook, and chill, the core FightBAC! food safety recommendations, but more guidance was needed to do these properly. Many consumers are still not fully aware of the importance of:

1. Maintaining a refrigerator temperature of 40°F or below
2. Using cooking and appliance thermometers
3. Properly cleaning fresh fruits and vegetables

The gaps in consumer knowledge are addressed in this new brochure. The brochure was developed through collaboration between Partnership members and government agencies that participate in FightBAC! including the FDA, the CDC, and the USDA.

(Source: Partnership for Food Safety Education, 2004, www.fightbac.org.)

When food workers fail to wash their hands after blowing their noses or using the toilet, they can "share" their germs very easily. Mucus and feces are favorite breeding areas of pathogens.

Food workers who have even small cuts on their hands must wear gloves because a wound could carry a pathogen. Foods must be covered and stored properly to keep dust, insects, and animals from reaching and possibly contaminating them. Water from unknown sources should not be used for cooking because it, too, can carry pathogens.

Temperatures during preparation and storage of food must be carefully observed. When infected foods are undercooked, the pathogen is not destroyed and can be passed to consumers (Table 10-2). Foods allowed to stand

Table 10-2 *Cooking Temperatures*

PRODUCT	FAHRENHEIT
Eggs and Egg Dishes	
Eggs	Cook until yolk and white are firm
Egg dishes	160°
Fresh Beef, Veal, Lamb	
Ground products like hamburger (prepared as patties, meatloaf, meatballs, etc.)	160°
Roasts, steaks, and chops	
Medium rare	145°
Medium	160°
Well done	170°
Fresh Pork	
All cuts including ground product	
Medium	160°
Well done	170°
Poultry	
Ground chicken, turkey	165°
Whole chicken, turkey	
Well done	180°
Whole bird with stuffing (stuffing must reach 165°)	180°
Poultry breasts, roasts	170°
Thighs, wings	Cook until juices run clear
Ham	
Fresh (raw)	160°
Fully cooked, to reheat	140°

Source: U.S. Department of Agriculture Food Safety and Inspection Service.

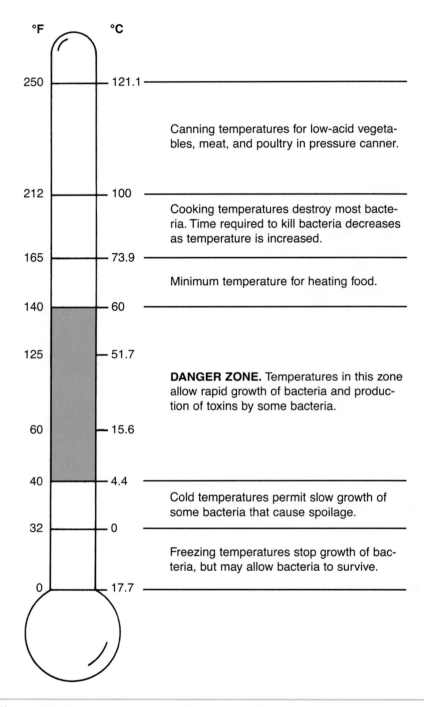

°F	°C	
250	121.1	
		Canning temperatures for low-acid vegetables, meat, and poultry in pressure canner.
212	100	
		Cooking temperatures destroy most bacteria. Time required to kill bacteria decreases as temperature is increased.
165	73.9	
		Minimum temperature for heating food.
140	60	
125	51.7	
		DANGER ZONE. Temperatures in this zone allow rapid growth of bacteria and production of toxins by some bacteria.
60	15.6	
40	4.4	
		Cold temperatures permit slow growth of some bacteria that cause spoilage.
32	0	
		Freezing temperatures stop growth of bacteria, but may allow bacteria to survive.
0	17.7	

Figure 10-1 *Temperatures of food for control of bacteria.*

at temperatures between 40° and 140°F provide an ideal breeding place for pathogens (Figure 10-1).

Leftover food should always be refrigerated as soon as the meal is finished, and covered when it is cold. It should not be allowed to cool to room temperature before it is refrigerated. Frozen food should be either cooked from the frozen state

Table 10-3 *To Prevent Food Poisoning*

- Keep kitchen and equipment thoroughly clean.
- Wash hands after blowing nose or using bathroom.
- Wear gloves if cooking with any hand wound.
- Cover and store foods to prevent microbes or animals from reaching it.
- Cook foods to appropriate temperatures.
- Limit standing time at temperatures between 40° and 140°F.
- Prevent known carriers from preparing foods.
- Select only packages and jars that were sealed by the manufacturer.
- Avoid bulging cans, foods that look or smell odd, and foods showing signs of mold.

or thawed in the refrigerator. (When cooked from the frozen state, cooking time will generally increase by at least 50%.) Frozen food should not be thawed at room temperature. Food must always be protected from dust, insects, and animals.

Carriers are people (or animals) capable of transmitting infectious (disease-causing) organisms. Often the carrier suffers no effects from the organism and therefore is unaware of the danger she or he represents. Food workers should be tested regularly to confirm that they are not carriers of communicable diseases.

Selection of food should be made with great care. Packages and jars should be properly sealed. Cans should not bulge. Foods that look or smell at all unusual and foods showing signs of mold should be left in the store. Only pasteurized milk and dairy products should be used (Table 10-3).

MISCELLANEOUS FOOD POISONINGS

Occasionally, food poisoning is caused by ingesting certain plants or animals that contain poison. Examples are plants such as poisonous mushrooms, rhubarb leaves, and fish from polluted water.

Poisoning also can result from ingesting cleaning agents, **insecticides,** or excessive amounts of a drug. Children may swallow cleaning agents or medicines. The cook may mistakenly use a poison instead of a cooking ingredient. Sometimes insecticides cling to fresh fruits and vegetables. It is essential that all potential poisons be kept out of the reach of young children and kept separate from all food supplies. Fresh fruits and vegetables should be thoroughly washed before being eaten.

FOOD ALLERGIES

An **allergy** is an altered reaction of the tissues of some individuals to substances that, in similar amounts, are harmless to other people. The substances causing **hypersensitivity** are called **allergens.** Some common allergens are pollen, dust, animal dander (bits of dried skin), drugs, cosmetics, and certain foods. This discussion will be limited to allergic reactions to foods. A food allergy occurs when the immune system reacts to a food substance, usually a protein. When such a reaction occurs, antibodies form and cause allergic symptoms. An altered

carrier
one who is capable of transmitting an infectious organism

EXPLORING THE WEB

Search the Web site of the Food Safety and Inspection Service of the U.S. Department of Agriculture, www.fsis.usda.gov. Look for information about eliminating pathogens and keeping food safe during preparation and storage. What helpful tips can you find? Create a fact sheet on maintaining the safety of food during preparation and storage in the home environment using the tips you find here.

insecticide
agent that destroys insects

allergy
sensitivity to specific substance(s)

hypersensitivity
abnormally strong sensitivity to certain substance(s)

allergens
substance-causing allergy

○ **urticaria**
hives; common allergic reaction

○ **dermatitis**
inflammation of the skin

○ **allergic reaction**
adverse physical reaction to specific substance(s)

○ **skin tests**
allergy tests using potential allergens on scratches on the skin

○ **elimination diet**
limited diet in which only certain foods are allowed; intended to find the food allergen causing reaction

reaction to a specific food that does not involve the immune system is called (the specific food) *intolerance.* Approximately 6–8% of children and 1–2% of adults are known to have food allergies; many of these allergies began in the first year of life.

Types of Allergic Reactions

Sometimes allergic reactions are immediate, and sometimes several hours elapse before signs occur. Allergic individuals seem most prone to allergic reactions during periods of stress. Typical signs of food allergies include hay fever, **urticaria,** edema, headache, **dermatitis,** nausea, dizziness, and asthma (which causes breathing difficulties).

Allergic reactions are uncomfortable and can be detrimental to health. When breathing difficulties are severe, they are life-threatening.

Allergic reactions to the same food can differ in two individuals. For example, the fact that someone gets hives from eating strawberries does not mean that an allergic reaction to strawberries will appear as hives in another member of the same family. Allergic reactions can even differ from time to time with the same individual.

Treatment of Allergies

The simplest treatment for allergies is to remove the item that causes the allergic reaction. However, because of the variety of allergic reactions, finding the allergen can be difficult.

When food allergies are suspected, it is wise for the patient to keep a food diary for several days and to record all food and drink ingested as well as allergic reactions and the time of their onset. Such records can help pinpoint specific allergens. Some common food allergens are listed in Table 10-4. It is common for other foods in the same class as the allergens to cause allergic reactions as well. Cooking sometimes alters the foods and can eliminate allergic reactions in some people.

Laboratory tests may be used to find the allergen or allergens. The RAST (radio allergosorbent test), for example, may be used to determine which compounds are causing allergic reactions. **Skin tests** are sometimes used to detect allergies. However, food allergies can be difficult to determine from skin tests.

After completion of the allergy testing, the client is usually placed on an **elimination diet.** For 1 or 2 weeks the client does not eat any of the tested compounds that gave a positive reaction. The client includes in the diet the foods that almost no one reacts to, such as rice, fresh meats and poultry,

Table 10-4 *Common Food Allergens*

Milk	Strawberries	Chocolate
Wheat	Tomatoes	Soybeans
Corn	Legumes	Pork
Eggs	Tree nuts	Fish
Citrus fruit	Peanuts	Shellfish

noncitrus fruits, and vegetables. Sometimes, these diets allow only a limited number of foods and can be nutritionally inadequate. If that is the case, vitamin and mineral supplements may be prescribed.

When relief is found from the allergic symptoms, the client is continued on the diet, and, gradually, other foods are added to the diet at a rate of only one every 4 to 7 days. Those foods most likely to produce allergic reactions are added last until an allergic reaction occurs. The allergy can then be pinpointed, and the offending foods eliminated from the diet. Knowing the cause of the allergy enables the client to lead a healthy, normal life, provided that eliminating these foods does not affect her or his nutrition.

If the elimination of the allergen results in a diet deficient in certain nutrients, suitable substitutes for those nutrients must be found. For example, if a client is allergic to citrus fruits, other foods rich in vitamin C to which the client is not allergic must be found. If the allergy is to milk, soybean milk may be substituted.

The client must be taught the food sources of the nutrient or nutrients lacking so that other foods can be substituted that are nutritionally equal to those causing the allergy. It is essential that the client be taught to read the labels on commercially prepared foods and to check the ingredients of restaurant foods carefully. Baked products, mixes, meat loaf, or pancakes may contain egg, milk, or wheat that may be responsible for the allergic reaction.

Sometimes, however, the allergies require such a restriction of foods that the diet does become nutritionally inadequate. As in all cases of allergy, and particularly in such cases, it is hoped that the client can become **desensitized** to the allergens so that a nutritionally balanced diet can be restored. The client is desensitized by eating a minute amount of food allergen after a period of complete **abstinence** from it. The amount of the allergen is gradually increased until the client can tolerate it.

EXPLORING THE WEB

Go to the Web site for the International Food Information Council Foundation, www.ific.org. Search for information on allergic reactions and foods. What types of illnesses can be caused by food allergies? How are these allergies detected? Can you locate a recipe source online for individuals with food allergies?

desensitize
to gradually reduce the body's sensitivity (allergic reaction) to specific items

abstinence
avoidance

SUPERSIZE **USA**

More and more children and teenagers are becoming obese. School cafeteria and vending machines are a logical place to begin changing students' eating habits. According to the Centers for Disease Control and Prevention, many schools are "making it happen" and have been successful in replacing soft drinks with water and juice, regular chips with low-fat or baked chips, candy with fruits, and fried foods with yogurt, thus giving students healthful choices. Students will soon consider healthful choices as the "norm" when those are all they see in the vending machines and the a la carte offerings. Couple these practices with concerns over keeping food safe and fresh, as well as offering allergy-free snack choices for students with peanut or other food intolerances. The role of the school nurse or dietitian is becoming more important and necessary.

(Source: Food and Nutrition Service, USDA; Centers for Disease Control Prevention, USDHHS; U.S. Department of Education. [2005, January]. *Making it happen! School nutrition success stories.* Retrieved May 4, 2006, from www.cdc.gov/Healthy Youth/Nutrition/Making-It-Happen.)

CONSIDERATIONS FOR THE HEALTH CARE PROFESSIONAL

Some clients will need simple instructions from the health care professional about avoiding microbial contamination of food supplies at home. Many, if not most, should be warned not to thaw food at room temperature. Others should be reminded that leftover foods should *not* be cooled at room temperature before being refrigerated.

Clients with food allergies will require careful training to avoid their specific allergens. They must be taught to read food labels carefully and to ask for the ingredients of foods in restaurants and at friends' homes. Role-playing is an effective way to help such clients.

SUMMARY

Infection or poisoning traced to food is usually caused by human ignorance or carelessness. The serving of safe meals is essentially the responsibility of the cook. Food should not be prepared by anyone who has or carries a contagious disease. All fresh fruits and vegetables should be washed before being eaten. Meats, poultry, fish, eggs, and dairy products should be refrigerated. Pork should always be cooked to the well-done stage. Food should be covered to prevent contamination by dust, insects, or animals. Garbage should also be covered so that it does not attract insects. Hands that prepare foods should be clean and free of cuts or wounds. Kitchen equipment should be spotless. Finally, the food itself should be safe. People should avoid foods containing natural poisons.

Food allergies can cause many different and unpleasant symptoms. Elimination diets are used to determine their causes. Some of the most common food allergens have been found to be milk, chocolate, eggs, tomatoes, fish, citrus fruit, legumes, strawberries, and wheat.

DISCUSSION TOPICS

1. Name four types of foodborne illness. If any class member has suffered from one, ask the person to describe the symptoms.

2. How does food become contaminated?

3. Why should foods be refrigerated?

4. What are allergies? What can cause them?

5. What are some common allergic reactions to food? How can they be avoided?

6. Do people inherit allergies? Explain.

7. Of what use is a food diary in relation to allergies? What are elimination diets, and when are they used?

8. What is the most difficult part of treating food allergies?

9. How can an allergic client be desensitized?

10. Is an elimination diet always nutritious? Explain.

11. Explain how eggs, wheat, or milk may be hidden in each of the following foods: mayonnaise, bread, rye crackers, potato salad, gravy, meatloaf, breaded veal cutlet, bologna, malted milk.

SUGGESTED ACTIVITIES

1. Ask a doctor or registered nurse to explain skin tests to the class. Discuss these tests after the lecture.

2. Ask someone with food allergies to speak to the class. Follow this talk with questions from the audience.

3. Visit a restaurant kitchen. Look for practices that may lead to potential food poisoning. Note the practices and uses of equipment designed to prevent food poisoning.

REVIEW

Multiple choice. Select the *letter* that precedes the best answer.

1. A microorganism is a(n)
   a. unit of measurement
   b. tiny animal or plant
   c. component of a microscope
   d. individual human cell

2. Salmonella bacteria are destroyed by heating foods to 140°F for a minimum of
   a. 2 minutes   c. 30 minutes
   b. 10 minutes   d. 2 hours

3. Someone who is capable of spreading an infectious organism but is not sick is called a
   a. food handler   c. transport
   b. carrier   d. fomite

4. When an organism is infectious, it is
   a. disease-causing   c. not contagious
   b. prone to infections d. always fatal

5. Most cases of food poisoning in the United States are caused by
   a. careless processing in commercial factories
   b. lack of government inspection
   c. careless handling of food in the kitchen
   d. house pets

6. Food poisoning symptoms generally include
   a. joint pain
   b. constipation
   c. abdominal upset and headache
   d. swelling of the feet

7. Salmonella infections and staphylococcal poisoning are caused by
   a. a virus   c. protozoa
   b. bacteria   d. worms

8. The deadliest of the bacterial food poisonings is
   a. staphylococcal   c. botulism
      poisoning
   b. salmonellosis   d. perfringens poison-
                            ing

9. The disease caused by a parasite sometimes found in pork is
   a. tularemia   c. avitaminosis
   b. dysentery   d. trichinosis

10. The disease caused by a protozoan and characterized by severe diarrhea is
    a. salmonellosis   c. dysentery
    b. botulism   d. infectious hepatitis

11. Foods may be contaminated by
    a. people   c. refrigeration
    b. overcooking them d. all of the above

12. The temperatures in the danger zone that encourage bacterial growth are from
    a. 0 to 32°F   c. 40° to 140°F
    b. 32° to 60°F   d. 125° to 212°F

13. Leftover foods should be
    a. put in the refrigerator immediately after meals
    b. cooled to room temperature before refrigerating
    c. cooled in the refrigerator for at least an hour before freezing
    d. stored unwrapped in the refrigerator

14. Frozen foods should be
    a. thawed at room temperature
    b. refrozen if not used immediately after thawing
    c. thawed in the refrigerator
    d. any of the above

15. An adverse physical reaction to a food is called a food
    a. refusal   c. symptom
    b. allergy   d. allergen

16. Substances that cause altered physical reactions are called
    a. symptoms   c. allergens
    b. allergies   d. abstinence

17. One of the typical symptoms of food allergies is
    a. diabetes mellitus c. hives
    b. colitis   d. atherosclerosis

18. The simplest treatment for a food allergy is
    a. a skin test
    b. avoiding all fruit
    c. elimination of the allergen
    d. the use of penicillin

19. In cases of food allergy, an elimination diet may be prescribed to
    a. desensitize the   c. avoid surgery
       patient
    b. avoid medication d. find the allergen

20. Some foods that frequently cause an allergic reaction are
    a. milk, eggs, and wheat c. canned pears and tapioca
    b. lamb, rice, and sugar d. rice and pears

CASE IN POINT

MEHALIA: EATING UNSAFE FOOD

Mehalia, a 23-year-old Native American and successful businesswoman, was in a hurry. She was to be a bridesmaid in her friend Stacey's wedding in two days and could squeeze her final dress fitting in during her lunchtime. On racing to the designer's, Mehalia stopped for a quick bite at Harry's Food Stand. Mehalia ordered a hot dog, house salad with the creamy house dressing, and a diet cola. On her way to the designer, Mehalia ate her hot dog and decided to save her salad until she got back to work. After all, it would only be an hour before she would be back at her desk.

Two-and-a-half hours later, Mehalia returned to work. She ate her warm salad while she dove into her pile of work that she had to complete before leaving for the day. Leaving work at 6 p.m. was not a bad thing, Mehalia decided. The traffic was not as heavy then, and she was able to reach home in record time. When Mehalia reached home, she took her dog, Molly, for a walk. During this time Mehalia started to feel some stomach cramping and pain and knew she had better get home quickly. She made it home just in time; she started to vomit and had a horrible headache. She noticed a neck and chest rash.

ASSESSMENT

1. What subjective complaints did Mehalia have?
2. What objective data can you gather from the case study?
3. What do you suspect is the problem?
4. Which food was most likely to have caused the problem?

DIAGNOSIS

5. Mehalia's abdominal pain and diarrhea could have been caused by_____.

PLAN/GOAL

6. What is the immediate goal for Mehalia?
7. What is the long range goal?

IMPLEMENTATION

8. What information does Mehalia need to tell her doctor when she calls for an appointment?
9. Is time a factor in Mehalia's symptoms?
10. What information could have helped Mehalia?
11. How could the information on the Department of Agriculture Web site, at www.usda.gov, have helped?

EVALUATION/OUTCOME CRITERIA

12. When the intervention is complete, how will Mehalia know it has been effective?

THINKING FURTHER

13. What teaching tips or fact sheets might help Mehalia better choose and handle her food in the future?

RATE THIS PLATE

Mehalia had never been so sick! She decided that she didn't want that to happen again. Mehalia was invited to a graduation party where everyone brought a dish, and the food was served buffet style. Mehalia had known all the guests for years and knew what wonderful cooks everyone was. The buffet consisted of the following items. Make a plate for Mehalia telling why you chose what you did. Rate the plate.

Ham, roast beef, turkey, and salami (meat tray over ice)
Cocktail rolls
Mayonnaise, mustard, pickles and olive tray
Meatballs kept warm in a crock pot
Potato salad
Green salad with dressing choices on the side
Macaroni salad
Warm nacho cheese dip with tortilla chips
Cheese ball with crackers
Previously baked crab dip
Gelatin fruit salad
Chocolate cake and ice cream

CASE IN POINT

MICHAEL: DISCOVERING A SHELLFISH ALLERGY

Michael is visiting his wife's family in Boston, Massachusetts. Michael and Robin had eloped and have been married for 1 year. He is not looking forward to the visit since this is the first time he will be meeting her parents. Robin and Michael's flight arrived at Logan Airport at 6 p.m. When Robin's parents picked Michael and Robin up, they suggested that they eat at their favorite restaurant, Anthony's Pier 4. Michael is from Iowa. He is a farm boy who loves his meat and potatoes. However, he is not shy about trying new foods. At Anthony's Pier 4, Michael tries lobster for the first time. It has a fresh sea taste that he loves. Michael also tried clams and oysters on the half shell. He was okay with the clams but did not like the appearance or taste of the oysters. After their meal, the family arrived home and spent some time getting to know one another. Michael and Robin were tired after their long flight from Los Angeles, so they turned in at 10 p.m. During the night Michael awoke with severe stomach pains, and he was dizzy and nauseated. He woke Robin up, and they decided to go to the local ER for help when Michael started to complain of difficulty breathing.

ASSESSMENT

1. What complaints did Michael have during the night?
2. What objective data could be gathered by the ER nurse?
3. What would you expect to be the problem?
4. Which foods were most likely the cause of the problem?

DIAGNOSIS

5. Michael's abdominal pain and nausea could have been caused by _____.
6. What information should be gathered during his initial assessment?

PLAN/GOAL

7. What is the immediate goal for Michael?
8. What is the long-range goal?

IMPLEMENTATION

9. In the ER what should Michael and Robin discuss with the physicians?
10. Does it appear that Michael may have a food allergy?
11. Is the doctor able to verify that this is an allergy?
12. What is the most likely recommendation for Michael?
13. What should Michael be cautioned about in the future about dining out?

EVALUATION/OUTCOME CRITERIA

14. When the intervention is complete, how will Michael know it has been effective?

THINKING FURTHER

15. What information could be obtained from the Food Allergy Network, www.foodallergy-network.com?

RATE THIS PLATE

Obviously, either Michael ate something that he was allergic to, or he contracted a foodborne illness. What should be eliminated from his plate? What would be a better choice? Rate the Plate with contamination in mind.

Oysters on the half shell

Lobster

Clams

Baked potato with chive butter

Caesar salad, made at the table with raw egg, olive oil, red wine vinegar, and lemon juice

Roll and butter

Wine

Coffee with cream

CHAPTER

11

DIET DURING PREGNANCY AND LACTATION

OBJECTIVES

After studying this chapter, you should be able to:

- Identify nutritional needs during pregnancy and lactation
- Describe nutritional needs of pregnant adolescents
- Modify the normal diet to meet the needs of pregnant and lactating women

Good nutrition during the 38–40 weeks of a normal pregnancy is essential for both mother and child. In addition to her normal nutritional requirements, the pregnant woman must provide nutrients and calories for the **fetus,** the **amniotic fluid,** the **placenta,** and the increased blood volume and breast, uterine, and fat tissue.

Studies have shown a relationship between the mother's diet and the health of the baby at birth. It is also thought that the woman who consumed a nutritious diet before pregnancy is more apt to bear a healthy infant than one who did not. Malnutrition of the mother is believed to cause growth and mental **retardation** in the fetus. Low-birth-weight infants (less than 5.5 pounds) have a higher mortality (death) rate than those of normal birth weight.

In The Media

CONSEQUENCES OF EXCESSIVE WEIGHT GAIN IN PREGNANCY

Research by Dr. Yvonne Linne of Stockholm, Sweden, showed that women who gain more than 35 pounds during pregnancy will more than likely remain overweight 15 years later. In the study, women who gained up to 35 pounds were more apt to return to within 4.5 pounds of their prepregnancy weight. Any higher weight gain and they were twice as likely to remain overweight after the birth. The target amount of weight gain for the average woman during pregnancy should be between 25 and 35 pounds.

(Source: Associated Press, May 2004.)

fetus
infant in utero

amniotic fluid
surrounds fetus in the uterus

placenta
organ in the uterus that links blood supplies of mother and infant

retardation
delayed in mental development

WEIGHT GAIN DURING PREGNANCY

Weight gain during pregnancy is natural and necessary for the infant to develop normally and the mother to retain her health. In addition to the developing infant, the mother's uterus, breasts, placenta, blood volume, body fluids, and fat must all increase to accommodate the infant's needs (Table 11-1).

The average weight gain during pregnancy is 25 to 35 pounds. During the first **trimester** of pregnancy, there is an average weight gain of only 2 to 4 pounds. Most of the weight gain occurs during the second and third trimesters of pregnancy, when it averages about 1 pound a week. This is because there is a substantial increase in maternal tissue during the second trimester, and the fetus grows a great deal during the third trimester.

Weight gain varies, of course. A pregnant **adolescent** who is still growing should gain more weight than a mature woman of the same size. Underweight women should gain 28 to 40 pounds. Women of average weight should avoid excessive weight gain and try to stay within the 25- to 35-pound average gain. If the woman is pregnant with twins, then the recommended weight gain is 35 to 45 pounds. Overweight women can afford to gain less than the average woman, but not less than 15 pounds.

No one should lose weight during pregnancy, because it could cause nutrient deficiencies for both mother and infant. On average, a pregnant adult requires no additional calories during the first trimester of pregnancy and only an additional 300 calories a day during the second and third trimesters.

trimester
3-month period; commonly used to denote periods of pregnancy

adolescent
person between the ages of 13 and 20

Table 11-1 *Components of Weight Gain during Pregnancy, with Approximate Amounts of Gain*

COMPONENT	AMOUNT OF GAIN
Fetus	7.5 pounds
Placenta	1 pound
Amniotic fluid	2 pounds
Uterus	2 pounds
Breasts	1–3 pounds
Blood volume	4 pounds
Maternal fat	4+ pounds

EXPLORING THE WEB

Visit the Web site of the American College of Obstetricians and Gynecologists at www.acog.org. Search the site for information regarding pregnancy and nutrition. What information can you find related to nutritional needs before, during, and after pregnancy? How does lactation affect caloric needs?

NUTRITIONAL NEEDS DURING PREPREGNANCY

Ideally when couples decide to have a child, they should make an appointment with their physician to discuss any health concerns or needed changes to the woman's diet. At that time the physician needs to emphasize the importance of the woman taking a folic acid supplement at least one month prior to conception. During the 1990s, researchers established a correlation between taking folic acid before pregnancy and during the first trimester and having babies with brain and spinal cord defects. The results of this research led the U.S. government to require the addition of folic acid to grain products. The U.S. Public Health Service and the March of Dimes recommend that all women of childbearing age take a multivitamin or 400 µg of folic acid daily.

Lifestyle and habits also need to be taken into consideration before becoming pregnant. Certain medications, smoking, illegal drugs, and alcohol can all be detrimental to the embryo. Good nutrition is essential before becoming pregnant and during pregnancy.

NUTRITIONAL NEEDS DURING PREGNANCY

Some specific nutrient requirements are increased dramatically during pregnancy, as can be seen in Table 11-2. These figures are recommended for the

Table 11-2 *RDA, DRI, and AI Needed during Pregnancy and Lactation*

Age	Weight (kg) (lb)	Height (cm) (in)	Protein (g)	FAT-SOLUBLE VITAMINS			WATER-SOLUBLE VITAMINS			
				Vitamin A (µg RE)	Vitamin D (µg)	Vitamin E (mg α-TE)	Vitamin K (AI)	Vitamin C (mg)	Thiamine (mg)	Riboflavin (mg)
11–14 years										
Not pregnant	46 101	157 62	46	700	5	11	75	56	1.4	1.0
Pregnant			60	750	5	15	75	80	1.5	1.6
Lactating			65	1,200	5	16	75	115	1.4	1.6
15–18 years										
Not pregnant	55 120	163 64	44	700	5	15	75	75	1.4	1.0
Pregnant			60	750	5	15	75	80	1.5	1.6
Lactating			65	1,300	5	16	90	120	1.4	1.6
19–24 years										
Not pregnant	58 128	164 65	46	700	5	15	90	75	1.4	1.1
Pregnant			60	770	5	15	90	85	1.5	1.6
Lactating			65	1,300	5	16	90	120	1.4	1.6
25 years +										
Not pregnant	63 138	163 64	50	700	5	15	90	75	1.4	1.1
Pregnant			60	770	5	15	90	85	1.5	1.6
Lactating			65	1,300	5	16	90	120	1.4	1.6

(continued)

general U.S. population; the physician may suggest alternative figures based on the client's nutritional status, age, and activities.

The protein requirement is increased by 20% for the pregnant woman over 25 and by 25% for the pregnant adolescent. Proteins are essential for tissue building, and protein-rich foods are excellent sources of many other essential nutrients, especially iron, copper, zinc, and the B vitamins.

Current research indicates there is no need for increased vitamin A during pregnancy. Excess vitamin A (more than 3,000 RE) has been known to cause birth defects such as hydrocephaly (enlargement of the fluid-filled spaces of the brain), microcephaly (small head), mental retardation, ear and eye abnormalities, cleft lip and palate, and heart defects. The required amount of vitamin D is 10 μg. The requirement for vitamin E is 15 mg α-TE. The amount of vitamin K required is given as AI of 75–90 μg depending upon age. See Chapter 7 for specifics about the need for fat-soluble vitamins.

The requirements for all the water-soluble vitamins are increased during pregnancy. Additional vitamin C is needed to develop collagen and to increase the absorption of iron. The B vitamins are needed in greater amounts because of their roles in metabolism and the development of red blood cells.

The requirements for the minerals calcium, iron, zinc, iodine, and selenium are all increased during pregnancy. Calcium is, of course, essential for the development of the infant's bones and teeth as well as for blood clotting and

Table 11-2 Continued

WATER-SOLUBLE VITAMINS				MINERALS							
Niacin (mg NE)	Vitamin B6	Folate (μg)	Vitamin B$_{12}$ (μg)	Calcium (mg)	Phosphorus (mg)	Magnesium (mg)	Fluoride (mg)	Iron (mg)	Zinc (mg)	Iodine (μg)	Selenium (μg)
15	1.4	150	2.0	1,300	1,055	200	2.0	15	12	150	45
17	2.2	400	2.2	1,300	1,055	200	2.0	30	15	175	65
20	2.1	280	2.6	1,300	1,055	200	2.0	15	19	200	75
15	1.5	180	2.0	1,300	1,055	300	2.9	15	12	150	50
17	2.2	400	2.2	1,300	1,055	335	2.9	30	15	175	65
20	2.1	280	2.6	1,300	1,055	300	2.9	15	19	200	75
15	1.6	180	2.0	1,000	580	255	3.1	15	12	150	55
17	2.2	400	2.2	1,000	580	290	3.1	30	15	175	65
20	2.1	280	2.6	1,000	580	255	3.1	15	19	200	75
15	1.6	180	2.0	1,000	580	265	3.1	15	12	150	55
17	2.2	400	2.2	1,000	580	300	3.1	30	15	175	65
20	2.1	280	2.6	1,000	580	265	3.1	15	19	200	75

◎ SUPERSIZE USA

"What to eat today? It is so great to go to the drive-by window at the fast-food restaurant each morning and pick up a large (44-ounce) soda to start the day along with an egg on an English muffin. For lunch with coworkers, the meal consists of a soda along with a grilled chicken salad with ranch dressing and bread sticks (pregnant women have to watch what they eat so they don't gain too much weight). Afternoon break is the time for a quick soda and a snack— perhaps pretzels. Salmon, roasted vegetables, fruit salad and a soda are for dinner." A picture perfect day of eating, or is it? Is anything wrong with this food picture for a pregnant woman?

Yes. There are too many empty calories in all the soda—80 ounces of soda equals 1,000 calories. Breakfast should include fruit or juice. Other healthy items missing from this eating plan are milk and whole-grain foods such as 100% whole wheat bread. Finally, there are not enough servings of fruits and vegetables.

muscle action. If the mother is not consuming adequate calcium in her diet, the baby will get its calcium from her bones.

The need for iron increases because of the increased blood volume during pregnancy. In addition, the fetus increases its hemoglobin level to 20 to 22 grams per 100 ml of blood. This is nearly twice the normal human hemoglobin level of 13 to 14 mg per 100 ml of blood.

The infant's hemoglobin level is reduced to normal shortly after birth as the extra hemoglobin breaks down. The resulting iron is stored in the liver and is available when needed during the infant's first few months of life, when the diet is essentially breast milk or formula. Therefore, an iron supplement is commonly prescribed during pregnancy. However, if the pregnant woman's hemoglobin remains at an acceptable level without a supplement, the physician will not prescribe one.

FULFILLMENT OF NUTRITIONAL NEEDS DURING PREGNANCY

To meet the nutritional requirements of pregnancy, the woman should base her diet on MyPyramid. Special care should be taken in the selection of food so that the necessary calories are provided by nutrient-dense foods.

One of the best ways of providing these nutrients is by drinking additional milk each day or using appropriate substitutes. The extra milk will provide protein, calcium, phosphorus, thiamine, riboflavin, and niacin. If whole milk is used, it will also contribute saturated fat and cholesterol and provide 150 calories per 8 ounces of milk. Fat-free milk contributes no fat and provides 90 calories per 8-ounce serving and thus is the better choice.

To be sure that the vitamin requirements of pregnancy are met, **obstetricians,** nurse midwives, and physician's assistants (PAs) may prescribe a prenatal vitamin supplement in addition to an iron supplement. However, it is *not* advisable for the mother to take any unprescribed nutrient supplement, as an excess of vitamins or minerals can be toxic to mother and infant.

◌ **obstetrician**
doctor who cares for the mother during pregnancy and delivery

The unusual cravings for certain foods during pregnancy do no harm unless eating them interferes with the normal balanced diet or causes excessive weight gain.

CONCERNS DURING PREGNANCY

Nausea

Sometimes nausea (the feeling of a need to vomit) occurs during the first trimester of pregnancy. This type of nausea is commonly known as **morning sickness,** but it can occur at any time. It typically passes as the pregnancy proceeds to the second trimester. The following suggestions can help relieve morning sickness:

- Eat dry crackers or dry toast before rising.
- Eat small, frequent meals.
- Avoid foods with offensive odors.
- Avoid liquids at mealtime.

In rare cases, the nausea persists and becomes so severe that it is life-threatening. This condition is called **hyperemesis gravidarum.** The mother may be hospitalized and given **parenteral nutrition.** This means the patient is given nutrients via a vein. This is discussed more fully in Chapter 22. Such cases are difficult, and the patients need emotional support and optimism from those who care for them.

Constipation

Constipation can result from relaxation of the cardiac sphincter and smooth muscles related to progesterone. Constipation and hemorrhoids can be relieved by eating high-fiber foods, getting daily exercise, drinking at least 13 glasses of liquid each day, and responding immediately to the urge to defecate.

Heartburn

Heartburn is a common complaint during pregnancy. As the fetus grows, it pushes on the mother's stomach, which may cause stomach acid to move into the lower esophagus and create a burning sensation there. Heartburn may be relieved by eating small, frequent meals, avoiding spicy or greasy foods, avoiding liquids with meals, waiting at least an hour after eating before lying down, and waiting at least 2 hours before exercising.

Excessive Weight Gain

If weight gain becomes excessive, the pregnant woman should reevaluate her diet and eliminate foods (except for the extra pint of milk) that do not fit within MyPyramid. Examples include candy, cookies, rich desserts, chips, salad dressings (other than fat-free), and sweetened beverages. In addition, she might

morning sickness
early morning nausea common to some pregnancies

hyperemesis gravidarum
nausea so severe as to be life-threatening

parenteral nutrition
nutrition provided via a vein

drink fat-free milk, if not doing so, which would reduce her calories, but not her intake of proteins, vitamins, and minerals. Except in cases in which the woman cannot tolerate lactose (the sugar in milk), it is not advisable to substitute calcium pills for milk because the substitution reduces the protein, vitamin, and mineral content of the diet.

A bowl of clean, crisp, raw vegetables such as broccoli or cauliflower tips, carrots, celery, cucumber, zucchini sticks, or radishes dipped in a fat-free salad dressing or salsa can provide interesting snacks that are nutritious, filling, satisfying, and low in calories. Fruits and custards made with fat free milk make nutritious, satisfying desserts that are not high in calories. Broiling, baking, or boiling foods instead of frying can further reduce the caloric intake.

Pregnancy-Induced Hypertension

Pregnancy-induced hypertension (PIH) was formerly called *toxemia* or *preeclampsia.* It is a condition that sometimes occurs during the third trimester. It is characterized by high blood pressure, the presence of albumin in the urine **(proteinuria),** and edema. The edema causes a somewhat sudden increase in weight. If the condition persists and reaches the **eclamptic** (convulsive) **stage,** convulsions, coma, and death of mother and child may occur. The cause of this condition is not known, but it occurs more frequently in first-time pregnancies, in multifetal pregnancies, in those women with morbid obesity, and among pregnant women on inadequate diets, especially protein-deficient diets. Pregnant adolescents have a higher rate of PIH than do pregnant adults.

Pica

Pica is the craving for nonfood substances such as starch, clay (soil), or ice. The reasons people get such a craving are not clear. Although both men and women are affected, pica is most common among pregnant women. Some believe it relieves nausea. Others think the practice is based on cultural heritage. The consumption of soil should be highly discouraged. Soil contains bacteria that would contaminate both mother and fetus. Ingesting soil can lead to an intestinal blockage, and substances in the soil would bind with minerals, preventing absorption by the body and thus leading to nutrient deficiencies. If any of the nonfood substances replaces nutrient-rich foods in the diet, this will result in multiple nutrient deficiencies. Eating laundry starch, in addition to a regular diet, will add unneeded calories and carbohydrates.

Anemia

Anemia is a condition caused by an insufficiency of red blood cells, hemoglobin, or blood volume. The patient suffering from it does not receive sufficient oxygen from the blood and consequently feels weak and tired, has a poor appetite, and appears pale. *Iron deficiency* is its most common form. During pregnancy, the increased volume of blood creates the need for additional iron. When this need is not met by the diet or by the iron stores in the mother's body, iron deficiency anemia develops. This may be treated with a daily iron supplement.

pregnancy-induced hypertension (PIH)
typically occurs during late pregnancy; characterized by high blood pressure, albumin in the urine, and edema

proteinuria
protein in the urine

eclamptic stage
convulsive stage of toxemia

pica
abnormal craving for nonfood substance

anemia
condition caused by insufficient number of red blood cells, hemoglobin, or blood volume

Folate deficiency can result in a form of megaloblastic anemia that can occur during pregnancy. It is characterized by too few red blood cells and by large immature red blood cells. The body's requirement for folic acid increases dramatically when new red blood cells are being formed. Consequently, the obstetrician might prescribe a folate supplement of 400–600 μg a day during pregnancy.

Alcohol, Caffeine, Drugs, and Tobacco

Alcohol consumption is associated with subnormal physical and mental development of the fetus. This is called **fetal alcohol syndrome (FAS).** Many infants with FAS are premature and have a low birth weight. Physical characteristics may include a small head, short eye slits that make eyes appear to be set far apart, a flat midface, and a thin upper lip. There is usually a growth deficiency (height, weight), placing the child in the lowest tenth of age norms. There is also evidence of central nervous system dysfunction, including hyperactivity, seizures, attention deficits, and microcephaly (small head) (Figure 11-1). Another condition caused by ingesting alcohol while pregnant is fetal alcohol effect (FAE). Children with FAE are born with less dramatic or no physical defects, but with many of the behavioral and psychosocial problems associated with FAS. Those with FAE are not able to lead normal lives due to deficits in intelligence and behavioral and social abilities. When the mother drinks alcohol, it enters the fetal blood- stream in the same concentration as it does the mother's. Unfortunately, the fetus does not have the capacity to metabolize it as quickly as the

fetal alcohol syndrome (FAS)
subnormal physical and mental development caused by mother's excessive use of alcohol during pregnancy

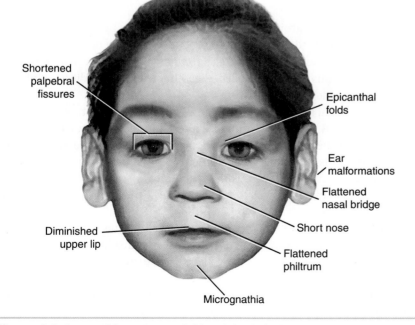

Shortened palpebral fissures

Epicanthal folds

Ear malformations

Flattened nasal bridge

Short nose

Diminished upper lip

Flattened philtrum

Micrognathia

Figure 11-1 *Facial features in a child with fetal alcohol syndrome.*

mother, so it stays longer in the fetal blood than it does in the maternal blood. Abstinence is recommended.

Caffeine is known to cross the placenta, and it enters the fetal bloodstream. Birth defects in newborn rats whose mothers were fed very high doses of caffeine during pregnancy have been observed, but there are no data on humans showing that moderate amounts of caffeine are harmful. As a safety measure, however, it is suggested that pregnant women limit their caffeine intake to 2 cups of caffeine-containing beverages each day, or less than 300 mg/day.

Drugs vary in their effects, but self-prescribed drugs, including vitamins and mineral supplements and dangerous illegal drugs, can all damage the fetus. Drugs derived from vitamin A can cause **fetal malformations** and **spontaneous abortions.** Illegal drugs can cause the infant to be born addicted to whatever substance the mother used and, possibly, to be born with the human immunodeficiency virus (HIV). If a pregnant woman is known to be infected with HIV, her physician may prescribe AZT in an attempt to prevent the spread of the disease to the developing fetus.

Tobacco smoking by pregnant women has for some time been associated with babies of reduced birth weight. The more the mother smokes, the smaller her baby will be, because smoking reduces the oxygen and nutrients carried by the blood. Other risks associated with smoking include SIDS (sudden infant death syndrome), fetal death, spontaneous abortion, and complications at birth. Smoking during pregnancy may also affect the intellectual and behavioral development of the baby as it grows up.

Because the substances discussed in this section may cause fetal problems, it is advisable that pregnant women avoid them.

DIET FOR THE PREGNANT WOMAN WITH DIABETES

Diabetes mellitus is a group of diseases in which one cannot use or store glucose normally because of inadequate production or use of insulin. This impaired metabolism causes glucose to accumulate in the blood, where it causes numerous problems if not controlled. (See Chapter 17 for additional information on diabetes mellitus.)

Some women have diabetes when they become pregnant. Others may develop **gestational diabetes** during pregnancy. In most cases, this latter type disappears after the infant is born; however, there is a 40% increased risk of developing type 2 diabetes later in life. Either type increases the risks of physical or mental defects in the infant, stillbirth, and **macrosomia** (birth weight over 9 pounds) unless blood glucose levels are carefully monitored and maintained within normal limits.

Every pregnant woman should be tested for diabetes between 16 and 28 weeks of gestation. Those found to have the disease must learn to monitor their diets to maintain normal blood glucose levels and to avoid both **hypoglycemia** and **hyperglycemia.**

In general, the nutrient requirements of the pregnant woman with diabetes are the same as for the normal pregnant woman. The diet should be planned with a registered dietitian or a certified diabetes educator, because it

○ **fetal malformations**
physical abnormalities of the fetus

○ **spontaneous abortion**
occurring naturally; miscarriage

○ **gestational diabetes**
diabetes occurring during pregnancy; usually disappears after delivery of the infant

○ **macrosomia**
birthweight over 9 pounds

○ **hypoglycemia**
subnormal levels of blood sugar

○ **hyperglycemia**
excessive amounts of sugar in the blood

will depend on the type of insulin and the time and number of injections. Clients with gestational diabetes and diabetic clients who do not normally require insulin to control their diabetes may require insulin during pregnancy to control blood glucose levels. Oral hypoglycemic agents have not been approved for use during pregnancy. Between-meal feedings help maintain blood glucose at a steady level. Artificial sweeteners have been researched extensively and found to be safe for use during pregnancy.

PREGNANCY DURING ADOLESCENCE

Teenage pregnancy is an increasing concern. The nutritional, physical, psychological, social, and economic demands on a pregnant adolescent are tremendous. With the birth of the infant, they increase. Young women who are themselves still in need of nurturing and financial support are suddenly responsible for helpless newborns. If the mother does not have sufficient help, the total effect on her and the child can be devastating.

The young woman may need prenatal health care, infant care, and psychological, nutritional, and economic counseling, as well as help in locating appropriate housing. And at this time, the young woman's family may or may not be supportive.

At such a time, nutritional habits can seem to some as being of slight importance. They are, however, of primary importance. An adolescent's eating habits may not be adequate to fulfill the nutritional needs of her own growing body. When she adds the nutritional burden of a developing fetus, both are put at risk. Adolescents are particularly vulnerable to pregnancy-induced hypertension and premature delivery. PIH can cause cardiovascular and kidney problems later. Premature delivery is a leading cause of death among newborns. Inadequate nutrition of the mother is related to both mental and physical birth defects.

These young women will need to know their own nutritional needs and the additional nutritional requirements of pregnancy (see Table 11-2). The government-funded WIC (Women, Infants, and Children) program can help with prenatal care, nutrition education, and adequate food for the best outcome possible. Pregnant teenagers will need much counseling and emotional support from caring, experienced people before nutritional improvements can be suggested.

LACTATION

A woman needs to decide whether to breast-feed before her infant is born. Almost all women can breast-feed; breast size is no barrier. **Lactation,** the production and secretion of breast milk for the purpose of nourishing an infant, is facilitated by an interplay of various hormones after delivery of the infant. Oxytocin and prolactin instigate the lactation process. Prolactin is responsible for milk production, and oxytocin is involved in milk ejection from the breast. The infant's sucking initiates the release of oxytocin, which causes the ejection of milk into the infant's mouth. This is called the let-down reflex. It is a supply-and-demand mechanism. The more an infant nurses, the more milk the mother produces.

It will take 2 to 3 weeks to fully establish a feeding routine; therefore, it is recommended that no supplemental feedings be given during this time. Human

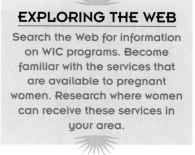

EXPLORING THE WEB

Search the Web for information on WIC programs. Become familiar with the services that are available to pregnant women. Research where women can receive these services in your area.

lactation
the period during which the mother is nursing the baby

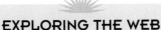 **lactation specialist**
Expert on breastfeeding

milk is formulated to meet the nutrient needs of infants for the first 6 months of life. Iron content in breast milk is very low, but it is very well absorbed; therefore no iron supplement is needed for breastfed babies.

Lactation Specialist

Lactation specialists are the experts on breastfeeding and help new mothers who may be having problems such as the baby not latching on properly. This could cause the breast to become sore and could be discouraging to first-time mothers. Since the best first food for babies is breast milk, a lactation specialist can teach the proper techniques for successful breastfeeding.

Benefits of Breastfeeding

There are many positive reasons to breast-feed. The primary benefit of breast milk is nutritional. Breast milk contains just the right amount of lactose, water, essential fatty acids, and amino acids for brain development, growth, and digestion. No babies are allergic to their mother's milk, although they may have reactions to something their mother eats. Human milk contains at least 100 ingredients not found in formula.

Breastfed babies have a lower incidence of ear infections, diarrhea, allergies, and hospital admissions. Breastfed babies receive immunities from their mothers for the diseases that the mother has had or has been exposed to. When a baby becomes ill, the bacteria causing the illness is transmitted to the mother while the baby is breastfeeding; the mother's immune system will start making antibodies for the baby.

Sucking at the breast promotes good jaw development because it is harder work to get milk out of a breast than a bottle, and the exercise strengthens the jaws and encourages the growth of straight, healthy teeth. Breastfeeding facilitates bonding between mother and child. The skin-to-skin contact helps a baby feel safe, secure, and loved. Pediatricians encourage mothers of premature babies to hold their babies on their chests—skin to skin. This is called "kangaroo care," which has been shown to soothe and calm a baby and help maintain the baby's temperature. Fathers too can participate in kangaroo care by placing their infants against their bare chests.

Benefits for mother include help in losing the pounds gained during pregnancy and stimulating the uterus to contract to its original size. Resting is important for a new mother, and breastfeeding gives her that opportunity. Breastfeeding is economical, always the right temperature and readily available—especially in the middle of the night.

There is no need to stop breastfeeding when returning to work; a breast pump can be used to express milk for feedings when the mother is not available. Breast milk will keep 8 to 10 hours at room temperature (66°–72°F), 8 days in the refrigerator, 3 to 4 months in the refrigerator freezer, and 12 months in a deep freezer. Previously frozen milk must be used within 24 hours after defrosting in the refrigerator. Breast milk should not be heated in the microwave or directly on the stove. Those methods of heating breast milk will kill its immune-enhancing ability.

Calorie Requirements during Lactation

The mother's calorie requirement increases during lactation. The caloric requirement depends on the amount of milk produced. Approximately 85 calories are required to produce 100 ml (3⅓ ounces) of milk. During the first 6 months, average daily milk production is 750 ml (25 ounces), and for this the mother requires approximately an extra 640 calories a day. During the second 6 months, when the baby begins to eat food in addition to breast milk, average daily milk production slows to 600 ml (20 ounces), and the caloric requirement is reduced to approximately 510 extra calories a day.

The Food and Nutrition Board suggests an increase of 500 calories a day during lactation. This is less than the actual need because it is assumed that some fat has been stored during pregnancy, which can be used for milk production. The precise number of calories the mother needs depends on the size of the infant and its appetite and on the size and activities of the mother. Each ounce of human milk contains 20 calories.

If the mother's diet contains insufficient calories, the quantity of milk will be reduced. Thus, lactation is not a good time to go on a strict weight loss diet. There will be some natural weight loss caused by the burning of the stored fat for milk production.

Nutrient Requirements during Lactation

In general, most nutrient requirements are increased during lactation. The amounts depend on the age of the mother (see Table 11-2). Protein is of particular importance because it is estimated that 10 grams of protein are secreted in the milk each day.

MyPyramid will be helpful in meal planning for the lactating mother. She should be sure to include sufficient fruits and vegetables, especially those rich in vitamin C. Extra fat-free milk will provide many of the additional nutrients and calories required during lactation. Chips, sodas, candies, and desserts provide little more than calories.

Vegetarians will need to be especially careful to be sure they have sufficient calories, iron, zinc, copper, protein, calcium, and vitamin D. A vitamin B_{12} supplement can be prescribed for them.

It is important that the nursing mother have sufficient fluids to replace those lost in the infant's milk. Water and real fruit juice are the best choices.

The mother should be made aware that she must reduce her caloric intake at the end of the nursing period to avoid adding unwanted weight.

Medicines, Caffeine, Alcohol, and Tobacco

Most chemicals enter the mother's milk, so it is essential that the mother check with her obstetrician before using any medicines or nutritional supplements. Caffeine can cause the infant to be irritable. Alcohol in excess, tobacco, and illegal drugs can be very harmful. Both illegal drugs, such as marijuana or heroin, and prescription medication, such as methadone and oxycodone, can cause the baby to be excessively drowsy and to feed poorly. Stimulant drugs can cause the baby to be irritable. The biggest concern is addiction of the mother and baby.

CONSIDERATIONS FOR THE HEALTH CARE PROFESSIONAL

Good nutrition during pregnancy can make the difference between a healthy, productive life and one shattered by health and economic problems—for both mother and child.

Most pregnant women will want the best nutrition for themselves and their children. They also will be concerned about their weight during and after pregnancy. It is essential that they receive advice from a properly trained health care professional. Articles in newspapers and magazines or in pamphlets from health food stores may or may not be correct and should not be taken at face value unless approved by a professional in the dietetic field.

Nutrition is currently a popular topic, and people are inclined to believe what is printed. It can be difficult to persuade people that the information they read is incorrect. As always, the health care professional must use great patience in reeducating those clients who may require it.

The pregnant teenager can present the greatest challenge. Her needs are vast, but her experience, and thus her perspective, is limited. Teaching pregnant adolescents about good nutrition may be difficult but, if successful, can help not only that particular client but also her child and her friends.

SUMMARY

A pregnant woman is most likely to remain healthy and bear a healthy infant if she follows a well-balanced diet. Research has shown that maternal nutrition can affect the subsequent mental and physical health of the child. Anemia and PIH are two conditions that can be caused by inadequate nutrition. Caloric and most nutrient requirements increase for pregnant women (especially adolescents) and women who are breast-feeding. The average weight gain during pregnancy is 25 to 35 pounds.

DISCUSSION TOPICS

1. Discuss the statement "A pregnant woman must eat for two."

2. Why is it especially important for a pregnant woman to have a highly nutritious diet?

3. Discuss weight gain during pregnancy from the first month through the ninth. Why is an excessive weight gain during pregnancy undesirable? Is pregnancy a good time to reduce? Explain.

4. Of what value are protein-rich foods during pregnancy?

5. It is common for an iron supplement to be prescribed during pregnancy. Why? What may happen if the mother-to-be does not receive an adequate supply of iron? How might such a condition affect her baby? Discuss the advisability of the pregnant woman's taking a self-prescribed iron or vitamin supplement in addition to that prescribed by the obstetrician.

6. Discuss why the obstetrician regularly checks the pregnant woman's blood pressure, urine, and weight during pregnancy.

7. What is morning sickness, and how can it be helped? If any class member has been pregnant, ask her questions regarding morning sickness. Can this be a truly serious problem? Explain.

8. Why is it a good idea for a pregnant woman to include a citrus fruit or melon with every meal?

9. Why is the average weight gain 25 to 35 pounds during pregnancy when the infant weighs approximately 7½ pounds?

10. Describe pica. Why is it undesirable?

11. Discuss the dangers to the fetus if the mother uses drugs.

12. How can the mother's diabetes affect the fetus?

SUGGESTED ACTIVITIES

1. Ask a dietitian to speak to the class on the importance of adequate nutrition before and during pregnancy. Ask the speaker questions regarding the effects of good and poor nutrition on the health of the mother, prenatal development, infant mortality, and the growth and development of the child. Ask the speaker's opinion regarding the use of alcohol, caffeine, and tobacco during pregnancy. During lactation.

2. Invite a nurse practitioner to speak to the class on the symptoms and dangers of PIH.

3. Invite a certified diabetes educator to speak to the class on the problems that can occur during the pregnancy of a diabetic mother.

REVIEW

Multiple choice. Select the *letter* that precedes the best answer.

1. The infant developing in the mother's uterus is called the
   a. sperm
   b. fetus
   c. placenta
   d. ovary

2. A common form of anemia is caused by
   a. pica
   b. an excess of vitamin A
   c. a lack of iron
   d. improper cooking of meat

3. High blood pressure, edema, and albumin in the urine are symptoms of
   a. nausea
   b. anemia
   c. pica
   d. pregnancy-induced hypertension

4. A common name given nausea in early pregnancy is
   a. morning sickness
   b. pica
   c. pregnancy-induced hypertension
   d. mortality

5. Folate and vitamin B_{12} requirements increase during pregnancy because of their roles in
   a. building strong bones and teeth
   b. fighting infections in the placenta
   c. building blood
   d. enzyme action

6. The average additional daily energy requirement for the pregnant woman during the last two trimesters is
   a. 100 calories
   b. 300 calories
   c. 500 calories
   d. 1,000 calories

7. The additional calories required during pregnancy can be met by
   a. eating steak each day
   b. drinking a malted milk each day
   c. using an additional pint of fat-free milk each day
   d. using an iron supplement

8. Craving nonfood substances during pregnancy is known as
   a. anemia
   b. megaloblastic anemia
   c. nausea
   d. pica

9. During pregnancy, the average weight gain is
   a. 15 to 24 pounds
   b. 25 to 35 pounds
   c. 11 to 24 kilograms
   d. 15 to 24 kilograms

10. The period during which a mother nurses her baby is known as
    a. pregnancy
    b. trimester
    c. lactation
    d. obstetrics

11. Some appropriate substitutes for milk include
    a. orange juice and tomato juice
    b. cheese and custard
    c. breads and cereals
    d. vegetables and fruit juices

12. The RDA/DRI for additional calories for a nursing mother is
    a. 100
    b. 300
    c. 500
    d. 1,000

13. The daily diet during pregnancy and lactation should
    a. be based on MyPyramid
    b. include at least 2 quarts of milk
    c. be limited to 1,900 calories
    d. all of the above

14. Appropriate snacks for pregnant and lactating women include
    a. fruits and raw vegetables
    b. potato chips and pretzels
    c. sodas
    d. hard candies

15. The duration of a normal pregnancy is
    a. 34–36 weeks   c. 38–40 weeks
    b. 36–38 weeks   d. 40–42 weeks

16. The fluid surrounding the fetus in the uterus is the
    a. parenteral fluid   c. amniotic fluid
    b. intracellular fluid   d. synovial fluid

17. During pregnancy, parenteral nutrition may be necessary for patients
    a. with excessive weight gain
    b. suffering from hyperemesis gravidarum
    c. who cannot tolerate milk
    d. who do not eat meat

18. Heartburn may be prevented by
    a. eating small, frequent meals
    b. lying down immediately after eating
    c. taking an aspirin
    d. increasing liquid at meals

19. Pregnancy-induced hypertension
    a. is relieved with salty food
    b. may occur when diets contain insufficient protein
    c. tends to be a precursor of iron deficiency
    d. causes megaloblastic anemia

20. Gestational diabetes
    a. tends to cause low-birth-weight babies
    b. always develops into type 1 insulin-dependent diabetes mellitus
    c. usually disappears after the baby is born
    d. presents no danger to mother or child

21. Maternal malnutrition
    a. has little effect on the fetus
    b. may cause an increase in the fetal hemoglobin level
    c. often causes macrosomia
    d. can lead to developmental or mental retardation

22. The need for iron increases during pregnancy because
    a. it prevents maternal goiter
    b. it is essential to bone development
    c. it is necessary to fetal metabolism
    d. of the increased blood volume

23. Nutrient-dense foods provide substantial amounts of
    a. vitamins, minerals, and proteins
    b. calories per gram of food
    c. carbohydrates, fats, and water
    d. sodium, chloride, and water

24. Excessive vitamin A should be avoided during pregnancy because it may
    a. cause birth defects
    b. cause gestational diabetes
    c. contribute to gallstones in the fetus
    d. reduce the mother's appetite

CASE IN POINT

SHAGMET: MANAGING A PREGNANCY AT 6 MONTHS

Shagmet, a 30-year-old accountant whose family emigrated to the United States from Nepal when she was 4, has two young boys, ages 3 and 2. She went through both pregnancies without difficulty. As soon as she thought she was pregnant, she had made a doctor's appointment, started her prenatal vitamins, and watched her diet. Her doctor recommended that she gain no more than 25 pounds with each pregnancy.

Now, Shagmet's husband, Germain, has taken a new position in Montana. Shagmet and Germain know that the change in lifestyle will be a challenge but are eager to sample what the West has to offer, especially in Big Sky country.

After the move, Shagmet has been totally involved in setting up her new home and getting her life back to a somewhat normal routine. She has been so busy that she has lost track of time. Now, after 4 months, she realizes she could not remember her last period and suspects she is pregnant. Because she has not had the time to find a new physician, she keeps putting it off. Her closest neighbor had said that the only good doctor was a 40-minute drive from their home.

After 6 months, Shagmet starts to feel guilty about not having a prenatal checkup. She knows she needs to establish a doctor-patient relationship, but she is embarrassed because she is so far along. She feels as if her diet was inadequate to feed two people, and she has not taken any vitamin supplements. Shagmet has been under a lot of stress with the move across country and has not been eating as healthy as she would have if she had not made the move. Shagmet finally makes a doctor's appointment.

ASSESSMENT

1. What objective information do you have about Shagmet?
2. What was the cause of Shagmet's situation?
3. What is the problem with the timing of the family move for Shagmet?

DIAGNOSIS

4. Shagmet's lack of attention to _____ is related to _____ as shown by her choice to _____.

PLAN/GOAL

5. What is your immediate goal for Shagmet?
6. What is your long-term goal for Shagmet?
7. What are your education goals for Shagmet?

IMPLEMENTATION

8. What major topics need to be discussed with Shagmet regarding a healthy pregnancy?
9. What topics need to be taught in regard to her lack of nutritional supplements?

EVALUATION/OUTCOME CRITERIA

10. At her next doctor's appointment, what will the doctor check to determine whether she has been compliant?

THINKING FURTHER

11. What teaching goals should be put in place as Shagmet nears her delivery date?

◎ RATE ⫶ PLATE

Shagmet has been getting the family's home and lives organized since the move, and she has not been preparing meals as she normally would. This is what she has chosen to eat for a hurry-up breakfast. Rate the plate.

4 oz orange juice

1 cinnamon roll

1 cup frosted flakes cereal

2 oz milk on cereal

2 cups coffee, black

What would you change, if anything, and why?

CASE IN POINT

MONICA: TEENAGE PREGNANCY

Monica was a blonde, blue-eyed 17-year-old high school junior. She was smart, had an A average, and had career ambitions after her graduation. Monica was liked by all her classmates and was active in sports and extracurricular activities. She even volunteered for the local Boys and Girls Club in her city.

Monica attended the junior prom with Eric. He was the captain of the football team and very handsome. After the prom, Monica and Eric attended the after-prom parties at the local hotel. They swam in the Olympic-size pool, partied, and stayed overnight.

During summer vacation Monica worked at Mc-Donald's. She had the 6 a.m. shift. Monica seldom ate breakfast, and the smell of the frying food at McDonald's made her sick to her stomach. She was exhausted by the time her shift ended and went home and slept. Monica missed her June and July periods. The over-the-counter pregnancy test she purchased declared that she was pregnant. Monica confided in her mother, and they made an appointment for her first prenatal visit. During the visit she was asked about her smoking and alcohol consumption and her eating habits. She was instructed to stop smoking. She was given prenatal vitamins and was told to increase her calories and iron intake. Monica made and kept her follow-up visits. She wanted to have a healthy baby, but she did not want to be fat. She gained 15 pounds during her pregnancy and smoked when the stress level got too much for her.

Monica's baby was born at 37 weeks gestation. He was 5 pounds 3 ounces and 18 inches long. He had periods of apnea in which he temporarily stopped breathing, so he had to wear an apnea monitor when he went home. Monica and her mother were instructed in infant CPR and were taught how to treat apnea at home.

ASSESSMENT

1. What objective data do you have about Monica?
2. What caused Monica to eat the way she did?
3. Which prenatal behaviors of Monica were helpful? Which were not?

DIAGNOSIS

4. Complete the following diagnosis statement: Monica's baby's risk for disproportionate growth was related to _____ .
5. Complete the following statement: Monica was at high risk for _____ secondary to _____ .
6. Complete the following diagnosis statement: Monica's deficient knowledge about a healthy pregnancy and infant health is demonstrated by her lack of compliance with _____ .

PLAN/GOAL

7. What is your plan for Monica's health after the birth?
8. What is your goal for the baby's health related to reducing the risk of SIDS and delayed development?

IMPLEMENTATION

9. What topics does Monica need to be taught about her baby's health and development? What does she need to know about apnea and SIDS? What does she need to learn about normal infant growth and development?
10. Who else needs to be present for the teaching?
11. As a teenage mother with a low-birth-weight baby, Monica needs what type of medical and nursing follow-up? Would home health care nursing visits help?
12. What is your primary concern for the baby?

EVALUATION/OUTCOME CRITERIA

13. At the next visit, what criteria will the nurse practitioner be using to see if Monica and her baby are healthy?

THINKING FURTHER

14. What other problems are likely for Monica's baby because he was a low-birth-weight baby?
15. What other issues make this situation more difficult for a teen mother to be successful?
16. What other types of support may be helpful to a teenage mother?

⦿ RATE THIS PLATE

Monica continued to work at McDonald's through her pregnancy. She continued her habit of not eating breakfast, but for lunch she had the following. Rate this plate.

Caesar salad without chicken and balsamic vinaigrette
Small order of French fries
32-oz diet soda

How many calories and how much protein and iron does this plate contain? Is that enough for a pregnant teen? Why or why not?

DIET DURING INFANCY

OBJECTIVES

After studying this chapter, you should be able to:

- State the effect inadequate nutrition has on an infant
- Discuss positive aspects of breastfeeding and bottle feeding
- Describe when and how foods are introduced into the baby's diet
- Describe inborn errors of metabolism and their dietary treatment

Food and its presentation are extremely important during the baby's first year. Physical and mental development are dependent on the food itself, and **psychosocial development** is affected by the time and manner in which the food is offered.

Infants react to their parents' emotions. If food is forced on a child, or withheld until the child is uncomfortable, or if the food is presented in a tense manner, the child reacts with tension and unhappiness. If the parent is relaxed, an infant's mealtime can be a pleasure for both parent and child (Figure 12-1).

Although babies have been fed according to prescribed time schedules in the past, it is preferable to feed infants **on demand.** Feeding on demand prevents the frustrations that hunger can bring and helps the child develop trust in people. The newborn may require more frequent feedings, but normally the demand schedule averages approximately every 4 hours by the time the baby is 2 or 3 months old.

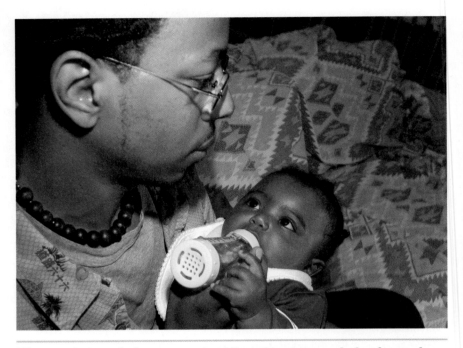

Figure 12-1 *Food is better accepted and digested in a happy and relaxed atmosphere.*

NUTRITIONAL REQUIREMENTS

psychosocial development
relating to both psychological and social development

on demand
feeding infants as they desire

The first year of life is a period of the most rapid growth in one's life. A baby doubles its birth weight by 6 months of age and triples it within the first year. This explains why the infant's energy, vitamin, mineral, and protein requirements are higher per unit of body weight than those of older children or adults. It is important to remember, however, that growth rates vary from child to child. Nutritional needs will depend largely on a child's growth rate.

During the first year, the normal child needs 98–108 calories per kilogram of body weight each day. This is approximately two to three times the adult requirement. Low-birth-weight infants and infants who have suffered from malnutrition or illness require more than the normal number of calories per kilogram of body weight. The nutritional status of infants is reflected by many of the same characteristics as those of adults (see Table 1-2).

The basis of the infant's diet is breast milk or formula. Either one is a highly nutritious, digestible food containing proteins, fats, carbohydrates, vitamins, minerals, and water.

It is recommended that infants up to 6 months of age have 2.2 grams of protein per kilogram of weight each day, and from 6 to 12 months, 1.56 grams of protein per kilogram of weight each day. This is satisfactorily supplied by human milk or by infant formulas (Figure 12-2).

Infants have more water per pound of body weight than do adults. Thus, they usually need 1.5 ml of water per calorie. This is the same ratio of water to calories as is found in human milk and in most infant formulas. Essential vitamins and minerals can be supplied in breast milk, formula, and food. Except for

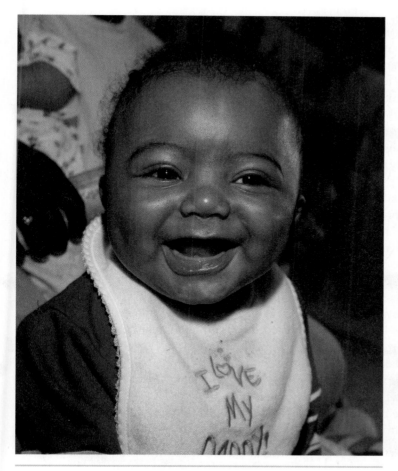

Figure 12-2 *A happy, healthy, well-fed infant.*

vitamin D, breast milk provides all the nutrients an infant needs for the first 4 to 6 months of life. An infant is born with a 3- to 6-month supply of iron. When the infant reaches 6 months of age, the pediatrician usually starts the infant on iron-fortified cereal.

Human milk usually supplies the infant with sufficient vitamin C. Iron-fortified formula is available, and its use is recommended by the American Academy of Pediatricians if the baby is not being breast-fed. The pediatrician can prescribe a vitamin D supplement for infants who are nursed and who are not exposed to sunlight on a regular basis. Newborns lack intestinal bacteria to synthesize vitamin K, so they are routinely given a vitamin K supplement shortly after birth. In addition, some pediatricians prescribe fluoride for breast-fed babies or for formula-fed babies living in areas where the water, such as well water, contains little fluoride.

Care must be taken that infants do not receive excessive amounts of either vitamin A or D because both can be toxic in excessive amounts. Vitamin A can damage the liver and cause bone abnormalities, and vitamin D can damage the cardiovascular system and kidneys.

BREASTFEEDING

Although babies will thrive whether nursed or formula-fed, breastfeeding provides advantages that formulas cannot match. Breastfeeding is nature's way of providing a good diet for the baby. It is, in fact, used as the guide by which nutritional requirements of infants are measured (Figure 12-3).

Mother's milk provides the infant with temporary **immunity** to many infectious diseases. It is economical, nutritionally perfect, and sanitary, and it saves time otherwise spent in shopping for or preparing formula. It is **sterile,** is easy to digest, and usually does not cause gastrointestinal disturbances or allergic reactions. Breastfed infants have fewer infections (especially ear infections) during the first few months of life than formula-fed babies. And because breast milk contains less protein and minerals than infant formula, it reduces the load on the infant's kidneys. Breastfeeding also promotes oral motor development in infants and decreases the infant's risk of obesity and diabetes.

The breast should be offered about every 2 hours in the first several weeks. As the infant grows and develops, a stronger sucking ability will allow more milk to be extracted at each feeding, and the frequency of nursing sessions will decrease. It is recommended that an infant nurse at each breast for approximately 10 to 15 minutes each session. Growth spurts occur at about 10 days, 2 weeks, 6 weeks, and 3 months. During this time, the infant will nurse more frequently to increase the supply of nutrients needed to support growth.

One can be quite confident the infant is getting sufficient nutrients and calories from breastfeeding if (1) there are six or more wet diapers a day, (2) there is normal growth, (3) there are one or two mustard-colored bowel movements a day, and (4) the breast becomes less full during nursing.

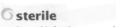

immunity
ability to resist certain diseases

sterile
free of infectious organisms

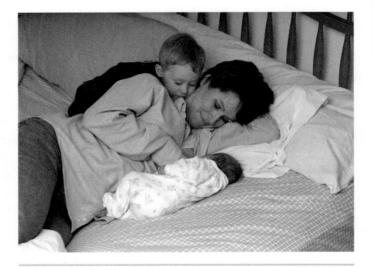

Figure 12-3 *Breastfeeding offers many nutritional benefits to the newborn.*

From the mother's perspective at least, the **bonding** that occurs during breastfeeding is unmatched. In addition, breastfeeding helps the mother's uterus return to normal size after delivery, controls postpartum bleeding, and also helps the mother more quickly return to her prepregnancy weight. Research has shown a correlation between breastfeeding and a decreased risk of breast cancer and osteoporosis in premenopausal women.

Breastfeeding had been on the decline for many years, but a growing number of mothers are now nursing their babies. If the mother works and cannot be available for every feeding, breast milk can be expressed earlier, refrigerated or frozen, and used at the appropriate time, or a bottle of formula can be substituted. Never warm the breast milk in a microwave because the antibodies will be destroyed.

⊙ **bonding**
emotional attachment

BOTTLE FEEDING

Many parents will choose to bottle-feed their babies. Some women fear they will be unable to produce enough breast milk. Some lack emotional support from their families, and some simply find breastfeeding foreign to their culture. Others who are employed or involved in many activities outside the home find bottle feeding more convenient. Either way of feeding is acceptable provided the infant is given love and attention during the feeding.

The infant should be cuddled and held in a semi-upright position during the feeding (Figure 12-4). It appears that babies fed this way are less inclined to

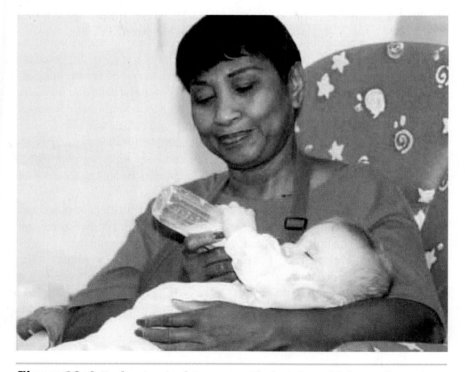

Figure 12-4 *Feeding is a good time to provide the infant with love and attention.*

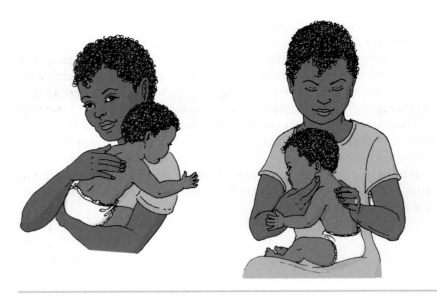

Figure 12-5 *To burp a baby, hold him or her in one of the two positions shown and gently stroke his or her back.*

⊙ **regurgitation**
vomiting

develop middle ear infections than those fed lying down. It is believed that the upright position prevents fluid from pooling at the back of the throat and entering tubes from the middle ear. During and after the feeding, the infant should be burped to release gas in the stomach, just as the breast-fed infant should be burped (Figure 12-5). Burping helps prevent **regurgitation**.

If the baby is to be bottle-fed, the pediatrician will provide information on commercial formulas and feeding instructions. Formulas are usually based on cow's milk because it is abundant and easily modified to resemble human milk. It must be modified because it has more protein and mineral salts and less milk sugar (lactose) than human milk. Formulas, such as soy formula, are developed so that they are similar to human milk in nutrient and caloric values.

When an infant is extremely sensitive or allergic to infant formulas, a synthetic formula may be given. Synthetic milk is commonly made from soybeans. Formulas with predigested proteins are used for infants unable to tolerate all other types of formulas.

Formulas can be purchased in ready-to-feed, concentrated, or powdered forms. Sterile or boiled tap water must be mixed with the concentrated and powdered forms. The most convenient type is also the most expensive.

If the type purchased requires the addition of water, it is essential that the amount of water added be correctly measured. Too little water will create too heavy a protein and mineral load for the infant's kidneys. Too much water will dilute the nutrient and calorie value so that the infant will not thrive, and also it could lead to brain edema or seizures.

Infants under the age of 1 year should not be given regular cow's milk. Because its protein is more difficult and slower to digest than that of human milk, it can cause gastrointestinal blood loss. The kidneys are challenged by its high protein and mineral content, and dehydration and even damage to the central nervous system can result. In addition, the fat is less bioavailable, meaning it is not absorbed as efficiently as that in human milk.

Formula may be given cold, at room temperature, or warmed, but it should be given at the same temperature consistently. To warm the formula for feeding, place the bottle in a saucepan of warm water or a bottle warmer. The bottles should be shaken occasionally to warm the contents evenly. Warming the bottle in the microwave is not advisable because milk can heat unevenly and burn the infant's mouth. The temperature of the milk can be tested by shaking a few drops on one's wrist. The milk should feel lukewarm.

Infants should not be put to bed with a bottle. Saliva, which normally cleanses the teeth, diminishes as the infant falls asleep. The milk then bathes the upper front teeth, causing tooth decay. Also, the bottle can cause the upper jaw to protrude and the lower to recede. The result is known as the baby bottle mouth or nursing bottle syndrome. It is preferable to feed the infant the bedtime bottle, cleanse the teeth and gums with some water from another bottle or cup, and then put the infant to bed.

SUPPLEMENTARY FOODS

The age at which infants are introduced to solid and semisolid food has varied considerably over the years. At the beginning of this century, doctors advocated that children be fed only breast milk during their first 12 months. By the 1950s, in response to parental demand, some pediatricians advised the introduction of solid food before the age of 1 month. Now, the general recommendation is that the infant's diet be limited to breast milk or formula until the age of 4 to 6 months and that breast milk or formula remain the major food source until the child is 1 year old. With the appropriate supplements of iron and vitamin D,

⊙ SUPERSIZE USA

We the USA have already supersized our population. Almost 50% of children 6–9 years old are overweight or are at risk of becoming overweight (Hedley et al., 2004). Educating parents about "what is the normal size portion for their child" will be the first step in the fight against obesity. Overweight and obese parents may struggle with portion control when everything seems to have been supersized—plates, serving bowls, silverware, and glasses. Food comes in large packages, and chicken really is a *big* bird before processing. This big bird will yield boneless chicken breasts that will weigh 9–12 ounces raw—and this is called a single serving—that is, by those that are overeating and are no longer able to discern a normal 3–4 ounce serving. The easiest way to master portion sizes is by buying meat already prepared in portion sizes or by asking the butcher to cut exactly what you need. Be sure and allow 1 ounce for shrinkage from cooking. Also, get out the measuring cups and spoons—keeping a set clean at all times just for measuring.

Here are some steps to preventing *supersizing children:*

- Breast-feed babies. Breastfeeding is the first step to preventing an overweight child.
- Select the right foods, and take the time to eat them. Kids fail to eat enough meats, fruits, and vegetables. Kids should have at least 15 to 20 minutes to eat.
- Set goals for activity—not only for kids, but for parents as well. Limit time for television, video games, and computers. The recommendation for exercise is 60 minutes per day.
- Work with other parents to remove junk food and soda from school vending machines.
- Do not reward children with food.

What age should babies be introduced solid foods 4 mos.—

1st solid Between 4 to 6 mos,

Rice Cereal Flakes

Honey should never before 2 — because could get botulism,

After 2 yrs. of age

Juice 4 oz DAY

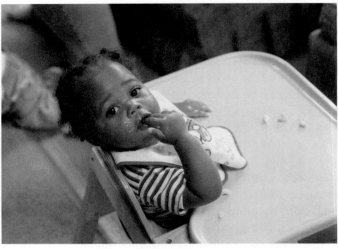

Figure 12-6 *Infants sometimes find more pleasure in touching their food while tasting it.*

and possibly vitamin C and fluoride, breast milk or formula fulfills the nutritional requirements of most children until they reach the age of 6 months.

The introduction of solid foods before the age of 4 to 6 months is not recommended. The child's gastrointestinal tract and kidneys are not sufficiently developed to handle solid food before that age. Further, it is thought that the early introduction of solid foods may increase the likelihood of overfeeding and the possibility of the development of food allergies, particularly in children whose parents suffer from allergies.

An infant's readiness for solid foods will be demonstrated by (1) the physical ability to pull food into the mouth rather than always pushing the tongue and food out of the mouth (extrusion reflex disappears by 4–6 months), (2) a willingness to participate in the process (Figure 12-6), (3) the ability to sit up with support, (4) having head and neck control, and (5) the need for additional nutrients. If the infant is drinking more than 32 ounces of formula or nursing 8 to 10 times in 24 hours, and is at least 4 months old, then solid food should be started.

Solid foods must be introduced gradually and individually. One food is introduced and then no other new food for 4 or 5 days. If there is no allergic reaction, another food can be introduced, a waiting period allowed, then another, and so on. The typical order of introduction begins with cereal, usually iron-fortified rice, then oat, wheat, and mixed cereals. Cooked and pureed vegetables follow, then cooked and pureed fruits, egg yolk and, finally, finely ground meats. Between 6 and 12 months, toast, zwieback, teething biscuits, and Cheerios can be added in small amounts. Honey should never be given to an infant because it could be contaminated with *Clostridium botulinum* bacteria. When the infant learns to drink from a cup, juice can be introduced (Figure 12-7). Juice should never be given from a bottle because babies will fill up on it and not get enough calories from other sources. Pasteurized apple juice is usually given first. It is recommended that only 4 ounces per day of 100% juice products be given because they are nutrient-dense.

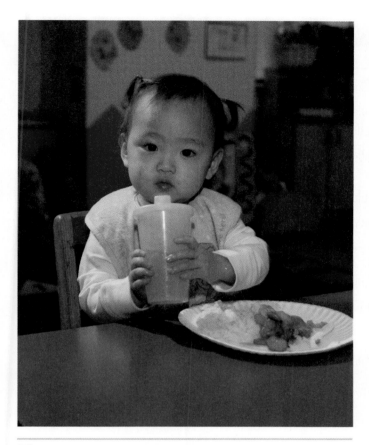

Handwritten notes:

All Food from My pyramid by age 1 yr except honey.

Why would you Not giving a child peanuts?
1) choking
2) allergic

Figure 12-7 *Juice should be served in a cup, not a bottle.*

Babies differ in the amount of food they eat from day to day. An infant will let you know when he or she is full by:

- Playing with the nipple on a bottle or a breast
- Looking around and no longer opening his or her mouth to solid food
- Falling asleep while eating
- Playing with food and not eating

Adults may try to overfeed infants when solid food is introduced. The guidelines in Table 12-1 may be helpful.

By the age of 1 year, most babies are eating foods from all of the MyPyramid groups and may have most any food that is easily chewed and digested. However, precautions must be taken to avoid offering foods on which the child can choke. Examples include hot dogs, nuts, whole peas, grapes, popcorn, small candies, and small pieces of tough meat or raw vegetables. Foods should be selected according to the advice of the health care provider or pediatrician. It is not necessary to use the commercially prepared "junior" foods. Table foods generally can be used, though they may need to first be mashed or run through a blender.

MyPyramid provides excellent help in determining the baby's menu. Its use will help supply the appropriate nutrients and develop good eating habits. It is particularly important at this time to avoid excess sugar and salt in the infant's

Table 12-1 *Guidelines to Prevent Overfeeding of Infants*

FEEDING	4–5 MONTHS	5–7 MONTHS
Early morning	Breast milk or 5–6 oz formula*	Breast milk or 5–6 oz formula*
Breakfast	Breast milk or 5–6 oz formula* 1–2 Tbsp infant cereal† (optional)	Breast milk or 5–6 oz formula* 3–4 Tbsp infant cereal†
Lunch	Breast milk or 5–6 oz formula*	Breast milk or 5–6 oz formula* 1–2 Tbsp vegetables
Late afternoon	Breast milk or 5–6 oz formula*	Breast milk or 5–6 oz formula*
Supper	Breast milk or 5–6 oz formula*	Breast milk or 5–6 oz formula* 3–4 Tbsp infant cereal† 1–2 Tbsp vegetables
Evening	Breast milk or 5–6 oz formula*	Breast milk or 5–6 oz formula* (optional)

Babies differ in the amounts of food they eat. Expect your baby's appetite to vary from day to day.

FEEDING	7–9 MONTHS	9–12 MONTHS
Breakfast	Breast milk or 6–8 oz formula* 4 Tbsp infant cereal† 2–3 Tbsp fruit	Breast milk or 6–8 oz formula* 4–6 Tbsp infant cereal† 2–3 Tbsp fruit
Lunch	Breast milk or 6–8 oz formula* 1–3 Tbsp meat or meat alternative 2–3 Tbsp vegetables 2–3 Tbsp fruit	Breast milk or 6–8 oz formula* 2–4 Tbsp infant cereal† 1–2 Tbsp meat or meat alternative 3–5 Tbsp vegetables 3–4 Tbsp fruit
Late afternoon	Breast milk or 6–8 oz formula*	Breast milk or 6–8 oz formula*
Supper	Breast milk or 6–8 oz formula* 4 Tbsp infant cereal† 2–3 Tbsp vegetables 2–3 Tbsp fruit	Breast milk or 6–8 oz formula* 2–3 Tbsp meat or meat alternative 3–5 Tbsp vegetables 2–3 Tbsp fruit
Evening	Breast milk or 6–8 oz formula* (optional)	Breast milk or 6–8 oz formula* (optional)

*If baby is not breast-fed, iron-fortified, commercial infant formula is recommended for the first 9 to 12 months.
†Iron-fortified infant cereal is recommended for babies during the first 2 years.

⊙ **weaning**
training an infant to drink from the cup
instead of the nipple

diet so that the child does not develop a taste for them and, consequently, over-use them throughout life.

Weaning actually begins when the infant is first given food from a spoon (Figure 12-8). It progresses as the child shows an interest in and an ability to drink from a cup. The child will ultimately discard the bottle or refuse the breast. If the child shows great reluctance to discard the bottle or still seeks the breast, the parents should be patient and discuss this with their health care provider.

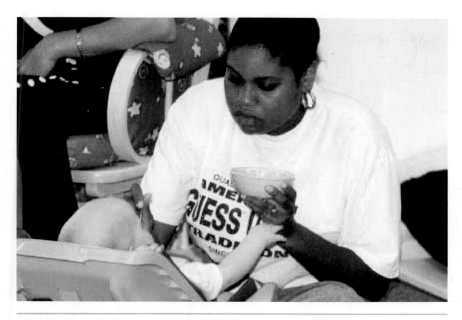

Figure 12-8 *Weaning an infant from the bottle actually begins when food is given with a spoon.*

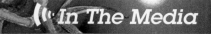

OVERFEEDING IN INFANCY MIGHT LEAD TO CHILDHOOD OBESITY

Nutrition Journal published the results of a small pilot study indicating that obese women fed their 4- to 5-month-old infants more energy-rich food, and spent less time feeding and interacting with them, than normal-weight women. The 24-hour observational study showed that obese mothers fed their babies an average of 19.7 calories per kilogram of body weight *more* than normal-weight mothers. The extra calories were from carbohydrates. The obese mothers also spent less time feeding their children and less time playing or interacting with them, and as a result their children got less exercise and spent more time sleeping. More research is needed in this area before solid conclusions can be drawn, but a good suggestion is for all parents to spend quality time feeding, enjoying, and playing with their infants to help them later develop active lifestyles and healthy eating behaviors.

(Source: NewsRX.com and *Women's Health Weekly*, 2005.)

SPECIAL CONSIDERATIONS FOR INFANTS WITH ALTERED NUTRITIONAL NEEDS

Premature Infants

An infant born before 37 weeks gestation is considered to be premature. These babies have special needs. The sucking reflex is not developed until 34 weeks gestation, and infants born earlier must be fed by total parenteral nutrition, tube

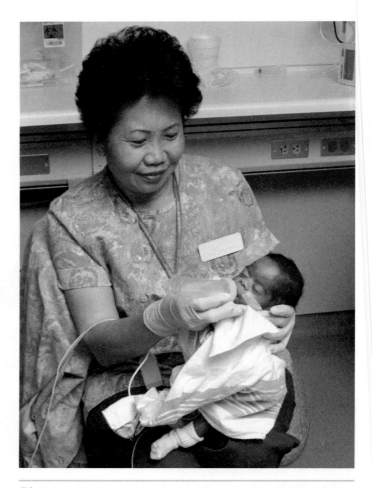

Figure 12-9 *This premature infant receives a specially designed formula to meet his nutritional needs; note placement of nasogastric tube.*

feedings, or bolus feedings (Figure 12-9). The best food for a premature infant is its mother's breast milk, which contains more protein, sodium, immunologic properties, and some other minerals than does the milk produced by mothers of full-term infants. Other concerns in preterm infants are low birth weight, underdeveloped lungs, immature GI tract, inadequate bone mineralization, and lack of fat reserves. Many specialized formulas are available for premature infants, but breast milk is best because its composition is made just for the baby, and it changes according to the baby's needs. Mothers of premature babies should be encouraged to pump their milk until the infant is able to nurse.

Cystic Fibrosis

Cystic fibrosis (CF) is an inherited disease. CF causes the body to produce abnormally thick, sticky secretions (mucus) within cells lining organs such as the lungs and pancreas. The thick mucus also obstructs the pancreas, preventing enzymes from reaching the intestines to help break down and digest food. Eighty-five percent of CF children have exocrine pancreatic insufficiency (PI) and are at nutritional risk due to decreased production of digestive enzymes. Malabsorption of fat is also associated with CF; therefore the recommendation is 35%–40% of total calorie intake to be fat. Digestive enzymes are taken in capsule form when food is eaten, and supplementation of fat-soluble vitamins should also be done at mealtime. There is also a water-miscible form of fat-soluble vitamins that can be administered if normal levels cannot be maintained with the use of only fat-soluble vitamins. It is not unusual for those having CF to be malnourished, even with supplementation, due to malabsorption of nutrients and increased needs. One possible solution would be nighttime tube feedings to supplement oral intake if adequate nutrition and weight cannot be maintained.

Failure to Thrive

Failure to thrive (FTT) can be determined by plotting the infant's growth on standardized growth charts (Figure 12-10); consideration must be made for genetic and ethnic variations. Weight for height is the first parameter affected when determining FTT. Later, height and head circumference are affected. Other signs might be slow development or lack of physical skills such as rolling over, sitting, standing, and walking. Mental and social skills will also be delayed. Babies grow the most in the first 6 months of life, and this is when their brain undergoes crucial development, which can affect the rest of their lives. Failure to thrive can have many causes, such as watered-down formula, congenital abnormalities, AIDS, lack of bonding, child abuse, or neglect.

SPECIAL CONSIDERATIONS FOR INFANTS WITH METABOLIC DISORDERS

Some infants are born with the inability to metabolize specific nutrients. These congenital disabilities are called **inborn errors of metabolism.** They are caused by **mutations** in the genes. There is great variation in the seriousness of the conditions caused by these defects. Some cause death at an early age, and some can be minimized so that life can be supported by adjustments in the normal diet. Among children born with these defects, there is, however, the common danger of damage to the central nervous system because of their abnormal body chemistry. This results in mental retardation and sometimes retarded growth. Early diagnosis of these inborn errors combined with diet therapy increases the chances of preventing retardation. Hospitals test newborns for some of these disorders as a matter of course. If there is a family history of a certain genetic disorder, genetic screening can be done. In addition, some of these abnormalities can be discovered by **amniocentesis.**

Galactosemia

Galactosemia is a condition, affecting 1 in 30,000 live births, in which there is a lack of the liver enzyme **transferase.** Transferase normally converts galactose to glucose. Galactose is the simple sugar resulting from the digestion of lactose, the sugar found in milk (see Chapter 4). When transferase is missing and

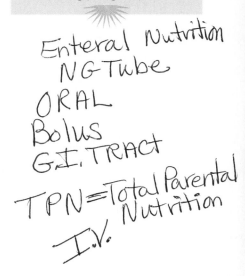

Enteral Nutrition
NG Tube
ORAL
Bolus
G.I. TRACT
TPN = Total Parental Nutrition
I.V.

⟲ **inborn errors of metabolism**
congenital disabilities preventing normal metabolism

⟲ **mutations**
changes in the genes

⟲ **amniocentesis**
a test to determine the status of the fetus in utero

⟲ **galactosemia**
inherited error in metabolism that prevents normal metabolism of galactose

⟲ **transferase**
liver enzyme that converts galactose to glucose

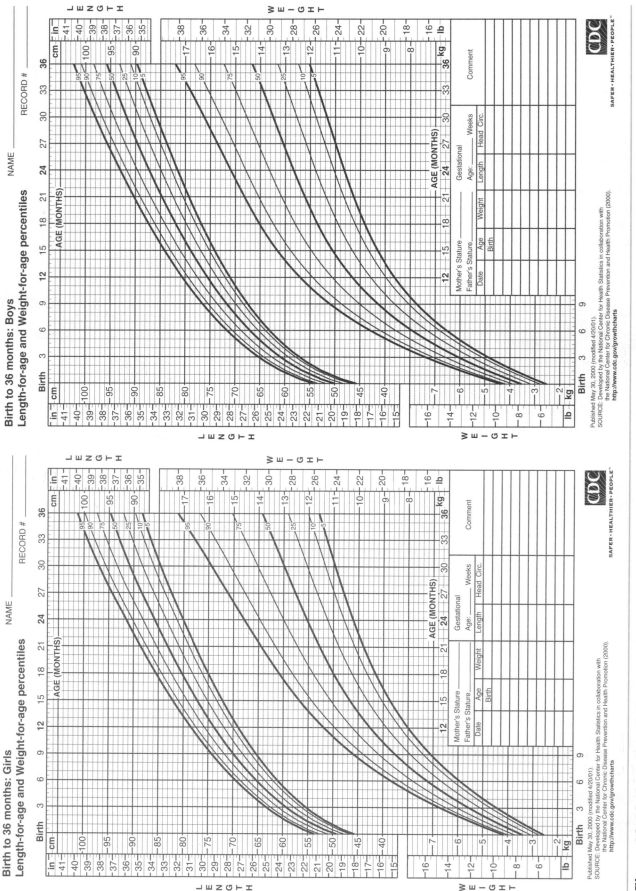

Figure 12-10 *Physical growth charts. (Courtesy of National Center for Health Statistics, U.S. Centers for Disease Control and Prevention, 2001)*

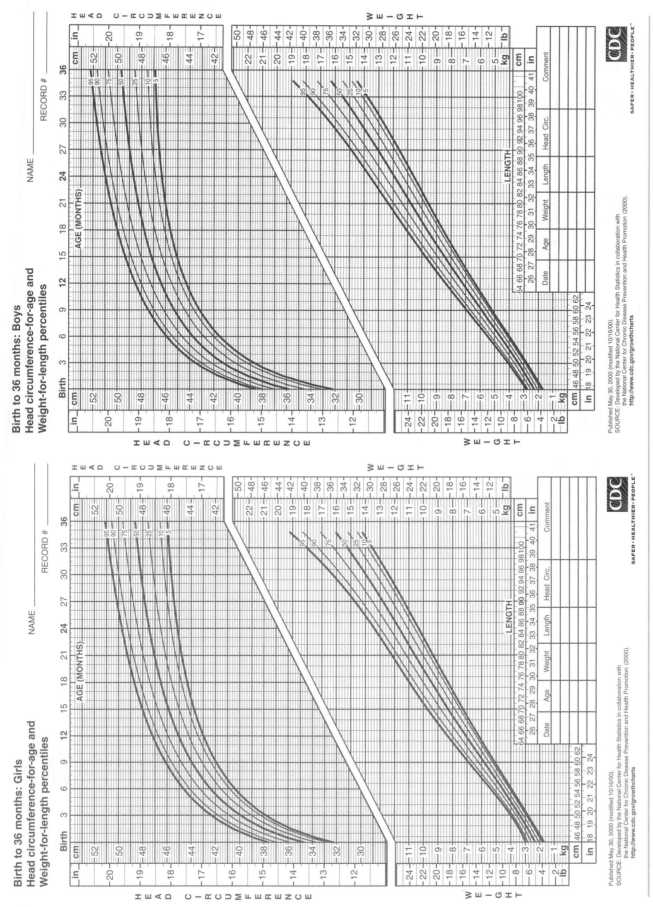

Figure 12-10 *Continued*

galactosuria
galactose in the urine

EXPLORING THE WEB

Visit the Galactosemia Information and Resources Web site, www.galactosemia.com. Search for content related to diet and the control of the disorder. How could you help parents of an infant with galactosemia begin to make the transition to solid foods for their baby? Create a list of safe foods that can be passed along to clients.

phenylketonuria (PKU)
condition caused by an inborn error of metabolism in which the infant lacks an enzyme necessary to metabolize the amino acid phenylalanine

phenylalanine hydroxylase
liver enzyme necessary to metabolize the amino acid phenylalanine

phenylalanine
amino acid

Lofenalac
commercial infant formula with 95% of phenylalanine removed

maple syrup urine disease (MSUD)
disease caused by an inborn error of metabolism in which the body cannot metabolize certain amino acids

leucine
an amino acid

isoleucine
an amino acid

valine
an amino acid

the infant ingests anything containing galactose, the amount of galactose in the blood becomes so excessive that it is toxic. The newborn suffers diarrhea, vomiting, and edema, and the child's liver does not function normally. Cataracts may develop, **galactosuria** occurs, and mental retardation ensues.

Diet Therapy. Diet therapy for galactosemia is the exclusion of anything containing milk from any mammal. During infancy, the treatment is relatively simple because parents can feed the baby lactose-free, commercially prepared formula and can provide supplemental minerals and vitamins. As the child grows and moves on to adult foods, parents must be extremely careful to avoid any food, beverage, or medicine that contains lactose. Nutritional supplements of calcium, vitamin D, and riboflavin must be given so that the diet is nutritionally adequate. This restricted diet may be necessary throughout life, but some physicians allow a somewhat liberalized diet as the child reaches school age. This may mean only small amounts of baked or processed foods that contain small amounts of milk. Even this restricted diet must be accompanied by careful and regular monitoring for galactosuria.

Phenylketonuria (PKU) *Lacks liver ENZYme*

In **phenylketonuria**, infants lack the liver enzyme **phenylalanine hydroxylase**, which is necessary for the metabolism of the amino acid **phenylalanine**. Infants seem to be normal at birth, but if the disease is not treated, most of them become hyperactive, suffer seizures between 6 and 18 months, and become mentally retarded. Public health law requires most hospitals today to screen newborns for phenylketonuria. PKU babies typically have light-colored skin and hair.

Diet Therapy. There is a special, nutritionally adequate, commercial infant formula available for PKU babies. It is called **Lofenalac.** It has had 95% of phe-nylalanine removed from its protein source. It provides just enough phenylalanine for basic needs but no excess. The specific amount depends on the infant's size and growth rate. Regular blood tests determine the adequacy of the amounts. Diets are carefully monitored for calorie and nutrient content and are adjusted frequently as needs change. Except for fats and sugars, there is some protein in all foods. Some of that protein is phenylalanine, so diets for the growing child eating normal food must be carefully planned. There are two varieties of synthetic milk available for older children. They are *Phenyl-free* and *PKU-1, -2,* or *-3.* None of these contains any phenylalanine. They can be used as beverages or in puddings and baked products. Diets should be monitored throughout life to avoid mental retardation and to control hyperactivity and aggressive behavior (Table 12-2).

Maple Syrup Urine Disease (MSUD) *— Urine Smells like Maple Syrup.*

Maple syrup urine disease (MSUD) is a congenital defect resulting in the inability to metabolize three amino acids: **leucine, isoleucine,** and **valine.** It is named for the odor of the urine of these infants and affects 1 in 100,000–300,000 live births. When the infant ingests food protein, there are increased blood levels of these amino acids, causing ketosis. Hypoglycemia, apathy, and convulsions occur

Table 12-2 *Acceptable and Nonacceptable Foods for Those with PKU*

FOODS ALLOWED FOR PEOPLE WITH PKU	FOODS NOT ALLOWED FOR PEOPLE WITH PKU
Special low-phenylalanine formulas	Meats
The following, which contain no phenylalanine:	Fish
Fats	Poultry
Sugars	Eggs
Jellies	Milk
Some candies	Cheese
The following, which contain some phenylalanine:	Nuts
Fruits	Dried beans and peas
Vegetables	Commercially prepared products made from regular flour
Cereals	

EXPLORING THE WEB

Visit the National PKU News Web site, www.pkunews.org. Read through the diet-related material. Prepare a list of acceptable safe foods for clients with PKU. Read through some of the personal stories and be prepared to share some support group references with the parents of an infant with PKU.

SPOTLIGHT on the Life Cycle

The Women, Infants, and Children (WIC) program is federally funded and provides monthly food vouchers for infant formula or milk, cereal, eggs, cheese, peanut butter, and juice for a mother who is breast-feeding. Infants and children who qualify are given monthly food vouchers until the age of 5. Eligibility depends on nutritional risk, history of miscarriage or premature birth, abnormal growth, anemia, and low income. Nutrition education is a component of the services provided.

[handwritten margin note: Women, Infants, Children Dietary Staff]

very early. Depending on the extent of the disease, if not treated promptly, the child can die from acidosis. Mild forms of the disease, if left untreated, will cause mental retardation and bouts of acidosis.

Diet Therapy. The diet must provide sufficient calories and nutrients, but with extremely restricted amounts of leucine, isoleucine, and valine. A special formula and low-protein foods are used. Diet therapy appears to be necessary throughout life.

CONSIDERATIONS FOR THE HEALTH CARE PROFESSIONAL

Although the physical and mental development of infants depends on the nutrients and calories they receive, their psychosocial development depends on *how and when* these nutrients and calories are provided. Some new parents will have a solid knowledge of the nutrition information needed but lack a real understanding of the importance of how and when food should be presented to infants. They may hold the infant during feedings but focus instead on the television or newspaper.

Other parents may know instinctively how important cuddling and attention are to an infant, but they lack accurate knowledge of infant nutrition.

Parents from both groups are apt to have opinions that may or may not be correct. The health care professional will help these parents most by listening carefully to them. The parents are more inclined to listen to advice when a two-way discussion follows.

SUMMARY

It is particularly important that babies have adequate diets so that their physical and mental development are not impaired. Breastfeeding is nature's way of feeding an infant, although formula feeding is quite acceptable. Cow's milk is usually used in formulas because it is most available and is easily modified to resemble human milk. The young child's diet is supplemented on the advice of the pediatrician. Added foods should be based on MyPyramid.

Inborn errors of metabolism cause various problems, ranging from mental retardation to death, if not properly treated. In these conditions, diet therapy is the primary tool in maintaining the patient's health.

Premature, CF, and FTT infants have special nutritional needs.

DISCUSSION TOPICS

1. Do any of the students know a woman who has breast-fed her baby? If so, what were her reactions to the experience?

2. Why is breastfeeding not always possible?

3. Discuss the possible effects of regularly propping the baby's bottle instead of holding the baby during feeding.

4. Why is a rigid time schedule for feeding a baby not advisable? Explain why feeding infants on demand the first few months can lead to a regular feeding schedule.

5. How may weaning be accomplished?

6. What is meant by inborn errors of metabolism? What causes them? How might they affect people?

7. Discuss PKU. Include its cause, symptoms, effects, and treatment.

SUGGESTED ACTIVITIES

1. Have a panel discussion on the advantages and disadvantages of breastfeeding. Invite lactation specialists, doctors, and parents as panelists.

2. Observe a demonstration of the actual feeding and burping of a baby.

3. Visit a store that carries prepared infant formulas and compare their prices and nutritional values.

4. Invite a physician or nurse practitioner to give a talk on inborn errors of metabolism.

REVIEW

Multiple choice. Select the *letter* that precedes the best answer.

1. The most rapid growth in a child's life occurs during
   a. its first month
   b. the month following weaning
   c. its first year
   d. its sixth year

2. The amount of protein needed by a child during its first year
   a. is greater during the first 6 months than during the second
   b. is greater during the second 6 months than during the first
   c. does not change from the first month to the twelfth
   d. increases on a weekly basis

[handwritten: Breast milk all except Vitamin D]

3. After the initial supplement of vitamin K following birth, breast milk provides all the nutrients an infant needs during the first 4 to 6 months except for
a. vitamin A   c. vitamin C.
b. vitamin B   **d. vitamin D** *(circled)*

4. The vitamin in question 3 might be provided
a. by injection
b. in diluted orange juice
c. by regular walks in the sunshine *(circled)*
d. in pasteurized apple juice

5. Breast-fed babies are more resistant to infection than are bottle-fed babies because mother's milk provides
a. a sterile environment   c. leucine
b. synthetic antibiotics   **d. immunity** *(circled)*

6. The development of emotional attachment to a child is called
a. transferase
b. bonding *(circled)*
c. psychosocial development
d. immunity

7. It is recommended that, at each feeding, an infant nurse at each breast for approximately
a. 3–5 minutes   **c. 10–15 minutes** *(circled)*
b. 5–10 minutes   d. 20 minutes

8. It can be said that infant formulas
a. are usually based on cow's milk *(circled)*
b. have the same protein content as cow's milk
c. contain fewer minerals than cow's milk
d. contain no sugar

9. Infants with sensitivities or allergies to cow's milk may be given
a. goat's milk
b. synthetic milk, often made from soybeans *(circled)*
c. formula with predigested carbohydrates
d. any of the above

10. By the age of 6 months, a child
a. may be introduced to a new formula
b. is usually completely weaned
c. is usually introduced to solid foods *(circled)*
d. is no longer given milk

Briefly answer the following questions.

1. Why should the mother give her baby special attention during feedings?

2. How is a bottle warmed? Is it always necessary to warm the bottle? Explain. Why is a microwave oven not recommended?

3. Why is it not advisable to give an 8-month-old child peanuts? *[handwritten: Choking Hazard Allergies]*

CASE IN POINT

RICARDO: OVERCOMING FAILURE TO THRIVE (FTT)

Toni was a 36-year-old Colombian woman who was having her sixth child. Ricardo was 8 pounds 6 ounces and 21 inches long at birth. Toni brought him home after 48 hours to a houseful of happy siblings. After being home for 3 days, Toni's husband left her for another woman. Toni's life was in an upheaval. What was she going to do with six children, no husband, and no job? How was she going to feed, clothe, and take care of them all by herself? Toni could only focus on finding out what had happened to her marriage and how she was to live in the future. Her oldest daughter tried to help with the younger children, but she was not at home during the day. Ricardo became cranky and did not eat well. He was on the bottle so Toni knew he was eating something. After 3 months of grieving for herself, Toni decided that she needed to get her life and her children's lives back on track. Toni took Ricardo to see the nurse practitioner (NP) at the family clinic. Toni told the nurse all about her husband's leaving the home and how difficult things had been for her and the kids. The NP noticed that Ricardo was small for his age; he was not smiling or tracking objects. The NP asked Toni to return weekly to monitor Ricardo closely.

After the 5-month appointment, the NP plotted Ricardo's growth. He weighed 10 pounds and measured 22 inches long. The NP told Toni that Ricardo was in trouble. He had failure to thrive. Toni was devastated.

ASSESSMENT

1. What data do you have about Toni?
2. What data do you have about Ricardo?
3. What factors contributed to Ricardo's problem?
4. Using the growth charts in Figure 12-10, determine a baby's normal weight and height at 5 months. What should Ricardo weigh, and how long should he be?
5. What should Ricardo be doing developmentally at 5 months?
6. How severe is Ricardo's failure to thrive?

DIAGNOSIS

7. Complete the following: Ricardo's failure to thrive is related to _____ .
8. Complete the following: Ricardo's imbalanced nutrition, less than body requirements, is secondary to _____ .
9. Complete the following: ineffective feeding is a result of _____ .

PLAN/GOAL

10. What is your immediate goal for Ricardo?
11. What is your longer-term goal for Ricardo?
12. What is your short-term goal for Toni?
13. What is your long-term goal for Toni?

IMPLEMENTATION

14. What changes need to occur for Ricardo to thrive?
15. What does the NP need to teach Toni?
16. How else can the NP help Toni?
17. Who else needs to be involved in Ricardo's care?

EVALUATION/OUTCOME CRITERIA

18. After the plan has been in place for 6 weeks, what changes should Toni see in Ricardo?
19. What will the NP measure and observe in Ricardo and Toni if the plan is successful?

THINKING FURTHER

20. Why is it important for infants to have a good start in life? Why is their nutrition so critical? What future complications can be avoided as a result?

◎ RATE THIS PLATE

Ricardo was picking up on his mother's stress and anxiety, and that affected his eating. Toni needs to take extra quiet time with Ricardo during feeding time. Also, she may consider offering him a bottle more often. He is old enough to start solid food, and so Toni offered Ricardo the following baby food items. Rate the plate.

2 Tbsp rice cereal made with formula

2 Tbsp green beans

2 Tbsp chicken

2 Tbsp peaches

Were Toni's choices good for starting on solid foods? How about the portion sizes? Would you change anything?

CASE IN POINT

CODY: ADJUSTING TO BOTTLE FEEDING

Paula was a 37-year-old New Yorker, married, and a television journalist. She and her husband, Aaron, were eagerly awaiting the birth of their first child. Paula knew it was going to be rough to juggle her career and take care of the baby. Her career was just taking off. Her boss was very flexible and supportive; he suggested that she work on background research while she was on maternity leave. He was willing to let her bring the baby to the office when she returned to work. Paula had been interviewing nannies so she could return to work. Cody was a good baby, but Paula had had no idea that breastfeeding was so time consuming. She nursed Cody successfully for 6 weeks while she tried to maintain her career.

In consultation with her doctor, she made the transition to bottle feeding and a nanny at 8 weeks instead of the 12th week as originally planned. Cody cried more with the bottle feeding, but he drank the formula. The nanny took care of Cody 5 hours a day when she started. Paula returned to full-time work at 12 weeks, and the nanny took care of Cody while both Paula and Aaron were at work. Paula enjoyed the time at home with Cody after she returned each day, and she was pleased that she had nursed him for 6 weeks.

ASSESSMENT

1. What data do you have about the problem?
2. What factor contributed the most to the change in Paula's breastfeeding plans?
3. What benefit did Cody receive from 6 weeks of breastfeeding?
4. What can you guess is the status of bonding between Paula and Cody?
5. What do you suspect will be the relationship between Cody and the nanny?

DIAGNOSIS

6. Why did Paula switch to bottle feeding earlier than she had planned?
7. Does the change from breastfeeding to bottle feeding remain nutritionally adequate?
8. Could Cody's problem with crying be emotionally related?

PLAN/GOAL

9. What is your primary goal for Cody?
10. What needs have to be met for Cody to develop?
11. What goals do you have for Paula?

IMPLEMENTATION

12. What are the advantages of breast milk over formula?
13. Other than nutritional intake, what else occurs when a mother is breast-feeding that is important to a child's development?

14. What else could Paula have done if she didn't have time to breast-feed but wanted Cody to get her breast milk?
15. What needs to be done after bottle feeding?
16. What criteria can Paula use to evaluate whether Cody is getting enough calories and nutrients?
17. Who can assist Paula in this transition?

EVALUATION/OUTCOME CRITERIA

18. After Paula had been back to work about 1 month, what criteria could she use to assure that Cody was happy and developing on time?

THINKING FURTHER

19. If income were not an issue, what other solutions were possible in this situation?
20. How can you use this information in other situations?

RATE THIS PLATE

Rate the plate for Cody. Cody is now 6 months old and is eating baby food. On Cody's luncheon plate are the following:

1/2 jar chicken (1/4 cup)
1/2 jar carrots (1/4 cup)
1 jar peaches (1/2 cup)
8 oz formula

CHAPTER

13

DIET DURING CHILDHOOD AND ADOLESCENCE

OBJECTIVES

After studying this chapter, you should be able to:

- Identify nutritional needs of children ages 1 to 12 and of adolescents
- State the effects of inadequate nutrition during the growing years
- Describe eating disorders that can occur during adolescence
- Discuss the consequences of obesity in childhood
- Evaluate the nutritive value of the fast-food products available in the United States today

Although specific nutritional requirements change as children grow, nutrition always affects physical, mental, and emotional growth and development. Studies indicate that the mental ability and size of an individual are directly influenced by nutrition during the early years. Children who have an inadequate supply of nutrients—especially of protein—and calories during their early years may be shorter and less intellectually able than children who receive an adequate diet.

CHILDREN AGES 1 TO 12

Eating habits develop during childhood. Once developed, poor eating habits will be difficult to change. They can exacerbate emotional and physical problems such as irritability, **depression, anxiety,** fatigue, and illness.

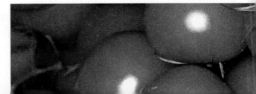

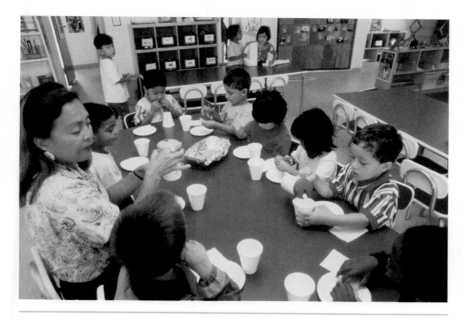

Figure 13-1 *Snacks are enjoyed with friends in the playroom.*

Because children learn partly by imitation, learning good eating habits is easier if the parents have good habits and are calm and relaxed about the child's. Nutritious foods should be available at snack time as well as at mealtime (Figure 13-1), and meals should include a wide variety of foods to ensure good nutrient intake.

Parents should be aware that it is not uncommon for children's appetites to vary. The rate of growth is not constant. As the child ages, the rate of growth actually slows. The approximate weight gain of a child during the second year of life is only 5 pounds. In addition, children's attention is increasingly focused on their environment rather than their stomachs. Consequently, their appetites and interest in food commonly decrease during the early years. Children between the ages of 1 and 3 undergo vast changes. Their legs grow longer; they develop muscles; they lose their baby shape; they begin to walk and talk; and they learn to feed and generally assert themselves (Figure 13-2). A 2-year-old child's statement "No!" is his or her way of saying "Let me decide!"

As children continue to grow and develop, they will increasingly and healthfully assert themselves. They want and need to show their growing independence. Parents should respect this need as much as possible. Children's likes and dislikes may change. New foods should be introduced gradually, in small amounts, and as attractively as possible. Allowing the child to assist in purchasing and preparing a new food is often a good way of arousing interest in the food and a desire to eat it.

Children should be offered nutrient-dense foods because the amount eaten often will be small. Fats should not be limited before the age of 2 years, but meals and snacks should not be fat-laden either. Whole milk is recommended until the age of 2, but low-fat or fat-free should be served from 2 on. The guideline for fat

depression
feelings of extreme sadness

anxiety
apprehension

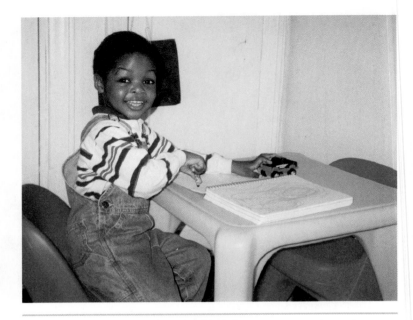

Figure 13-2 *A healthy 3-year-old at play.*

intake is 30%–35% of calories from fat for 2–3-year-olds, and 25%–35% of calories from fat for 4–18-year-olds, with no more than 7% from saturated fats. It is recommended that children not salt their food at the table or have foods prepared with a lot of salt.

Young children are especially sensitive to and reject hot (temperature) foods, but they like crisp textures, mild flavors, and familiar foods. They are wary of foods covered by sauce or gravy. Parents should set realistic goals and expectations about the amount of food a child needs. A good rule of thumb for preschool children is 1 tablespoon for each year of age. Table 13-1 details serving sizes according to age. Calorie needs will depend on rate of growth, activity level, body size, metabolism, and health.

Children can have food jags, such as eating only one or two foods, or rituals, such as not letting foods touch on the plate, or using a different spoon for each food eaten. Choking is prevalent in young children. To prevent choking, do not give children under 4 years of age peanuts, grapes, hot dogs, raw carrots, hard candy, or thick peanut butter.

A child needs a snack every 2 to 3 hours for continued energy. Children often prefer finger foods for snacks. Snacks should be nutrient dense and as nutritious as food served at mealtime. Cheese, Cheerios, fruit, milk, and unsweetened cereals make good snacks.

Mealtime should be pleasant, and food should not be forced on the child. *The parent's primary responsibility is to provide nutritious food in a pleasant setting, and the child's responsibility is to decide how much food to eat or whether to eat,* according to child expert Ellyn Satter (1995). When a child is hungry, he or she will eat. Forcing a child to eat can cause disordered eating and, ultimately, chronic overeating, **anorexia nervosa,** or **bulimia** (discussed later in this chapter).

anorexia nervosa
psychologically induced lack of appetite

bulimia
condition in which patient alternately binges and purges

Table 13-1 *Food Plan for Preschool and School-Age Children Based on MyPyramid*

FOOD GROUP	NO. OF SERVINGS	AGE 1–2	APPROXIMATE SERVING SIZE*		
			AGE 3–4	AGE 5–6	AGE 7–12
Milk, yogurt, and cheese	3	½–¾ cup or 1 oz	¾ cup or 1½ oz	1 cup or 2 oz	1 cup or 2 oz
Meat, poultry, fish, dry beans, eggs, and nuts	2 or more	1 oz or 1–2 Tbsp	1½ oz or 3–4 Tbsp	1½ oz or ½ cup	2 oz or ½ cup
Vegetables	3 or more	1–2 Tbsp	3–4 Tbsp	½ cup	½ cup
Fruits	2 or more	1–2 Tbsp or ½ cup juice	3–4 Tbsp or ½ cup juice	½ cup or ½ cup juice	½ cup or ½ cup juice
Bread, cereal, rice, and pasta	6 or more	½ slice or ½ cup	1 slice or ½ cup	1 slice or ¾ cup	1 slice or ¾ cup

Adapted from Food and Nutrition Service, U.S. Department of Agriculture: *Meal pattern requirements and offer versus serve manual,* FNS-265, 1990.

*Use as a starting point. Increase serving size as energy yields dictate, but maintain variety in the diet by making sure all food groups are still appropriately represented.

Calorie and Nutrient Needs

The *rate* of growth diminishes from the age of 1 until about 10; thus the caloric requirement per pound of body weight also diminishes during this period. For example, at 6 months, a girl needs about 54 calories per pound of body weight, but by the age of 10, she will require only 35 calories per pound of body weight.

Nutrient needs, however, do not diminish. From the age of 6 months to 10 years, nutrient needs actually *increase* because of the increase in body size. Therefore, it is especially important that young children are given nutritious foods *that they will eat.*

MyPyramid (Figure 13-3) is a good foundation for developing meal plans that, with adjustments, will suit all family members. A variety of foods should be offered and, when possible, the child should be offered some choices of foods. Such a choice at the table helps the child's psychosocial development.

In general, the young child will need 2 to 3 cups of low-fat or fat-free milk each day, or the equivalent in terms of calcium. However, excessive use of milk should be avoided because it can crowd out other, iron-rich foods and possibly cause iron deficiency. The selections of the other food groups are the same for adults, but the portions will be smaller. The use of sweets should be minimized because the child is apt to prefer them to nutrient-rich foods. Sweetened fruit juices, especially, should be limited. Children also need water and fiber in their diets. They need to drink 1 ml of water for each calorie. If food valued at 1,200 calories is eaten, then five 8-ounce glasses of water are needed. Fiber needs are calculated according to age. After age 3, a child's fiber needs are "age + 5 grams" and no more than "age + 10 grams." A child who eats more fiber than that might be too full to eat enough other foods to provide all the calories needed for growth and development. Fiber should be

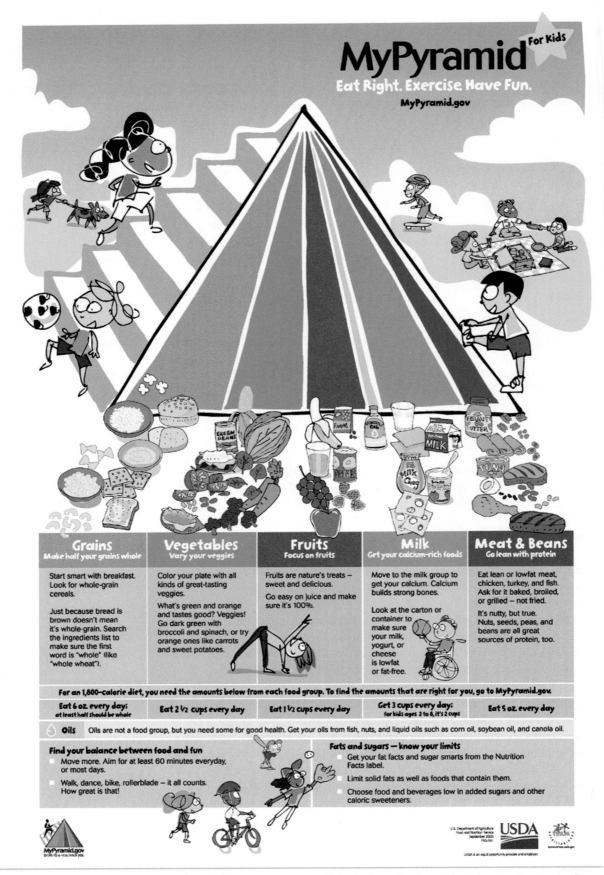

Figure 13-3 *MyPyramid for Kids. (Courtesy of the U.S. Department of Agriculture Food and Nutrition Service, September 2005. Retrieved January 19, 2006, from http://teamnutrition.usda.gov/Resources/mpk_poster2.pdf.)*

added slowly, if not already in the diet, and fluids must also be increased. Childhood is a good time to develop the lifelong good habit of getting enough dietary fiber to prevent constipation and diseases such as colon cancer and diverticulitis.

Childhood Obesity

Normal stature and weight for children can be determined using standardized growth charts (Figure 13-4). Expected growth patterns will fall between the 5th and 95th percentile; children whose weight falls outside those parameters need special evaluation and attention. Childhood obesity has become an epidemic. Overweight has doubled in the last 20 to 30 years, and one in five children is now overweight. The definition of overweight is a child at or above the 95th percentile of body mass index (BMI) by sex and age. Children are considered obese when their body fat exceeds lean muscle mass. Type 2 diabetes mellitus, rarely seen before in children, is now being diagnosed in children as young as 10; it is related to diet and weight. The causes of obesity are complex, but genetics does play a role. If one parent is obese, there is a 50% risk that his or her children will be obese. If both parents are obese, the risk increases to 80%. Playing a major role are the family eating habits, lifestyle habits, and exercise patterns. Obese children have an 85% chance of becoming obese adults if they are obese after the age of 10.

Obese children and adults have similar health and social problems. Obese children with asthma are more likely to have more severe problems than their normal-weight peers. Obese children also may have increased blood pressure, heart rate, cardiac output, type 2 diabetes, sleep apnea, and hyperlipidemia. Older children and adolescents may develop hip and knee problems from obesity, but more important is the social stigma attached to obesity.

What can be done to help the children? The best thing to do for overweight children is to turn off the TV and computer and get them moving. Walking is exercise, but it must be brisk and for at least 60 minutes per day. Along with walking, the best activities to encourage are step aerobics, bicycling, swimming, skating, running, and sports such as tennis and racquetball, if a child cannot participate in team sports (Figure 13-5). Children are natural-born triathletes—encourage them to get up and try several different activities.

Weight control boils down to calories consumed must equal calories burned. All foods are fattening if consumed beyond needs. Portion control and snacking appear to be a big issue with obese children. Children should not be put on "diets." Children continue to grow; therefore, if weight can be maintained by exercise and portion control until growth catches up, the problem of obesity will no longer exist.

An obese child, like a child of normal weight, may need a snack after school. Make that snack a healthy choice such as fruit, vegetables (use salsa as a dip), low-fat popcorn, a single serving of cereal, or an individual bag of pretzels. Single-serving sizes are ideal because an obese child may have trouble consuming a correct portion if given a large bag. Help children avoid "drinking" their daily caloric needs in sodas and other sweetened drinks.

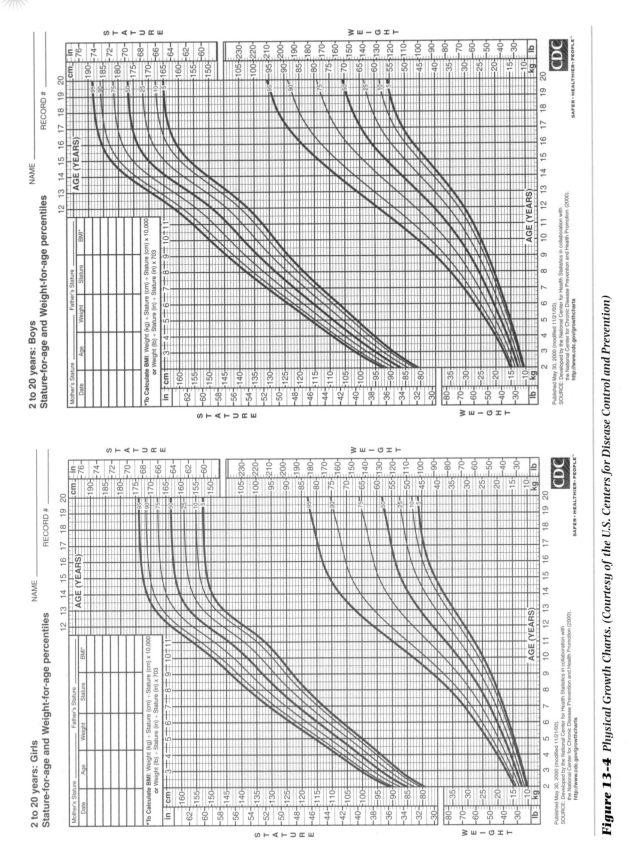

Figure 13-4 *Physical Growth Charts. (Courtesy of the U.S. Centers for Disease Control and Prevention)*

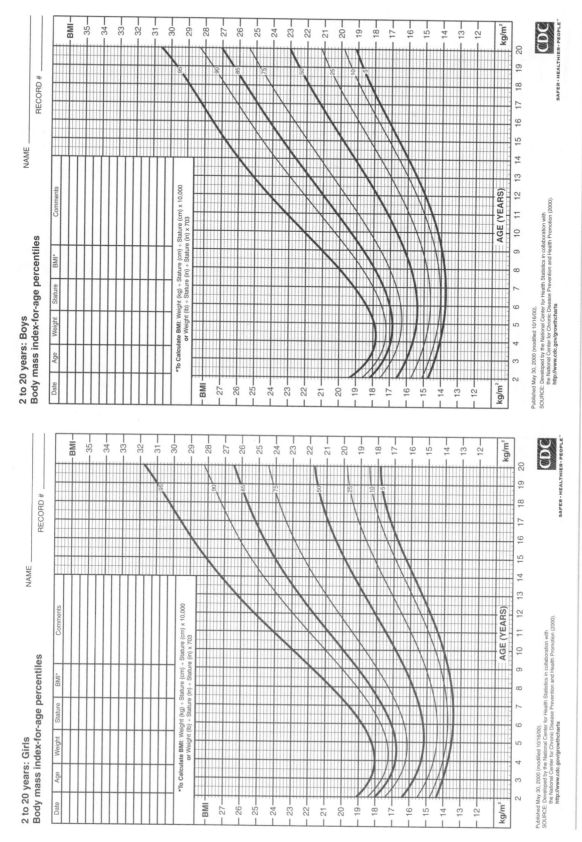

Figure 13-4 *(Continued)*

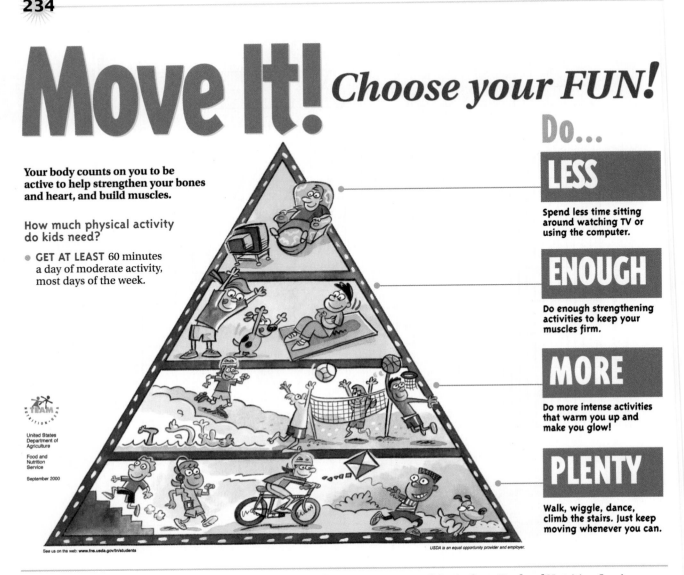

Move It! *Choose your FUN!*

Do...

LESS
Spend less time sitting around watching TV or using the computer.

ENOUGH
Do enough strengthening activities to keep your muscles firm.

MORE
Do more intense activities that warm you up and make you glow!

PLENTY
Walk, wiggle, dance, climb the stairs. Just keep moving whenever you can.

Your body counts on you to be active to help strengthen your bones and heart, and build muscles.

How much physical activity do kids need?

- **GET AT LEAST** 60 minutes a day of moderate activity, most days of the week.

United States Department of Agriculture
Food and Nutrition Service
September 2000

See us on the web: www.fns.usda.gov/tn/students

USDA is an equal opportunity provider and employer.

Figure 13-5 *Children's activity pyramid. (Courtesy of the U.S. Department of Agriculture Food and Nutrition Service, September 2000. Retrieved January 19, 2006, from http://teamnutrition.usda.gov/Resources/moveit.pdf.)*

What Can Parents Do to Help?

- Provide only healthy, nourishing food for meals and snacks. If it is not available a child cannot eat it.
- Limit TV and computer time. Remove TV sets from your child's bedroom.
- Get moving yourself. Exercise benefits everyone.
- Never tell a child he cannot have a food because "he is too fat."
- Learn correct portions, even if this means weighing and measuring (see Table 13-1).

◎ SUPERSIZE USA

Vending machines are everywhere! Vending machines are neither good nor bad—what is good or bad are the choices the person makes by pressing the buttons to get a snack or drink. How often does your child buy something from a vending machine? What was the last thing purchased? Compare the last purchase with the lists below. Which category was the purchase under?

Good Choices	Bad Choices
Water	Breakfast pastries
Baked chips	Chips (nacho cheese)
Dried fruit	Candy bars
100% juice (no sugar added)	Cookies
Nutrition bars	Doughnuts
Nuts	Sandwich crackers
Pretzels	Sausage meats and jerky
Skim milk	Whole milk
Tea (unsweetened or diet)	Snack cakes
Vegetables	Soda
Yogurt	Sugary juice or punch

The bad choices contain too much sugar and saturated and trans fats. As a once-in-awhile treat they are OK, but not on a daily basis.

(Source: www.forbes.com.)

- Remember, there is nothing a child cannot eat; it is just how often and how much will be consumed of a particular food. There are no good or bad foods.

- Never provide food for comfort or as a reward.

- Eat only at the table and at designated times.

- Give water to drink rather than calorie-laden fruit juice. If a child won't drink water, then a small amount of juice can be mixed with water to give flavor. Use ¼ cup juice to 8–12 ounces of water. This glass of water-juice will contain about 30 calories versus 120–180 for 100% juice.

- Eat slowly—it takes 20 minutes for the brain to get the message that the stomach is full. Make it a game—set a timer and see who can make the meal last for 20 minutes.

- Use the 20-minutes technique if your child wants a calorie-dense snack such as cookies, chocolate, candy bars, or other calorie-dense foods. The child must set the timer, sit at the table with a portion-controlled serving, pay attention to the treat, and make it last for 20 minutes. Holding it in the mouth and rolling it around on the tongue will satisfy taste buds quicker than swallowing immediately and may contribute to satiety sooner.

- Learn to determine whether your child is really hungry or just bored, tired, or lonely. It takes 3 to 4 hours for a stomach to completely empty after a significant meal, so if that amount of time has elapsed then your child is truly hungry.

⬐ Make sure your child gets enough sleep (8–10 hours per night), as sleep deprivation has been linked to obesity.

⬐ Change any unhealthy habits you may possess. You are your child's teacher.

Preventing and reversing childhood obesity will also decrease the incidence of obesity-linked type 2 diabetes.

EXPLORING THE WEB

Search the Web for topics related to childhood obesity. What types of programs exist that claim to be able to help children lose weight? Are these programs healthy for the child from a nutritional standpoint? Are there better, healthier recommendations that parents can use to help prevent or reduce obesity in their children? What additional resources are available for parents whose children are overweight?

Childhood Type 2 Diabetes

As a result of the increase of childhood obesity, there is a parallel increase in diabetes, particularly type 2. Type 2 diabetes is normally found only in adults, usually after the age of 40, and is associated with weight. Most obese children will develop type 2 diabetes between the ages of 10 and 14.

Children with type 2 diabetes should see a certified diabetes educator to learn what to eat to control their diabetes. The diabetes educator will also prescribe daily exercise and attention to fiber intake, both of which help control blood glucose.

Increasing nutrition and exercise knowledge of parents and children appears to be the only way to prevent obesity and childhood type 2 diabetes.

Osteoporosis and Cardiovascular Disease

Children and adolescents live in the moment. This creates problems associated with osteoporosis and cardiovascular diseases. Adherence to sound nutrition principles during childhood and adolescence are needed to protect the heart and bones.

Calcium must be consumed at the DRI level until the age of 30. Fat intake should follow the American Heart Association recommendations of 7% saturated fat, 8% polyunsaturated fat, and 15% monounsaturated fat while keeping total fat to ≤ 35% of daily calories.

The typical diet of a teenager contains too much saturated fat and soda and not enough milk. These habits lead to adult health problems. Motivating children and teens to change their habits will be a challenge, but needs to be done.

ADOLESCENTS

In general, a person between the ages of 13 and 20 is considered an **adolescent**. Adolescence is a period of rapid growth that causes major changes. It

○ **adolescent**
person between the ages of 13 and 20

tends to begin between the ages of 10 and 13 in girls and between 13 and 16 in boys. The growth rate may be 3 inches a year for girls and 4 inches for boys. Bones grow and gain density, muscle and fat tissue develop, and blood volume increases. Sexual maturity occurs. Boys' voices change; girls experience the onset of menses; and both may experience **acne.** Acne is not caused by specific foods but by overactivity of the sebaceous glands of the skin.

These changes are obvious and have a tremendous effect on an adolescent's psychosocial development. No two individuals will develop in the same way. One girl may become heavier than she might like; another may be thin; a boy may not develop the muscle or the height he desires; some may develop serious complexion problems. It can be a time of great joy, but it also can be a time when counseling is needed.

◌ **acne**
pimples

Food Habits

Adolescents, especially boys, typically have enormous appetites. When good eating habits have been established during childhood and there is nutritious food available, the teenager's food habits should present no serious problem.

Adolescents are imitators, like children, but instead of imitating adults, adolescents prefer to imitate their **peers** and do what is popular. Unfortunately, the foods that are popular often have low nutrient density such as potato chips, sodas, and candy. These foods provide mainly carbohydrates and fats and very little protein, vitamins, and minerals, except for salt, which is usually provided in excess. Adolescents' eating habits can be seriously affected by busy schedules, part-time jobs, athletics, social activities, and the lack of an available adult to prepare nutritious food when adolescents are hungry or have time to eat.

When the adolescent's food habits need improvement, it is wise for the adult to tactfully inform her or him of nutritional needs and of the poor nutrition quality of the foods she or he is eating. The adolescent has a natural desire for independence and may resent being told what to do.

Before attempting to change an adolescent's food habits, carefully check her or his food choices for nutrient content. It is too easily assumed that because the adolescent chooses the food, the food is automatically a poor choice in regard to nutrient content. It might be a good choice. An adolescent who has a problem maintaining an appropriate weight may need some advice regarding diet.

◌ **peer group**
group of people approximately one's own age

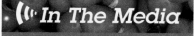

CALIFORNIA BANS SODA IN PUBLIC HIGH SCHOOLS

California Governor Schwarzenegger signed legislation to ban carbonated soda in state high schools as part of an effort to stem obesity. The new law allows milk, drinks with at least 50% fruit or vegetable juice, and drinking water without sweetener. The ban will begin in 2007 and be in full effect by 2009. The ban is already in existence in the elementary schools. Another bill signed by the governor will boost spending on fruits and vegetables in school meals.

(Source: MSNBC News. Retrieved January 19, 2006, from www.msnbc.msn.com/id/ 93554361.)

Calorie and Nutrient Needs

Because of adolescents' rapid growth, calorie requirements naturally increase. Boys' calorie requirements tend to be greater than girls' because boys are generally bigger, tend to be more physically active, and have more lean muscle mass than do girls.

Except for vitamin D, nutrient needs increase dramatically at the onset of adolescence. Because of menstruation, girls have a greater need for iron than do boys. The DRIs for vitamin D, vitamin C, vitamin B_{12}, calcium, phosphorus, and iodine are the same for both sexes. The DRIs for the remaining nutrients are higher for boys than they are for girls.

SPECIAL CONSIDERATIONS FOR THE ADOLESCENT RELATED TO NUTRITION CONCERNS

Adolescence is a stressful time for most young people. They are unexpectedly faced with numerous physical changes; an innate need for independence; increased work and extracurricular demands at school; in many cases, jobs; and social and sexual pressures from their peers. For many teens, such stress can cause one or more of the following problems.

Anorexia Nervosa

In general, adolescent boys in the United States are considered well nourished. Studies show, however, that girls sometimes have diets deficient in calories and protein, iron, calcium, vitamin A, or some of the B vitamins.

These deficiencies can be due to poor eating habits caused by concern about weight. A moderate concern about weight is understandable, and possibly even beneficial, provided it does not cause diets to be deficient in essential nutrients or lead to a potentially fatal condition called anorexia nervosa.

Anorexia nervosa, commonly called *anorexia,* is a psychological disorder more common to women than men. It can begin as early as late childhood, but usually begins during the teen years or the early twenties. It causes the client to drastically reduce calories, causing altered metabolism, which results in hair loss, low blood pressure, weakness, **amenorrhea,** brain damage, and even death.

The causes of anorexia are unclear. Someone with this disorder (an anorexic) has an inordinate fear of being fat. Some anorexics have been overweight and have irrational fears of regaining lost weight. Some young women with demanding parents perceive this as their only means of control. Some may want to resemble slim fashion models and have a distorted body image, where they see themselves as fat even though they are extremely thin. Some fear growing up. Many are perfectionistic overachievers who want to control their body. It pleases them to deny themselves food when they are hungry.

amenorrhea
the stoppage of the monthly menstrual flow

(• In The Media

MARY-KATE OLSEN SEEKS TREATMENT FOR EATING DISORDER

In 2005, television star Mary-Kate Olsen entered a treatment center for an eating disorder, reported to be anorexia nervosa. Anorexia nervosa is a psychiatric disorder with physiological consequences; the disorder is characterized by self-starvation and excessive weight loss. Clients with anorexia nervosa are typically in denial about having an eating disorder, so the biggest step toward recovery is acknowledging there is a problem.

The executive director of an eating disorder clinic in Tucson, Arizona, stated that western society has placed demands on women to stay thin, and the pressure is even more intense in Hollywood (*USA Today,* 2004 by Cesar G. Soriano). Health care professionals can be proactive in encouraging parents and teens to adopt realistic self-images and weight expectations and to seek professional assistance immediately if a problem is suspected.

These young women usually set a maximum weight for themselves and become expert at "counting calories" to maintain their chosen weight. They also often exercise excessively to control or reduce their weight. If the weight declines too far, the anorexic will ultimately die.

Treatment requires:

1. Development of a strong and trusting relationship between the client and the health care professionals involved in the case.
2. That the client learn and accept that weight gain and a change in body contours are normal during adolescence.
3. Nutritional therapy so the client will understand the need for both nutrients and calories and how best to obtain them.
4. Individual and family counseling so the problem is understood by everyone.
5. Close supervision by the health care professional.
6. Time and patience from all involved.

Bulimia

Bulimia is a syndrome in which the client alternately binges and purges by inducing vomiting and using laxatives and diuretics to get rid of ingested food. Bulimics are said to fear that they cannot stop eating. They tend to be high achievers who are perfectionistic, obsessive, and depressed. They generally lack a strong sense of self and have a need to seem special. They know their binge-purge syndrome is abnormal but also fear being overweight. This condition is more common among women than men and can begin any time from the late teens into the thirties.

A bulimic usually binges on high-calorie foods such as cookies, ice cream, pastries, and other "forbidden" foods. The binge can take only a few moments or can run several hours—until there is no space for more food. It occurs when the person is alone. Bulimia can follow a period of excessive dieting, and stress usually increases the frequency of binges.

Bulimia is not usually life-threatening, but it can irritate the esophagus and cause electrolyte imbalances, malnutrition, dehydration, and dental caries.

Treatment usually includes limiting eating to mealtimes, portion control, and close supervision after meals to prevent self-induced vomiting. Diet therapy helps teach the client basic nutritional facts so that he or she will be more inclined to treat the body with respect. Psychological counseling will help the client to understand his or her fears about food. Group therapy also can be helpful.

Both bulimia and anorexia can be problems that will have to be confronted throughout the client's life.

Overweight

Overweight during adolescence is particularly unfortunate because it is apt to diminish the individual's **self-esteem** and, consequently, can exclude her or him from the normal social life of the teen years, further diminishing self-esteem. Also, it tends to make the individual prone to overweight as an adult.

> **EXPLORING THE WEB**
>
> Search the Web for information related to anorexia and bulimia. What nutritional deficits do these disorders cause? What effects will these deficits have on the body? What are the signs and symptoms that would indicate the presence of these disorders? What resources are available for parents of children or young clients suffering from these disorders?

ᗡ **self-esteem**
feelings of self-worth

Although numerous studies have been done, the cause of overweight is difficult to determine. Heredity is believed to play a role. Just as one inherits height, color of hair, or artistic talents, it appears that one may inherit the tendency (or lack of it) to overweight. Overfeeding during infancy and childhood also can be a contributing factor. Then, once a person is overweight, the overweight itself contributes further to the problem.

For example, if a teenager becomes the center of his classmates' jokes, he or she may prefer to spend time alone, perhaps watching television, and finding comfort in food. This behavior adds more calories, reduces activity, and, thus, worsens the condition.

The problem of overweight during adolescence is especially difficult to solve until the individual involved makes the independent decision to change lifestyle habits. After making such a decision, the teenager should see a physician to ensure that his or her health is good. The health care provider can play an important role by offering guidance on changing eating habits, increasing exercise, and adopting a healthier lifestyle.

Fast Foods

fast foods
restaurant food that is ready to serve before orders are taken

Many Americans have become extremely fond of **fast foods**. Many others are highly critical of their nutrient content. Examples of these foods—most of which are favorites of teenagers—include hamburgers, cheeseburgers, French fries, milkshakes, pizza, sodas, tacos, chili, fried chicken, and onion rings. Many fast-food companies have the nutrient content of their products available to help the public make better choices.

Generally speaking, fast foods are excessively high in fat and sodium, as well as calories, and contain only limited amounts of vitamins and minerals (other than sodium) and little fiber. In Table 13-2, the nutrient content of some varieties of fast foods are shown compared with the DRIs for a 16-year-old girl. This shows the potential for problems with a diet that regularly consists of these foods to the exclusion of others.

Nevertheless, these foods are more nutritious than sodas, cakes, and candy. When used with discretion in a balanced diet, they are not harmful. However, teens often use fast foods as a snack to hold them over until dinner, and this results in consumption of many extra calories.

Alcohol

fermentation
changing of sugars and starches to alcohol

In a process called **fermentation**, sugars and starches can be changed to alcohol. Enzyme action causes this change. Alcohol is typically made from fruit, corn, rye, barley, rice, or potatoes. It provides 7 calories per gram but almost no nutrients.

Alcohol is a substance that can have serious side effects. Initially, it causes the drinker to feel "happy" because it lowers inhibitions. This feeling affects the drinker's judgment and can lead to accidents and crime. Ultimately, alcohol is a depressant; continued drinking leads to sleepiness, loss of consciousness, and, when too much is consumed in a short period, death.

alcoholism
chronic and excessive use of alcohol

Abuse (overuse) of alcohol is called **alcoholism**. Alcoholism can destroy the lives of families and devastate the drinker's nutritional status and thus

Table 13-2 *Nutrient and Calorie Contents of Some Fast Foods Compared with DRIs for a 16-Year-Old Female*

	WEIGHT (OZ)	CALORIES	PROTEIN (g)	FAT (g)	CALCIUM (mg)	IRON (mg)	SODIUM (mg)	VITAMIN A (RE)	THIAMINE (mg)	RIBOFLAVIN (mg)	NIACIN (mg)	VITAMIN C (mg)
Hamburger	3½	250	12	11	56	2.2	463	14	0.23	0.24	3.8	1
French fries	2	160	2	8	10	0.4	108	0	0.09	0.01	1.6	5
Chocolate milkshake	10	335	9	8	374	0.9	314	59	0.13	0.63	0.4	0
Pizza	4	300	15	9	220	1.6	700	106	0.34	0.29	4.2	2
Soda	12	160	0	0	11	0.2	18	0	0	0	0	0
Doughnut	2	210	3	12	22	1.0	192	5	0.12	0.12	1.1	0
Potato chips	2	315	3	21	15	0.6	300	0	0.09	0	2.4	24
Chocolate bar with peanuts	1½	225	6	16	75	0.6	30	12	1.0	1.0	2.1	0
DRI/RDA for 16-year-old girl		2,200	44	73	1,200	15	500	800	1.1	1.3	15	60

⟲ **cirrhosis**
generic term for liver disease
characterized by cell loss

health. It affects absorption and normal metabolism of glucose, fats, proteins, and vitamins. When thiamine and niacin cannot be absorbed, the cells cannot use glucose for energy. Blood cells, which depend on glucose for energy, are particularly affected. Over time, if alcohol abuse continues, fat will accumulate in the liver, leading to **cirrhosis**. Alcohol causes kidneys to excrete larger than normal amounts of water, resulting in an increased loss of minerals. In a poor nutritional state, the body is less able to fight off disease.

In addition, excessive, long-term drinking can cause high blood pressure and can damage the heart muscle. It is associated with cancer of the throat and the esophagus and can damage the reproductive system.

The risks to the drinker are obvious. When a pregnant or lactating woman drinks, however, she puts the fetus or the nursing infant at risk as well. Alcohol can lower birth weight and cause fetal alcohol syndrome or fetal alcohol effect, with related developmental disorders (see Chapter 11).

Unfortunately, many teenagers ignore the dangers of alcohol and use it in an effort to appear adult. In addition to the damage to their own health and the accidents and the random acts of violence caused by their drinking, their behavior inspires younger children to emulate them. The health professional is in a good position to spread the message that alcohol is a substance and can cause severe economic and family problems, as well as addiction, disease, and death.

Marijuana

Marijuana use continues to increase among teenagers. Marijuana increases appetite, especially for sweets. One marijuana cigarette is as harmful as four or five tobacco cigarettes because the marijuana smoke is held in the lungs for a longer period of time. As marijuana is smoked, the lungs absorb the fat-soluble active ingredient, delta-9-tetrahydrocannabinol (THC), and store it in the fat (Indiana Prevention Resource Center, 1992). Experts believe that the use of marijuana can lead to the use of other drugs such as cocaine. Common street names for marijuana include grass, weed, pot, and dope.

Cocaine

Cocaine is highly addictive and extremely harmful. It causes restlessness, heightened self-confidence, euphoria, irritability, insomnia, depression, confusion, hallucinations, loss of appetite, and a tendency to withdraw from normal activities. Cocaine can cause cardiac irregularities, heart attacks, and cardiac arrests resulting in death. Weight loss is very common, mostly because it decreases appetite; addicts would give up food for the drug. The smokable form of cocaine is *crack*, which is more addictive than any other drug. It is estimated that half of all crimes against property committed in major cities are related to the use of crack cocaine and the addict's need for money to buy the drug.

Tobacco

Cigarette smoking is addictive. Cigarette smoking by teenagers is very prevalent. Teenagers smoke to "be cool," to look older, because they think it will help them lose weight, or because of peer pressure. Smoking can influence appetite, nutrition status, and weight. Smokers need the DRI for vitamin C plus 35 mg, because smoking alters the metabolism. Low intakes of vitamin C, vitamin A, beta-carotene, folate, and fiber are common in smokers. Smoking increases the risk of lung cancer and heart disease.

Other Addictive Drugs

Methamphetamine is the most potent form of amphetamine. Amphetamines cause heart, breathing, and blood pressure rates to increase. The mouth is usually dry, and swallowing is difficult. Urination is also difficult. Appetite is depressed. The users' pupils are dilated, and reflexes speed up. As the drug wears off, feelings of fatigue or depression are experienced. Street names include crank, speed, crystal, meth, zip, and ice.

Inhalants are chemicals whose fumes are inhaled into the body and produce mind-altering effects. Some inhalants are gasoline, lighter fluid, tool-cleaning solvents, model airplane glue, typewriter correction fluid, and permanent ink in felt-tip pens. Inhalants are both physically and psychologically addictive. Individuals who inhale may risk depression and apathy, nosebleeds, headaches, eye pain, chronic fatigue, heart failure, loss of muscle control, and death.

Nutrition for the Athlete

Good nutrition during the period of life when one is involved in athletics can prevent unnecessary wear and tear on the body as well as maintain the athlete in top physical form. The specific nutritional needs of the athlete are not numerous, but they are important. The athlete needs additional water, calories, thiamine, riboflavin, niacin, sodium, potassium, iron, and protein.

The body uses water to rid itself of excess heat through perspiration. This lost water must be regularly replaced during the activity to prevent dehydration. Plain water is the recommended liquid because it rehydrates the body more quickly than sweetened liquids or the drinks that contain electrolytes. The "electrolyte" drinks are useful to replenish fluids after an athletic event but not during one. Salt tablets are not recommended, because despite the loss of salt and potassium through perspiration, the loss is not equal to the amount contained in the tablets. If there is an insufficient water intake, these salt tablets can increase the risk of dehydration.

The increase in calories depends on the activity and the length of time it is performed. The requirement could be double the normal, up to 6,000 calories per day. Because carbohydrates, not protein, are used for energy, the normal diet proportions of 50% to 55% carbohydrate, 30% fat, and 10% to 15% protein are advised.

There is an increased need for B vitamins because they are necessary for energy metabolism. They are provided in the breads, cereals, fruits, and vegetables needed to bring the calorie count to the total required. Some extra protein is used during training, when muscle mass and blood volume are increasing. This amount is included in the DRI for age and is provided in the normal diet. Protein needs are not increased by physical activity. In fact, excess protein can cause increased urine production, which can lead to dehydration.

EXPLORING THE WEB

Search for information regarding adolescents and drug use. Choose one particular drug and research the nutritional deficits that may occur with the use of this substance. What are the signs and symptoms that may indicate a child is using this substance? What resources are available to help the child stop using the drug?

The minerals sodium and potassium are needed in larger amounts because of loss through perspiration. This amount of sodium can usually be replaced just by salting food to taste, and orange juice or bananas can provide the extra potassium.

A sufficient supply of iron is important to the athlete, particularly to the female athlete. Iron-rich foods eaten with vitamin C-rich foods should provide sufficient iron. The onset of menstruation can be delayed by the heavy physical activity of the young female athlete, and amenorrhea may occur in those already menstruating.

When weight is a concern of the athlete, such as with wrestlers, care should be taken that the individual does not become dehydrated by refusing liquids in an effort to "make weight" for the class.

When weight must be added, the athlete will need an additional 2,500 calories to develop 1 pound of muscle mass. The additional foods eaten to reach this amount of calories should contain the normal proportion of nutrients. A high-fat diet should be avoided because it increases the potential for heart disease. Athletes should reduce calories when training ends.

In general, the athlete should select foods using MyPyramid. The pregame meal should be eaten 3 hours before the event and should consist primarily of carbohydrates and small amounts of protein and fat. Concentrated sugar foods are not advisable because they may cause extra water to collect in the intestines, creating gas and possibly diarrhea.

Glycogen loading (carboloading) is sometimes used for long activities. To increase muscle stores of glycogen, the athlete begins 6 days before the events. For 3 days, the athlete eats a diet consisting of only 10% carbohydrate and mostly protein and fat as she or he performs heavy exercise. This depletes the current store of glycogen. The next 3 days, the diet is 70% carbohydrate, and the exercise is very light so that the muscles become loaded with glycogen. This practice may cause an abnormal heartbeat and some weight gain.

Currently, it is recommended that the athlete exercise heavily and eat carbohydrates as desired. Then, during the week before the competition, exercise should be reduced. On the day before competition, the athlete should eat a high-carbohydrate diet and rest.

After the event, the athlete may prefer to drink fruit juices until relaxed and then satisfy the appetite with sandwiches or a full meal. Many athletes will use "power drinks" or "energy drinks," which are not any better than soda and contain mostly sugar and empty calories.

There are no magic potions or diet supplements that will increase an athlete's prowess, as may be touted by health food faddists. *Steroid* drugs should not be used to build muscles (Figure 13-6). They can affect the fat content of the blood, damage the liver, change the reproductive system, and even alter facial appearance. Good diet, good health habits, and practice combined with innate talent remain the essentials for athletic success.

glycogen loading (carboloading)
process in which the muscle store of glycogen is maximized; also called carboloading

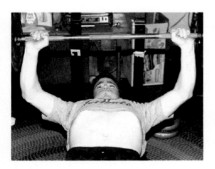

Figure 13-6 *Building muscles requires using them—NOT steroid drugs.*

CONSIDERATIONS FOR THE HEALTH CARE PROFESSIONAL

The health care professional who works with young children may encounter poor appetites and eating habits in her or his clients. Compounding this problem will be the anxiety of the clients' parents. They will understandably be concerned about their children's appetites and physical conditions. The health care professional can be most helpful to all concerned by exhibiting patience and understanding and by listening to parents and client.

The problems of adolescent clients, perhaps particularly those with disordered eating, can be especially challenging. For example, telling an anorexic client to eat could be counterproductive. Health care professionals working with such clients should consult with the client's psychological counselor. Parents of clients with disordered eating must be included in both nutritional and family counseling.

SUMMARY

Children's nutritional needs vary as they grow and develop. The rate of growth slows between the ages of 1 and 10, and the child's calorie requirement per pound of body weight slows accordingly. However, nutrient needs gradually increase during these years. During adolescence, growth is rapid, and nutritional and calorie requirements increase substantially. Anorexia nervosa, bulimia, and obesity are problems of weight control that can occur during adolescence. Fast foods are acceptable when used with discretion in a balanced diet. Alcohol can be a serious problem for adolescents, and it is essential that adolescents understand its potential dangers. The nutritional needs of athletes are similar to those of nonathletes except for increased needs for calories, B vitamins, sodium, potassium, and iron.

DISCUSSION TOPICS

1. Discuss how parents' anxieties about children's food habits may affect those habits.

2. In what ways does overweight affect an adolescent's self-esteem?

3. Why can it be especially difficult for a parent to influence her or his adolescent's attitudes about food?

4. Discuss the nutrient content of some fast foods. Explain why they can be useful additions to the diet and also why they should not be used exclusively.

5. What could result if a 30-year-old lawyer continued to eat as he did as a 17-year-old football player?

6. Describe anorexia nervosa. Ask if anyone in the class knows anyone who has suffered from it. Ask that individual for descriptions of the person's attitude, physical condition, possible causes, and today's condition.

7. Discuss how snack foods can affect one's overall nutrition.

8. Describe a "typical" bulimic client. What role does stress often play in bulimia? Why do bulimics often binge on cakes, cookies, and ice cream? How does bulimia upset one's electrolyte balance? How does it irritate the esophagus? How can it cause dental caries? What could happen in uncontrolled bulimia?

SUGGESTED ACTIVITIES

1. List your favorite snack foods. List nutritious snack foods. Check the calorie values of these foods and compare lists for nutrition and taste. Discuss possible improvements in your list of favorite snacks.

2. Plan a talk for fourth-grade students on the importance of good food habits. Begin with an outline, and develop it into a narrative that 9-year-old children will understand. If possible, ask permission of a fourth-grade teacher to deliver this talk to the class.

3. Role-play a situation in which your younger sister, who is considerably overweight, has just asked you how she can lose weight. Ask her why she wants to lose weight, how much weight she wants to lose, if she is willing to change her eating habits for the rest of her life, what her favorite foods are, when she eats, the amounts she eats, where she eats, and with whom she eats.

4. Invite a registered dietitian to speak to the class on any or all of the following: carbohydrate loading, fast foods, anorexia nervosa, bulimia, overweight in adolescence.

5. Invite a counselor who specializes in adolescent eating disorders to speak to the class.

6. Hold a panel discussion on alcohol and drugs. Assign the following topics to individual class members. They should prepare themselves by doing outside research before the panel discussion.

What is alcohol?
What are some commonly abused drugs?
Why do people use alcohol or drugs?
How do alcohol and drugs affect the human body?
How can alcohol and drug abuse affect one's nutritional status?
What are the dangers of drinking or using drugs during pregnancy?

REVIEW

Multiple choice. Select the *letter* that precedes the best answer.

1. Anorexia nervosa
   a. is characterized by binges and purges
   b. causes severe acne
   c. is a psychological disorder
   d. typically causes overweight

2. A child's eating habits
   a. can reflect his or her desire to assert self
   b. seldom change after the child reaches the age of 1 year
   c. usually improve when parents force the child to try new foods
   d. have no relation to the child's growth rate

3. Children's appetites
   a. vary
   b. are static
   c. are irrelevant to their nutritional status
   d. are entirely dependent on the size of the child

4. Of the following foods, children are most apt to prefer
   a. carrot-zucchini casserole
   b. creamed carrots with peas
   c. raw carrot sticks
   d. carrot and pineapple gelatin salad

5. A psychological disorder that causes people to drastically and chronically reduce caloric content of their food is called
   a. bulimia   c. anorexia nervosa
   b. amenorrhea   d. metabolic psychosis

6. Children's iron requirement is high because iron is needed for
   a. healthy bones and teeth
   b. fighting infections
   c. prevention of night blindness
   d. carrying oxygen

7. As a child grows, his or her calorie requirement per pound of body weight
   a. remains unchanged
   b. increases
   c. becomes less
   d. doubles each year

8. Meatloaf is a good source of
   a. protein   c. calcium
   b. vitamin C   d. all of the above and more

9. Low-nutrient-dense foods provide
   a. carbohydrate and fat
   b. proteins, minerals, and vitamins
   c. no calories
   d. fiber

10. Although adolescent boys usually need more calories than adolescent girls, the girls usually need more
    a. protein   c. iron
    b. vitamin C   d. vitamin D

CASE IN POINT

MEGAN: IDENTIFYING ANOREXIA NERVOSA

Megan is an active 12-year-old Caucasian girl. She loves to play hard and is an avid reader. She has been growing like a weed and seems to have just the right amount of love and caring from her family. She is proud to be "almost as tall as her grandmother." She is 5 feet tall and weighs 70 pounds. Megan can wear some of her summer shorts from 3 years ago. They may be short, but they fit her waist and hips.

When Megan sat down to a meal with her family, she would eat slowly and oftentimes not finish her meals, saying she was too full. Her grandmother noticed, at mealtime, that her dad would make sure her little sister ate well, but when telling Megan to finish her meal, her mother would step in and say, "If she isn't hungry, don't force her."

Megan oftentimes complains of bone pain. Her parents call it growing pains, and there is a history of severe arthritis in her family. Megan's complexion is very pale. After school Megan comes home and eats a piece of fruit and then says she is not hungry at mealtime. Once when at her grandmother's house, Megan said she was hungry but was not going to allow herself to eat. Her grandmother informed her parents of this right away. Since that statement, both parents and the grandmother are watching Megan's eating habits.

ASSESSMENT

1. What objective information do you have about Megan?
2. What subjective information do you have about Megan?
3. Which psychological issues are having an effect on Megan's understanding of proper nutrition?
4. What are the psychological needs of preteens?
5. What would lead you to believe Megan may be having appearance issues?

DIAGNOSIS

6. Complete the following statement: Megan's imbalanced nutrition is secondary to _____ .
7. What signs of anorexia nervosa does Megan exhibit?

PLAN/GOAL

8. What is the major nutritional goal for Megan?
9. What is the priority for Megan's physical development?

IMPLEMENTATION

10. What should Megan and her mother be taught about good nutrition?
11. What needs to be taught about anorexia nervosa? Who else needs this information?
12. Would a counselor be of assistance to Megan and her mother?
13. What can be done to prevent anorexia nervosa in her sister? Does anorexia nervosa have an age limit?

EVALUATION/OUTCOME CRITERIA

14. What criteria could be used to demonstrate that her anorexia nervosa was under control?
15. Can anorexia nervosa be cured?

THINKING FURTHER

16. How can parents, teachers, and coaches help the young preteens who have eating disorders?
17. Will Megan's younger sister be at risk for anorexia nervosa?

⊙ RATE THIS PLATE

Megan is at the age for growth spurts for girls. She has grown tall, but her calories have been taken up with growing tall and not increasing her fat stores. Megan is also active and burns up calories. She is tiny and probably has a small stomach. She may have made the comment about not eating, since fruit after school fills her up and she decided to wait for dinner. She needs nutrient-dense foods. Rate the plate.

Chicken thigh
Mashed potatoes
Broccoli
Chocolate pudding
Lemonade

Are any of these foods nutrient dense? If so, which one(s)? If any of these is not, how could the food be made nutrient dense?

CASE IN POINT

MADISON: ESTABLISHING HEALTHY PRETEEN EATING HABITS

Madison is a 10-year-old African American girl. She loves playing the piano and composing her own music. She is an avid computer wiz, taking after her father. She has designed all the family birthday cards and loves playing video games. When she comes home from school, she has a sweet snack, finishes her homework, and goes straight to the piano to practice. She spends hours at the keyboard, and by mealtime she says she is hungry.

Madison is 48 inches tall and weighs 98 pounds. Knowing that the family has a tendency to be heavier, her mother, Amy, is concerned about Madison's weight; Amy has been on and off Weight Watchers program for 15 years. Amy feels Madison should have more physical activity and needs to stop snacking on cupcakes and sweets. Madison is due for a preschool checkup. Amy is planning to ask the doctor for help with Madison's weight.

ASSESSMENT

1. What objective data do you have about Madison?
2. Using Figure 13-4, what percentile weight and height is Madison for a 10-year-old girl?
3. How do diet, activity, heredity, and family lifestyle impact her current weight?
4. How significant is this problem?

DIAGNOSIS

5. Complete the following diagnostic statement: Imbalanced nutrition: more than body requirements related to _____ .
6. Complete the following diagnostic statement: Deficient knowledge related to _____ .

PLAN/GOAL

7. State two reasonable, measurable goals for Madison.
8. What referral might be helpful for Madison?

IMPLEMENTATION

9. What information does the dietitian need to know to help Madison?
10. Who needs to be involved in the plan for it to be successful?
11. What are the two big changes that need to occur to help Madison stop gaining weight?
12. What strategies could you suggest so Madison would be successful but have fun in the process?

13. How can playing out doors with friends be helpful?
14. How can her family help?

EVALUATION/OUTCOME CRITERIA

15. How often should Madison be weighed?
16. What outcome is reasonable in 3 months? In 6 months?

THINKING FURTHER

17. Why is it important to intervene with Madison's weight now? What are the future consequences of a lifetime of being overweight? Why is this a community health issue in America now?
18. What would the internet be able to provide?
19. Check out National School lunch menus at www.schoolmenu.com.

◎ RATE ᴛʜɪꜱ PLATE

On Madison's plate is:

4 oz chicken breast

1 cup mashed potatoes

Biscuit with 1 tsp butter

1/2 cup green beans

1 cup 2% milk

How would you rate this plate? Check the serving sizes in Table 13-1.

CHAPTER

14

DIET DURING YOUNG AND MIDDLE ADULTHOOD

KEY TERMS

calorie requirement
energy imbalance
hypertension
lean muscle mass
nutrient requirement
obesity

OBJECTIVES

After studying this chapter, you should be able to:

- Identify the nutritional needs of young adults and the middle-aged
- Explain sensible, long-range weight control for this age group
- Discuss the importance of exercise in weight control
- Discuss diet-related diseases that can be prevented by good nutrition at this age: osteoporosis, heart disease, diabetes

Adulthood can be broadly divided into three periods: young, middle, and late adulthood. The first two periods will be discussed in this chapter. Late adulthood is discussed in Chapter 15.

Young adulthood is a time of excitement and exploration. The age range runs from about 18 to 40 years of age. Individuals are alive with plans, desires, and energy as they begin searching for and finding their places in the mainstream of adult life. They appear to have boundless energy for both social and professional activities. They are often interested in exercise for its own sake and may participate in athletic events as well.

The middle period ranges from about 40 to 65 years of age. This is a time when the physical activities of young adulthood typically begin to decrease, resulting in lowered caloric requirement for most individuals. During these years, people seldom have young children to supervise, and the strenuous physical labor of some occupations may be delegated to younger people. Middle-aged people may tire more easily than they did when they were younger. Therefore, they

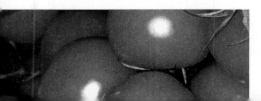

249

may not get as much exercise as they did in earlier years. Because appetite and food intake may not decrease, there is a common tendency toward weight gain during this period.

During young to middle adulthood, the beginnings of osteoporosis may also be evident. A diet rich in calcium, vitamin D, and fluoride is thought to help prevent osteoporosis.

The onset of rheumatoid arthritis (RA) usually occurs between the ages of 30 to 50 and will affect approximately 1% of the population (2.1 million), women outnumbering men three to one. RA affects the wrists, joints of the fingers other than those closest to the fingernail, hips, knees, ankles, elbows, shoulders, and necks. Although researchers have determined that diet changes have no effect on rheumatoid arthritis, it is still important to maintain a healthy diet that includes adequate calcium and protein. A multiple vitamin containing vitamin D and a calcium supplement should be taken daily. Omega-3 fatty acids have been helpful in reducing inflammation, but a physician should be consulted before taking this supplement.

NUTRITIONAL REQUIREMENTS

Growth is usually complete by the age of 25. Consequently, except during pregnancy and lactation, the essential nutrients are needed only to maintain and repair body tissue and to produce energy. During these years, the **nutrient requirements** of healthy adults change very little.

The iron requirement for women throughout the childbearing years remains higher than that for men. Extra iron is needed to replace blood loss during menstruation and to help build both the infant's and the extra maternal blood needed during pregnancy. After menopause, this requirement for women matches that of men.

Protein needs for adults are thought to be 0.8 gram per kilogram of body weight. To determine the specific amount, one must divide the weight in pounds by 2.2 to obtain the weight in kilograms and then multiply the weight in kilograms by 0.8.

The current requirement for calcium for adults from 19 to 50 is 1,000 mg, and for vitamin D, 5 μg. Both calcium and vitamin D are essential for strong bones, and both are found in milk. Bone loss begins slowly, at about the age of 35 to 40, and can lead to osteoporosis later. Therefore, it is wise for young people, especially women, who are more prone to osteoporosis than men, to consume foods that provide more than the requirements for these two nutrients. Three glasses of milk a day nearly fulfill the requirement for each of these nutrients. Increasing this amount could prevent osteoporosis. Fat-free milk or foods made from fat-free milk should be consumed to limit the amount of fat in the diet.

CALORIE REQUIREMENTS

Calorie requirements begin to diminish after the age of 25, as basal metabolism rates decrease (Table 14-1). After 25 years, a person will gain weight if the total calories are not reduced according to actual need, which will be determined by activity, BMI (REE), and amount of **lean muscle mass.** Those who are more active will require more calories than those who are less active.

---

nutrient requirement
amount of specific nutrient needed by the body

calorie requirement
number of calories required daily to meet energy needs

lean muscle mass
percentage of muscle tissue

Table 14-1 *Median Weights and Heights and Recommended Daily Energy Intake for Adults*

CATEGORY	AGE (YEARS) OR CONDITION	WEIGHT (kg)	(lb)	HEIGHT (cm)	(in)	REE (calories/day)	AVERAGE ENERGY ALLOWANCE CALORIES Multiples of REE	per kg	per day
Males	19–24	72	160	177	70	1,780	1.67	40	2,900
	25–50	79	174	176	70	1,800	1.60	37	2,900
	51+	77	170	173	68	1,530	1.50	30	2,300
Females	19–24	58	128	164	65	1,350	1.60	38	2,200
	25–50	63	138	163	64	1,380	1.55	36	2,200
	51+	65	143	160	63	1,280	1.50	30	1,900

Reprinted with permission from *Recommended Dietary Allowances: 10th Edition.* Copyright © 1989 by the National Academy of Sciences. Courtesy of the National Academy Press, Washington, D.C.

◎ SUPERSIZE USA

Pizza is probably the food most consumed by young and middle-aged adults. Especially popular is the buffet—all the salad and pizza, pasta, cinnamon sugar pizza strips, and dessert pizza you can eat. Wow, what a feast! Let's see how much can be eaten in one sitting. That is the way that most people approach a buffet. This is how we as Americans have supersized ourselves. How should a buffet be handled?

Tune in on hunger upon arrival—how hungry are you? Head for the salad bar first, and choose vegetables, ignoring the cheese, eggs, pasta, bacon bits, seeds, and regular dressing. Having a vegetable salad will help fill you almost up; so will having a glass of water or milk before the meal. At this point, tune in to "full." Are you full yet? If not, then the pizza buffet awaits. Choose one slice of a pizza topped with vegetables (mushrooms, peppers) over a pizza topped with sausage or pepperoni. Walk back to your seat. Eat slowly and enjoy. Ask yourself again, are you still hungry? If you're comfortable, then it's time to stop eating. The pizza will be there the next time you want it. Some adults can eat two to three times their caloric needs in one sweep of the pizza buffet, so instead of piling on the food at the first pass and feeling compelled to clear your plate, choose smaller portions and walk back up to the buffet if you are still hungry. How do you handle pizza buffets?

SPECIAL CONSIDERATIONS RELATED TO NUTRITION CONCERNS

It is especially important to maintain good eating habits during young and middle adulthood. Women, who may be concerned about weight, cost of food, or time, can easily develop nutrient deficiencies. For example, a woman who settles for a piece of pie at lunchtime while her husband eats a hamburger and salad is being very foolish. If she continues to eat like this, she will jeopardize her health.

A hamburger can have 250 to 400 calories. The salad will contain less than 50 calories without dressing, and the dressing could be limited to 1 tablespoon, or approximately 100 calories, for a total intake of about 400 to

550 calories. Pies average 100 calories per 1-inch slice. Most slices are about 3½ inches. A scoop of ice cream on the pie would bring the total to at least another 100 calories.

Although the calorie intakes of the husband and wife would be comparable, the nutrient intakes would differ. The wife's would be inadequate. If the woman is of childbearing age and plans to have children, she or her children could suffer from such habits.

In general, people today are concerned about nutrition and want to limit fats, cholesterol, sugar, salt, and calories and increase fiber. Many know the sources of these items; others do not. Unfortunately, both groups tend to select their food because of convenience and flavor rather than nutritional content. It is easier to drive through a fast-food restaurant or heat a prepared frozen dinner in the microwave and complete the meal with ice cream than it is to shop for individual food items, cook them, and wash up after the meal. Consequently, many people ingest more fats, sugar, salt, and high-calorie foods and less fiber and other nutrients than they should.

WEIGHT CONTROL

Weight control is one of the top concerns of U.S. adults. Whether for reasons of vanity, health, or both, most people are interested in controlling their weight. It is advisable, because overweight can introduce health problems. Cases of diabetes mellitus, metabolic syndrome, and **hypertension** are more numerous among the overweight than among those of normal weight. Overweight individuals are poor risks for surgery, and their lives are generally shorter than are those of people who are not overweight. They are prone to social and emotional problems because overweight and **obesity** can reduce self-esteem.

The causes of overweight are not always known, but the most common cause appears to be **energy imbalance.** In other words, if one is overweight, chances are that more calories have been taken in than were needed for energy.

An intake of 3,500 calories more than the body needs for maintenance and activities will result in a weight gain of 1 pound. An individual who overeats by only 200 calories a day can gain 20 pounds in 1 year. Obviously, when nutrient requirements remain static but calorie requirements decrease, people must select their foods carefully to fulfill their nutrient requirements. (See Table 14-2.) Genetics and, rarely, a hypothyroid condition, can also contribute to overweight.

Individuals who are overweight simply because of energy imbalance can solve the problem by eating less and increasing physical exercise. Exercise will increase the number of calories burned. However, unless the exercise is sufficient to burn more calories than the ingested food contains, exercise alone will not solve the problem. By far the most effective method of weight loss is increased exercise combined with reduced calories. This will help tone the muscles as excess fat is lost. Exercise may also increase lean muscle mass in such a way that weight loss will not be necessarily significant; in this case, a decrease in clothing size may be a better indicator of fat loss.

When weight reduction is to be undertaken, the client should confirm with his or her physician that he or she is in good health. Then, with the help of a registered dietitian, a healthy eating plan should be developed that will fit the dieter's lifestyle. A healthy eating plan is easiest to follow when it is based on

○ **hypertension**
higher than normal blood pressure

○ **obesity**
excessive body fat, 20% above average

○ **energy imbalance**
eating either too much or too little for the amount of energy expended

Table 14-2 *2,000-calorie Daily Menu*

BREAKFAST

½ cup orange juice	50 calories	
1 cup dry cereal	100	
½ cup fat-free milk	43	
2 tsp sugar	35	
2 slices toast	150	
½ Tbsp margarine	50	
1 cup black coffee	0	428 calories
	428	

LUNCH

Roast beef sandwich:		
3 oz roast beef	200	
2 slices toast	150	
1 Tbsp mayonnaise	100	
lettuce	10	
1 cup fat-free milk	85	
1 orange	75	620 calories
	620	

DINNER

2 oz broiled fish	150	
1 baked potato	100	
1½ Tbsp margarine	150	
½ cup green peas	50	
tossed salad with 1 Tbsp dressing	150	
1 cup fat-free milk	86	
¾ cup ice cream	200	
1 oatmeal cookie	100	986 calories
	986	2,034

((• *In The Media*

GOOD FOR THE HEART = GOOD FOR THE HEAD

Eating a low-fat diet high in antioxidants, maintaining a normal weight, exercising regularly, not smoking, and not drinking excessively during adulthood have been shown to delay or prevent Alzheimer's disease. Maintaining social connections and keeping the brain active with lifetime learning will also help to protect against Alzheimer's disease. Nearly half of those that live past the age of 85 will develop this devastating disease. Protection and prevention are essential.

(Source: Adapted from the *New York Times*, March 2005.)

MyPyramid. This plan will aid the dieter in obtaining needed nutrients, will help change previously unsatisfactory eating habits, and will allow him or her to adapt, and thus enjoy, home, party, or restaurant meals. For additional information about weight loss diets, see Chapter 16.

CONSIDERATIONS FOR THE HEALTH CARE PROFESSIONAL

The young and middle years of life are busy. Most people feel they have too many things to do and too little time to accomplish them. Most have families, jobs, and social obligations and, thus, more responsibilities.

EXPLORING THE WEB

Search the Web for information related to diet and disease or disorders. What conditions are directly affected by diet? Can these conditions be prevented by changing one's nutritional status? How can this be done? What resources are available for individuals experiencing a nutrition-related disorder?

◉ SUPERSIZE USA

"French fries are a staple in my diet! I love French fries, and I understand that they are the most consumed vegetable in the USA. I don't doubt that, because I do my share of consuming; it is so easy to drive through and get dinner. Supersize those fries—of course! I sometimes wonder if I should vary my vegetable intake, but isn't a potato good for you? It has vitamins, fiber (more if they are fries with the skin left on), and minerals. I have noticed that my weight has increased each year since high school graduation. I recently had my first lipid profile run, and the doctor said that the numbers were too high, except the HDL, which was too low. That started me thinking—since French fries are my vegetable of choice, could there be anything bad for me in them? How are they cooked? Are they high in sodium? What kind of carbohydrates do they contain? Do potatoes have any substances that could be detrimental to my health?"

French fries may be cooked in hydrogenated or partially hydrogenated fat that contains trans-fatty acids, which are as detrimental to the body as saturated fats (fats that are solid at room temperature). Unless ordered otherwise, French fries are salted by the employee in the fast-food restaurant without measuring the quantity of salt. Potatoes are starchy vegetables because they have a high content of carbohydrates and calories. French fries also contain a chemical called acrylamide, which is known to cause cancer in laboratory rats and mice. Weight gain after graduation from high school can lead to overweight and obesity, which has been shown as a leading factor in diseases such as heart disease and type 2 diabetes.

SUMMARY

Although calorie requirements diminish after the age of 25, most nutrient requirements do not. Consequently, food must be selected with increasing care as one ages to ensure that nutrient requirements are met without exceeding the calorie requirement.

Overweight can cause health problems. If it is caused by energy imbalance, a program of weight loss, which includes exercise, should be undertaken. The diet should be based on MyPyramid, and eating habits should be taught so that the lost weight will not be regained later.

DISCUSSION TOPICS

1. Why do calorie requirements tend to diminish after the age of 25? Why do nutrient requirements not diminish at the same time?

2. How can only an extra 200 calories a day result in overweight?

3. Why does a 40-year-old carpenter require more calories than a 40-year-old architect?

4. Why are middle-aged adults more inclined to overweight than young adults?

5. Why is 35-year-old Vera putting on weight even though she doesn't eat any more than she did as a 17-year-old cheerleader?

6. What are the health and psychological consequences of overweight?

SUGGESTED ACTIVITIES

1. Keep a food diary for a day and check off each food under MyPyramid headings, as shown in the form below.

	Fat/ Sweet	Dairy	Meats	Veg.	Fruit	Bread/ Cereal
Recommended no. of servings a day	Use sparingly	2–3	2–3	3–5	2–4	6–11
Breakfast						
Lunch						
Dinner						
Total						

a. Total the entries in the vertical columns. Which columns have the highest totals?
b. Discuss the shortages or excesses and the possible dangers of each.
c. Discuss realistic ways of improving your diet.
d. Repeat this exercise in a week. Evaluate for improvements.

REVIEW

Multiple choice. Select the *letter* that precedes the best answer.

1. The number of calories one needs each day is called one's
   a. nutrient requirement
   b. calorie intake
   c. calorie requirement
   d. nutritional requirement

2. Overweight during middle age is often due to
   a. obesity
   b. hypertension
   c. adipose tissue
   d. energy imbalance

3. The measure of energy in foods eaten is one's
   a. calorie requirement
   b. calorie intake
   c. nutrient requirement
   d. energy imbalance

4. Because of menstruation and pregnancy during the young and middle years, women have a greater need than men for
   a. proteins   c. iodine
   b. B vitamins   d. iron

5. Calorie requirements
   a. increase with age
   b. decrease with age
   c. remain unchanged throughout adult life
   d. none of the above

6. To lose 1 pound of weight, one must reduce calorie intake by
   a. 1,000 calories   c. 3,500 calories
   b. 800 calories   d. none of the above

7. Daily protein needs of adults are thought to be
   a. 0.5 gram per kilogram of body weight
   b. 0.8 gram per kilogram of body weight
   c. 10 grams per kilogram of body weight
   d. 8 mg per day regardless of body weight

8. Exercise
   a. is more important to men than to women
   b. has no effect on muscles after the age of 40
   c. eliminates the need for postmenopausal women to drink milk
   d. helps to burn calories as it tones the muscles

9. Nutrient requirements during adult life generally
   a. increase with age
   b. decrease with age
   c. change very little
   d. none of the above

10. Women's calorie requirements as compared with men's are generally
    b. lower
    a. higher
    c. the same
    d. none of the above

CASE IN POINT

ANATOLI: LOSING WEIGHT AT 38

Anatoli was a 38-year-old man originally from Romania. He has been working for 10 to 12 hours a day, 5 to 6 days a week, for 20 years. He has worked for General Motors and has decided to return to school to get a degree in engineering. His wife and daughters support his decision 100% because they know how hard Anatoli has worked. Before returning to school as a full-time student, Anatoli has decided to drop about 25 pounds of unwanted fat. Since high school he had developed bad eating habits, making many trips to the fast-food restaurants, and had lost interest in anything physical. He has 3 months before school starts, and he hopes to develop healthier eating habits.

ASSESSMENT

1. What do you know about Anatoli?
2. What value has he acted on for 20 years?
3. What values does he want to act on in the future?
4. What do you suspect Anatoli had been eating?
5. Suppose Anatoli is 6 feet 2 inches tall and weighs 235 pounds. What is his ideal weight?

DIAGNOSIS

6. What are possible causes of Anatoli's weight problem?
7. What education is needed to help Anatoli lose weight?

PLAN/GOAL

8. What is a reasonable goal for weight loss for Anatoli before he starts school? Assume a loss of 1 to 2 pounds per week.

IMPLEMENTATION

9. What are the two most important changes that Anatoli needs to make to lose weight?
10. How could a 24-hour food diary help?
11. What does he need to do about exercise?
12. How can his family help?
13. How can strategies like packing his lunch help?
14. Would he be more successful losing weight alone or in a group?

EVALUATION/OUTCOME CRITERIA

15. One month after starting the above plan, what changes will be in place?

16. If the plan is successful, what changes will Anatoli report in 3 months?

THINKING FURTHER

17. Even though Anatoli's short-term goal is to lose weight, how could he maintain his new habits so he won't regain the weight?
18. Why is it important to control excess weight in middle age?
19. To stay at his ideal weight, what does he need to adjust with age according to Table 14-1?

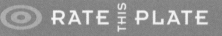

RATE THIS PLATE

Anatoli has decided to change his eating habits to shed some unwanted weight. Anatoli has chosen the following for lunch at a restaurant with his family:

2 4-oz grilled tarragon chicken breasts
Steamed broccoli
1 cup rice pilaf
Trip to the salad bar—his plate includes the following:
    Lettuce
    Spinach
    Chopped eggs
    Onions
    Chopped ham
    Carrots
    Mushrooms
    Celery
    Sunflower seeds
    Cottage cheese
    Potato salad
2 ladles blue cheese dressing, about 4 Tbsp

CASE IN POINT

SUEATA: KEEPING AN EYE ON WEIGHT

Sueata was a 35-year-old Indian woman and mother of four boys. The youngest boy was in school, and she was looking forward to a little time to herself. She was used to being busy all day doing laundry, running errands, making meals, and chauffeuring the boys to their after-school sports. She would miss her afternoons with her youngest, James. They played one-on-one basketball, kickball, and soccer until the older boys were out of school. Meals were always light and simple at Sueata's house. Lots of salads, vegetables, and cold baked chicken were the order of the day, so that all the boys could eat with their different schedules. Within a month, Sueata had settled into a new routine of doing crafts and cooking hot meals. She finally had the opportunity to do some "girl" things, as she called them, and she loved it. She also took great pride in having a hot meal on the table and even served dessert. She had lunch out with her friends and invited neighbors and friends over for casual dinners. She was thoroughly enjoying herself, except for one thing. Within 3 months, she had gained 8 pounds. She let it slide. When that figure was up to 15 pounds, Sueata decided she had better do something about it.

ASSESSMENT

1. What information do you have about Sueata's activity and eating habits?
2. How did Sueata's habits change after James was in school?
3. How has the change affected her?
4. How long should Sueata expect to take to lose the 15 pounds she gained?

DIAGNOSIS

5. Write a diagnosis for Sueata's alteration in nutrition.
6. Write a diagnosis for Sueata's activity-level change.

PLAN/GOAL

7. What is a reasonable, measurable goal for Sueata's weight loss?

IMPLEMENTATION

8. List some strategies that match Sueata's new priorities.
9. What can the boys do to help her lose weight?
10. How can she enjoy her new routine without gaining weight?
11. How can the Web site Shape Up America!, www.shapeup.org, be helpful to Sueata?

EVALUATION/OUTCOME CRITERIA

12. What criteria would Sueata use to determine the success of the plan?
13. What is the safe, reasonable weight loss in the first month? In 3 months?

THINKING FURTHER

14. How can she maintain weight control for the rest of her life?

◎ RATE ≡ PLATE

Sueata had been very active and has since changed her lifestyle, and not for the better. Sueata loved her new freedom and lifestyle except for the weight gain. She prepared the following meal. Rate the plate.

Baked chicken and rice (made with cream of chicken soup)
Sautéed mixed fresh vegetables in butter
Homemade rolls and butter
Peach cobbler

Is this meal conducive to weigh loss? If not, how would you change it to make it more weight loss friendly? What else should Sueata add to her daily routine to lose those 15 pounds?

CHAPTER

15

DIET DURING
LATE ADULTHOOD

OBJECTIVES

After studying this chapter, you should be able to

🦶 Explain the nutritional and calorie needs of people 65 and over

🦶 Explain the development of given chronic diseases

🦶 Identify physiological, economic, and psychosocial problems that can affect an older adult's nutrition

Currently, the fastest-growing age group in the United States is that of people age 85 and older. The average life expectancy in this country is now 80.1 years for women and 74.8 years for men (Hoyert, Kung, & Smith, 2005). It is expected that by the year 2030 there will be 65 million people in the United States 80 years and older. Consequently, **gerontology,** the study of aging, is of increasing importance.

The rate of aging varies. Each person is affected by heredity, emotional and physical stress, and nutrition. Research continues to reveal more about the causes of aging and the role of nutrition in the aging process.

THE EFFECTS OF AGING

As people age, **physiological,** psychosocial, and economic changes occur that affect nutrition.

Physiological Changes

The body's functions slow with age, and the ability of the body to replace worn cells is reduced. The metabolic rate slows; bones become less dense; lean muscle mass is reduced; eyes do not focus on nearby objects as they once did, and some grow cloudy from cataracts; poor **dentition** is common; the heart and kidneys become less efficient; and hearing, taste, and smell are less acute. If poor nutrition has been chronic, the immune system may be compromised.

Osteoarthritis and its debilitating effects are of great concern to the elderly. Arthritis can limit the ability to perform activities of daily living (ADLs). The role that diet plays in arthritis has been of increasing interest to researchers. Excessive weight, certain vitamin deficiencies, and the type of diet being followed may influence some types of arthritis. Eating a healthy, well-balanced diet that includes the "5 a day" fruits and vegetables, along with grain products, and sugar and salt in moderation, may be beneficial for arthritis sufferers. Your physician or dietitian may also recommend taking a multiple vitamin daily.

There appears to be no direct connection between a specific kind of food and a specific symptom of arthritis. Neither is there a special diet that is consistently beneficial for arthritis sufferers; however, the best advice is to eat a healthy diet that includes a variety of foods and to exercise.

Digestion is affected because the secretion of hydrochloric acid and enzymes is diminished. This in turn decreases the intrinsic factor synthesis, which leads to a deficiency of vitamin B_{12}. The tone of the intestines is reduced, and the result may be constipation or, in some cases, diarrhea.

Psychosocial Changes

Feelings do not decrease with age. In fact, psychosocial problems can increase as one grows older. Age does not diminish the desire to feel useful and appreciated and loved by family and friends. Retirement years may not be "golden" if one suffers a loss of self-esteem from feelings of uselessness. Grief over the loss of a spouse or close friend, combined with the resulting loneliness, can be devastating. Physical disabilities that develop in the senior years and prevent one from going out independently can destroy a social life. Becoming a fifth wheel in a grown child's home or a resident of a nursing home can lead to severe depression. Problems such as these can diminish a person's appetite and ability to shop and cook.

Economic Changes

Retirement typically results in decreased income. Unless one has carefully prepared for it, this can affect one's quality of life by reducing social activities, adding worry about meeting bills, and causing one to select a less than healthy diet by choosing foods on the basis of cost rather than nutrient content.

Sidestepping Potential Problems

Healthy eating habits throughout life, an exercise program suited to one's age, and social activities that please can prevent or delay physical deterioration and psychological depression during the senior years. The benefits can be said to be circular. The first two contribute largely to one's physical condition, and social activities can prevent or diminish depression, which, if unchecked, can also depress

gerontology
the study of aging

physiological
relating to bodily functions

dentition
arrangement, type, and number of teeth

EXPLORING THE WEB

Visit the National Institute on Aging's Web site at www.niapublications.org for guidelines on good nutrition throughout life. What are some of the challenges and concerns facing older adults in relation to healthy eating?

appetite. They give purpose to the day, joy to the heart, and zest to the appetite. Whenever an elderly person is depressed, the patient's nutrition and lifestyle should be carefully reviewed.

Food-drug interactions must be monitored closely in the elderly. Frequently, specific foods will prevent, decrease, or enhance the absorption of a particular drug. Dairy products should not be consumed within 2 hours of taking the antibiotic tetracycline, or it will not be absorbed. A person taking a blood clot-reducing drug such as coumadin or warfarin (often called blood thinners) needs to consume vitamin K-rich food in moderation since vitamin K counteracts blood thinners. Even vitamin supplements can cause interactions. The antioxidant vitamins are not to be taken with blood clot-reducing medications because they also have a tendency to thin the blood.

Drug-drug interactions as well as food-drug interactions can contribute to decreased nutritional status. These interactions could affect appetite as well as absorption of nutrients from the food eaten. Careful monitoring is recommended. (See Appendix E.)

NUTRITIONAL REQUIREMENTS

Although the nutritional needs of growth disappear with age, the normal nutritional needs for maintaining a constant state of good health remain throughout life. Good nutrition can speed recovery from illness, surgery, or broken bones and generally can improve the spirits and the quality, and even the length, of life.

Despite the physical changes the body undergoes after the age of 51 or so, only a few of the DRIs, and AIs for people in that age category are less than those for younger people.

The protein requirement remains at the average 50 grams per day for women and 63 grams for men. This is based on the estimated need of 0.8 gram per

⊙ SUPERSIZE USA

Eating out is my favorite thing to do, especially for breakfast. Actually, I could have breakfast three times a day, if possible. The last time I went out, I ordered two eggs, over medium, home fries with onions, sausage patty, and raisin toast. What I received was three eggs (standard serving at this restaurant), two patties of sausage, approximately a half pound of potatoes with one-eighth cup of onions, and one Texas-size slice of raisin toast. The restaurant had *supersized* my breakfast without even asking me. I was with a friend, and as we talked, I continued to eat; and eventually with enough talking, I finished everything on the plate. Was I that hungry—*no.* What could I have done, had I known beforehand that the servings were so huge, to eliminate being tempted to eat too much? What questions should I have asked my waitress before ordering? In such instances, how should I manage the rest of the day in terms of eating?

I could have insisted that the waitress bring me just what I ordered.
I could have asked for a carry-out container and put the extra food in it.
It would have been wise to question my waitress about serving sizes and cooking methods.
In such instances, the rest of the day I should eat very lightly. I could have a salad for lunch and then have a light dinner. And I need to listen closely to my hunger and full signals the rest of the day.

Table 15-1 *Median Weights and Heights and Recommended Daily Energy Intake for Adults*

CATEGORY	AGE (YEARS) OR CONDITION	WEIGHT (kg)	(lb)	HEIGHT (cm)	(in)	REE (calories/day)	AVERAGE ENERGY ALLOWANCE CALORIES Multiples of REE	per kg	per day
Males	25–50	79	174	176	70	1,800	1.60	37	2,900
	51+	77	170	173	68	1,530	1.50	30	2,300
Females	25–50	63	138	163	64	1,380	1.55	36	2,200
	51+	65	143	160	63	1,280	1.50	30	1,900

Source: *Recommended Dietary Allowances: Tenth Edition.* Copyright © 1989 by the National Academy of Sciences. Courtesy of the National Academy Press, Washington, D.C.

kilogram of body weight. After age 65, it may be advisable to increase one's daily protein intake to 1.0 gram per kilogram of body weight. In general, vitamin requirements do not change after the age of 51, except for a slight decrease in the DRIs for thiamine, riboflavin, and niacin. The need for these three vitamins depends largely on the calorie intake, and calorie requirement is reduced after the age of 51. The need for iron is decreased after age 51 in women because of menopause.

The calorie requirement decreases approximately 2% to 3% a decade because metabolism slows and activity is reduced (see Table 15-1). If the calorie intake is not reduced, weight will increase. This additional weight would increase the work of the heart and put increased stress on the **skeletal system**. It is important that the calorie requirement not be exceeded and just as important that the nutrient requirements be fulfilled to maintain good nutritional status. An exercise plan appropriate for one's age and health can be helpful in burning excess calories and toning and strengthening the muscles.

⚲ **skeletal system**
body's bone structure

FOOD HABITS

If the established food habits of the older person are poor, such habits will undoubtedly have been a long time in the making. These habits will not be easy to change. Poor food habits that begin during old age can also present problems. Decreased income during retirement, lack of transportation, physical disability, and inadequate cooking facilities may cause difficulties in food selection and preparation. Anorexia caused by grief, loneliness, boredom, depression, or difficulty in chewing can decrease food consumption. Dementia and Alzheimer's may cause the elderly to think they have eaten when they may not have.

Studies indicate that many senior citizens consume diets deficient in protein; vitamins C, D, B_6, B_{12}, and folate; and the minerals calcium, zinc, iron, and sometimes calories.

An elderly client's diet plan should be based on MyPyramid and the nutrients should be checked against the DRIs and AIs. Older persons' needs can vary considerably, depending on their conditions, so each person should be examined by a physician to determine specific requirements. If the client consumes less that 1,500 calories a day, a multivitamin-mineral supplement is recommended.

Variety and nutrient-dense foods should be encouraged, as should water. Water is important to help prevent constipation, to maintain urinary volume, to prevent dehydration, and to prevent urinary tract infections (UTIs). When there is serious protein and calorie malnutrition (PEM), the reason may be economic or

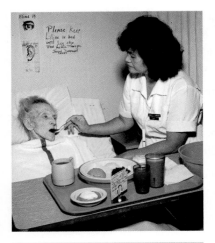

Figure 15-1 *Older adults may have health problems that affect their ability to feed themselves.*

⊙ **food faddists**

people who have certain beliefs about particular foods or diets

EXPLORING THE WEB

Search the Web for information on food fads. What makes the elderly vulnerable to food fads? Are these types of diets and fads geared toward the elderly population? Why? What advice would you provide to an elderly client inquiring about one of these fads?

psychosocial. Elderly people who have long hospital stays can develop PEM in the hospital. They may dislike the food, drugs may dull the appetite, and they may be lonely and depressed. Sometimes poor or missing teeth can make eating protein foods difficult (Figure 15-1). In such cases, protein-rich supplements can be used.

If overweight is a problem, it may be caused by overeating, lack of exercise, drugs, or alcohol.

Any adjustment in food habits will require great tact, and plans for changes must be based on the individual's total situation.

FOOD FADS

Some older people are consciously or unconsciously searching for eternal life, if not youth. Consequently, they are frequently susceptible to the claims of **food faddists** who seek to profit from their ignorance. Senior citizens spend money on unnecessary vitamins, minerals, and special honey, molasses, bread, milk, and other foods that may be guaranteed by the salesperson to prevent or cure various diseases. This money could be much more effectively used on ordinary foods from MyPyramid that would cost considerably less.

APPROPRIATE DIETS

The diets of older adults should be planned around MyPyramid (Table 15-2). When special health problems exist, the normal diet should be adapted to meet individual needs (see Section 3, Medical Nutrition Therapy).

The federal government provides the states with funds to serve hot meals at noon in senior centers across the country. These senior centers become social clubs and are immensely beneficial to the elderly. They provide companionship in addition to nutritious food. Frequently the noon meal at "the center" becomes the focal point of an older person's day.

The federal government also provides transportation for those who are otherwise unable to reach the senior center for the meal. When individuals are completely homebound, arrangements can be made for the meals to be delivered to their homes. Some communities have Meals-on-Wheels projects. Participating people pay according to ability. In addition, food stamps are available and can sometimes be used for the Meals-on-Wheels programs.

((⸱ In The Media

AS OBESITY EPIDEMIC PEAKS, OUR GRANDPARENTS ARE STARVING TO DEATH

Our preoccupation is on obesity, but our attention needs to be focused on any intentional and unintentional weight loss in the elderly, which can result in premature disability and death. Weight loss in the elderly should send up a red flag about health problems. According to the National Health and Nutrition Examination Survey, 16% of Americans over the age of 65 eat less than 1,000 calories per day, putting them at severe risk of malnutrition. The less the elderly eat, the less they are able to eat. When they develop a disease such as COPD or cancer or suffer a hip fracture, they are set up for anorexia, emaciation, and malnutrition. Decreased food intake must be taken seriously before they enter the downward spiral to death.

(Source: Adapted from an article in the newsletter, *Aging Successfully*, March 2004.)

Table 15-2 *2,200-calorie Daily Menu*

BREAKFAST

½ cup orange juice	50 calories	
1 cup dry cereal	100	
½ cup fat-free milk	43	
2 tsp sugar	35	
2 slices whole-grain bread, toasted	150	
½ Tbsp margarine	50	
1 Tbsp jelly	50	
1 cup black coffee	0	478 calories
	478	

LUNCH

¾ cup macaroni and cheese	300	
1 tomato, sliced	25	
½ cup green beans	25	
1 cup fat-free milk	85	
⅔ cup custard	200	635 calories
	635	

DINNER

½ cup pineapple juice	75	
3 oz broiled hamburger	240	
½ cup rice	100	
½ cup shredded lettuce	10	
1 Tbsp salad dressing	75	
1 cup fat-free milk	85	
Fresh fruit	100	685 calories
	685	

SNACKS

1 banana	100	
5 dried prunes	100	
2 oatmeal cookies	200	400 calories
	400	2,198

SPECIAL CONSIDERATIONS FOR THE CHRONICALLY ILL OLDER ADULT

It is estimated that 85% of people over 65 have one or more chronic diseases or physical problems. Examples include osteoporosis, arthritis, cataracts, cancer, diabetes mellitus, hypertension, heart disease, and periodontal disease. The branch of medicine that is involved with diseases of older adults is called **geriatrics.**

geriatrics
the branch of medicine involved with diseases of the elderly

Osteoporosis

osteoporosis
condition in which bones become brittle because there have been insufficient mineral deposits, especially calcium

Osteoporosis is a condition in which the amount of calcium in bones is reduced, making them porous. It is estimated that 28 million older adults have osteoporosis, and 80% of these are women. A bone density scan can be done with a special X-ray to determine if one has osteoporosis. It is typically unnoticed at its onset, which occurs at approximately age 45, and it may not be noticed at all until a fracture occurs. One of its symptoms is a gradual reduction in height.

estrogen
hormone secreted by the ovaries

Doctors are not certain of its cause. It is thought that years of a sedentary life coupled with a diet deficient in calcium, vitamin D, and fluoride contribute to it, as does **estrogen** loss, which occurs after menopause. Physicians are recommending estrogen replacement therapy (ERT) to help prevent osteoporosis. Some doctors are also advising clients to consume 1,500 mg of calcium, which would require the daily consumption of over 1 quart of milk or its equivalent. Calcium tablets, preferably calcium carbonate, could be used instead, but the client would also require supplementary vitamin D if sunshine were unavailable year-round or if the client were homebound. A diet with sufficient calcium and vitamin D plus an appropriate exercise program begun early in the adult years is thought to help prevent this disease.

periodontal disease
disease of the mouth and gums

Another possible cause of osteoporosis may be a diet containing excessive amounts of phosphorus, which can speed bone loss. It is known that Americans are ingesting increasing amounts of phosphorus. Sodas and processed foods contain phosphorus, and their consumption is increasing as milk consumption is decreasing in the United States. Some believe that **periodontal disease** may be a harbinger of osteoporosis. Periodontal disease is characterized by bone loss in the jaw, which can lead to loosened teeth and infection in the gums.

SPOTLIGHT on Life Cycle

The National Institutes of Health report the following statistics relating to osteoporosis:

- Osteoporosis is a major public health threat for 28 million Americans, 80% of whom are women.
- In the United States today, 10 million individuals already have osteoporosis, and 18 million more have low bone mass, placing them at increased risk for this disease.
- One of out every two women and one in eight men over 50 will have an osteoporosis-related fracture in their lifetime.
- More than 2 million American men suffer from osteoporosis, and millions more are at risk. Each year, 80,000 men suffer a hip fracture, and one-third of these men die within a year.
- Osteoporosis can strike at any age.
- Osteoporosis is responsible for more than 1.5 million fractures annually, including approximately 300,000 hip fractures, 700,000 vertebral fractures, 250,000 wrist fractures, and more than 300,000 fractures at other sites.
- Estimated national direct expenditures (hospitals and nursing homes) for osteoporosis and related fractures are $14 billion each year.
- Individuals over age 50 consume 1,200 mg of calcium per day.

(Source: The National Institute of Health Osteoporosis and Related Bone Diseases National Resource Center. Retrieved December 1, 2005, from http://www.osteo.org/osteo.html.)

Arthritis

Arthritis is a disease that causes the joints to become painful and stiff. It results in structural changes in the cartilage of the joints. A client with arthritis should be especially careful to avoid overweight because the extra weight adds stress to joints that are already painful. If the client is overweight, a weight reduction program should be instituted.

The regular use of aspirin by these clients may cause slight bleeding in the stomach lining and subsequent anemia, so their diets may require additional iron. Arthritis can greatly complicate a client's life because it may partially or completely immobilize the client so much that shopping, moving around, and cooking become difficult.

Aspirin and other anti-inflammatory drugs do help relieve the pain of arthritis, but there is as yet no cure. Clients should be well informed of this to prevent them from wasting their money on so-called miracle cures recommended by health food faddists or quacks.

arthritis
chronic disease involving the joints

Cancer

Research about the role of nutrition in cancer development continues. The American Cancer Society has indicated that diets consistently high in fat or low in fiber and vitamin A may contribute to cancer (see Chapter 21).

Diabetes Mellitus

Diabetes mellitus is a chronic disease. It develops when the body does not produce sufficient amounts of insulin or does not use it effectively for normal carbohydrate metabolism. Diet is very important in the treatment of diabetes. Chapter 17 discusses this treatment in detail.

Hypertension

Hypertension, or high blood pressure, can lead to strokes. It is associated with diets high in salt or possibly low in calcium. Most Americans ingest from two to six times the amount of salt needed each day. It is thought that the earlier a person reduces salt intake, the better that person's chances of avoiding hypertension, particularly if there is a family history of it. Hypertension is discussed in detail in Chapter 18.

hypertension
higher than normal blood pressure

Heart Disease

Heart attack and stroke are the major causes of death in the United States. They occur when arteries become blocked (occluded), preventing the normal passage of blood. These **occlusions** (blockages) are caused by blood clots that form and are unable to pass through an unnaturally narrowed artery. Arteries are narrowed by **plaque**, a fatty substance containing cholesterol that accumulates in the walls of the artery. This condition is called **atherosclerosis.** It is believed that excessive cholesterol and saturated fats in the diet over many years

occlusions
blockages

plaque
fatty deposit on the interior of artery walls

atherosclerosis
a form of arteriosclerosis affecting the intima (inner lining) of the artery walls

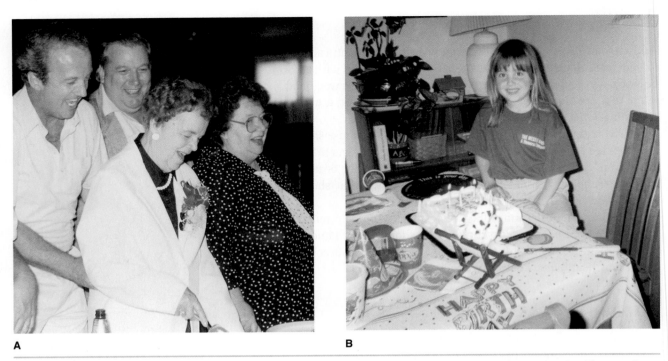

A　　　　　　　　　　　　　　　　　　　　　　　　**B**

Figure 15-2 *Celebrating one's eightieth birthday (A) is as much fun as celebrating one's eighth (B) when health is good.*

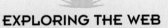

EXPLORING THE WEB

Search the Web for information on exercises that are appropriate for the elderly. What information can you find? Create a list of references of safe and effective exercises for the elderly. What benefits can these exercises bring to the elderly client? If an elderly client is active, what effect does that have on his or her nutritional needs?

contribute to this condition. The therapeutic diet appropriate for atherosclerosis is discussed in Chapter 18.

Effects of Nutrition

Current research about the role of nutrition in preventing or relieving these chronic diseases continues. The effects of nutrition are cumulative over many years. The effects of a lifetime of poor eating habits cannot be cured overnight. When diets have been poor for a long time, prevention of these chronic diseases may not be possible. It may be possible, however, to use nutrition to help stabilize the condition of a client who has one of these diseases. The prevention of many of the diseases of the elderly should begin in one's youth (Figure 15-2).

CONSIDERATIONS FOR THE HEALTH CARE PROFESSIONAL

It is essential that the health care professional remember that each client is an individual with individual needs. It is easy for someone working exclusively with geriatric clients to group them together, but doing so diminishes the quality of the care they receive and adds to their unhappiness. The 80-year-old client is just as pleased to see a smile on the face of a nurse as is an 18-year-old client. The 70-year-old overweight arthritic client deserves as much help with a weight loss program as the 45-year-old client. The 85-year-old client suffering from senility still enjoys a bright hello and a gentle pat on the back. People's feelings must never be forgotten. The incapacitation that can accompany old age is a terrible indignity, and these clients deserve special care.

SUMMARY

The elderly are becoming an increasingly large segment of the U.S. population, and their nutritional needs are of growing concern. It is becoming apparent that many of the chronic diseases of the elderly could be delayed or avoided by maintaining good nutrition throughout life. Most nutrient requirements do not decrease with age, but calorie requirements do. When food habits of senior citizens must be changed, adjustments require great tact and patience on the part of the dietitian. Older people are easily attracted to food fads that promise good health and prolonged life.

DISCUSSION TOPICS

1. Why does the iron requirement usually diminish for women after the age of 50?
2. Why might elderly people suffer from anorexia?
3. How might arthritis affect one's eating habits?
4. In what ways can emotional stress affect eating habits? What kinds of emotional stress do the elderly sometimes suffer?
5. Why are older people inclined to believe food faddists' stories?
6. What is osteoporosis?
7. Why do calorie requirements diminish as people age?

SUGGESTED ACTIVITIES

1. Arrange a talk on nutrition for senior citizens at a congregate meal site.
2. If possible, visit a nursing home at mealtime. Write your evaluation of the food and a description of client reactions to it and to you, the visitor.
3. Describe an appropriate response to your 65-year-old aunt, who has just become captivated by a salesperson in a local health food store and has announced that she is buying a 6-month supply of vinegar-honey tablets that are guaranteed to prevent arthritis.

REVIEW

Multiple choice. Select the *letter* that precedes the best answer.

1. Gerontology is of increasing interest because it is
   a. the branch of medicine involved with diseases of older people
   b. the study of nutrition
   c. hoped that experimentation in this field will explain the causes of aging
   d. the study of heart disease
2. After the age of 51, nutrient requirements generally
   a. increase   c. remain unchanged
   b. decrease   d. none of the above
3. After the age of 51, calorie requirements generally
   a. increase   c. remain unchanged
   b. decrease   d. none of the above
4. The iron requirement for women after the age of approximately 51 generally
   a. increases   c. remains unchanged
   b. decreases   d. none of the above
5. As the metabolic rate slows with age,
   a. the calorie requirement is increased
   b. the calorie requirement is decreased
   c. there is a decreased need for vitamins A, D, and K
   d. cataracts can develop
6. Osteoporosis is a disease that causes
   a. poor appetite
   b. a reduction in the number of red blood cells
   c. joints to become painful and stiff
   d. bones to become porous
7. Arthritis is a disease that causes
   a. poor appetite
   b. a reduction in the number of red blood cells
   c. joints to become painful and stiff
   d. bones to become porous
8. Hypertension is related to diets high in
   a. cholesterol   c. calcium
   b. vitamin D   d. salt
9. Diets high in cholesterol content are thought to contribute to
   a. diabetes mellitus c. heart disease
   b. hypertension   d. cataracts

CASE IN POINT

CHESTER: TREATING BONE DENSITY LOSS

Chester and Mildred have been married for 54 years. They have enjoyed retirement in their Florida home. Since their forties, they have tried to eat right, exercise, and be proactive about their health. Since Mildred had her hysterectomy, Chester has made sure she takes her estrogen. Mildred has been concerned about Chester recently because he cracked a molar and had to have a replacement. When the dentist saw the X-rays, he commented that Chester had lost some bone density in his jaw. The dentist also noticed that two of Chester's teeth were loose. Chester told Mildred that the dentist gave him a questionnaire to fill out with questions like "Have you noticed a loss of height?"

ASSESSMENT

1. What do you know about Chester's health?
2. What did the dentist suspect about Chester?
3. How significant is this problem?
4. How common is this problem in the elderly?

DIAGNOSIS

5. Write a diagnosis for Chester's alteration in health maintenance and its cause.
6. Write a diagnosis for Chester's deficient knowledge and the type of education he needs.

PLAN/GOAL

7. What needs to change in Chester's diet?

IMPLEMENTATION

8. What additions or alterations in Chester's diet would prevent further osteoporosis? What are the best sources of calcium?
9. What information does Chester need to make this change?
10. Who can help him learn?
11. Why doesn't Mildred show any of these signs?
12. How can regular exercise help?
13. How could information from the Web site, National Osteoporosis Foundation, www.nof.org, help Chester?

EVALUATION/OUTCOME CRITERIA

14. In 6 months, when the dentist examines Chester again, what will Chester report?
15. How long will it take before the dentist can measure an improvement on an X-ray?

THINKING FURTHER

16. How could a DEXA scan help measure improvement?
17. How could alendronate (Fosamax) help?
18. Why is it important to intervene with a person at any age who suffers from osteoporosis?
19. How can you use this lesson in other situations?

◎ RATE THIS PLATE

Chester's problem has been first noticed by his dentist. He needs to get a DEXA scan to determine whether he has osteopenia or osteoporosis. Even though Chester has eaten "right" since his forties, it was too late then to lay down bone density. That should have happened prior to his thirties. He hasn't drunk much milk after age 40 because it caused flatulence (gas) and that was embarrassing. Rate the plate.

Homemade potato soup

Crackers

Peanut butter

Fresh pear

Water with lemon

Will this meal give Chester a serving of calcium? How many milligrams of calcium is considered a serving? What changes, if any, could be made to this meal to add needed calcium?

CASE IN POINT

WALTER: MAINTAINING HEALTH IN ADVANCED AGE

Walter is a 97-year-old man living in a home with his only son, Mel. Walter was married at 23 to Evie, whom he dearly loved. Walter and Evie had a good life, and they were prosperous. Walter was a CPA for a large company. Evie was a stay-at-home mom who did everything for Mel and Walter. When Mel's marriage failed, he moved back home. He had an upstairs apartment in the family's large home. After 40 years of marriage, Evie had a cerebral hemorrhage and died. This left Walter and Mel devastated. They were lost without Evie. Walter had never had to cook or clean or do laundry. Mel learned to cook and take care of his dad. Walter kept active; he rode a stationary bike every day for 30 minutes. He attributes his good health to drinking good beer and being German. Walter was very active in the community and at 85 volunteered at the local senior citizens' center preparing taxes during the tax season.

Mel started to notice that at 93 his dad was sleeping longer and becoming forgetful. Mel would make lunch for his dad before leaving for work, and Walter often forgot to look for lunch in the refrigerator. Walter would become morbid about his will and what Mel was to do about the house after his death. He would make Mel go over every document of his estate planning to make sure he understood. Mel noticed that at 96 his dad was not taking care of his physical self, not bathing or brushing his teeth. He would sit for hours in front of the TV with his eyes closed. Or after breakfast he would go back to bed and stay in bed all day. Mel became concerned because he saw his father becoming more emaciated and more confused. Walter complained of many different pains, so much so that Mel stopped listening. Mel noticed that his dad had some red sores around his mouth and took his dad to the doctor.

ASSESSMENT

1. What do you know about Walter and his health?
2. What do you know is a barrier in Walter's life to maintaining health?
3. What nutrients are missing from Walter's diet? Why are they missing?
4. How significant is the problem? What are the long-term consequences of the problem?

DIAGNOSIS

5. Complete the following statement: Imbalanced nutrition: less than body requirements related to _____ .
6. What nutrition education does Mel need to help Walter?

PLAN/GOAL

7. What are your goals for Walter's diet?

IMPLEMENTATION

8. Identify how each of the following resources can help Walter solve this problem and prevent further problems.
   a. His son Mel
   b. His grandchildren
   c. His church
   d. Local agencies
9. What are the sources of vitamins C, D, B_6, B_{12}, and folate?
10. How can the NP help?

EVALUATION/OUTCOME CRITERIA

11. At Walter's next NP appointment, what changes would the NP expect to note? What would the NP expect Mel to report?

THINKING FURTHER

12. Why it is so important in older persons to assure there is a balance between nutrition, medication, and chronic illness.
13. How can you use this lesson in other situations?

◎ RATE ⸽ PLATE

Some of Walter's lack of energy could be directly related to not eating. Let's see if we entice Walter to eat this lunch.

2 oz. cheddar cheese, sliced

6 crackers

1/2 blueberries

1/2 cup strawberries

1 container of vanilla pudding

What do you think of Mel's choices for his father's lunch? Are the choices good or does any food need to be changed or added? Which food could help the red sores at the corner of the mouth that Walter is experiencing? Rate the plate.

Section Three

MEDICAL

NUTRITION

THERAPY

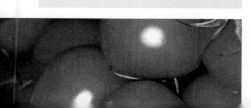

CHAPTER
16

DIET AND
WEIGHT CONTROL

OBJECTIVES

After studying this chapter, you should be able to:

- Discuss the causes and dangers of overweight
- Discuss the causes and dangers of underweight
- Identify foods suitable for high-calorie diets and those suitable for low-calorie diets

One needs to understand some commonly used terms before discussing weight control. The term *normal weight* can mean average, desired, or standard. **Normal weight** is that which is appropriate for the maintenance of good health for a particular individual at a particular time. The following is a simple method of determining one's ideal body weight. It is known as the "rule of thumb" method.

1. Males assume 106 pounds for the first 5 feet (60 inches) and add 6 pounds for each inch over 60.
2. Females assume 100 pounds for the first 5 feet (60 inches) and add 5 pounds for each inch over 60.
3. Large-boned individuals of both sexes *increase* the first sum by 10%.
4. Small-boned individuals of both sexes *decrease* the first sum by 10%.

This method is quick, but one must remember that it is only an estimate.

    Overweight can be defined as weight 10% to 20% above average. **Obesity** can be defined as excessive body fat, with weight 20% above average. **Underweight** is weight 10% to 15% below average.

⊙ normal weight
average weight for size and age

⊙ overweight
weight 10%–20% above average

⊙ obesity
excessive body fat, 20% above average

⊙ underweight
weight 10%–15% below average

⊙ metabolic
based on metabolism

⊙ caliper
mechanical device used to measure percentage of body fat by skinfold measurement

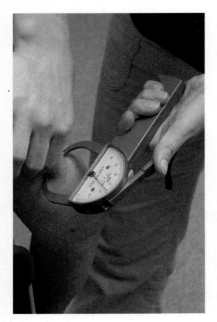

Figure 16-1 *A caliper measures skinfold thickness.*

The medical standard used to define obesity is the body mass index (BMI). It is used to determine whether a person is at health risk from excess weight. The BMI is obtained by dividing weight in kilograms by height in meters squared. Fewer health risks are associated with a BMI range of 19 to 25 than with BMI above or below that range. A BMI between 25 and 30 indicates overweight, while a BMI over 30 indicates obesity. Table 16-1 presents a range of BMIs using English units, so one needn't do the metric conversion.

The *distribution* of fat is another indicator of possible health problems. Fat in the abdominal cavity (*visceral fat*) has been shown to be associated with a greater risk for hypertension, coronary heart disease, type 2 diabetes, and certain types of cancer than has fat in the thigh, buttocks, and hip area. A pear-shaped body has a lower risk for disease than does the apple-shaped body. A waist-to-hip ratio also can give an indication of risk. This is determined by dividing the waist measurement by the hip measurement. A ratio greater than 1.0 in men and 0.8 in women indicates risk for the same diseases as given above. There also appears to be an increased risk of **metabolic** complications for men with a waist circumference of 40 inches and women with a waist circumference of 35 inches, according to the American Heart Association.

Body weight is composed of fluids, organs, fat, muscle, and bones, so large variation exists among people. In addition to height, one needs to consider age, physical condition, heredity, gender, and general frame size (small, medium, or large) in determining desired weight. For example, a 6-foot 2-inch man with a 44-inch chest, 36-inch-long arms, and 8½-inch wrists will weigh more than a 6-foot 2-inch man with a 40-inch chest, 35-inch-long arms, and 7½-inch wrists because he has more body tissue. Table 16-2 gives lists of acceptable weights according to age, sex, and height for adults that reflect realistic weight goals.

Some people can weigh more than is indicated on Table 16-2 and still be in good physical condition. Professional football players, because of the amount of lean muscle mass they develop, are examples. However, when they retire and reduce their physical activity, that same muscle can change to fat. If their weights remain the same, they then will be considered overfat because the proportion of fat will have become too high. Some can weigh what Table 16-2 indicates they should weigh and yet be overfat because too great a percentage of the weight is made up of fat.

Body fat is measured with a **caliper.** Using a caliper correctly requires practice and skill. Because the fat under the skin on the stomach and on the upper arm is representative of the percentage of overall body fat, it is usually measured when knowledge of the percentage of body fat is required. If it is more than 1½ inches, one is considered overweight. If it is under ½ inch, one is considered underweight (Figure 16-1).

A moderate amount of fat is a necessary component of the body. It protects organs from injury and acts as insulation. The final determination of desirable weight depends on common sense.

OVERWEIGHT AND OBESITY

Obesity and overweight have become epidemic. Sixty-four percent of Americans are overweight or obese. Data from the National Center for Health Statistics show that 30% of adults 20 years old and older are obese. The

Table 16-1 *Body Mass Index*

ARE YOU AT A HEALTHY WEIGHT?

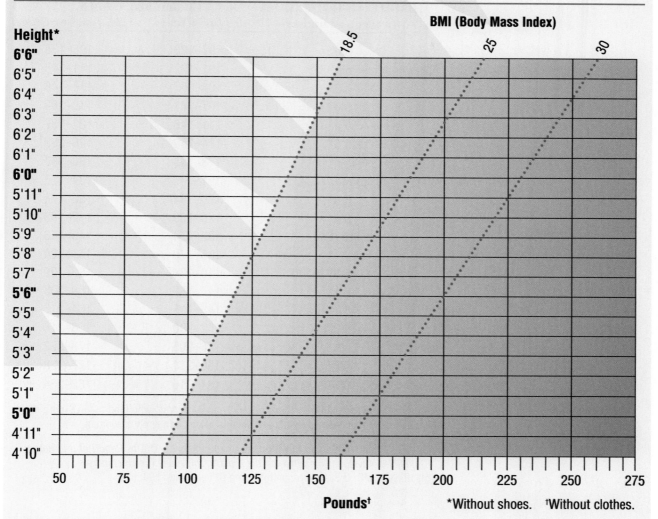

BMI measures weight in relation to height. The BMI ranges shown above are for adults. They are not exact ranges of healthy and unhealthy weights. However, they show that health risk increases at higher levels of overweight and obesity. Even within the healthy BMI range, weight gains can carry health risks for adults.

Directions: Find your weight on the bottom of the graph. Go straight up from that point until you come to the line that matches your height. Then look to find your weight group.

☐ **Healthy Weight** BMI from 18.5 up to 25 refers to healthy weight.

☐ **Overweight** BMI from 25 up to 30 refers to overweight.

■ **Obese** BMI 30 or higher refers to obesity. Obese persons are also overweight.

Source: *Report of the Dietary Guidelines Advisory Committee on the Dietary Guidelines for Americans,* 2000.

Table 16-2 USDA Acceptance Weights for Adults		
HEIGHT WITHOUT SHOES (in feet and inches)	**WEIGHT WITHOUT CLOTHES** (in pounds), BY AGE*	
	19 to 34 Years	**35 Years or Older**
5'0"	97–128	108–138
5'1"	101–132	111–143
5'2"	104–137	115–148
5'3"	107–141	119–152
5'4"	111–146	122–157
5'5"	114–150	126–162
5'6"	118–155	130–167
5'7"	121–160	134–172
5'8"	125–164	138–178
5'9"	129–169	142–183
5'10"	132–174	146–188
5'11"	136–179	151–194
6'0"	140–184	155–199
6'1"	144–189	159–205
6'2"	148–195	164–210
6'3"	152–200	168–216
6'4"	156–205	173–222
6'5"	160–211	177–228
6'6"	164–216	182–234

*The higher weights in the ranges generally apply to men, who tend to have more muscle and bone than women; the lower weights more often apply to women.

Source: From The Human Nutrition Information Service, USDA. *Report of the Dietary Guidelines Advisory Committee on the Dietary Guidelines for Americans—1990.* Hyattsville, MD: U.S. Government Printing Office, June 1990, p. 8.

diabetes mellitus
chronic disease in which the body lacks the normal ability to metabolize glucose

hypertension
higher than normal blood pressure

energy imbalance
eating either too much or too little for the amount of energy expended

percentage of overweight children and teens has tripled in the last 25 years and currently is 16%. Overweight puts extra strain on the heart, lungs, muscles, bones, and joints, and it increases the susceptibility to **diabetes mellitus** and **hypertension**. It increases surgical risks, shortens the life span, causes psychosocial problems, and is associated with heart disease and some forms of cancer.

Causes

There is no one cause for excess weight, but poor diet and inactivity appear to be leading factors. Genetic, physiological, metabolic, biochemical, and psychological factors can also contribute to it. **Energy imbalance** is a significant cause of overweight. People eat more than they need. Excess weight can accumulate during and after middle age because people reduce their level of activity and metabolism slows with age. Consequently, weight accumulates unless calorie intake is reduced. **Hypothyroidism** is a possible, but rare, cause of obesity. In this condition, the basal metabolic rate (BMR) is low, thereby reducing the number of calories needed for energy. Unless corrected with medication, this condition can result in excess weight.

There are two popular theories about weight loss: the fat cell theory and the set-point theory. According to the **fat cell theory,** obesity develops when the size of fat cells increases. When their size decreases, as during a reducing diet, the individual is driven to eat in order for the fat cells to regain their former size. Therefore, it is difficult to lose weight and keep it off.

According to the **set-point theory,** everyone has a set point or natural weight at which the body is so comfortable that it does not allow for deviation. This is said to be the reason why some people cannot lose weight below a "set point" or why, if they do, they quickly regain to that "set point." The only way to lower a set point is through exercising three to five times a week.

Healthy Weight

Not everyone fits the USDA weight table shown in Table 16-2 or the "healthy weight target," which is a BMI of 19 to 25. For anyone with a BMI of 25 or higher, a more realistic approach would be a reduction of one or two BMI points to reduce health problems and disease risks. After this loss has been maintained for 6 months, further lowering of the BMI needs to be attempted. A "healthy weight" may be the weight at which one is eating nutritiously, is exercising, has no health problems, and is free from disease.

○ **hypothyroidism**
condition in which the thyroid gland secretes too little thyroxine and T3; body metabolism is slower than normal

○ **fat cell theory**
belief that fat cells have a natural drive to regain any weight lost

○ **set-point theory**
belief that everyone has a natural weight ("set point") at which the body is most comfortable

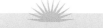

EXPLORING THE WEB

Search the Web for additional information on fat cell theory at www.americanheart.org, www.mypyramid.gov, or www.cdc.gov and set point theory. Outline the key points of each theory. What information can you find that may disprove each theory? What would an individual need to do to change his or her weight based upon these theories?

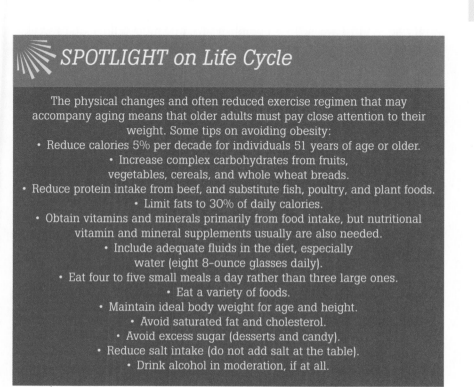

SPOTLIGHT on Life Cycle

The physical changes and often reduced exercise regimen that may accompany aging means that older adults must pay close attention to their weight. Some tips on avoiding obesity:
- Reduce calories 5% per decade for individuals 51 years of age or older.
- Increase complex carbohydrates from fruits, vegetables, cereals, and whole wheat breads.
- Reduce protein intake from beef, and substitute fish, poultry, and plant foods.
- Limit fats to 30% of daily calories.
- Obtain vitamins and minerals primarily from food intake, but nutritional vitamin and mineral supplements usually are also needed.
- Include adequate fluids in the diet, especially water (eight 8-ounce glasses daily).
- Eat four to five small meals a day rather than three large ones.
- Eat a variety of foods.
- Maintain ideal body weight for age and height.
- Avoid saturated fat and cholesterol.
- Avoid excess sugar (desserts and candy).
- Reduce salt intake (do not add salt at the table).
- Drink alcohol in moderation, if at all.

DIETARY TREATMENT OF OVERWEIGHT AND OBESITY

Obviously, if a significant cause of overweight is overeating, the solution is to reduce portion size and caloric intake. This is seldom easy. To accomplish it, one must undertake a weight reduction (low-calorie) diet. For the diet to be effective, one must have a genuine desire to lose weight.

The simplest and, therefore, perhaps the best weight reduction diet is a normal diet based on MyPyramid but with the calorie content controlled.

Exchange lists provide another excellent method to healthfully control the calorie value of the diet. These lists were originally developed by the American Diabetes Association and the American Dietetic Association for use with diabetic patients. They are organized to provide specific numbers of calories and nutrients according to six lists and are discussed in detail in Chapter 17.

Counting fat grams is another way sometimes used to lower calorie intake. Each gram of fat contains 9 calories, so the reduction of only a few grams of fat per day may result in weight loss. However, for optimal absorption of fat-soluble vitamins, one requires that at least 10% of daily caloric intake come from fats, and 20%–35% is the recommended amount for adults. Therefore, in diets limiting fats to 30% of total calories, one must consume 3 grams of fat per 90 calories; in those limiting fats to 20% of total calories, one must consume 2 grams of fat per 90 calories; and in those limiting fats to 10% of total calories, one needs 1 gram of fat per 90 calories. See Table 16-3 to calculate individual fat-gram allowances.

A reduction of 3,500 calories will result in a weight loss of 1 pound. Physicians frequently recommend that no more than 1 or 2 pounds of weight be lost in 1 week. To accomplish this, one must reduce one's weekly calories (or expend more through exercising) by 3,500–7,000, or daily intake by 500–1,000. Diets should not be reduced below 1,200 calories a day or the dieter will not receive the necessary nutrients. The diet should consist of 10% to 20% protein, 45% to 65% carbohydrate, and 20%-35% or less of fat. In other words, normal proportions of nutrients but in reduced amounts. The number of meals and snacks each day should be determined by the dieter's needs and desires, but the total number of calories must not be exceeded.

There is no magic way of losing weight and maintaining the reduced weight, but there is a key to it. That *key is changing eating habits.* In fact, unless eating habits are truly changed, it is likely that the lost weight will be regained. The cost of slimness is eating less than one might prefer and exercising most days of the week for 90 minutes.

Food Selection

The dieter must learn to "eat smart." Daily calorie counting is not necessary if one learns the calorie and fat-gram values of favorite foods and considers them before indulging. Some foods are good choices on weight loss diets because of their low-calorie and low-fat-gram values, and some foods should be used in moderation

Table 16-3 *Figuring Your Fat-Gram Allowance*

Step 1: Determine how many calories you need to maintain your ideal weight. Start by finding your ideal weight in Table 16-2.

Step 2: a. To find your calorie needs, multiply your ideal weight by 15 if you are moderately active or by 20 if you are very active.

b. From that total, subtract the following according to your age:

Age 25–34, subtract 0

Age 35–44, subtract 100

Age 45–54, subtract 200

Age 55–64, subtract 300

Age 65+, subtract 400

Step 3: To find your fat-gram allowance, multiply your daily calories by the percentage of fat desired (10%, 20%, or 30%); then divide by 9 calories/g.

SUGGESTED DAILY FAT INTAKE TABLE

CALORIES	30%	20%	10%
1,200	40 g	26 g	13 g
1,400	47 g	31 g	16 g
1,600	53 g	36 g	18 g
1,800	60 g	40 g	20 g
2,000	67 g	44 g	22 g
2,200	73 g	49 g	24 g
2,400	80 g	53 g	27 g

*The maximum amount of fat you can eat every day and still keep your blood cholesterol at a safe level.

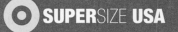

SUPERSIZE USA

"The kids love to eat at the fast-food restaurant, and it is so easy to take them several times a week. My 5-year-old son loves the cheeseburgers and fries and is now ordering an adult meal. He is husky and keeps getting bigger and bigger. I give them a good breakfast (cereal and juice), and they purchase the school lunch. I do have after-school snacks for the kids. His skinny sister likes chips, so I try to have them for her. I do keep carrots in the refrigerator for him. What can I do to prevent my son from getting heavier? What can I do to help him lose weight?"

Eat at home! Learn to cook a variety of food serving lots of vegetables, fruits, and low-fat meat. Eat out only once a month and order a kid-size meal when you do. Watch your portion sizes—serve meals on a small plate. Only keep healthy snacks in the house. Your daughter can benefit from eating fruit as a snack, and both could have popcorn. The habits they learn now will last a lifetime. As a family, you need to exercise. Ride bikes or go inline skating after dinner. Go to the YMCA or YWCA to swim. Walk and talk. ***Walk!***

Table 16-4 *Foods to Allow or to Use in Moderation on a Low-Calorie Diet*

FOODS TO ALLOW	FOODS TO USE IN MODERATION	
Fat-free milk, low-fat buttermilk, low-fat yogurt	Cream soups	Jellies and jams
Low-fat cottage cheese and other fat-free-milk cheeses	Cream sauces	Processed meats
Eggs, except prepared with fat	Cream in any form	Salad dressing
Lean beef, lamb, veal, pork, chicken, turkey, fish	Gravies	Cakes
Clear soup	Rich desserts	Cookies
Whole-grain or enriched bread	Sweet drinks and sodas	Pastries
All vegetables	Alcoholic beverages	Oily fish
Fresh fruits and those canned in their own juice or in water	Candy	Whole milk
Coffee or tea, without milk and sugar	Fried foods	Butter
Pepper, herbs, garlic, and onions	Cheese	Sugar
	Nuts	

because of their high calorie and high-fat-gram values (see Table 16-4). The low-calorie, low-fat-gram foods should be used during weight loss and thereafter.

Substitutions of foods with very low calorie contents, preferably nutrient dense, should be made for those with high-calorie contents whenever possible. The following are examples:

- Fat-free milk for whole milk
- Evaporated fat-free milk for evaporated milk
- Yogurt or low-fat sour cream for regular sour cream
- Lemon juice and herbs for heavy salad dressings
- Fat-free salad dressings for regular salad dressings
- Fruit for rich appetizers or desserts
- Consommé or bouillon instead of cream soups
- Water-packed canned foods rather than those packed in oil or syrup

There are many low-calorie, fat-free, low-fat, sugar-free, and dietetic foods on the market. A food that is said to be fat-free or sugar-free is not calorie-free. The food label must be read to determine if the product can fit into a healthy eating plan for weight reduction. Diet soda can act as a diuretic and can make one hungry, and it should be used in moderation. Ice water with lemon or lime slices makes a pleasant calorie-free drink and helps prevent dehydration.

Some foods that can be eaten with relative disregard for caloric content (provided they are served without additional calorie-rich ingredients) are listed in Table 16-5.

Cooking Methods

Broiling, grilling, baking, roasting, poaching, or boiling are the preferred methods because no additional fat is added, unlike frying. Skimming fat from the tops of soups and meat dishes will reduce their fat content, as will trimming fat

Table 16-5 *Low-Calorie Foods That May Be Used Freely on a Weight-Loss Diet*

Plain tea or tea with lemon	Cauliflower
Cantaloupe	Broccoli
Strawberries	Celery
Lettuce	Cucumbers
Cabbage	Red and green peppers
Asparagus	Bean sprouts
Tomatoes	Mushrooms
Zucchini	Spinach

from meats before cooking. The addition of extra butter or margarine to foods should be avoided, and should be replaced with fat-free seasonings such as fruit juice, vinegar, and herbs and spices.

Exercise

Exercise, particularly aerobic exercise, is an excellent adjunct to any weight loss program. Aerobic exercise uses energy from the body's fat reserves as it increases the amount of oxygen the body takes in. Examples are dancing, jogging, bicycling, skiing, rowing, and power walking. Such exercise helps tone the muscles, burns calories, increases the BMR so food is burned faster, lowers the set point, and is fun for the participant. Any exercise program must begin slowly and increase over time to avoid physical injuries.

Exercise alone can only rarely replace the actual diet, however. The dieter should be made aware of the number of calories burned by specific exercises so as to avoid overeating after the workout. General daily guidelines for exercise are 30 minutes to prevent chronic diseases, 60–90 minutes to prevent weight gain, and over 90 minutes to maintain weight loss. Children should exercise or be active 60 minutes every day.

Behavior Modification for Weight Loss

Behavior modification means change in habits. The fundamental behavior modifications for a weight loss program are the development of a new and healthy eating plan and an exercise program that can be used over the long term. These are both major lifestyle changes, and one may need to participate in a support group or undergo psychological counseling in order to successfully adapt to these changes.

It is important that one learn the difference between hunger and appetite. **Hunger** is the physiological need for food that is felt 4 to 6 hours after eating a full meal. **Appetite** is a learned psychological reaction to food caused by pleasant memories of eating it. For example, after eating a full meal one is unlikely to be hungry. Yet when dessert is served, appetite causes one to want to eat it. One must learn to listen to one's body and recognize the

((In The Media

WALK SLOWLY FOR WEIGHT LOSS

Leisurely walking along with low-impact cardiovascular activity appears to be the best formula for obese people seeking to get into shape and stay healthy, according to a University of Colorado at Boulder study. People who walk a mile at a leisurely pace burn more calories than if they walk a mile at their normal pace. Brisk walking dramatically increases the knee joint forces, which can lead to a variety of problems including joint injuries and arthritis. By leisurely walking, obese people reduce the load on their knee joints by up to 25%.

(Source: Adapted from Browning & Kram, *Obesity Research*, May 2005.)

○ **hunger**
physiological need for food

○ **appetite**
learned psychological reaction to food caused by pleasant memories of eating

difference between hunger and appetite. Additional behavior modifications are given below.

1. Weigh regularly (for example, once a week), but do not weigh yourself daily.

2. Don't wait too long between meals.

3. Join a support group and go to meetings during and after the weight loss.

4. Eat slowly.

5. Use a small plate, and fill it two-thirds with fruits, vegetables, and whole-grain products and just one-third with meat products.

6. Use low-calorie garnishes.

7. Eat whole, fresh foods that are low calorie and nutrient dense. Avoid processed foods.

8. Treat yourself with something other than food.

9. Anticipate problems (e.g., banquets and holidays). "Undereat" slightly before and after.

10. "Save" some calories for snacks and treats.

11. If something goes wrong, don't punish yourself by eating.

12. If there is no weight loss for 1 week, realize that lean muscle mass is being produced from exercising or there may be retention of water.

13. If a binge does occur, don't punish yourself by continuing to binge. Stop it! Go for a walk, to a movie, to a museum. Call a friend.

14. Adapt family meals to suit your needs. Don't make a production of your diet. Avoid the heavy-calorie items. Limit yourself to a spoonful of something too rich for a weight loss diet. Substitute something you like that is low in calories.

15. Take small portions.

16. Eat vegetables and bread without butter or margarine.

17. Include daily exercise. Park further from work and walk.

Patience and encouragement are needed throughout the adoption of a healthful diet and exercise regime. Temptation is everywhere, and the dieter should be forewarned. Just one piece of chocolate cake could set the diet back for half a day (400 to 500 calories) and lower resistance to future temptation. Breaking the diet one day will make it seem easy to break it a second day, and so on. Fresh vegetables and drinks of water may be used to harmlessly prevent or soothe the hunger pains that are bound to appear. The human body needs at least 8 glasses of water each day, and water can give one a feeling of being full. A short walk or a few minutes of exercise may help to turn the dieter's thoughts from food.

Fad Diets

Many of the countless fad diets regularly published in magazines and books are **crash diets.** This means they are intended to cause a very rapid rate of weight

EXPLORING THE WEB

Visit the U.S. Department of Health & Human Services at www.smallstep.gov to help lose weight and make lifelong changes. This site will link to the U.S. Department of Agriculture, www.mypyramid.gov.

 crash diets
fad-type diets intended to reduce weight very quickly; in fact they reduce water, not fat tissue

reduction. Often **fad diets** require the purchase of expensive foods. Others are part of a weight loss plan including exercise with special equipment. Expensive food items and equipment can add to the burden of dieting.

A crash diet usually does result in an initial rapid weight loss. However, the weight loss is caused by a loss of body water and lean muscle mass rather than body fat. Sudden weight loss of this type is followed by a **plateau period:** that is, a period in which weight does not decrease. Disillusionment is apt to occur during this period and may cause the dieter to go on an eating binge. This can result in regaining the weight that was lost and sometimes more. This weight gain in turn causes the dieter to try another weight loss diet, creating a **yo-yo effect**.

Some popular reducing diets severely limit the foods allowed, providing a real danger of nutrient deficiencies over time, and their restricted nature makes them boring. Some provide too much cholesterol and fat, contributing to atherosclerosis. Some contain an excess of protein, which puts too great a demand on the kidneys. Rapid weight loss can cause the formation of gallstones that could result in the need for surgery.

These diets ultimately fail because they defeat the dual purpose of the dieter, which is to lose weight and prevent its returning. Both can be accomplished only if eating habits are changed, and crash diets do not do this.

Surgical Treatment of Obesity

When obesity becomes **morbid** (damaging to health) and dieting and exercising are not working, surgery could be indicated. Two of the surgical procedures used are the **gastric bypass** and **stomach banding**. Both procedures reduce the size of the stomach.

In gastric bypass, most of the stomach is stapled off, creating a pouch in the upper part. The pouch is attached directly to the **jejunum** so that the food eaten bypasses most of the stomach (Figure 16-2). In stomach banding, the stomach is also stapled but to a slightly lesser degree than in gastric bypass. The food moves to the duodenum, but the outlet from the upper stomach is somewhat restricted (Figure 16-2). In both procedures the reduced stomach capacity limits the amount of food that can be eaten, and fewer nutrients are absorbed. Consequently weight is lost.

These procedures are done only on morbidly obese clients who meet certain strict criteria. A psychological evaluation will also be given to determine if the client is ready to change his or her lifestyle and adhere to healthier eating and an exercise routine. If not, the surgery will not be a success. Also, extensive nutrition counseling with a dietitian will take place before and after the surgery.

Some obese people may feel that this surgery would be a quick fix, but it is not. There can be complications such as bleeding, infections, gastritis, gallstones, and iron, vitamin B_{12}, and calcium deficiencies. Another common complication is "dumping syndrome," which can cause nausea and vomiting, diarrhea, bloating, and dizziness. Dumping occurs when foods quickly pass into the intestines without absorption of any nutrients. This happens after partial stomach removal or small intestine removal, where food (chyme) dumps directly into the large intestine.

fad diets
currently popular weight-reducing diets; usually nutritionally inadequate and not useful or permanent methods of weight reduction

plateau period
period in which there is no change in weight

yo-yo effect
refers to crash diets; the dieter's weight goes up and down over short periods because these diets do not change eating habits

EXPLORING THE WEB

Search the Web for fad diets and crash diets. List the variety of diets you find. What are these diets doing to one's body in reality? What nutrients are lacking in these diets? What potential harmful effects could these diets have? What advice would you provide to someone inquiring about these types of diets?

morbid
damaging to health

gastric bypass
surgical reduction of the stomach

stomach banding
surgical reduction of stomach, but to a lesser degree than a bypass

jejunum
the middle section comprising about two-fifths of the small intestine

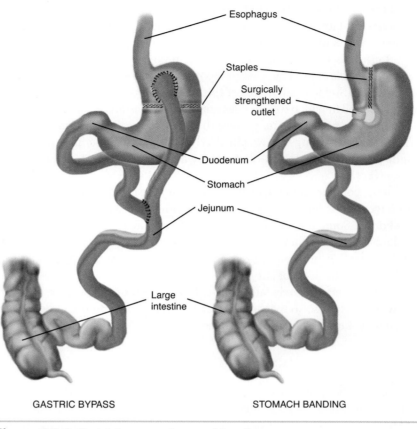

Esophagus

Staples

Surgically
strengthened
outlet

Duodenum

Stomach

Jejunum

Large
intestine

GASTRIC BYPASS   STOMACH BANDING

Figure 16-2 Gastric bypass and stomach banding.

Pharmaceutical Treatment of Obesity

The use of any weight loss medication, whether by prescription or over the counter, should be considered very carefully. Miracles are still in short supply.

Amphetamines (pep pills) have been prescribed for the treatment of obesity because they depress the appetite. However, it has been learned that their effectiveness is reduced within a relatively short time. The dosage must be regularly increased, they cause nervousness and insomnia, and they can become habit forming. Consequently, they are rarely prescribed now. Over-the-counter diet pills are available. They are intended to reduce appetite but are not thought to be effective. In addition to caffeine and artificial sweeteners, they contain **phenylpropanolamine,** which can damage blood vessels and should be avoided.

Some people believe that **diuretics** and laxatives promote weight loss. They do, but only of water. They do not cause a reduction of body fat, which is what the dieter is seeking. An excess of either could be dangerous because of possible upsets in fluid and electrolyte balance. In addition, laxatives can become habit-forming. They should not be used on any frequent or regular basis without the supervision of a physician.

Although there is no magic pill to help those with excess weight reduce, the wish for one remains, and pharmaceutical companies continue the search.

amphetamines
drugs intended to inhibit appetite

phenylpropanolamine
constituent of diet pills; can damage blood vessels

diuretics
substances used to increase the amount of urine excreted

Two medications that have recently been approved by the Food and Drug Administration (FDA) are sibutramine (Meridia) and orlistat (Xenical). Sibutramine helps to suppress the appetite and is used in conjunction with a reduced-calorie diet. It is indicated for those with a body mass index (BMI) of at least 30. Orlistat works in the digestive system where it blocks about one-third of the fat in food from being digested. It is recommended that a reduced-calorie diet with no more than 30% from fat be followed when taking orlistat.

UNDERWEIGHT

Dangers

Underweight can cause complications in pregnancy and cause various nutritional deficiencies. It may lower one's resistance to infections and, if carried to the extreme, can cause death.

Causes

Underweight can be caused by inadequate consumption of nutritious food because of depression, disease, anorexia nervosa, bulimia, or poverty, or it can be genetically determined. It also can be caused by excessive activity, the tissue wasting of certain diseases, poor absorption of nutrients, infection, or **hyperthyroidism**. For further discussion of anorexia nervosa and bulimia, see Chapter 13.

Treatment

Underweight is treated by a high-calorie diet or by a high-calorie diet combined with psychological counseling if the condition is psychological in origin as, for example, in depression or anorexia nervosa. In many cases, a high-calorie diet will be met with resistance. It can be as difficult for an underweight person to gain weight as it is for an overweight person to lose it.

The diet should be based on MyPyramid so that it can be easily adapted from the regular, family menus or to a soft-textured diet. The total number of calories prescribed per day will vary from person to person, depending on the person's activity, age, size, gender, and physical condition.

If the individual is to gain 1 pound a week, 3,500 calories in addition to the individual's basic normal weekly calorie requirement are prescribed. This means an extra 500 calories must be taken in each day. If a weight gain of 2 pounds per week is required, an additional 7,000 calories each week, or an additional 1,000 calories per day, are necessary. This diet cannot be immediately accepted at full-calorie value. Time will be needed to gradually increase the daily calorie value. In this diet, there is an increased intake of foods rich in carbohydrates, some fats, and protein. Vitamins and minerals are supplied in adequate amounts. If there are deficiencies of some vitamins and minerals, supplements are prescribed.

Nearly all nutritious foods are allowed in the high-calorie diet, but easily digested foods (carbohydrates) are recommended. Because an excess of fat can be distasteful and spoil the appetite, fatty foods must be used with discretion. Fried foods are not recommended. Bulky foods should be used sparingly. Bulk takes up stomach space that could be better used for more concentrated, high-calorie

 hyperthyroidism
condition in which the thyroid gland secretes too much thyroxine and T3; the body's rate of metabolism is unusually high

Table 16-6 *High-Calorie and High-Protein Shakes and Spreads*

HIGH-CALORIE SHAKE: 6-OZ SERVING

½ cup vanilla ice cream   1 Tbsp vegetable oil
½ cup corn syrup   1 tsp chocolate syrup
2 Tbsp whole milk

Place ingredients in blender and blend at high speed until smooth. Drink immediately.

Calories, 530; protein, 4 g; sodium, 165 mg; potassium, 180 mg; phosphorus, 135 mg

HIGH-CALORIE, HIGH-PROTEIN SHAKE: 8-OZ SERVING

¼ cup Egg Beaters   2 Tbsp corn syrup, honey, or sugar
½ cup whipping cream   ½ tsp vanilla, if desired†
½ cup vanilla ice cream*

Beat Egg Beaters until frothy. Add other ingredients and beat until well blended. Refrigerate. This recipe may be made by the quart and stored for 2–3 days.

*Strawberry ice cream may be substituted.

†Substitute ½ tsp maple, black walnut, rum, or chocolate flavoring for vanilla.

Calories, 685; protein, 14 g; sodium, 155 mg; potassium, 325 mg; phosphorus, 225 mg

PEANUT BUTTER SNACK SPREAD: ⅓ CUP SERVING

1 Tbsp instant dry milk   1 Tbsp honey
1 tsp water   3 heaping Tbsp peanut butter
1 tsp vanilla

Combine dry milk, water, and vanilla, stirring to moisten. Add honey and peanut butter, stirring slowly until liquid blends with peanut butter. Spread between graham crackers or soda crackers. The spread can also be formed into balls, chilled, and eaten as candy. Keeps well in refrigerator, but is difficult to spread when cold.

Calories, 440; protein, 17 g

foods. See Table 16-6 for high-calorie and high-protein shakes and spread that could be used to increase caloric intake.

Persons requiring this diet frequently have poor appetites, so meals need to be especially appetizing. Favorite foods should be served, and portions of all foods should be small to avoid discouraging the clients. Many of the extra calories needed may be gotten as snacks between meals, unless these snacks reduce the client's appetite for meals and consequently reduce daily calorie total. Some clients do better if the number of meals is reduced, thereby increasing the appetite for each meal served. When the causes of underweight are psychological, therapy is required before the diet is begun, and the dietitian and therapist may well need to consult one another before and during treatment. Foods to be avoided in a high-calorie diet are foods the client dislikes, fatty foods, and bulky, low-calorie foods.

CONSIDERATIONS FOR THE HEALTH CARE PROFESSIONAL

Even for the most determined clients, a successful weight loss program will be charged with anxiety. There will be days of disappointment. It will take a long time to reach the ultimate goal. The health care professional will need to supply psychological support and nutritional advice when disappointing results create the need for emotional support. It is essential that the health care professional see the problems, support the client, and then effectively lead her or him back to the diet. The key words for the health care professional are *support* and *encouragement*.

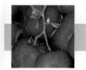

SUMMARY

Excessive weight endangers health and should be lost by the use of a reduced-calorie diet based on MyPyramid. Such a diet helps the dieter change eating habits and avoid regaining the lost weight. Excess weight is usually caused by energy imbalance. Exercise is beneficial to weight loss regimens but rarely can replace the reduced-calorie diet. Fad diets are expensive and boring and may lead to nutritional deficiencies. They ultimately fail because they do not change eating habits. Underweight is also dangerous to health, and psychological counseling as well as a high-calorie diet may be required for proper treatment. Behavior modification must be an essential component of any weight loss or weight gain regimen.

DISCUSSION TOPICS

1. Discuss *overweight*, *obesity*, and *underweight*. Tell how someone may be overweight according to the weight charts and still be considered to be in good physical condition. What factors contribute to the determination of one's correct weight?

2. What are some causes of overweight? Discuss why some people eat more than they need. Discuss how overeating can be prevented or changed.

3. Explain why changing eating habits is essential to an effective weight loss program.

4. Name 10 foods that may be used without concern about calories during a weight loss program. Explain why.

5. Describe the use of exercise during a weight loss program. Could it be used in lieu of the diet? Why?

6. Describe one or two popular reducing diets. Could such a diet have any effect on the nutrition of those people who subscribe to it? If so, what? Ask if anyone in the class has used such a diet. If anyone has, ask that person to describe the diet, the physical effects felt during the diet, and the ultimate result.

7. Explain why a high-calorie diet could be unpleasant for a client.

8. Discuss the causes and dangers of underweight.

SUGGESTED ACTIVITIES

1. Using Appendix D, look for caloric values of 10 favorite foods. Make two lists. On the left, list which of the 10 foods would be suitable for a high-calorie diet. On the right side, list those foods suitable for a low-calorie diet.

2. Make a list of foods eaten yesterday. Circle those foods that would not be suitable for a low-calorie diet. Explain why.

3. Keep a record of your food intake for 3 days (one of the days must be on a weekend), and using the MyPyramid Web site, www.mypyramid.gov, input your food for each day and print all reports available. Add your total calories for each day and divide them by 3 to get your average caloric intake. Were your calories identical or close to your caloric needs as indicated on your personnal profile? What will be the consequences if you continue to eat your average number of calories?

REVIEW

Multiple choice. Select the *letter* that precedes the best answer.

1. The general types of foods that should be limited in the low-calorie diet are
   a. fatty foods
   b. foods the client likes
   c. breads and cereals
   d. coffee and tea

2. The low-calorie diet may be prescribed for
   a. obesity
   b. anorexia nervosa
   c. hyperthyroidism
   d. severe allergies

3. A proper weight reduction plan allows for loss of
   a. 1 to 2 pounds per day
   b. 1 to 2 pounds per week
   c. 3 to 5 pounds per week
   d. 15 to 20 pounds per month

4. Popular crash diets
   a. are always effective and totally harmless
   b. are useful for teenagers
   c. result in a slow, even loss of weight
   d. are potentially hazardous

5. Normal weight
   a. is always the same for two people of the same sex and height
   b. does not change during one's lifetime
   c. may be greater than the amounts indicated on the weight charts
   d. all of the above

6. The most common cause of overweight is
   a. hypothyroidism
   b. hyperthyroidism
   c. energy imbalance
   d. all of the above

7. The dysfunction of the thyroid gland in which the basal metabolic rate is lowered and the need for calories is reduced is called
   a. hypothyroidism
   b. hyperthyroidism
   c. energy imbalance
   d. all of the above

8. The dysfunction of the thyroid gland in which the basal metabolic rate is raised and the need for calories is increased is called
   a. hypothyroidism
   b. hyperthyroidism
   c. energy imbalance
   d. goiter

9. To lose 2 pounds per week, one must reduce weekly calories by
   a. 500
   b. 1,000
   c. 3,500
   d. 7,000

10. To lose 1 pound per week, one must reduce weekly calories by
    a. 500
    b. 1,000
    c. 3,500
    d. 7,000

11. The key to losing weight and maintaining the reduced weight is
    a. skipping lunch
    b. fasting 1 day each week
    c. changing eating habits
    d. assiduously counting calories each meal

12. Strawberries, low-fat yogurt, poached egg, and whole wheat toast would
    a. be allowed on a calorie-restricted diet
    b. not be allowed on a low-calorie diet
    c. constitute a poor breakfast for someone on a high-calorie diet
    d. not be a nutritious breakfast for someone on a weight-control diet

13. Baking, roasting, broiling, boiling, and poaching are recommended for
    a. low-calorie diets only
    b. high-calorie diets only
    c. both high- and low-calorie diets
    d. none of the above

14. Fad diets are not recommended as reducing diets because they
    a. usually cause illness
    b. alter eating habits excessively
    c. do not alter eating habits
    d. require an excessive amount of time before weight loss occurs

15. Someone on a weight reduction diet with the goal of losing 80 pounds
    a. will undoubtedly have a BMI of 20 or less
    b. can eat fat-free foods with abandon
    c. should avoid all carbohydrates
    d. should not weigh himself daily

CASE IN POINT

CAMERON: LOSING WEIGHT AT 40

Cameron is a 40-year-old man of Dutch descent and the father of two. He has been divorced for 6 years. Cameron wants to start dating again. He misses having an adult to talk to as a friend. However, he is embarrassed by the extra weight he has gained. He is about 5 feet 11 inches tall and currently weighs 230 pounds. He knows he is overweight, and he has not been faithful about exercising. Cameron is not a good cook, but he can make basic meals. A typical dinner is some meat, vegetables, fruit, and milk. He lets the kids have candy or sweets only on special occasions. He makes sure they eat breakfast together before school. In warm weather, breakfast is cold cereal and sometimes juice. Even the little kids can make that breakfast themselves. In the winter, breakfast is oatmeal and hot chocolate. Cameron is proud of his kids. They are athletic and are always busy after school with one sport or another throughout the school year.

Cameron passed his physical with his doctor and told the doctor of his plan to get back in shape and lose the weight he has acquired. The doctor told him to avoid fad weight loss pills and advertised quick weight loss plans. The doctor gave him a couple of pamphlets on safe weight loss programs that he wanted Cameron to consider. The doctor asked Cameron to check back in 3 months so that he could monitor his progress.

ASSESSMENT

1. What do you know about Cameron and his current priorities? What is a new priority he wants to add to his life?

2. Use the rule of thumb to determine Cameron's ideal weight.

3. How long will it take him to reach his ideal weight if he loses 1 or 2 pounds a week?

4. What major changes does Cameron need to make to lose weight?

5. Use the BMI to determine whether he is at risk for health problems at his current weight.

DIAGNOSIS

6. What would be the best method for Cameron to lose weight and keep it off?

7. Was Cameron eating nutritiously?

8. What changes do you think Cameron needs to make in his diet?

9. Complete the following diagnostic statement: Imbalanced nutrition: more than body requirements, related to _____ .

PLAN/GOAL

10. What are some reasonable, measurable goals for Cameron? Over what period of time?

IMPLEMENTATION

11. What are the advantages and disadvantages of each of the following methods of weight loss for Cameron?
    a. Weight Watchers
    b. Jenny Craig
    c. Slimfast and low-fat diet

12. What are the advantages and disadvantages of each of the following exercises
    a. Self-guided plan
    b. Health club near home
    c. Hospital-based facility

13. Looking at the options in questions 11 and 12 and taking into consideration Cameron's priorities, what type of program would you recommend for Cameron?

14. How can the children help? How can Cameron spend time with his children and get some exercise?

15. What low-calorie foods can Cameron keep at work and at home that he can eat when he is hungry between meals?

EVALUATION/OUTCOME CRITERIA

16. What does Cameron need to learn to drink to help with his weight loss?

17. What habit does Cameron need to develop to help maintain his weight loss?

THINKING FURTHER

18. In 3 months when Cameron returns to the doctor, what changes will Cameron be able to report, and what will the doctor be able to measure?

19. If Cameron follows your program, how long will it take before he will have lost enough weight to consider dating?

◎ RATE ≣ PLATE

Cameron may have thought he was well, but the dietitian may feel otherwise. Cameron doesn't take his lunch, preferring to go out with the guys. Ordering is no problem. Rate the plate.

Caesar salad with chicken strips and caesar salad dressing (about 1/4 cup)

2 bread sticks (dipped in garlic-flavored butter)

Diet soda with 2 refills

What questions should Cameron ask his waitress before ordering lunch? What decisions should Cameron make with the answers to his questions? Does this meal need changing, and if so, how would you modify it?

CASE IN POINT

ANNETTE: STAYING HEALTHY FOLLOWING GASTRIC BYPASS SURGERY

Annette is a 60-year-old Italian-born woman who is 5 feet 2 inches tall and weighs 250 pounds. She had been heavy all her life but ballooned to over 200 in the last 5 years. Annette loved pasta of any kind, especially in alfredo sauces. She would eat bagels and cream cheese, and she would butter the bagel before using the cream cheese. She had peanut butter and jelly sandwiches with butter and loved ice cream for desserts. She had fruit and vegetables occasionally but preferred her pastas. She had tried numerous fad diets. The grapefruit diet, the Mayo diet, and the cucumber diet. She generally lost 20 or more pounds on each diet but would gain all the weight back plus 10 pounds more. Foods were her means of stress reduction and her source of comfort.

Recently, Annette went to the doctor because of swelling in her lower limbs. She complained of shortness of breath on exertion and was experiencing headaches. She had trouble sleeping at night and cried at the drop of a hat. Her doctor placed her on hypertensive medication and an antidepressant. Annette asked her doctor about gastric bypass surgery. She reluctantly agreed to have Annette screened for surgery. She discussed with Annette the necessary lifestyle, dietary, and exercise changes she would have to make for the surgery to be successful.

Annette was scheduled for the surgery after 2 months of research on her part and assessment by physicians to ensure it was safe. After surgery, she was placed on a rigorous, closely supervised recovery program. Her sister had to agree to move in with her for this period to be her recovery coach. Annette attended classes about the meaning of food, how to eat, weight loss, exercise, and behavior modification.

ASSESSMENT

1. What do you know about Annette?
2. What was her new priority?
3. What is her ideal weight?
4. How many pounds does she need to lose?
5. How long should it take to be done safely?
6. What is her current risk for health problems on the basis of her BMI?
7. What are her known health problems?
8. At what weight will her health risk be reasonable?
9. How long will it take to reach that reasonable health-risk weight?

DIAGNOSIS

10. Write a complete nursing diagnostic statement for Annette's nutrition problem.
11. Write a complete nursing diagnostic statement for Annette's deficient knowledge.
12. Write a diagnosis for her activity intolerance.

PLAN/GOAL

13. Write at least three goals for Annette that are reasonable and measurable.

IMPLEMENTATION

14. Use Table 16-3 to calculate the number of grams of fat and calories that Annette can consume on a 30% fat diet.
15. What topics are essential in Annette's nutrition classes?
16. Use the food items Annette liked to eat and list low-calorie, low-fat alternatives.
17. What are some behavior modification hints or tips related to where and when she eats that would help her?
18. Annette was instructed to turn in her home scale to the doctor's office and to see her every Friday morning to weigh in and have her blood pressure checked. What is the rationale for these directions?
19. How would the information at the obesity Web site, www.nhlbi.nih.gov, be helpful to Annette?

EVALUATION/OUTCOME

20. What changes should the doctor see, hear, and be able to measure that are indicative of success?

THINKING FURTHER

21. Why is it important for Annette to persevere at weight reduction?
22. What are some of the serious potential complications of this surgery?

◎ RATE THIS PLATE

Annette took a very life-altering step when she had gastric bypass surgery. Immediately after surgery, Annette was on liquids for several days and was only able to consume 2 tablespoons at a time. It has been awhile, and her stomach can now hold about 1 cup. It is imperative that Annette eat enough protein to promote healing and to prevent the body from using lean muscle mass instead of fat for energy. She has met with a dietitian and is now planning her meals. Rate the plate.

2 oz chicken

1/4 cup sweet potatoes

1/4 cup macaroni salad

1/4 cup milk

1 piece hard candy

Check the Internet to determine if this plate is correct.

CHAPTER 17

DIET AND DIABETES MELLITUS

OBJECTIVES

After studying this chapter, you should be able to:

- Describe diabetes mellitus and identify the types
- Describe the symptoms of diabetes mellitus
- Explain the relationship of insulin to diabetes mellitus
- Discuss appropriate nutritional management of diabetes mellitus

Diabetes mellitus is the name for a group of serious and chronic (long-standing) disorders affecting the metabolism of carbohydrates. These disorders are characterized by **hyperglycemia** (abnormally large amounts of glucose in the blood). According to the American Diabetes Association, 18.2 million people in the United States have diabetes. An estimated 13 million have been diagnosed with the disease. Unfortunately, 5.2 million remain undiagnosed (The American Diabetes Association (ADA)). It is a major cause of death; blindness; heart and kidney disease; amputations of toes, feet, and legs; and infections.

Hundreds of years ago, a Greek physician named it *diabetes*, which means "to flow through," because of the large amounts of urine generated by victims. Later, the Latin word *mellitus*, which means "honeyed," was added because of the amount of glucose in the urine.

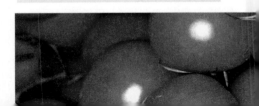

Diabetes insipidus is a different disorder. It also generates large amounts of urine, but it is "insipid," not sweet. This is a rare condition, caused by a damaged pituitary gland. It is not discussed in this chapter.

The body needs a constant supply of energy, and glucose is its primary source. Carbohydrates provide most of the glucose, but about 10% of fats and up to nearly 60% of proteins can be converted to glucose if necessary.

The distribution of glucose must be carefully managed for the maintenance of good health. Glucose is transported by the blood, and its entry into the cells is controlled by hormones. The primary hormone is **insulin.**

Insulin is secreted by the beta cells of the islets of Langerhans in the pancreas. When there is inadequate production of insulin or the body is unable to use the insulin it produces, glucose cannot enter the cells and it accumulates in the blood, creating hyperglycemia. This condition can cause serious complications.

Another hormone, **glucagon,** which is secreted by the alpha cells of the islets of Langerhans, helps release energy when needed by converting glycogen to glucose. Somatostatin is a hormone produced by the delta cells of the islets of Langerhans and the hypothalamus. All actions of this hormone are inhibitory. It inhibits the release of insulin and glucagons.

The amount of glucose in the blood normally rises after a meal. The **pancreas** reacts by providing insulin. As the insulin circulates in the blood, it binds to special insulin receptors on cell surfaces. This binding causes the cells to accept the glucose. The resulting reduced amount of glucose in the blood in turn signals the pancreas to stop sending insulin.

ETIOLOGY

The **etiology** (cause) of diabetes is not confirmed. Although it appears that diabetes may be hereditary, environmental factors also may contribute to its occurrence. For example, viruses or obesity may precipitate the disease in people who have a genetic predisposition.

The World Health Organization indicates that the prevalence of the disease is increasing worldwide, especially in areas showing improvement in living standards.

SYMPTOMS

The abnormal concentration of glucose in the blood of diabetic clients draws water from the cells to the blood. When hyperglycemia exceeds the **renal threshold,** the glucose is excreted in the urine **(glycosuria).** With the loss of the cellular fluid, the client experiences **polyuria** (excessive urination), and **polydipsia** (excessive thirst) typically results.

The inability to metabolize glucose causes the body to break down its own tissue for protein and fat. This response causes **polyphagia** (excessive appetite), but at the same time a loss of weight, weakness, and fatigue occur. The body's use of protein from its own tissue causes it to excrete nitrogen.

Because the untreated diabetic client cannot use carbohydrates for energy, excessive amounts of fats are broken down, and consequently the liver produces **ketones** from the fatty acids. In healthy people, ketones are

diabetes mellitus
chronic disease in which the body lacks the normal ability to metabolize glucose

hyperglycemia
excessive amounts of sugar in the blood

insulin
secretion of the islets of Langerhans in the pancreas gland; essential for the proper metabolism of glucose

glucagon
hormone from alpha cells of pancreas; helps cells release energy

pancreas
gland that secretes enzymes essential for digestion and insulin, which is essential for glucose metabolism

etiology
cause

renal threshold
kidneys' capacity

glycosuria
excess sugar in the urine

polyuria
excessive urination

polydipsia
abnormal thirst

polyphagia
excess hunger

ketones
substances to which fatty acids are broken down in the liver

ketonemia
ketones collected in the blood

ketonuria
ketone bodies in the urine

acidosis
condition in which excess acids accumulate or there is a loss of base in the body

diabetic coma
unconsciousness caused by a state of acidosis due to too much sugar or too little insulin

vascular system
circulatory system

retinopathy
damage to small blood vessels in the eyes

neuropathy
nerve damage

type 1 diabetes
diabetes occurring suddenly between the ages of 1 and 40; clients secrete little, if any, insulin and require insulin injections and a carefully controlled diet

type 2 diabetes
diabetes occurring usually after age 40; onset is gradual and production of insulin gradually diminishes; can usually be controlled by diet and exercise

subsequently broken down to carbon dioxide and water, yielding energy. In diabetic clients, fats break down faster than the body can handle them. Ketones collect in the blood (**ketonemia**) and must be excreted in the urine (**ketonuria**). Ketones are acids that lower blood pH, causing **acidosis.** Acidosis can lead to **diabetic coma,** which can result in death if the client is not treated quickly with fluids and insulin.

In addition to the symptoms previously mentioned, diabetic clients suffer from diseases of the **vascular system.** Atherosclerosis (a condition in which there is a heavy buildup of fatty substances inside artery walls, reducing blood flow) is a major cause of death among diabetic clients. Damage to the small blood vessels can cause retinal degeneration. **Retinopathy** is the leading cause of blindness in the United States. Nerve damage (**neuropathy**) is not uncommon, and infections, particularly of the urinary tract, are frequent problems.

CLASSIFICATION

The types of diabetes are prediabetes, type 1, type 2, and gestational. Prediabetes means that the cells in the body are not using insulin properly. The diagnosis is made by a fasting blood glucose which is more than 110 but less than 126 mg/dl. One's lifestyle will determine when prediabetes will advance to type 2.

Type 1 diabetes develops when the body's immune system destroys the pancreatic beta cells. These are the only cells in the body that make the hormone insulin that regulates blood glucose. Type 1 diabetes is usually diagnosed in children and young adults. It can account for 5% to 10% of all cases of newly diagnosed diabetes. Some risk factors include genetics, autoimmune status, and environmental factors.

Type 2 diabetes was previously called adult-onset diabetes because it usually occurred in adults over the age of 40. Type 2 is associated with obesity, and obesity has become an epidemic, which has drastically increased the incidence of type 2 diabetes among adolescents and young adults. A family history of diabetes, prior history of gestational diabetes, impaired glucose tolerance, older age, physical inactivity, and race and ethnicity can predispose one to type 2 diabetes. African Americans, Hispanic and Latino Americans, Native Americans, some Asian Americans, and Native Hawaiians and other Pacific Islanders are at particularly high risk for type 2 diabetes. It is not uncommon for the client to have no symptoms of diabetes and to be totally ignorant of his or

((• *In The Media*

RAISING AWARENESS OF DIABETES

Actor Mark Consuelos, having many family members with diabetes, has taken on the role as a spokesperson for diabetes awareness. He, along with sponsors, launched the Taking Diabetes Freedom to the Streets tour. This is a 22-city tour, and attendees are asked to take the Diabetes Freedom pledge as the first step in committing to a healthier lifestyle through regular exercise, proper nutrition, and frequent blood glucose monitoring. The pledge is a commitment to manage diabetes or help others manage their condition.

(Source: *Diabetes Health,* November 2005.)

her condition until it is discovered accidentally during a routine urine or blood test or after a heart attack or stroke. In type 2 diabetes, hypertension may be present as part of the metabolic syndrome (i.e., obesity, hyperglycemia, and **dyslipidemia**) that is accompanied by high rates of cardiovascular disease. The American Diabetes Association recommends that blood pressure be controlled at 130/80 mm Hg for diabetics.

Type 2 diabetes can usually be controlled by diet and exercise, or by diet, exercise, and an **oral diabetes medication.** Table 17-1 shows six

○ **dyslipidemia**
increased lipid in the blood

○ **oral diabetes medications**
oral hypoglycemic agents, medications that may be given to type 2 diabetics to lower blood glucose

Table 17-1 *Types of Oral Diabetes (Glucose-Lowering) Medications*

Meglitinide	Repaglinide (Prandin)
	Nateglinide (Starlix)
Thiazolidinedione	Pioglitazone (Actos)
	Rosiglitazone (Avandia)
Combination drugs	Glyburide and metformin (Glucovance)
	Glipizide and metformin (Metaglip)
Nonsulfonylurea	Metformin (Glucophage)
	Melformin and a time-released controlling polymer (Glucophage XR)
Alpha-glucosidase inhibitor	Acarbose (Precose)
	Miglitol (Glycet)
Second-generation sulfonylureas	Glyburide (DiaBeta, Micronase, Glynase Prestabs)
	Glipizide (Glucotrol, Glucotrol XL)
	Glimepride (Amaryl)

SPOTLIGHT on Life Cycle

The National Diabetes Education Program of the U.S. Department of Health and Human Services (National Institutes of Health, 2005) is spreading the word that lifestyle changes can be especially effective in preventing type 2 diabetes in adults aged 60 and older. The National Institutes of Health (NIH) reports that about 40% of adults ages 40 to 74 (approximately 41 million people) have prediabetes, a recognized risk for developing type 2 diabetes, heart disease, and stroke. Studies show that while adults over 60 are at increased risk for type 2 diabetes, the combination of losing a small amount of weight and increasing physical activity is especially effective in reducing that risk among this age group. The NIH is committed to getting the word out to middle-aged and older adults that modest lifestyle changes can yield big rewards in preventing or delaying the onset of type 2 diabetes. Steps for older adults include:

- Finding out if they are at risk for type 2 diabetes
- Learning what actions they can take to prevent the disease
- Losing a small amount of weight by following a low-fat, low-calorie meal plan
- Getting 30 minutes of physical activity five times per week

These lifestyle interventions worked particularly well in people aged 60 and older, reducing the development of diabetes by 71%.

(Source: National Institutes of Health (2005). Data compiled and retrieved December 2, 2005, from http://www.ndep.nih.gov/campaigns/tools.htm#fsPrev.)

types of oral glucose-lowering medications in order from newest and most frequently used to oldest and least frequently used. The goals of medical nutrition therapy for clients with type 2 diabetes include maintaining healthy glucose, blood pressure, and lipid levels. Also, because approximately 80% of type 2 clients are overweight, these clients may be placed on weight reduction diets after their blood glucose levels are within acceptable range. Thus, monitoring their weight loss also becomes part of their therapy. Exenatide (Byetta) injection is the first in a new class of drugs for the treatment of type 2 diabetes. The drugs are called incretin mimetics. When food is eaten, incretin hormones are released from cells located in the small intestine. In the pancreas, incretins will act on the beta cells to increase glucose-dependent insulin secretions to ensure an appropriate insulin response after a meal. This medication is used in conjunction with the nonsulfonylurea metformin to help clients lower their HgbA1c to less than 7%. **HbgA1c** is a blood test to determine how well blood glucose has been controlled for the last three months. The American Diabetes Association prefers the outcome be less than 6%.

Gestational diabetes can occur between the sixteenth and twenty-eighth week of pregnancy. If it is not responsive to diet and exercise, insulin injection therapy will be used (Figure 17-1). It is recommended that a dietitian or a diabetic educator be consulted to plan an adequate diet that will control blood sugar for mother and baby.

Concentrated sugars should be avoided. Weight gain should continue, but not in excessive amounts. Usually, gestational diabetes disappears after the infant is born. However, diabetes can develop 5 to 10 years after the pregnancy (see Chapter 11).

Secondary diabetes occurs infrequently and is caused by certain drugs or by a disease of the pancreas.

TREATMENT

The treatment of diabetes is intended to:

1. Control blood glucose levels
2. Provide optimal nourishment for the client
3. Prevent symptoms and thus delay the complications of the disease

Treatment is typically begun when blood tests indicate hyperglycemia or when other previously discussed symptoms occur. Normal blood glucose levels (called fasting blood sugar, FBS) are from about 70 to 110 mg/dl.

Treatment can be by diet alone or by a diet combined with insulin or an oral glucose-lowering medication plus regulated exercise and the regular monitoring of the client's blood glucose levels.

The physician and dietitian can provide essential testing, information, and counseling and can help the client delay potential damage. The ultimate responsibility, however, rests with the client. When a person with diabetes uses nicotine, eats carelessly, forgets insulin, ignores symptoms, and neglects appropriate blood tests, she or he increases the risk of developing permanent tissue damage.

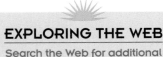

HgbA1c
a blood test to determine how well blood glucose has been controlled for the last 3 months

gestational diabetes
diabetes occurring during pregnancy; usually disappears after delivery of the infant

EXPLORING THE WEB

Search the Web for additional information on gestational diabetes. What are the presenting signs and symptoms of gestational diabetes? What are the dangers of gestational diabetes to the mother and to the fetus if left untreated? Are there factors that put certain women at a higher risk for developing gestational diabetes? If yes, what are these risks?

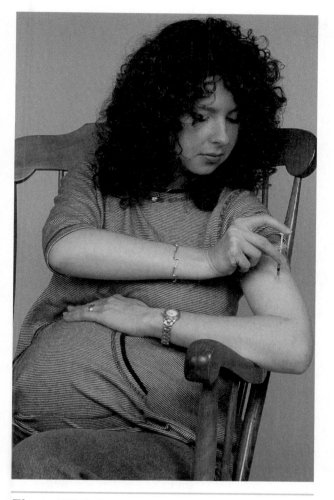

Figure 17-1 *A pregnant woman can develop diabetes during her pregnancy that may need to be managed by insulin injections.*

NUTRITIONAL MANAGEMENT

The dietitian will need to know the client's diet history, food likes and dislikes, and lifestyle at the onset. The client's calorie needs will depend on age, activities, lean muscle mass, size, and REE.

It is recommended that carbohydrates provide 50% to 60% of the calories. Approximately 40% to 50% should be from complex carbohydrates (starches). The remaining 10% to 20% of carbohydrates could be from simple sugar.

Research provides no evidence that carbohydrates from simple sugars are digested and absorbed more rapidly than are complex carbohydrates, and they do not appear to affect blood sugar control. It is the *total amount of carbohydrates eaten* that affects blood sugar levels rather than the type. Being able to substitute foods containing sucrose for other carbohydrates increases flexibility in meal planning for the diabetic.

◎ SUPERSIZE **USA**

Diabetes is just one of the many health risks associated with obesity. Where you live geographically may have an impact on your chance of becoming overweight. Does your state rank in the top 12 states for obesity? Obesity was based on the 2004 percentage of adults within the state whose body mass index reading fell within the obese range. Check the following list of states, ranking from highest percentage to lowest percentage of obese adults.

Mississippi	29.5%
Alabama	28.9%
West Virginia	27.6%
Tennessee	27.2%
Louisiana	27.0%
Kentucky	25.8%
Texas	25.8%
Indiana	25.5%
Michigan	25.4%
South Carolina	25.1%
Missouri	24.9%
Oklahoma	24.9%

(Source: *The Journal Gazette*, October 23, 2005.)

Fats should be limited to 30% of total calories, and proteins should provide from 15% to 20% of total calories. Lean proteins are advisable because they contain limited amounts of fats.

Regardless of the percentages of energy nutrients prescribed, the foods ultimately eaten should provide sufficient vitamins and minerals as well as energy nutrients.

The client with type 1 diabetes needs a nutritional plan that balances calories and nutrient needs with insulin therapy and exercise. It is important that meals and snacks be composed of similar nutrients and calories and eaten at regular times each day. Small meals plus two or three snacks may be more helpful in maintaining steady blood glucose levels for these clients than three large meals each day.

The client with type 1 diabetes should anticipate the possibility of missing meals occasionally and carry a few crackers and some cheese or peanut butter to prevent **hypoglycemia,** which can occur in such a circumstance.

The client with type 2 diabetes may be overweight. The nutritional goal for this client is not only to keep blood glucose levels in the normal range but to lose weight as well. Exercise can help attain both goals.

◔ hypoglycemia
subnormal levels of blood sugar

Carbohydrate Counting

Carbohydrate counting is the newest method for teaching a diabetic client how to control blood sugar with food. The starch and bread category, milk, and fruits have all been put under the heading of "carbohydrates." This means that these three food groups can be interchanged within one meal. One would still have the same number of servings of carbohydrates, but it would not be the typical number of starches or fruits and milk that one usually eats. For example, one is to have four carbohydrates for breakfast (2 breads, 1 fruit, and 1 milk). If there is no milk available, a bread or fruit must be eaten in place of the milk. The exchange lists are utilized in carbohydrate counting as well as in traditional meal planning. Protein, approximately 3 to 4 ounces, is eaten for lunch and dinner. One or two fat exchanges are recommended for each meal. Two carbohydrates should be eaten for an evening snack. These are only beginning guidelines. A dietitian or diabetic educator can help tailor this to the individual client.

Diets Based on Exchange Lists

The method of diet therapy most commonly used for diabetic clients is that based on **exchange lists.** These lists were developed by the American Diabetes Association in conjunction with the American Dietetic Association and are summarized in Table 17-2 and included completely in Table 17-3.

Under this plan, foods are categorized by type and included in the lists in Table 17-3.

The foods within each list contain approximately equal amounts of calories, carbohydrates, protein, and fats. This means that any one food on a particular list can be substituted for any other food on that *particular list* and still provide the client with the prescribed types and amounts of nutrients and calories.

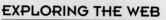

EXPLORING THE WEB

Search the Web for additional information and resources for carbohydrate counting. Are there tools that make this easy for the diabetic client?

exchange lists
lists of foods with interchangeable nutrient and calorie contents; used in specific forms of diet therapy

Table 17-2 *Summary of Exchange Lists*				
GROUP/LIST	**CARBOHYDRATE (grams)**	**PROTEIN (grams)**	**FAT (grams)**	**CALORIES**
Carbohydrate Group				
Starch	15	3	1 or less	80
Fruit	15	—	—	60
Milk				
Fat-free	12	8	0–3	90
Reduced fat (2%)	12	8	5	120
Whole	12	8	8	150
Other carbohydrates	15	varies	varies	varies
Vegetables	5	2	—	25
Meat and Meat Substitute Group				
Very lean	—	7	0–1	35
Lean	—	7	3	55
Medium fat	—	7	5	75
High fat	—	7	8	100
Fat Group	—	—	5	45

Source: *Exchange List for Meal Planning.* The American Diabetes Association and The American Dietetic Association, 1995.

Table 17-3 *Exchange Lists for Meal Planning*

STARCH EXCHANGE LIST

One starch exchange equals 15 g carbohydrate, 3 g protein, 0–1 g fat, and 80 calories

Bread/Starches

Bagel	½ (1 oz)
Bread, reduced calorie	2 slices (1½ oz)
Bread, white, whole wheat, pumpernickel, rye	1 slice (1 oz)
Bread sticks, crisp, 4 in. long × ½ in.	2 (⅔ oz)
English muffin	½
Hotdog or hamburger bun	½ (1 oz)
Pita, 6 in. across	½
Raisin bread, unfrosted	1 slice (1 oz)
Roll, plain, small	1 (1 oz)
Tortilla, corn, 6 in. across	1
Tortilla, flour, 7–8 in. across	1
Waffle, 4½ in. square, reduced fat	1

Beans, Peas, and Lentils *(Count as 1 starch exchange, plus 1 very lean meat exchange.)*

Beans and peas (garbanzo, pinto, kidney, white, split, black-eyed)	½ cup
Lima beans	⅔ cup
Lentils	½ cup
Miso*	3 Tbsp

* = 400 mg or more sodium per exchange.

Cereals and Grains

Bran cereals	½ cup
Bulgur	½ cup
Cereals	½ cup
Cereals, unsweetened, ready to eat	¼ cup
Cornmeal (dry)	3 Tbsp
Couscous	⅓ cup
Flour (dry)	3 Tbsp
Granola, low fat	¼ cup
Grape-Nuts	¼ cup
Grits	½ cup
Kasha	½ cup
Millet	¼ cup
Muesli	¼ cup
Oats	½ cup

(continues)

Table 17-3 *Continued*

Cereals and Grains *continued*

Pasta	½ cup
Puffed cereal	1½ cups
Rice milk	½ cup
Rice, white or brown	⅓ cup
Shredded wheat	½ cup
Sugar-frosted cereal	½ cup
Wheat germ	3 Tbsp

Crackers and Snacks

Animal crackers	8
Graham crackers, 2½-in. square	3
Matzoh	¾ oz
Melba toast	4 slices
Oyster crackers	24
Popcorn (popped, no fat added or low-fat microwave)	3 cups
Pretzels	¾ oz
Rice cakes, 4 in. across	2
Saltine-type crackers	6
Snack chips, fat-free (tortilla, potato)	15–20 (¾ oz)
Whole wheat crackers, no fat added	2–5 (¾ oz)

Starchy Vegetables

Baked beans	⅓ cup
Corn	½ cup
Corn on cob, medium	1 (5 oz)
Mixed vegetables with corn, peas, or pasta	1 cup
Peas, green	½ cup
Plantain	½ cup
Potato, baked or boiled	1 small (3 oz)
Potato, mashed	½ cup
Squash, winter (acorn, butternut)	1 cup
Yam, sweet potato, plain	½ cup

Starchy Foods Prepared with Fat

(Count as 1 starch exchange, plus 1 fat exchange.)

Biscuit, 2½ in. across	1
Chow mein noodles	½ cup
Corn bread, 2-in. cube	1 (2 oz)
Crackers, round butter type	6

(continues)

Table 17-3 *Continued*

Starchy Foods Prepared with Fat *continued*

Croutons	1 cup
French-fried potatoes	16–25 (3 oz)
Granola	¼ cup
Muffin, small	1 (1½ oz)
Pancake, 4 in. across	2
Popcorn, microwave	3 cups
Sandwich crackers, cheese or peanut butter filling	3
Stuffing, bread (prepared)	⅓ cup
Taco shell, 6 in. across	2
Waffle, 4½-in. square	1
Whole wheat crackers, fat added	4–6 (1 oz)

MEAT AND SUBSTITUTES LIST

Very Lean Meat and Substitutes List

(One exchange equals 0 g carbohydrate, 7 g protein, 0–1 g fat, and 35 calories.)

• One very lean meat exchange is equal to any one of the following items.

Poultry: Chicken or turkey (white meat, no skin), Cornish hen (no skin)	1 oz
Fish: Fresh or frozen cod, flounder, haddock, halibut, trout; tuna fresh or canned in water	1 oz
Shellfish: Clams, crab, lobster, scallops, shrimp, imitation shellfish	1 oz
Game: Duck or pheasant (no skin), venison, buffalo, ostrich	1 oz
Cheese with 1 gram or less fat per ounce:	
Nonfat or low-fat cottage cheese	¼ cup
Fat-free cheese	1 oz
Other: Processed sandwich meat with 1 gram or less fat per ounce, such as deli thin, shaved meats, chipped beef,* turkey ham	1 oz
Egg whites	2
Egg substitutes, plain	¼ cup
Hotdogs with 1 gram or less fat per ounce*	1 oz
Kidney (high in cholesterol)	1 oz
Sausage with 1 gram or less fat per ounce	1 oz

• Count as one very lean meat and one starch exchange.

Beans, peas, lentils (cooked)	½ cup

* = 400 mg or more sodium per exchange.

(continued)

Table 17-3 *Continued*

Lean Meat and Substitutes List
(One exchange equals 0 g carbohydrate, 7 g protein, 3 g fat, and 55 calories.)
• One lean meat exchange is equal to any one of the following items.

Beef: USDA select or choice grades of lean beef trimmed of fat, such as round, sirloin, and flank steak; tenderloin; roast (rib, chuck, rump); steak (T-bone, porterhouse, cubed); ground round	1 oz
Pork: Lean pork, such as fresh ham; canned, cured, or boiled ham; Canadian bacon*; tenderloin, center loin chop	1 oz
Lamb: Roast, chop, leg	1 oz
Veal: Lean chop, roast	1 oz
Poultry: Chicken, turkey (dark meat, no skin), chicken (white meat, with skin), domestic duck or goose (well drained of fat, no skin)	1 oz
Fish:	
Herring (uncreamed or smoked)	1 oz
Oysters	6 medium
Salmon (fresh or canned), catfish	1 oz
Sardines (canned)	2 medium
Tuna (canned in oil, drained)	1 oz
Game: Goose (no skin), rabbit	1 oz
Cheese:	
4.5%-fat cottage cheese	¼ cup
Grated parmesan	2 Tbsp
Cheeses with 3 grams or less fat per ounce	1 oz
Other:	
Hot dogs with 3 grams or less fat per ounce*	1½ oz
Processed sandwich meat with 3 grams or less fat per ounce, such as turkey pastrami or kielbasa	1 oz
Liver, heart (high in cholesterol)	1 oz

Medium-Fat Meat and Substitutes List
(One exchange equals 0 g carbohydrate, 7 g protein, 5 g fat, and 75 calories.)
• One medium-fat meat exchange is equal to any one of the following items.

Beef: Most beef products fall into this category (ground beef, meatloaf, corned beef, short ribs, prime grades of meat trimmed of fat, such as prime rib)	1 oz
Pork: Top loin, chop, Boston butt, cutlet	1 oz
Lamb: Rib roast, ground	1 oz

(continued)

Table 17-3 *Continued*

Medium-Fat Meat and Substitutes List *continued*

Veal: Cutlet (ground or cubed, unbreaded)	1 oz
Poultry: Chicken (dark meat, with skin), ground turkey or ground chicken, fried chicken (with skin)	1 oz
Fish: Any fried fish product	1 oz
Cheese: With 5 grams or less fat per ounce	
Feta	1 oz
Mozzarella	1 oz
Ricotta	¼ cup (2 oz)
Other:	
Eggs (high in cholesterol, limit to 3 per week)	1
Sausage with 5 grams or less fat per ounce	1 oz
Soy milk	1 cup
Tempeh	¼ cup
Tofu	4 oz or ½ cup

High-Fat Meat and Substitutes List

(One exchange equals 0 g carbohydrate, 7 g protein, 8 g fat, and 100 calories.)
Remember these items are high in saturated fat, cholesterol, and calories and may raise blood cholesterol levels if eaten on a regular basis.

• One high-fat meat exchange is equal to any one of the following items.

Pork: Spareribs, ground pork, pork sausage	1 oz
Cheese: All regular cheeses, such as American,* cheddar, Monterey Jack, Swiss	1 oz
Other: Processed sandwich meats with 8 grams or less fat per ounce, such as bologna, pimento loaf, salami	1 oz
Sausage, such as bratwurst, Italian, knockwurst, Polish, smoked	1 oz
Hotdog (turkey or chicken)*	1 (10/lb)
Bacon	3 slices (20 slices/lb)

• Count as one high-fat meat plus one fat exchange.

Hotdog (beef, pork, or combination)*	1 (10/lb)
Peanut butter (contains unsaturated fat)	2 Tbsp

* = 400 mg or more sodium per exchange.

FRUIT EXCHANGE LIST

Fruit *(One fruit exchange equals 15 g carbohydrate and 60 calories.)*
The weight includes skin, core, seeds, and rind.

Apple, unpeeled, small	1 (4 oz)
Applesauce, unsweetened	½ cup

(continued)

Table 17-3 *Continued*

Fruit continued

Apples, dried	4 rings
Apricots, fresh	4 whole (5½ oz)
Apricots, dried	8 halves
Apricots, canned	½ cup
Banana, small	1 (4 oz)
Blackberries	¾ cup
Blueberries	¾ cup
Cantaloupe, small	⅓ melon (11 oz) or 1 cup cubes
Cherries, sweet, fresh	12 (3 oz)
Cherries, sweet, canned	½ cup
Dates	3
Fruit cocktail	½ cup
Grapefruit, large	½ (11 oz)
Grapefruit sections, canned	¾ cup
Grapes, small	17 (3 oz)
Honeydew melon	1 slice (10 oz) or 1 cup cubes
Kiwi	1 (3½ oz)
Mandarin oranges, canned	¾ cup
Mango, small	½ cup
Nectarine, small	1 (5 oz)
Orange, small	1 (6½ oz)
Papaya	½ fruit (8 oz) or 1 cup cubes
Peach, medium, fresh	1 (6 oz)
Peaches, canned	½ cup
Pear, large, fresh	½ (4 oz)
Pears, canned	½ cup
Pineapple, fresh	¾ cup
Pineapple, canned	½ cup
Plums, small	2 (5 oz)
Prunes, dried	3
Raisins	2 Tbsp
Raspberries	1 cup
Strawberries	1¼ cup whole berries
Tangerines, small	2 (8 oz)
Watermelon	1¼ cup cubes

(continued)

Table 17-3 Continued

Fruit Juice

Apple juice/cider	½ cup
Cranberry juice cocktail	⅓ cup
Cranberry juice cocktail, reduced calorie	1 cup
Fruit juice blends, 100% juice	⅓ cup
Grape juice	⅓ cup
Grapefruit juice	½ cup
Orange juice	½ cup
Pineapple juice	½ cup
Prune juice	⅓ cup

MILK EXCHANGE LIST

Fat-free and very low-fat milk

Each item on this list contains 12 g of carbohydrate, 8 g of protein, a trace of fat, and 90 calories. One exchange is equal to any one of the following items:

Fat-free milk	1 cup
½% milk	1 cup
Low-fat milk (1%)	1 cup
Low-fat buttermilk	1 cup
Evaporated fat-free milk	½ cup
Dry nonfat milk	⅓ cup
Plain nonfat yogurt	¾ cup
Nonfat or low-fat fruit-flavored yogurt sweetened with aspartame	1 cup

Low-Fat Milk

Each item on this list contains 12 g of carbohydrate, 8 g of protein, 5 g of fat, and 120 calories. One exchange is equal to any one of the following items:

Reduced-fat milk (2%)	1 cup
Plain low-fat yogurt (with added nonfat milk solids)	¾ cup

Whole Milk

Each item on this list contains 12 g of carbohydrate, 8 g of protein, 8 g of fat, and 150 calories. One exchange is equal to any one of the following items:

Whole milk	1 cup
Evaporated whole milk	½ cup
Whole plain yogurt	8 oz

(continued)

Table 17-3 *Continued*

FAT EXCHANGE LIST

Each item on this list contains 5 g of fat and 45 calories.
One exchange is equal to any one of the following items:

Unsaturated

Avocado	⅛ medium or 1 oz
Margarine	1 tsp
Margarine, diet	1 Tbsp
Mayonnaise	1 tsp
Mayonnaise, reduced calorie	1 Tbsp
Nuts and seeds:	
Almonds, dry roasted	6 whole
Cashews, dry roasted	6 whole
Pecans	2 whole
Peanuts	10 nuts
Peanut butter	2 tsp
Seeds, pine nuts, sunflower, (without seeds)	1 Tbsp
Oil (canola, corn, cottonseed, safflower, soybean, sunflower, olive, peanut)	1 tsp
Olives, ripe, black	8 large
Olives, green, stuffed	10 large
Salad dressing, mayonnaise type	2 tsp
Salad dressing, mayonnaise type, reduced calorie	1 Tbsp
Salad dressing (all varieties)	1 Tbsp
Salad dressing, reduced calorie	2 Tbsp

Saturated

Butter	1 tsp
Bacon	1 slice
Chitterlings, boiled	½ oz
Coconut, shredded	2 Tbsp
Cream (light, coffee, table)	2 Tbsp
Cream, sour	2 Tbsp
Cream (half and half)	2 Tbsp
Cream cheese	1 Tbsp
Salt pork	1 in. × 1 in. × ¼ in. if eaten rather than used as a flavoring

(continued)

Table 17-3 *Continued*

OTHER CARBOHYDRATES EXCHANGE LIST

One exchange equals 15 g carbohydrate, or 1 starch, or 1 fruit, or 1 milk.

Food	Serving Size	Exchanges per Serving
Angel food cake, unfrosted	¹⁄₁₂ cake	2 carbohydrates
Brownie, small, unfrosted	2 in. square	1 carbohydrate, 1 fat
Cake, unfrosted	2 in. square	1 carbohydrate, 1 fat
Cake, frosted	2 in. square	2 carbohydrates, 1 fat
Cookie, fat-free	2 small	1 carbohydrate
Cookie or sandwich cookie with cream filling	2 small	1 carbohydrate, 1 fat
Cranberry sauce, jellied	¼ cup	1½ carbohydrates
Cupcake, frosted	1 small	2 carbohydrates, 1 fat
Doughnut, plain cake	1 medium (1½ oz)	1½ carbohydrates, 2 fats
Doughnut, glazed	3¾ in. across (2 oz)	2 carbohydrates, 2 fats
Fruit juice bars, frozen, 100% juice	1 bar (3 oz)	1 carbohydrate
Fruit snacks, chewy (pureed fruit concentrate)	1 roll (¾ oz)	1 carbohydrate
Fruit spreads, 100% fruit	1 Tbsp	1 carbohydrate
Gelatin, regular	½ cup	1 carbohydrate
Gingersnaps	3	1 carbohydrate
Granola bar	1 bar	1 carbohydrate, 1 fat
Granola bar, fat-fee	1 bar	2 carbohydrates
Honey	1 Tbsp	1 carbohydrate
Hummus	⅓ cup	1 carbohydrate, 1 fat
Ice cream	½ cup	1 carbohydrate, 2 fats
Ice cream, light	½ cup	1 carbohydrate, 1 fat
Ice cream, fat-free, no sugar added	½ cup	1 carbohydrate
Jam or jelly, regular	1 Tbsp	1 carbohydrate
Milk, chocolate, whole	1 cup	2 carbohydrates, 1 fat
Pie, fruit, 2 crusts	⅙ pie	3 carbohydrates, 2 fats
Pie, pumpkin or custard	⅛ pie	1 carbohydrate, 2 fats
Potato chips	12–18 (1 oz)	1 carbohydrate, 2 fats
Pudding, regular (made with low-fat milk)	½ cup	2 carbohydrates
Pudding, sugar-free (made with low-fat milk)	½ cup	1 carbohydrate
Salad dressing, fat-free*	¼ cup	1 carbohydrate
Sherbet, sorbet	½ cup	2 carbohydrates
Spaghetti or pasta sauce, canned*	½ cup	1 carbohydrate, 1 fat
Sugar	1 Tbsp	½ carbohydrate
Sweet roll or Danish	1 (2½ oz)	2½ carbohydrates, 2 fats
Syrup, light	2 Tbsp	1 carbohydrate
Syrup, regular	1 Tbsp	1 carbohydrate
Syrup, regular	¼ cup	4 carbohydrates

(continued)

Table 17-3 *Continued*		
Food	**Serving Size**	**Exchanges per Serving**
Tortilla chips	6–12 (1 oz)	1 carbohydrate, 2 fats
Vanilla wafers	5	1 carbohydrate, 1 fat
Yogurt, frozen, low fat, fat-free	⅓ cup	1 carbohydrate, 0–1 fat
Yogurt, frozen, fat-free, no sugar added	½ cup	1 carbohydrate
Yogurt, low fat with fruit	1 cup	3 carbohydrates, 0–1 fat

* = 400 mg or more sodium per exchange.

Source: The American Diabetes Association and the American Diabetic Association.

The amounts of nutrients and calories on one list are not the same as those on any other list. Each list includes serving size by volume or weight and the calorie value of each food item, in addition to the grams of carbohydrates, and, when appropriate, proteins and fats. The number of calories needed will determine the number of items prescribed from any particular list. These lists also can be used to control calorie content of diets and are thus appropriate for low-calorie diets.

The total energy requirements for adult diabetic clients who are not overweight will be the same as for nondiabetic individuals. When clients are overweight, a reduction in calories will be built into the diet plans, typically allowing for a weight loss of 1 pound a week.

The diet is given in terms of exchanges rather than as particular foods. For example, the menu pattern for breakfast may include 1 fruit exchange, 1 meat exchange, 2 bread exchanges, and 2 fat exchanges. The client may choose the desired foods from the exchange lists for each meal but must adhere to the specific exchange lists named and the specific number of exchanges on each list. Vegetables (nonstarchy) are relatively free and can be eaten in amounts up to 1½ cups cooked or 3 cups raw. If more than this amount is eaten at one meal, count the additional amount as one more carbohydrate. Snacks are built into the plan. In this way, the client has variety in a simple yet controlled way.

When there are changes in one's physical condition, such as pregnancy or lactation, or in one's lifestyle, the diet will need to be modified. A change in job or in working hours can affect nutrient and calorie requirements. When such changes occur, the client should be advised to consult her or his physician or dietitian so that calorie and insulin needs can be promptly adjusted.

SPECIAL CONSIDERATIONS FOR THE DIABETIC CLIENT

Fiber

The therapeutic value of fiber in the diabetic diet has become increasingly evident. High-fiber intake appears to reduce the amount of insulin needed because it lowers blood glucose. It also appears to lower the blood cholesterol and triglyceride levels. High fiber may mean 25 or 35 grams of dietary fiber a day. Such high amounts can be difficult to include. High-fiber foods should be increased very gradually, as an abrupt increase can create intestinal gas and discomfort. When increasing fiber in the diet one must also increase intake of water. An increased fiber intake can affect mineral absorption.

Alternative Sweeteners

sucralose
a sweetener made from a molecule of sugar

aspartame
artificial sweetener made from amino acids; does not require insulin for metabolism

Sucralose is the newest sweetener to gain approval by the FDA. Sucralose is made from a sugar molecule that has been altered in such a way that the body will not absorb it. **Aspartame** is the generic name for a sweetener composed of two amino acids, phenylalanine and aspartic acid. The FDA removed the sweetener saccharine from its list of products that could cause cancer. Research indicates that all these sweeteners are safe. All have been approved by the FDA, and their use has been endorsed by the American Diabetes Association.

Dietetic Foods

The use of diabetic or dietetic foods is generally a waste of money and can be misleading to the client. Often the containers of foods will contain the same ingredients as containers of foods prepared for the general public, but the cost is typically higher for the dietetic foods. There is potential danger for diabetic clients who use these foods if they do not read the labels on the food containers and assume that because they are labeled "dietetic," they can be used with abandon. In reality, their use should be in specified amounts only, because these foods will contain carbohydrates, fats, and proteins that must be calculated in the total day's diet.

It is advisable for the diabetic client to use foods prepared for the general public but to avoid those packed in syrup or oil. The important thing is for the diabetic client to *read the label* on all food containers purchased.

Alcohol

Although alcohol is not recommended for diabetic clients, its limited use is sometimes allowed if approved by the physician. However, some diabetic clients who use hypoglycemic agents cannot tolerate alcohol. When used, alcohol must be included in the diet plan.

Exercise

Exercise helps the body use glucose by increasing insulin receptor sites and stimulating the creation of glucagon. It lowers cholesterol and blood pressure and reduces stress and body fat as it tones the muscles. For clients with type 2 diabetes, exercise helps improve weight control, glucose levels, and the cardiovascular system.

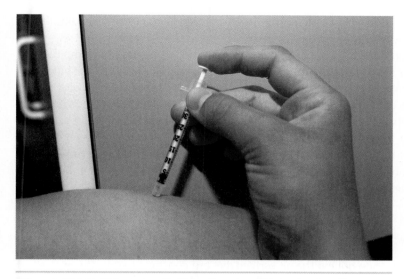

Figure 17-2 *This young diabetic client is self-injecting insulin.*

However, for clients with type 1 diabetes, exercise can complicate glucose control. As it lowers glucose levels, hypoglycemia can develop. Exercise must be carefully discussed with the client's physician. If done, it should be on a regular basis, and it must be considered carefully as the meal plans are developed so that sufficient calories and insulin are prescribed.

Insulin Therapy

Clients with type 1 diabetes must have injections of insulin every day to control their blood glucose levels (Figure 17-2). This insulin is called **exogenous insulin** because it is produced outside the body. **Endogenous insulin** is produced by the body.

Exogenous insulin is a protein. It must be injected, because, if swallowed, it would be digested and would not reach the bloodstream as the complete hormone. After insulin treatment is begun, it is usually necessary for the client to continue it throughout life.

Human insulin is the most common insulin given to clients. This insulin does not come from humans but is made synthetically by a chemical process in a laboratory. Human insulin is preferred because it is very similar to insulin made by the pancreas. Animal insulin comes from cows or pigs and is called beef or pork insulin. These insulins are rarely used because they contain antibodies that make them less pure than human insulin.

Various types of insulin are available. They differ in the length of time required before they are effective and in the length of time they continue to act. This latter category is called insulin action. Consequently, they are classified as very rapid-, rapid-, intermediate-, and long-acting. Those most commonly used are intermediate-acting types that work within 2 to 8 hours and are effective for 24 to 28 hours. For type 1 diabetes, insulin is often given in two or

exogenous insulin
insulin produced outside the body

endogenous insulin
insulin produced within the body

more injections daily and may contain more than one type of insulin. Injections are given at prescribed times.

More insulin-dependent diabetic clients are using insulin-pump therapy for better blood glucose control. Pumps deliver insulin two ways: the basal rate and a premeal bolus. The basal rate is a small amount of short-acting insulin delivered continuously throughout the day. This insulin keeps blood glucose in check between meals and during the night. Premeal boluses of short-acting insulin are designed to cover the food eaten during a meal. This allows more flexibility as to when meals are eaten. Insulin pumps are not for everyone. An endocrinologist and diabetes educator can determine the best candidates for pump therapy.

Insulin Reactions

 insulin reaction
hypoglycemia leading to insulin coma caused by too much insulin or too little food

 coma
state of unconsciousness

When clients do not eat the prescribed diet but continue to take the prescribed insulin, hypoglycemia can result. This is called an **insulin reaction,** or *hypoglycemic episode,* and may lead to **coma.** Symptoms include headache, blurred vision, tremors, confusion, poor coordination, and eventual unconsciousness. Insulin reaction is dangerous because if frequent or prolonged, brain damage can occur. (The brain must have sufficient amounts of glucose in order to function.) The physician should be consulted if an insulin reaction occurs or seems imminent.

Conscious clients may be treated by giving them a glucose tablet, a sugar cube, or a beverage containing sugar followed by a complex carbohydrate. If the client is unconscious, intravenous treatment of dextrose and water is given. It is advisable for the diabetic client to carry identification explaining the condition so that people do not think he or she is drunk when, in reality, the person is experiencing an insulin reaction.

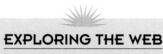

EXPLORING THE WEB

Search the Web for additional information on insulin therapies. What different types of therapies exist? Are there any experimental therapies currently being used and researched? What are some of the trial findings for these therapies?

CONSIDERATIONS FOR THE HEALTH CARE PROFESSIONAL

It is important to point out to the diabetic client that one can live a near-normal life if the diet is followed, medication is taken as prescribed, and time is allowed for sufficient exercise and rest. The importance of eating all of the prescribed food must be emphasized. It is important for meals to be eaten at regular times so that the insulin-glucose balance can be maintained. It is imperative that the client learn to read carefully all labels on commercially prepared foods.

Adjustments must be made in shopping, cooking, and eating habits so that the diet plan can be followed. Family meals can be simply adapted for the diabetic diet. The diabetic client soon learns which exchange lists are to be included at each meal and at snack times and the foods within each exchange list. (See Table 17-3 for the exchange lists, Table 17-4 for free foods, and Table 17-5 for seasonings that can be used.)

Table 17-4 *Free Foods Allowed on the Exchange List*

FREE FOOD LIST

A *free food* is any food or drink that contains less than 20 calories or less than 5 g of carbohydrate per serving. Foods with a serving size listed should be limited to three servings per day. Be sure to spread them out throughout the day. Eating all three servings at one time could affect your blood glucose level. Foods listed without a serving size can be eaten as often as you like.

Fat-Free or Reduced-Fat Foods

Cream cheese, fat-free	1 Tbsp
Creamers, nondairy, liquid	1 Tbsp
Creamers, nondairy, powdered	2 tsp
Mayonnaise, fat-free	1 Tbsp
Mayonnaise, reduced fat	1 tsp
Margarine, fat-free	4 Tbsp
Margarine, reduced fat	1 tsp
Miracle Whip, nonfat	1 Tbsp
Miracle Whip, reduced fat	1 tsp
Nonstick cooking spray	
Salad dressing, fat-free	1 Tbsp
Salad dressing, fat-free, Italian	2 Tbsp
Salsa	¼ cup
Sour cream, fat-free, reduced fat	1 Tbsp
Whipped topping, regular light	2 Tbsp

Drinks

Bouillon, broth, consommé*	
Bouillon or broth, low sodium	
Carbonated or mineral water	
Club soda	
Cocoa powder, unsweetened	1 Tbsp
Coffee	
Diet soft drinks, sugar-free	
Drink mixes, sugar-free	
Tea	
Tonic water, sugar-free	

Sugar-Free or Low-Sugar Foods

Candy, hard, sugar-free	1 candy
Gelatin dessert, sugar-free	
Gelatin, unflavored	
Gum, sugar-free	
Jam or jelly, low-sugar or light	2 tsp
Syrup, sugar-free	2 Tbsp
Sugar substitutes, alternatives, or replacements that are approved by the Food and Drug Administration (FDA) are safe to use. Common brand names include:	

    Equal (aspartame)
    Sprinkle Sweet (saccharin)
    Sweet One (acesulfame K)
    Sweet-10 (saccharin)
    Sugar Twin (saccharin)
    Sweet 'n Low (saccharin)

Condiments

Catsup	1 Tbsp
Horseradish	
Lemon juice	
Lime juice	
Mustard	
Pickles, dill*	1½ large
Soy sauce, regular or light*	
Taco sauce	1 Tbsp
Vinegar	

* = 400 mg or more of sodium per exchange.

Source: The American Diabetes Association and the American Dietetic Association.

Table 17-5 *Useful Seasonings*

Read the label, and choose those seasonings that do not contain sodium or salt.

Basil (fresh)	Garlic	Oregano
Celery seeds	Garlic powder	Paprika
Cinnamon	Herbs	Pepper
Chili powder	Hot pepper sauce	Pimento
Chives	Lemon	Spices
Curry	Lemon juice	Soy sauce
Dill	Lemon pepper	Soy sauce, low sodium ("lite")
Flavoring extracts	Lime	Wine, used in cooking (¼ cup)
(vanilla, almond,	Lime juice	Worcestershire sauce
walnut, peppermint,	Mint	
lemon, butter, etc.)	Onion powder	

Source: The American Diabetes Association and the American Dietetic Association.

SUMMARY

The diabetic diet is used in treating diabetes, a metabolic disease caused by the improper functioning of the pancreas that results in inadequate production or utilization of insulin. If the condition is left untreated, the body cannot use glucose properly, and then serious complications, even death, can occur. Treatment includes diet, medication, and exercise. Diabetic diets are prescribed by the physician or dietitian in consultation with the client.

DISCUSSION TOPICS

1. Explain why diabetes is a serious disease.

2. What is insulin? What is its use? Why can it not be taken orally?

3. What is the function of oral diabetes medication? For which type of diabetes is it usually prescribed?

4. Explain the differences between type 1 and type 2 diabetes.

5. Describe the symptoms of type 1 diabetes. Include the following terms: hyperglycemia, renal threshold, glycosuria, polydipsia, polyuria, polyphagia, ketones, ketonuria, and acidosis.

6. Explain why it is essential that diabetic clients read labels on food.

7. Why are "dietetic" foods not recommended for diabetic clients?

8. Discuss how an insulin reaction might occur.

9. How would pregnancy affect the diet of a client with type 1 diabetes? How would lactation affect the diet of a client with type 1 diabetes?

10. Discuss the effects of exercise on glucose utilization.

SUGGESTED ACTIVITIES

1. Ask a physician or dietitian or diabetic educator to speak to the class on diabetes and its treatment.

2. Ask a diabetic educator to explain and demonstrate carbohydrate counting.

3. Visit a local supermarket and compare regular and "dietetic" containers of food in terms of cost, calories, and nutrient content.

4. Invite someone with type 1 diabetes to talk to the class about his or her condition.

5. Invite someone with type 2 diabetes to talk to the class about his or her condition.

REVIEW

Multiple choice. Select the *letter* that precedes the best answer.

1. Diabetes mellitus is a metabolic disorder
   a. caused by malfunction of the thyroid gland
   b. for which a low-fiber diet may be ordered
   c. in which glucose accumulates in the blood
   d. that is contagious

2. The metabolism of glucose
   a. depends on insulin secreted by the islets of Langerhans
   b. depends on enzymes present in pancreatic juice
   c. is totally dependent on the acid content of the stomach
   d. is directly related to secretions from the thyroid gland

3. Type 1 diabetes mellitus is treated by the
   a. administration of insulin
   b. exclusion of foods that contain glucose
   c. administration of thyroxine
   d. use of a low-fat diet

4. The physician may recommend as part of the nutritional management of diabetes that the diet
   a. consist of 40% to 50% proteins
   b. consist of no more than 30% carbohydrates
   c. contain 15% to 20% proteins
   d. exclude all simple sugars

5. Diets based on the exchange lists
   a. are appropriate for clients with type 1 diabetes
   b. are not appropriate for clients with type 2 diabetes
   c. eliminate all carbohydrates
   d. should not be used by nondiabetic persons who want to control their calories

6. When an excessive amount of glucose accumulates in the blood, the condition
   a. is called hypoglycemia
   b. leads to glycosuria
   c. is known as acidosis
   d. always leads to coma

7. Diabetic coma
   a. is called alkalosis
   b. is caused by inadequate insulin
   c. is caused by an excessive amount of insulin
   d. causes polyuria

8. Type 2 diabetes
   a. usually occurs before the age of 40
   b. usually occurs after the age of 40
   c. usually requires insulin
   d. cannot be controlled by diet and a glucose-lowering medication

9. Glucose-lowering medications
   a. have exactly the same effect as insulin
   b. cannot be used for clients over 40
   c. stimulate the pancreas to produce insulin
   d. are only used for clients with type 1 diabetes mellitus

10. Diabetic diets based on the exchange lists regulate amounts of
    a. carbohydrate
    b. calories
    c. protein and fat
    d. all of the above

CASE IN POINT

MARIE-CLAIRE: MANAGING NEW-ONSET TYPE 2 DIABETES

Marie-Claire, a 36-year-old female of French background, is a busy mother of two older teens. She loves sports and prides herself on her appearance. She works out at the gym 3 nights a week. Marie-Claire has noticed that she is drinking a lot more water than she normally would and is always hungry. She attributes this to an unusually hot summer and to playing softball in the middle of the day. She has tried to curb her appetite and finds it difficult to do. But she continues to lose weight, so she thinks everything is fine. Marie-Claire had worked in human resources for a local recreational vehicle company, somewhat far from home. Because of the distance from home, she applied and has been hired at a new company just 10 miles from her home. Before starting her position, she has a preemployment physical. The NP doing the assessment listens to Marie-Claire and requests that she have a fasting blood sugar drawn. The results are high, 290. After more testing, Marie-Claire is told she has type 2 diabetes. She is to report to a dietitian within 3 days, bringing with her a diet history for those 3 days. She is started on glipizide metformin (Metaglip) for her blood glucose control.

ASSESSMENT

1. What do you know about Marie-Claire so far?
2. Using the rule of thumb in Chapter 16, what is Marie-Claire's ideal weight? At 5 feet 6 inches and 152 pounds, does she need to lose weight?
3. What are you looking for when reviewing her food diary?

DIAGNOSIS

4. Write a diagnostic statement for Marie-Claire.

PLAN/GOAL

5. What are reasonable, measurable goals for Marie-Claire?

IMPLEMENTATION

6. The dietitian recommends a 1,800 calorie diet for Marie-Claire. What distribution of categories would, as her nurse, you select for milk, bread, meat, fat, vegetables, and fruit?
7. After Marie-Claire learns the exchange system, what else does she need to do to manage her diabetes?
8. What would the advantages of the carbohydrate-counting system be compared with those of the exchange system?
9. How would the Web site of the American Diabetes Association, www.diabetes.org, help Marie-Claire?

EVALUATION/OUTCOME CRITERIA

10. At her 2-month follow-up visit with the diabetes team, what should Marie-Claire's HgbA1c be?
11. What should she be able to write out or describe?
12. What should her weight be?
13. Why would it be important to check her blood pressure and lipid levels?

THINKING FURTHER

14. Why is it important for all diabetic clients to maintain a normal blood glucose level?
15. What are the potentially serious health consequences of diabetic clients not controlling their diabetes?

◎ RATE THIS PLATE

Marie-Claire has seen a diabetes educator and decided that carbohydrate counting would be the easiest way to plan her menus. What do you think of her lunch? On an 1,800-calorie diet plan, Marie-Claire is allowed 4 carbohydrate choices per meal.

Sandwich made of:
2 slices 100% whole wheat bread
3 oz sliced roast beef
1 Tbsp reduced-fat mayonnaise
2 slices tomato
2 large pieces of leaf lettuce
1/4 cup raw mini carrots
1 oz baked potato chips
1/2 cup sugar-free chocolate pudding

CASE IN POINT

BRIAN: MANAGING NEW-ONSET TYPE 1 DIABETES

Brian, a 17-year-old African American high school junior was in his first semester of school when he developed an insatiable appetite. In addition, no matter how much he ate, he did not gain weight. During the night he noticed that he had to go to the bathroom "a lot" and had little to void. His mother became concerned when Brian told her about his nights and the fact that he was always thirsty. His mother noticed that he was becoming terribly thin, and she knew how much he was eating. After telling his mother that he seemed to always be tired, she decided to take him to their doctor. The doctor took a history and tested his urine and blood and then admitted Brian to the hospital with a diagnosis of type 1 diabetes.

ASSESSMENT

1. List all the subjective information you have about Brian related to diabetes.
2. What objective data do you have about Brian?
3. What tests are necessary to confirm the diagnosis of diabetes?

DIAGNOSIS

4. What education will be needed for Brian's diagnosis?
5. What other diagnoses, either actual or potential, apply to Brian?

PLAN/GOAL

6. Complete the following goal statement: Brian will verbalize his self-care measures related to _____.
7. Complete the following goal statement: Brian will verbalize and demonstrate diabetic survival skills and information by _____.

IMPLEMENTATION

The doctor has prescribed a mixed insulin injection for Brian twice a day, a diabetic diet, and exercise.

8. What topics are essential for Brian to learn?
9. What skills does he need to master before he goes home?
10. Who else needs to be in class with Brian?
11. What information does Brian's mother need to know about emergency situations?
12. What does Brian need to know about exercise?

EVALUATION/OUTCOME CRITERIA

13. What should Brian's fasting blood sugar be at his 2-week follow-up appointment?
14. What should he be able to verbalize and demonstrate?
15. What should happen to his weight?

THINKING FURTHER

16. Why is it essential for Brian to manage his diabetes?
17. What challenges does Brian face in balancing between being a carefree teenager and managing a serious chronic disease?

◎ RATE THIS PLATE

Brian was admitted to the hospital to regulate his blood glucose and to start him on insulin. While he is in the hospital, he will also receive basic diabetic education and then return as an outpatient for further education. He has had basic carbohydrate counting with the dietitian and is now home and is helping his mom plan his meals. He is on a 2,400-calorie ADA diet. Rate the plate.

2 pork chops
1 1/2 cups mashed potatoes with gravy
1/2 cup cooked greens
2 slices bread with butter
16 oz skim milk
1 cup ice cream with ½ cup fresh peaches

Did Brian get enough carbohydrates? How many does he need? Is this plate correct? If not, how would you change it?

CHAPTER 18

DIET AND CARDIOVASCULAR DISEASE

OBJECTIVES

After studying this chapter, you should be able to:

🖎 Identify factors that contribute to heart disease

🖎 Explain why cholesterol and saturated fats are limited in some
cardiovascular conditions

🖎 Identify foods to avoid or limit in a cholesterol-controlled diet

🖎 Explain why sodium is limited in some cardiovascular conditions

🖎 Identify foods that are limited or prohibited in sodium-controlled diets

Cardiovascular disease (CVD) affects the heart and blood vessels. It is the
leading cause of death and permanent disability in the United States today. The
grief and economic distress it causes are staggering. Organizations, especially
the American Heart Association, are promoting programs designed to alert
people to the risk factors for cardiovascular disease and thereby reduce its frequency. A group of risk factors have been identified and are known as the metabolic syndrome, previously known as syndrome X. These risk factors apply to
children as well as adults.

🖎 Abdominal obesity
🖎 High blood lipids such as high triglycerides, low HDL, and high LDL
🖎 High blood pressure

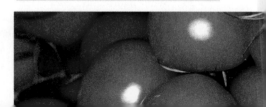

🗡 Insulin resistance

🗡 Elevated highly sensitive C-reactive protein in the blood

Those diagnosed with metabolic syndrome are at increased risk of coronary heart disease, stroke, peripheral vascular disease, and type 2 diabetes.

Cardiovascular disease can be acute (sudden) or chronic. **Myocardial infarction,** or **MI,** is an example of the acute form. Chronic heart disease develops over time and causes the loss of heart function. If the heart can maintain blood circulation, the disease is classified as **compensated heart disease.** Compensation usually requires that the heart beat unusually fast. Consequently, the heart enlarges. If the heart cannot maintain circulation, the condition is classified as **decompensated heart disease,** and congestive heart failure (CHF) occurs. The heart muscle **(myocardium),** the valves, the lining **(endocardium),** the outer covering **(pericardium),** or the blood vessels may be affected by heart disease.

ATHEROSCLEROSIS

Arteriosclerosis is the general term for **vascular disease** in which arteries harden (become thickened), making the passage of blood difficult and sometimes impossible. **Atherosclerosis** is the form of arteriosclerosis that most frequently occurs in developed countries. It is believed to begin in childhood and is considered one of the major causes of heart attack.

Atherosclerosis affects the inner lining of arteries (the intima), where deposits of **cholesterol,** fats, and other substances accumulate over time, thickening and weakening artery walls. These deposits are called **plaque** (Figure 18-1). Plaque deposits gradually reduce the size of the **lumen** of the artery and, consequently, the amount of blood flow. The reduced blood flow causes an inadequate supply of nutrients and oxygen delivery to and waste removal from the tissues. This condition is called **ischemia.**

The reduced oxygen supply causes pain. When the pain occurs in the chest and radiates down the left arm, it is called **angina pectoris** and should be considered a warning. When the lumen narrows so that a blood clot **(thrombus)** occurs in a coronary artery and blood flow is cut off, a heart attack occurs. The dead tissue that results is called an **infarct.** The heart muscle that should have received

cardiovascular disease (CVD)
disease affecting heart and blood vessels

myocardial infarction (MI)
heart attack; caused by the blockage of an artery leading to the heart

compensated heart disease
heart disease in which the heart is able to maintain circulation to all body parts

decompensated heart disease
heart disease in which the heart cannot maintain circulation to all body parts

myocardium
heart muscle

endocardium
lining of the heart

pericardium
outer covering of the heart

arteriosclerosis
hardening of the arteries

vascular disease
disease of the blood vessels

atherosclerosis
a form of arteriosclerosis affecting the intima (inner lining) of the artery walls

cholesterol
fatlike substance that is a constituent of body cells; is synthesized in the liver; also found in animal foods

plaque
fatty deposit on the interior of artery walls

lumen
the hollow area in a tube

ischemia
reduced blood flow causing an inadequate supply of nutrients and oxygen to, and wastes from, tissues

angina pectoris
pain in the heart muscle due to inadequate blood supply

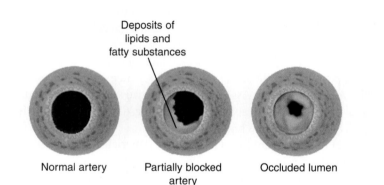

Deposits of
lipids and
fatty substances

Normal artery   Partially blocked artery   Occluded lumen

Figure 18-1 *Progression of atherosclerosis.*

thrombus
blood clot

infarct
dead tissue resulting from blocked artery

cerebrovascular accident (CVA)
either a blockage or bursting of blood vessel leading to the brain

peripheral vascular disease (PVD)
narrowed arteries some distance from the heart

hyperlipidemia
excessive amounts of fats in the blood

serum cholesterol
cholesterol in the blood

the blood is the myocardium. Thus, such an attack is commonly called an acute myocardial infarction (MI). Some clients who experience an MI will require surgery to bypass the clogged artery. The procedure is a coronary artery bypass graft (CABG), which is commonly referred to as bypass surgery.

When blood flow to the brain is blocked in this way or blood vessels burst and blood flows into the brain, a stroke, or **cerebrovascular accident (CVA)**, results. When it occurs in tissue some distance from the heart, it is called **peripheral vascular disease (PVD)**.

Risk Factors

Hyperlipidemia, hypertension (high blood pressure), and smoking are major risk factors for the development of atherosclerosis. Other contributory factors are believed to include obesity, diabetes mellitus, male sex, heredity, personality type (ability to handle stress), age (risk increases with years), and sedentary lifestyle. Although some of these factors are beyond one's control, some factors are not.

It is known that dietary cholesterol and triglycerides (fats in foods and in adipose tissue) contribute to hyperlipidemia. Foods containing saturated fats and trans fats increase **serum cholesterol,** whereas unsaturated fats tend to reduce it.

Lipoproteins carry cholesterol and fats in the blood to body tissues. Low-density lipoprotein (LDL) carries most of the cholesterol to the cells, and elevated blood levels of LDL are believed to contribute to atherosclerosis. High-density lipoprotein (HDL) carries cholesterol from the tissues to the liver for eventual excretion. It is believed that low serum levels of HDL can contribute to atherosclerosis.

Diet can alleviate hypertension (discussed later in this chapter), reduce obesity, and help control diabetes mellitus. A sedentary lifestyle can be changed. Exercise can help the client lose weight, lower blood pressure, and increase the HDL ("good") cholesterol level. Exercise must be done in consultation with the physician and be increased gradually. Also, one can stop smoking. In sum, a person can considerably reduce the risk of atherosclerosis and thus an MI, CVA, and PVD.

MEDICAL NUTRITION THERAPY FOR HYPERLIPIDEMIA

Medical nutrition therapy is the primary treatment for hyperlipidemia. It involves reducing the quantity and types of fats and often calories in the diet. When the amount of dietary fat is reduced, there is typically a corresponding reduction in the amount of cholesterol and saturated fat ingested and a loss of weight. In overweight persons, weight loss alone will help reduce serum cholesterol levels.

The American Heart Association categorizes blood cholesterol levels of 200 mg/dl or less to be desirable, 200 to 239 mg/dl to be borderline high, and 240 mg/dl and greater to be high.

In an effort to prevent heart disease, the American Heart Association has developed guidelines in which it is recommended that adult diets contain less than 200 mg of cholesterol per day and that fats provide no more than 20%–35% of calories, with a maximum of 7% from saturated fats and trans fat, a maximum of 8% from polyunsaturated fats, and a maximum of 15% to 20%

of monounsaturated fats. Carbohydrates should make up 50% to 55% of the calories, and proteins from 12% to 20% of them. Currently, it is believed that nearly 40% of the calories in the average U.S. diet come from fats.

A fat-restricted diet can be difficult for the client to accept. A diet very low in fat will seem unusual and highly unpalatable (unpleasant-tasting) to most clients. It takes approximately 2 or 3 months to adjust to a low-fat diet. If the physician will allow it, the change in the nutrient makeup of the diet should be made gradually (Table 18-1).

Table 18-1 *Foods to Include and Foods to Avoid on Fat-Restricted Diets*	
FOODS TO INCLUDE	**FOODS TO AVOID**
Breads and Cereals	
Whole-grain breads and rolls	Breads made with egg or cheese, croissants
Plain buns, bagels, pita bread	Bakery products
Cereals without coconut	Butter crackers
Saltines, matzos, rusks	
Rice, pasta	
Vegetables and Fruits	
Any fresh fruit or vegetable, except coconut	Coconut oil, palm oil
Meats, Poultry, and Fish	
After trimming fat and removing skin before eating:	Fatty or prime-grade meats, pastrami, spareribs,
Fish, but limited shrimp or lobster	sausage, bacon, lunch meats, domestic ducks
Lean beef, pork, lamb, veal	and geese, organ meats
Egg whites, yolks (2–3 per week)	
Dairy	
Fat-free milk or low-fat milk	Milk with more than 1% fat, cream, nondairy creamers
Dry curd or low-fat cottage cheese	Most cheese, especially processed or blue
Buttermilk	
Puddings made with fat-free milk	
Low-fat cheese	
Other Foods	
Oils (canola, olive, peanut)	Butter
Syrup	Lard
Gelatin	Bakery desserts
Jelly	Ice creams
Honey	Fried foods
Fat-free broths	Commercially prepared meals; salad dressings
Margarine made from liquid corn, sesame, olive,	Cream soups
or sunflower oil (in limited amounts)	Cream sauces; gravies
Limited nuts (walnuts, almonds)	
Limited home-made salad dressings	
Sherbet	
Hard candy	

Information about the fat content of foods and methods of preparation that minimize the amount of fat in the diet are essential to the client. The client must be taught to select whole, fresh foods and to prepare them without the addition of any fat. Only lean meat should be selected, and all visible fat must be removed. Fat-free milk and fat-free milk cheeses should be used instead of whole milk and natural cheeses. Desserts containing whole milk, eggs, and cream are to be avoided.

In a fat-controlled diet, one must be particularly careful when using animal foods. Cholesterol is found only in animal tissue. Organ meats, egg yolks, and some shellfish are especially rich in cholesterol and should be used in limited quantities, if at all. Saturated fats are found in all animal foods and in coconut, chocolate, and palm oil. They tend to be solid at room temperature. Polyunsaturated fats are derived from plants and some fish and are usually soft or liquid at room temperature. Soft margarine containing mostly liquid vegetable oil is substituted for butter, and liquid vegetable oils are used in cooking.

Studies indicate that water-soluble fiber, such as that found in oat bran, legumes, and fruits, bind with cholesterol-containing substances and prevent their reabsorption by the blood. It is thought that 25 to 35 grams of soluble fiber a day will effectively reduce serum cholesterol by as much as 15%. This is a large amount of fiber and must be introduced gradually to the diet along with increased fluids or the client will suffer from flatulence. Table 18-2 lists foods to limit on a low-cholesterol diet.

Some clients will find the diabetic exchange lists useful for controlling the fat content of their diets. When fat-controlled diets are severely restricted, limiting calorie intake to 1,200, they may be deficient in fat-soluble vitamins. Consequently, a vitamin supplement may be needed.

Table 18-2 *Foods to Limit on a Low-Cholesterol Diet*

Fats on meats and fish	Natural cheeses
Lard	Commercially fried foods
Organ meats	Commercially prepared baked
Bacon	goods
Lunch meats	Commercially prepared meatloaf
Prime-grade meats marbled	Commercially prepared mayonnaise
with fat	Quiche Lorraine
Duck	Chicken à la king
Skin on chicken and turkey	Cheeseburgers
Crab meat	Chicken livers
Shrimp	Custard
Lobster	Soufflé
Egg yolks	Lemon meringue pie
Butter	Cheesecake
Cream	Ice cream
Whole milk	Eggnog

Table 18-3 *Sample Menus for a Fat-Controlled Diet*		
BREAKFAST	**LUNCH**	**DINNER**
Orange juice	Tomato juice	3 oz salmon
Oatmeal	Uncreamed cottage	Baked sweet potato
1 Tbsp sugar and	cheese on fruit salad	Baked acorn squash
1 cup fat-free milk	2 slices wheat toast with	with 1 Tbsp honey
1 slice whole wheat toast	2 Tbsp honey	Lettuce salad
1 Tbsp jelly	Angel food cake	1 slice whole wheat
Coffee	1 cup fat-free milk	bread
	Tea	1 Tbsp jelly
		Canned peaches
		1 cup fat-free milk
		Tea

If appropriate blood lipid levels cannot be attained within 3 to 6 months by the use of a fat-restricted diet alone (see Table 18-3 for menus), the physician can prescribe a cholesterol-lowering drug such as atorvastatin (Lipitor) or simvastatin (Zocor). Food and/or drug interactions can occur with cholesterol-lowering drugs, as well as with other cardiac drugs. For example, Zocor and Lipitor interact with grapefruit and its juice; therefore total avoidance is necessary.

MYOCARDIAL INFARCTION

Myocardial infarction is caused by the blockage of a coronary artery supplying blood to the heart. The heart tissue denied blood because of this blockage dies (see Figure 18-2). Atherosclerosis is a primary cause, but hypertension, abnormal blood clotting, and infection such as that caused by rheumatic fever (which damages heart valves) are also contributory factors.

After the attack, the client is in shock. This causes a fluid shift, and the client may feel thirsty. The client should be given nothing by mouth (NPO), however, until the physician evaluates the condition. If the client remains nauseated after the period of shock, IV infusions are given to prevent dehydration.

After several hours, the client may begin to eat. A liquid diet may be recommended for the first 24 hours. Following that, a low-cholesterol–low-sodium diet is usually given, with the client regulating the amount eaten.

Foods should not be extremely hot or extremely cold. They should be easy to chew and digest and contain little roughage so that the work of the heart will be minimal. Both chewing and the increased activity of the gastrointestinal tract that follow ingestion of high-fiber foods cause extra work for the heart. The percentage of energy nutrients will be based on the particular needs of the client but, in most cases, the types and amounts of fats will be limited. Sodium is usually limited to prevent fluid accumulation. Some physicians will order a restriction on the amount of caffeine for the first few days after an MI. The dual goal is to allow the heart to rest and its tissue to heal.

EXPLORING THE WEB

Search the Web for additional information on cholesterol-lowering drugs. Create a table of these drugs and list the side effects of each drug, including any foods or medications that drug reacts with and any contraindications for use of the drug.

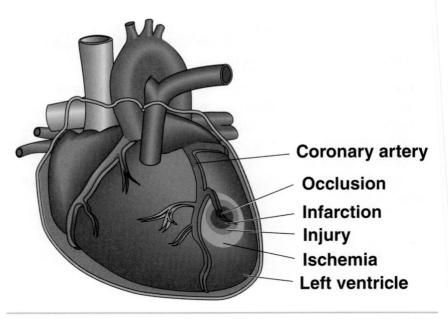

- Coronary artery
- Occlusion
- Infarction
- Injury
- Ischemia
- Left ventricle

Figure 18-2 *When a coronary artery is occluded, the heart muscle dies.*

CONGESTIVE HEART FAILURE

Congestive heart failure (CHF) is an example of decompensation, or severe heart disease. Heart failure is caused by conditions that damage the heart muscle, including **coronary artery disease (CAD)**, heart attack, **cardiomyopathy**, valve disease, heart defects present at birth, diabetes mellitus, and chronic renal disease. Heart failure can also occur if several diseases or conditions are present. In this situation, when damage is extreme and the heart cannot provide adequate circulation, the amount of oxygen taken in is insufficient for body needs. Shortness of breath is common, and chest pain can occur on exertion.

Because of the reduced circulation, tissues retain fluid that would normally be carried off by the blood. Sodium builds up, and more fluid is retained, resulting in **edema**. In an attempt to compensate for this pumping deficit, the heart beats faster and enlarges. This adds to the heart's burden. In advanced cases when edema affects the lungs, death can occur.

With the inadequate circulation, body tissues do not receive sufficient amounts of nutrients. This insufficiency can cause malnutrition and underweight, although the edema can mask these problems. In some cases a fluid restriction may be ordered.

Diuretics to aid in the excretion of water and sodium and a sodium-restricted diet are typically prescribed. Because diuretics can cause an excessive loss of potassium, the client's blood potassium should be carefully monitored to prevent **hypokalemia**, which can upset the heartbeat. Fruits, especially oranges, bananas, and prunes, can be useful in such a situation because they are excellent sources of potassium and contain only negligible amounts of sodium (Table 18-4). When necessary, the physician will prescribe supplementary potassium.

○ **congestive heart failure (CHF)**
a form of decompensated heart disease

○ **coronary artery disease (CAD)**
severe narrowing of the arteries that supply blood to the heart

○ **cardiomyopathy**
damage to the heart muscle caused by infection, alcohol, or drug abuse

○ **edema**
the abnormal retention of fluid by the body

○ **diuretics**
substances used to increase the amount of urine excreted

○ **hypokalemia**
low level of potassium in the blood

Table 18-4 *Potassium-Rich Foods*

FRUITS

Apricots	Dates	Kiwifruit
Oranges	Figs	Peaches
Bananas	Raisins	Pineapple
Avocados	Honeydew melon	Prunes
Cantaloupe	Grapefruit	Strawberries

VEGETABLES

Asparagus	Squash
Broccoli	Tomatoes
Cabbage	Spinach
Green beans	Potatoes, sweet potatoes, yams
Pumpkin	

((In The Media

DARK CHOCOLATE MAY REDUCE BLOOD PRESSURE AND IMPROVE INSULIN RESISTANCE

A daily bar-sized serving of flavonol-rich dark chocolate might lower your blood pressure and improve insulin resistance, according to a report in *Hypertension* (a journal published by the American Heart Association). Flavonoids are natural antioxidants found in many plant foods.

The study control group was fed white chocolate, which has no flavonoids. The researchers concluded that flavonoid-rich foods should be part of an overall healthy diet, with small amounts of dark chocolate being included, as well as fruits, vegetables, and whole grains.

(Source: Meisel, P. (2005). Hypertension, diabetes: Chocolate with a single remedy? *Hypertension*, 46(2), 398–405.

HYPERTENSION

When blood pressure is chronically high, the condition is called **hypertension** (HTN). In 90% of hypertension cases, the cause is unknown, and the condition is called **essential**, or **primary, hypertension.** The other 10% of the cases are called **secondary hypertension** because the condition is caused by another problem. Some causes of secondary hypertension include kidney disease, problems of the adrenal glands, and use of oral contraceptives.

The blood pressure commonly measured is that of the artery in the upper arm. This measurement is made with an instrument called the sphygmomanometer. The top number is the systolic pressure, taken as the heart contracts. The lower number is the diastolic pressure, taken when the heart is resting. The pressure is measured in millimeters of mercury (mm Hg). Hypertension can be diagnosed when, on several occasions, the systolic pressure is 140 mm Hg or more and the diastolic pressure is 90 mm Hg or more. The blood pressure categories are:

- Normal—less than 120/less than 80 mm Hg
- Prehypertension—120–139/80–88 mm Hg
- Stage 1 hypertension—140–159/90–99 mm Hg
- Stage 2 hypertension—160/100 mm Hg

Hypertension contributes to heart attack, stroke, heart failure, and kidney failure. It is sometimes called the *silent disease* because sufferers can be asymptomatic (without symptoms). Its frequency increases with age, and it is more prevalent among African Americans than others.

Heredity and obesity are predisposing factors in hypertension. Smoking and stress also contribute to hypertension. Weight loss usually lowers the blood pressure and, consequently, clients are often placed on weight reduction diets.

○ **hypertension**
higher than normal blood pressure

○ **essential hypertension**
high blood pressure with unknown cause; also called primary hypertension

○ **primary hypertension**
high blood pressure resulting from an unknown cause

○ **secondary hypertension**
high blood pressure caused by another condition such as kidney disease

SUPERSIZE USA

"Love, love, love Chinese buffets! Lunch is eaten out since I am on the road as a sales representative. I have discovered that Chinese buffets are a good place to eat because I can get a lot of food and even desserts. I usually eat at the buffets at least three times a week. During my yearly checkup, my doctor told me that my blood pressure was really high. She also commented on the weight that I had gained. What could be causing my blood pressure to be high? What can I do to lower my blood pressure? Is there anything in the Chinese food that could raise my blood pressure and cause me to gain weight?"

Sodium intake and increased weight could be causing high blood pressure. To lower it, lose weight, exercise, and do not salt your food at the table. Chinese food may contain MSG (monosodium glutamate). If you desire Chinese food, ask that the food be prepared with no MSG and order food in a clear sauce; brown sauces have soy sauce in them, which is high in sodium.

Excessive use of ordinary table salt also is considered a contributory factor in hypertension. Table salt consists of over 40% sodium plus chloride. Both are essential in maintaining fluid balance and thus blood pressure. When consumed in normal quantities by healthy people, they are beneficial.

When the fluid balance is upset and sodium and fluid collect in body tissue, causing edema, extra pressure is placed on the blood vessels. A sodium-restricted diet, often accompanied by diuretics, can be prescribed to alleviate this condition. When the sodium content in the diet is reduced, the water and salts in the tissues flow back into the blood to be excreted by the kidneys. In this way, the edema is relieved. The amount of sodium restricted is determined by the physician on the basis of the client's condition.

Previous research focused primarily on sodium as a primary factor in the development of hypertension, but as research continues, the effects of chloride also are receiving increasing scrutiny. In addition, the particular roles of calcium and magnesium in relation to hypertension are being studied. Knowing that sodium raises blood pressure and that potassium lowers blood pressure, the NIH (National Institutes of Health) created the DASH (Dietary Approaches to Stop Hypertension) eating plan. The DASH plan has been clinically shown to reduce high blood pressure while increasing the serving of fruits and vegetables to 8 to 12 servings per day, depending upon calorie intake. See Appendix C-1. Many fruits and vegetables are high in potassium levels, which will lower blood pressure. The newest guideline for potassium intake is 4.7 grams, or 4,700 mg, per day to lower blood pressure. It is recommended that a physician be consulted if the DASH eating plan is undertaken and one is already on blood pressure–lowering medication.

DIETARY TREATMENT FOR HYPERTENSION

As indicated above, weight loss for the obese client with hypertension usually lowers blood pressure, and thus a calorie-restricted diet might be prescribed. A sodium-restricted diet frequently is prescribed for clients with hypertension. Certain ethnic groups, such as African Americans with new onset of HTN and those already diagnosed with HTN, should limit sodium intake to 1,500 mg/day. A discussion of this diet follows. When diuretics are prescribed together with a sodium-restricted diet, the client may lose potassium via the urine and, thus, be advised to increase the amount of potassium-rich foods in the diet (see Table 18-4).

Sodium-Restricted Diets

A sodium-restricted diet is a regular diet in which the amount of sodium is limited. Such a diet is used to alleviate edema and hypertension. Most people obtain far too much sodium from their diets. It is estimated that the average adult consumes 7 grams of sodium a day. A committee of the Food and Nutrition Board recommends that the daily intake of sodium be limited to no more than 2,300 mg (2.3 grams), and the Board itself set a safe minimum at 500 mg/day for adults (see Table 8-6). Sodium is found in food, water, and medicine.

It is impossible to have a diet totally free of sodium. Meats, fish, poultry, dairy products, and eggs all contain substantial amounts of sodium naturally. Cereals, vegetables, fruits, and fats contain small amounts of sodium naturally. Water contains varying amounts of sodium. However, sodium often is added to foods during processing and cooking and at the table. The food label should indicate the addition of sodium to commercial food products. In some of these foods, the addition of sodium is obvious because one can taste it, as in prepared dinners, potato chips, and canned soups. In others, it is not. The following are examples of sodium-containing products frequently added to foods that the consumer may not notice.

- Salt (sodium chloride)—used in cooking or at the table and in canning and processing.

- **Monosodium glutamate** (called **MSG** and sold under several brand names)—a flavor enhancer used in home, restaurant, and hotel cooking and in many packaged, canned, and frozen foods.

- Baking powder—used to leaven quick breads and cakes.

- Baking soda (sodium bicarbonate)—used to leaven breads and cakes; sometimes added to vegetables in cooking or used as an "alkalizer" for indigestion.

- Brine (table salt and water)—used in processing foods to inhibit growth of bacteria; in cleaning or blanching vegetables and fruits; in freezing and canning certain foods; and for flavor, as in corned beef, pickles, and sauerkraut.

- Disodium phosphate—present in some quick-cooking cereals and processed cheeses.

- Sodium alginate—used in many chocolate milks and ice creams for smooth texture.

- Sodium benzoate—used as a preservative in many condiments such as relishes, sauces, and salad dressings.

- Sodium hydroxide—used in food processing to soften and loosen skins of ripe olives, hominy, and certain fruits and vegetables.

- Sodium propionate—used in pasteurized cheeses and in some breads and cakes to inhibit growth of mold.

- Sodium sulfite—used to bleach certain fruits in which an artificial color is desired, such as maraschino cherries and glazed or crystallized fruit; also used as a preservative in some dried fruit, such as prunes.

Because the amount of sodium in tap water varies from one area to another, the local department of health or the American Heart Association affiliate should be consulted if this information is needed. Softened water always has additional sodium. If the sodium content of the water is high, the client may have to use bottled water.

Some over-the-counter medicines contain sodium. A client on a sodium-restricted diet should obtain the physician's permission before using any medication or salt substitute. Many salt substitutes contain potassium, which can affect the heartbeat.

⌕ monosodium glutamate (MSG)

a flavor enhancer containing large amounts of sodium

⛭ SPOTLIGHT on Life Cycle

Clinical evidence indicates that mild sodium restriction can lower blood pressure. A no-added salt (4 grams of sodium) diet provides a wide variety of foods, limiting foods naturally high in salt such as bacon, lunch meat, dill pickles, chips, or foods with visible salt such as pretzels. The 4-gram-sodium diet also limits the use of salt at the table (removal of the salt shaker) but does allow for some salt in cooking. This diet is more appetizing and better tolerated by the older individual who may have many other restrictions or whose taste acuity is diminished.

The amount of sodium allowed depends on the client's condition and is prescribed by the physician. In extraordinary cases of fluid retention, a diet with 1 gram a day can be ordered. A mild restriction limits sodium to 2 grams a day. A moderate restriction limits sodium to 3–4 grams a day.

Adjustment to Sodium Restriction

Sodium-restricted diets range from "different" to "tasteless" because most people are accustomed to salt in their food. It can be difficult for the client to understand the necessity for following such a diet, particularly if it must be followed for the remainder of his or her life. If the physician allows, it will help the client adjust if the sodium content of the diet can be reduced gradually.

It is helpful, too, to remind the client of the numerous herbs, spices, and flavorings allowed on sodium-restricted diets (Table 18-5). Clients will also find it useful to practice ordering from a menu so as to learn to choose those foods lowest in sodium content.

Table 18-5 *Foods to Allow and Foods to Avoid on 1–2-gram Sodium-Restricted Diets*

FOODS PERMITTED ON MOST SODIUM-RESTRICTED DIETS	FOODS TO LIMIT OR AVOID
Fruit juices without additives	Tomato juice and vegetable cocktail
Fresh fruits	Canned vegetables
Fresh vegetables (except for those on the "Avoid" list)	Sauerkraut
Dried peas or beans	Frozen vegetables if prepared with salt
Fat-free milk	Dried, breaded, smoked, or canned fish or meats
Puffed-type cereals	Cheeses; salted butter or margarine
Regular, cooked cereals without added salt, sugar, or flavorings	Salt-topped crackers or breads
Plain pasta	Salty foods such as potato chips, salted nuts, peanut butter, pretzels
Rice	Canned fish, meats, or soups
Unsalted, uncoated popcorn	Ham, salt pork, corned beef, lunch meats, smoked or canned fish
Fresh fish	Prepared relishes, salad dressings, catsup, soy sauce
Fresh unsalted meats	Bouillon, baking soda, baking powder, MSG
Unsalted margarine	Commercially prepared meals
Oil	Fast foods
Vinegar	
Spices containing no salt, herbs, lemon juice	
Unsalted nuts	
Hard candy	
Jams, jellies, honey	
Coffee, tea	

((In The Media

LINK BETWEEN SALT SENSITIVITY AND RISK OF DEATH

A sensitivity to salt increases the risk of death as much as high blood pressure, according to a study by the National Heart, Lung, and Blood Institute. Unfortunately there is no easy way to test for salt sensitivity.

Since salt sensitivity increases the risk of death even for those with normal blood pressure, it is advisable that all Americans with normal blood pressure follow the recommendation of having no more than 2,400 mg of sodium a day. Research estimates that about 26% of Americans with normal blood pressure and about 58% of those with hypertension are salt sensitive.

Only 10% of dietary sodium comes from salt added to food at the table; therefore, to reduce salt intake, Americans should be careful about the sodium content in prepared, preserved, and processed foods.

(Source: Adapted from National Institutes of Health News Release, February 2001.)

CONSIDERATIONS FOR THE HEALTH CARE PROFESSIONAL

Clients with heart conditions serious enough to require hospitalization can be frightened, depressed, or angry. Most will be told they must reduce the fats, sodium, and, sometimes, the amount of calories in their diets, which could make them feel overwhelmed. The health care professional will find various moods among these clients. Most will need nutritional advice. Some will want it. Some will be against the new diets. The most important thing the health care professional can do is help the cardiac client want to learn how to help himself or herself via nutrition.

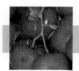

SUMMARY

Cardiovascular disease represents the leading cause of death in the United States. It may be acute, as in myocardial infarction, or chronic, as in hypertension and atherosclerosis. Hypertension may be a symptom of other disease. Weight loss, if the client is overweight, and a salt-restricted diet are typically prescribed.

Atherosclerosis is a vascular disease in which the arteries are narrowed by fatty deposits, reducing blood flow. Angina pectoris, myocardial infarction, or stroke can result. Because cholesterol is associated with atherosclerosis, a low-cholesterol diet or a fat-restricted diet might be prescribed.

By maintaining one's weight and activities at a healthy level, limiting salt and fat intake, and avoiding smoking, one reduces the risks of heart disease.

DISCUSSION TOPICS

1. Why are sodium-restricted diets prescribed for clients with hypertension or heart failure?
2. What precautions might one take to prevent hypertension? To prevent atherosclerosis? Explain your answers.
3. What may occur in severe myocardial infarction? What causes myocardial infarction?

4. What are diuretics? How could they be harmful? How could this danger be avoided?

5. What is edema? How is it related to cardiovascular disease?

6. Are sodium-restricted diets nutritious? Why?

7. Why is it impossible to prepare a diet absolutely free of salt?

8. Why might a sodium-restricted diet be unpleasant for a client?

9. Why are potato chips and peanuts not allowed on sodium-restricted diets?

10. For what heart condition might a fat-controlled diet be ordered?

11. What is cholesterol? How is it associated with atherosclerosis?

12. Why is fat-free milk allowed on low-fat diets when whole milk is not?

13. What is hyperlipidemia? How is it related to atherosclerosis?

14. Discuss known risk factors for the development of atherosclerosis. Which could be avoided? Explain.

SUGGESTED ACTIVITIES

1. Make a list of the foods eaten yesterday. Circle those foods that would not be allowed on a low-cholesterol diet and suggest satisfactory substitutions. Underline those not allowed on moderate sodium-restricted diets. Are any both circled and underlined?

2. Visit a local supermarket. List the foods containing sodium compounds. Suggest substitutes for these foods for clients on sodium-restricted diets.

3. Marita Jiminez was placed on a fat-restricted diet containing no more than 70 grams of fat. She wants to order the following breakfast. Would this be acceptable? Explain your answer and, if necessary, suggest alternative foods that would be acceptable.

   Sliced avocado
   Poached egg with ham in cheese sauce on English muffin
   Coffee with cream

4. Justin Chen has been told that he has atherosclerosis and must follow a low-cholesterol diet. He is visiting his aunt who is serving the following meal. Which of the foods can Justin eat, and which must he avoid? Why? Can he eat certain parts of any of the foods? If so, which? Why?

   Cream of broccoli soup
   Roast chicken
   Mashed potatoes with gravy
   Lima beans with butter
   Green salad with vinegar and oil dressing
   Rolls and butter
   Milk
   Angel food cake with whipped cream and strawberries

5. Susan Smith has developed hypertension and has been placed on a mild sodium-restricted diet. She has planned the following dinner for her daughter's graduation party. Which of the foods can she eat, and which must she avoid? Explain.

   Fresh fruit cup
   Baked ham
   Potato chips
   Fresh frozen broccoli chunks baked in canned cream of chicken soup
   Homemade coleslaw
   Rolls and butter
   Pickles and olives
   Chocolate cake with peppermint ice cream

REVIEW

Multiple choice. Select the *letter* that precedes the best answer.

1. Sodium
   a. is an essential vitamin
   b. regulates metabolism
   c. adds flavor to foods
   d. is found in sugar

2. Sodium is commonly found in
   a. sugar
   b. fresh fruits
   c. baking soda and baking powder
   d. coffee and tea

3. A client with angina pectoris might be advised to follow a diet
   a. that contains limited sodium
   b. in which the calories are increased
   c. containing minimum amounts of proteins
   d. in which saturated fats are limited

4. Herbs, spices, and flavorings may
   a. be used in sodium-restricted diets
   b. never be used in sodium-restricted diets
   c. increase sodium in the diet
   d. be used only in the mild sodium-restricted diet

5. A sodium-restricted diet may be ordered for clients with
   a. angina pectoris
   b. lipidemia
   c. congestive heart failure
   d. atherosclerosis

6. When water accumulates in body tissues,
   a. the condition is called edema
   b. a fat-restricted diet may be prescribed
   c. it is a definite symptom of myocardial infarction
   d. salt is completely eliminated from the diet

7. It is thought that excessive fats in the blood over time contribute to
   a. congestive heart failure
   b. hypokalemia
   c. plaque
   d. edema

8. Table salt
   a. is 100% sodium
   b. is over 40% sodium
   c. contains only negligible amounts of sodium
   d. must be restricted in fat-restricted diets

9. In a low-cholesterol diet
   a. eggs are used freely
   b. fat-free milk is used instead of whole milk
   c. organ meats are permitted
   d. vegetable oils are not permitted

10. Cholesterol
    a. has no connection to lipoproteins
    b. is found in food and in body tissue
    c. is the primary cause of congestive heart failure
    d. is commonly found in fruits and vegetables

11. Foods allowed in a low-fat diet include
    a. cheese
    b. cooked vegetables
    c. sausage
    d. all soups

12. When preparing foods for the low-fat diet,
    a. small amounts of fat can be added
    b. visible fats must be removed from meats
    c. fat-free milk is never used
    d. butter is substituted for vegetable oil

13. On the low-cholesterol diet, saturated fats are
    a. reduced
    b. eliminated
    c. increased
    d. unchanged from the amount in the regular diet

14. Saturated fats are usually
    a. solid at room temperature
    b. liquid at room temperature
    c. found in fruits
    d. derived from plants

15. Polyunsaturated fats are usually
    a. solid at room temperature
    b. liquid at room temperature
    c. found in animal foods
    d. derived from dairy products

16. When the heart muscle reacts with pain because of inadequate blood supply after activity, the condition is called
    a. cerebral accident
    b. edema
    c. hypertension
    d. angina pectoris

17. Some examples of blood lipids are
    a. triglycerides
    b. lumens
    c. diuretics
    d. plaques

18. Examples of foods particularly rich in potassium are
    a. milk and ice cream
    b. beef and lamb
    c. whole-grain breads and cereals
    d. bananas and oranges

CASE IN POINT

KADIM: EATING HEALTHY FOR HIS HEART

Kadim is a 29-year-old African American stock exchange manager for a large corporation. He has been feeling tightening in his chest for 3 days and now has shortness of breath and pain radiating down his left arm. Kadim thinks he is having a heart attack. He calls the EMS, who takes him to the hospital immediately. Kadim is admitted to the cardiac intensive care unit. He is placed on a cardiac monitor and is given nasal oxygen. The admitting nurse finds out that there is a history of heart attacks in young males in Kadim's family. His blood pressure is 210/110. His blood work shows a cholesterol of 320, elevated triglycerides, and markedly elevated LDL. As his team of physicians and nurses get Kadim stabilized, the dietitian places him on a low-cholesterol, low-fat, low-sodium diet. The doctor suggests that Kadim participate in a cardiac rehabilitation program to learn about exercise and his new diet. Kadim knew he was a candidate for a heart attack but decides to play the odds, hoping they would be in his favor. After all, he did eat well and exercised regularly before he started with his firm.

ASSESSMENT

1. What subjective data do you have about Kadim and his health?
2. What objective data do you have?
3. How significant is his problem?
4. What are the potential consequences if Kadim ignores his doctor's advice?

DIAGNOSIS

5. Write a diagnostic statement about Kadim's lack of knowledge regarding his cardiac condition and his new diet.
6. What education is needed to help achieve lower cholesterol?

PLAN/GOAL

7. What are several reasonable goals for Kadim?

IMPLEMENTATION

8. What dietary issues does Kadim need to learn to comply with his new diet?
9. What cardiac topics does Kadim need to learn to understand his new diet?
10. What two food categories can Kadim use that have almost no restriction in his new diet?
11. What other risk factors does Kadim have, and what does he need to do about them?
12. How could the information at the American Heart Association Web site, www.americanheart.org, be helpful to Kadim?

EVALUATION/OUTCOME CRITERIA

13. If diet and exercise are successful, what changes will be measurable in 3 to 6 months?
14. What will the dietitian be able to assess in an interview with Kadim?
15. If the diet is insufficient to lower his cholesterol in 6 months, what is the doctor likely to do?

FURTHER THINKING

16. What are the possible consequences for noncompliance for Kadim?

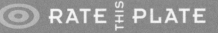 RATE THIS PLATE

Kadim was ready to begin his weight loss and, hopefully, behavior modification. Kadim has a good start on healthy eating with a meal that contained meat, vegetables, fruit, and milk. He decided that he should plan menus by the week. Here is one of his dinners. Rate the plate.

8 oz chicken breast baked with cream of mushroom soup
1 cup mashed potatoes with the juices from the chicken as gravy
Tossed salad with cucumber, tomato, and grated cheese on top (about 2 Tbsp)
Low-fat Italian dressing, about 4 Tbsp
Green beans with bacon bits
Baked apple with butter, brown sugar, and raisins in the center
8 oz 2% milk

The kids loved the dinner. Rate the plate for portions, additions, fat, and calories.

CASE IN POINT

JOYCE: WATCHING WEIGHT FOLLOWING A HEART ATTACK

Joyce is a 62-year-old retired schoolteacher from a Turkish family. Five years ago she had three episodes of chest pain at school that were so bad that she was transported to the emergency department via ambulance. The first year after retirement she had a heart attack and required a coronary artery bypass graft. She had triple bypass surgery. Joyce was sufficiently frightened to stop smoking at this time. Joyce was placed on a low-sodium diet. Today she is calling her doctor because she is having trouble breathing and has noticed severe lower-limb edema. In fact, she can push on her shin and leave an indentation of about an inch.

When the dietitian sees Joyce in the emergency room, she inquires about Joyce's diet history. Unfortunately, Joyce has not stayed with the low-sodium diet. Upon request, Joyce tells the dietitian that for breakfast she usually has an egg with bacon and toast with butter and a diet cola. For lunch she eats out and has macaroni and cheese or a salad with creamy dressings. Sometimes she has a luncheon meat sandwich and a diet cola. For dinner Joyce will eat a steak with mashed potatoes and gravy and some carrots and another diet cola. Joyce typically has five diet colas a day.

ASSESSMENT

1. What do you know about Joyce's health?
2. How significant is her health problem?
3. What would the consequences be if Joyce decided to ignore the doctor's advice?
4. What do you know about Joyce's willingness to comply?
5. List all the foods Joyce ate that contained sodium or are usually restricted on a low-sodium diet.
6. What needs to be changed in her food choices?

DIAGNOSIS

7. Write a diagnostic statement based on Joyce's condition.
8. What does Joyce need to understand about CHF and low-sodium diets?
9. Why does Joyce continue to retain fluid?

PLAN/GOAL

10. What are reasonable, measurable goals for Joyce?

IMPLEMENTATION

11. What are the main topics to teach Joyce about her diet?
12. Modify Joyce's food choices to reflect a low-sodium diet.
13. What food categories can Joyce eat without restrictions?

14. What else does Joyce need in order to control the edema?

EVALUATION/OUTCOME CRITERIA

15. At her 2-week doctor's appointment, what changes can the doctor observe and measure as evidence of the effectiveness of the diet?

THINKING FURTHER

16. Can this disease be cured?
17. Why is managing the disease a constant challenge?

◎ RATE THIS PLATE

It is discovered during the interview with the dietitian that Joyce does not do much cooking at home—her stove and oven are not working, but she has a toaster oven and microwave. The dietitian recommends that Joyce lose weight. She eats most of her meals out. Joyce loves to eat, so portion control is an issue. Rate the plate.

8 oz filet mignon
Baked potato with butter and sour cream
Green beans with bacon
2 rolls with butter
Peach cobbler with ice cream

What changes would you recommend for Joyce to make when ordering her meal, if any? What are some questions she should ask the server? What do you think of her portion control?

CHAPTER

19

DIET AND RENAL DISEASE

OBJECTIVES

After studying this chapter, you should be able to:

- Describe, in general terms, the work of the kidneys

- Discuss common causes of renal disease

- Explain why protein is restricted for renal clients

- Explain why sodium and water are sometimes restricted for renal clients

- Explain why potassium and phosphorus are sometimes restricted for renal clients

The kidneys are intricate and efficient processing systems that excrete wastes, maintain volume and composition of body fluids, and secrete certain hormones. To accomplish these tasks, they filter the blood, cleansing it of waste products, and recycle other, usable, substances so that the necessary constituents of body fluids are constantly available (Figure 19-1).

Each kidney contains approximately 1 million working parts called **nephrons.** Each nephron contains a filtering unit, called a **glomerulus,** in which there is a cluster of specialized capillaries (tiny blood vessels connecting veins and arteries). Approximately 180 liters of ultrafiltrate is processed each day. As the filtrate passes through the nephrons, it is concentrated or diluted to meet the body's needs. In this way, the kidneys help maintain both the composition and the volume of body fluids and, consequently, they maintain fluid balance, acid-base balance, and electrolyte balance.

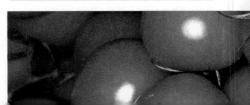

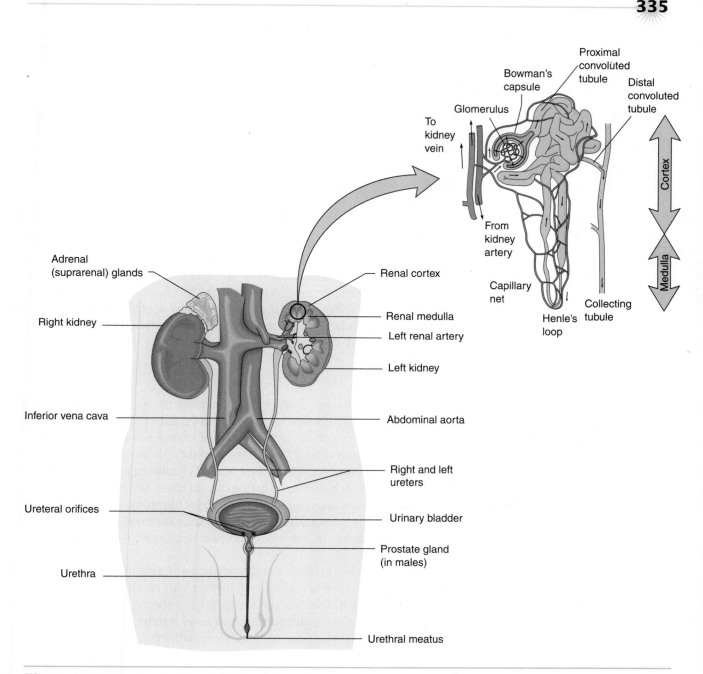

Figure 19-1 *The urinary system with inset of a nephron.*

The liquid waste is sent via two tubes called **ureters** from the kidneys to the urinary bladder, from which they are excreted in approximately 1.5 liters of urine per day. These waste materials include end products of protein metabolism (**urea, uric acid, creatinine,** ammonia, and sulfates), excess water and nutrients, dead renal cells, and toxic substances. When the urinary output is less than 500 ml/day, it is impossible for all the daily wastes to be eliminated. This condition is called **oliguria.** When the kidneys are unable to adequately eliminate nitrogenous waste (end products of protein metabolism), renal failure

⊙ nephron
unit of the kidney containing a glomerulus

⊙ glomerulus
filtering unit in the kidneys

⊙ ureters
tubes leading from the kidneys to the bladder

urea
chief nitrogenous waste product of protein metabolism

uric acid
one of the nitrogenous waste products of protein metabolism

creatinine
an end (waste) product of protein metabolism

oliguria
decreased output of urine to less than 500 ml/day

cysts
growths

renal stones
kidney stones

acute renal failure (ARF)
suddenly occurring failure of the kidneys

chronic renal failure
slow development of kidney failure

uremia
condition in which protein wastes are circulating in the blood

dialysis
mechanical filtration of the blood; used when the kidneys are no longer able to perform normally

nephritis
inflammatory disease of the kidneys

glomerulonephritis
inflammation of the glomeruli of the kidneys

nephrosclerosis
hardening of renal arteries

polycystic kidney disease
rare, hereditary kidney disease causing cysts or growths on the kidneys that can ultimately cause kidney failure in middle age

can result. The recycled materials are reabsorbed (taken back) by the blood. They include amino acids, glucose, minerals, vitamins, and water.

The kidneys synthesize and secrete certain hormones as needed. For example, it is the kidneys that make the final conversion of vitamin D. Active vitamin D promotes the absorption of calcium and the metabolism of calcium and phosphorus. The kidneys indirectly stimulate bone marrow to reproduce red blood cells by producing the hormone erythropoietin.

RENAL DISEASES
Etiology of Renal Disease

Kidney disorders can be initially caused by infection, degenerative changes, diabetes mellitus, high blood pressure **cysts, renal stones,** or trauma (surgery, burns, poisons). When these conditions are severe, renal failure may develop. It may be acute or chronic. **Acute renal failure (ARF)** occurs suddenly and may last a few days or a few weeks. It can be caused by another medical problem such as a serious burn, a crushing injury, or cardiac arrest. It can be expected in some of these situations, so preventive steps should be taken.

Classification of Renal Disease

Chronic kidney disease develops slowly, causing the number of functioning nephrons to diminish. When renal tissue has been destroyed to a point at which the kidneys are no longer able to filter the blood, excrete wastes, or recycle nutrients as needed, uremia occurs. **Uremia** is a condition in which protein wastes that should normally have been excreted are instead circulating in the blood. Symptoms include nausea, headache, convulsions, and coma. Severe renal failure can result in death unless **dialysis** is begun or a kidney transplant is performed.

Nephritis is a general term referring to the inflammatory diseases of the kidneys. Nephritis can be caused by infection, degenerative processes, or vascular disease.

Glomerulonephritis is an inflammation affecting the capillaries in the glomeruli. It may occur acutely in conjunction with another infection and be self-limiting, or it may lead to serious renal deterioration.

Nephrosclerosis is the hardening of renal arteries. It is caused by arteriosclerosis and hypertension. Although it usually occurs in older people, it sometimes develops in young diabetic clients.

Polycystic kidney disease is a relatively rare, hereditary disease. Cysts form and press on the kidneys. The kidneys enlarge and lose function. Al-

EXPLORING THE WEB

Choose one of the renal disorders discussed and thoroughly research the disorder using the Internet. Investigate the causes of the disorder, the presenting signs and symptoms of the disorder, how the disorder is diagnosed, and the treatment choices for the disorder. What role does nutrition play in the prevention, cause, or treatment of the disorder?

though people with this condition have normal kidney function for many years, renal failure may develop near the age of 50.

   Nephrolithiasis is a condition in which stones develop in the kidneys. The size of the stones varies from that of a grain of sand to much larger. Some remain at their point of origin, and others move. Although the condition is sometimes asymptomatic, symptoms include hematuria (blood in the urine), infection, obstruction and, if the stones move, intense pain. The stones are classified according to their composition—calcium oxalate, uric acid, **cystine**, calcium phosphate, and magnesium ammonium phosphate (known as struvite). They are associated with metabolic disturbances and immobilization of the client.

nephrolithiasis
kidney development of stones

cystine
a nonessential amino acid

SPECIAL CONSIDERATIONS FOR CLIENTS WITH RENAL DISEASES
Dietary Treatment of Renal Disease

Dietary treatment is intended to slow the buildup of waste in the bloodstream. Decreasing waste in the bloodstream will control symptoms of fluid retention, hyperkalemia, and nausea and vomiting. The goal is to reduce the amount of excretory work demanded of the kidneys while helping them maintain fluid, acid-base, and electrolyte balance. Clients require sufficient protein to prevent malnutrition and muscle wasting. Too much, however, can contribute to uremia. Typically, the client with chronic renal failure will have protein and sodium, and possibly potassium and phosphorus, restricted.

   It is essential that renal clients receive sufficient calories—25 to 50 calories per kilogram of body weight—unless they are overweight. Energy requirements should be fulfilled by carbohydrates and fat. The fats must be unsaturated to prevent or check hyperlipidemia. If the energy requirement is not met by carbohydrates and fat, ingested protein or body tissue will be metabolized for energy. Either would increase the work of the kidneys because protein increases the amount of nitrogen waste the kidneys must handle. The diet may limit protein to as little as 40 grams for predialysis clients. The specific amount of protein allowed is calculated according to the client's **glomerular filtration rate (GFR)** and weight.

   Fluids and sodium may be limited to prevent edema, hypertension, and congestive heart failure. Calcium supplements may be prescribed. In addition, vitamin D may be added and phosphorus limited, to prevent osteomalacia (softening of the bones due to excessive loss of calcium). Phosphorus appears to be retained in clients with kidney disorders, and a disproportionately high ratio of phosphorus to calcium tends to increase calcium loss from bones.

   Potassium may be restricted in some clients because **hyperkalemia** tends to occur in **end-stage renal disease (ESRD)**. Excess potassium can cause cardiac arrest. Because of this danger, renal clients should not use salt substitutes or low-sodium milk because the sodium in these products is replaced with potassium. Potassium restriction can be especially difficult for a renal client, who probably must limit sodium intake. Potassium is particularly

glomerular filtration rate (GFR)
the rate at which the kidneys filter the blood

hyperkalemia
excessive amounts of potassium in the blood

end-stage renal disease (ESRD)
the stage at which the kidneys have lost most or all of their ability to function

high in fruits—one of the few foods a client on a sodium-restricted diet may eat without concern.

Renal clients often have an increased need for vitamins B, C, and D, and supplements are often given. Vitamin A should not be given because the blood level of vitamin A tends to be elevated in uremia. If a client is receiving antibiotics, a vitamin K supplement may be given. Otherwise, supplements of vitamins E and K are not necessary. Iron is commonly prescribed because anemia frequently develops in renal clients. It is sometimes necessary to increase the amount of simple carbohydrates and unsaturated fats to ensure sufficient calories.

Dialysis

Dialysis is done by either **hemodialysis** or **peritoneal dialysis.** The most common is hemodialysis. Hemodialysis requires permanent access to the bloodstream through a fistula. Fistulas are unusual openings between two organs. They are often created near the wrist and connect an artery and a vein. Hemodialysis is done three times a week for approximately 3 to 5 hours each visit (Figure 19-2).

⊙ **hemodialysis**
cleansing the blood of wastes by circulating the blood through a machine that contains tubing of semipermeable membranes

⊙ **peritoneal dialysis**
removal of waste products from the blood by injecting the flushing solution into the abdomen and using the client's peritoneum as the semipermeable membrane

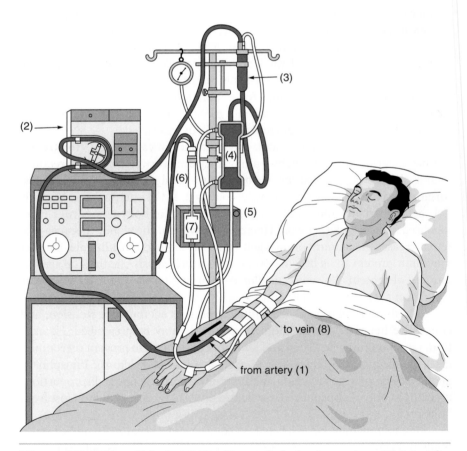

Figure 19-2 *Hemodialysis. (1) Blood leaves the body via an artery. (2) Arterial blood passes through the blood pump. (3) Blood is filtered to remove any clots. (4) Blood passes through the dialyzer. (5) Blood passes into the venous blood line. (6) Blood is filtered to remove any clots. (7) Blood flows through the air detector. (8) Blood returns to the client through the venous blood line.*

Peritoneal dialysis uses the peritoneal cavity as a semipermeable membrane and is less efficient than hemodialysis. Treatments usually last about 10 to 12 hours a day, three times a week (Figure 19-3). Some clients also use continuous ambulatory peritoneal dialysis (CAPD). The dialysis fluid is exchanged four or five times daily, making this a 24-hour treatment. Clients on CAPD have a more normal lifestyle than do clients on either hemodialysis or peritoneal dialysis. Some complications associated with CAPD include peritonitis, hypotension, and weight gain.

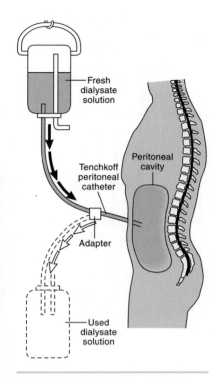

Figure 19-3 *Peritoneal dialysis.*

SPOTLIGHT on Life Cycle

A study has shown that nighttime dialysis for children improves their overall sense of well-being. Usually clients requiring hemodialysis go to a dialysis clinic several times per week for up to 5 hours each visit; for children, this often means missing school days and after-school activities such as sports or drama club. Home dialysis improves client well-being at reduced cost while bringing other benefits. Family schedules are less interrupted and families may feel they have more control of their lives. There is an improvement in the child's clinical status, school attendance and performance, and a small but consistent improvement in quality of life for these clients.

(Source: Adapted from Medline/Reuters, October 14, 2005.)

Diet during Dialysis

Dialysis clients may need additional protein, but the amount must be carefully controlled to prevent the accumulation of protein waste between treatments.

A client on hemodialysis requires 1.0 to 1.2 grams of protein per kilogram of body weight to make up for losses during dialysis. A client on peritoneal dialysis will require 1.2 to 1.5 grams of protein per kilogram of body weight. The protein needs for clients on CAPD are 1.2 grams per kilogram of body weight. Seventy-five percent of this protein should be high biological value (HBV) protein, which is found in eggs, meat, fish, poultry, milk, and cheese.

Potassium is usually restricted for dialysis clients. Healthy people ingest from 2,000 to 6,000 mg per day. The daily intake allowed clients in renal failure is 3,000 to 4,000 mg. End-stage renal disease further reduces intake allowed to 1,500 to 2,500 mg a day. The physician will prescribe the milligrams of potassium needed by the client. Table 19-1 lists low-, medium-, and high-potassium fruits and vegetables.

Clients are taught to regulate their intake by making careful choices. Milk is normally restricted to ½ cup a day because it is high in potassium and high in methionine, an essential amino acid. A typical renal diet could be written as "80-3-3," which means 80 grams of protein, 3 grams of sodium, and 3 grams of potassium a day. There may be a phosphorus restriction also. And there is often a need for supplements of water-soluble vitamins, vitamin D, calcium, and iron.

The ability of the kidney to handle sodium and water in ESRD must be assessed often. Usually, the diet contains 3 grams of sodium, which is the equivalent of a no-added-salt diet. Sodium and fluid needs may increase with perspiration, vomiting, fever, and diarrhea. The fluid content of foods, other

Table 19-1 *Potassium Content of Selected Fruits and Vegetables*

LOW POTASSIUM (less than 150 mg/serving*)	MEDIUM POTASSIUM (150–250 mg/serving*)	HIGH POTASSIUM (over 250 mg/serving*)
Applesauce	Apple juice	Avocado, ½ fruit
Berries: blackberries, blueberries, boysenberries, gooseberries, raspberries, strawberries	Apple, raw, 1 large	Banana, ½ fruit
	Apricots, raw, 2 medium, canned	Dried fruits: figs, apricots, dates, prunes, raisins
Cranberries	Cherries, raw (15) or canned	Kiwifruit
Cranberry sauce	Figs, raw, 2 medium	Mango
Figs, canned	Grapefruit juice	Melons: cantaloupe, ¼ medium; casaba,
Fruit cocktail, canned	Peach, raw, 1 medium	¾ cubed; honeydew ⅛ medium;
Grapes, canned or raw	Pear, raw, 1 medium	watermelon, 2 cups, cubed
Grape juice	Pineapple juice, raw or canned	Nectarine, 1 medium
Lemon or lime, 1 medium	Plums, raw, 2 medium	Orange, navel
Mandarin oranges, canned	Tangerine	Orange juice, fresh, frozen, canned
Peach, pear, or apricot nectar	Grapefruit sections	Prune juice, canned or bottled
Peaches, canned	Pineapple spears	Tangelo
Pears, canned		Papaya
Plums, canned		Raisins, seedless
Rhubarb		
Bamboo shoots	Asparagus	Artichoke
Bean sprouts	Beets	Beet greens
Beans, green, wax, snap	Broccoli	Dried beans and peas: kidney, lima,
Cabbage	Brussels sprouts	garbanzo, navy, and pinto beans;
Cauliflower	Carrots, cooked	blackeyed peas
Celery	Corn, canned or 1 small ear	Potato, ½ cup baked, boiled, or fried
Cucumber	Greens: collard, mustard, kale,	Pumpkin
Eggplant, cooked	dandelion, beet, turnip greens	Spinach
Hominy grits, cooked	Mixed vegetables	Sweet potato or yams
Leek	Okra	Tomato, raw or canned
Lettuce: cos, romaine, iceberg, leaf, endive, watercress (1 cup shredded)	Peas, green	Unsalted tomato juice
	Rutabaga	Winter squash: acorn, butternut,
Mushrooms	Summer squash: yellow crookneck, white scallop, zucchini	hubbard, spaghetti
Onion: green, red, yellow, white		
Peppers, sweet or hot		
Radishes, raw		
Turnips		
Water chestnuts, canned		
Watercress, chopped		

*All portions are ½ cup unless otherwise noted.

than liquids, is not counted in fluid restriction. Clients on fluid restriction must be taught to measure their fluid intake and urine output, examine their ankles for edema, and weigh themselves regularly.

Diet after Kidney Transplant

After kidney transplant, there may be a need for extra protein or for the restriction of protein. Carbohydrates and sodium may be restricted. The appropriate amounts of these nutrients will depend largely on the medications given at that time.

Additional calcium and phosphorus may be necessary if there was substantial bone loss before the transplant. There may be an increase in appetite after transplants. Fats and simple carbohydrates may be limited to prevent excessive weight gain.

Dietary Treatment of Renal Stones

Because the causes of renal stones have not been confirmed, treatment of them may vary. In general, however, large amounts of fluid—at least half of it water—are helpful in diluting the urine, as is a well-balanced diet. Once the stones have been analyzed, specific diet modifications may be indicated.

Calcium Oxalate Stones. About 80% of the renal stones formed contain calcium oxalate. Recent studies provide no support for the theory that a diet low in calcium can reduce the risk of calcium oxalate renal stones. In fact, higher dietary calcium intake may decrease the incidence of renal stones for most people. Dietary intake of excessive animal protein has been shown to be a risk factor for stone formation in some clients.

Stones containing oxalate are thought to be partially caused by a diet especially rich in oxalate, which is found in beets, wheat bran, chocolate, tea, rhubarb, strawberries, and spinach. Evidence also indicates that deficiencies of pyridoxine, thiamine, and magnesium may contribute to the formation of oxalate renal stones.

EXPLORING THE WEB

Search the Web for additional information on kidney dialysis, kidney transplant, and renal stones. Research the role diet plays in the treatment of these disorders. Could diet play a preventive role in these disorders? What is the morbidity and mortality of these disorders? Find some good resource material for clients with these disorders.

((• In The Media

COMEDIAN TO HELP FIGHT KIDNEY DISEASE

In 2005, comedian George Lopez received a donated kidney from his wife, Ann. George suffered from a genetic condition that caused his kidneys to deteriorate and needed the transplant to survive. "One in nine American adults has chronic kidney disease and most don't know it," stated Fred Brown, chairman of the National Kidney Foundation (NKF). "Latinos are a group that is at high risk for kidney disease. My wife and I look forward to helping the NKF raise public awareness about the importance of screening and early detection in the fight against kidney disease," says Lopez.

(Source: Adapted from the National Kidney Foundation, www.kidney.org/news/newsroom/newsitem.cFm?id=270, October 4, 2005.)

Table 19-2 Purine-Rich Foods	
AVOID	**LIMIT**
Liver	Meats
Kidneys	Fish
Sweetbreads	Poultry
Brains	Meat soups
Heart	
Anchovies	
Sardines	
Meat extracts	
Bouillon	
Broth	

purines
end products of nucleoprotein
metabolism

Uric Acid Stones. When the stones contain uric acid, purine-rich foods are restricted (Table 19-2). **Purines** are the end products of nucleoprotein metabolism and are found in all meats, fish, and poultry. Organ meats, anchovies, sardines, meat extracts, and broths are especially rich sources of them. Uric acid stones are usually associated with gout, GI diseases that cause diarrhea, and malignant disease.

Cystine Stones. Cystine is an amino acid. Cystine stones may form when the cystine concentration in the urine becomes excessive because of a hereditary metabolic disorder. The usual practice is to increase fluids and recommend an alkaline-ash diet.

Struvite Stones. Struvite stones are composed of magnesium ammonium phosphate. They are sometimes called infection stones because they develop following urinary tract infections caused by certain microorganisms. A low-phosphorus diet is often prescribed.

CONSIDERATIONS FOR THE HEALTH CARE PROFESSIONAL

The client with renal disease has a lifelong challenge. Anger and depression are common among these clients. These feelings complicate management of the disease if they contribute to the client's unwillingness to learn about his or her nutritional needs. These complications then add to the client's problems.

The health care professional can be extremely helpful if he or she can develop a trusting relationship with the client. Such a relationship can be established by listening to the client's complaints, needs, and concerns and responding with sincere understanding and sympathy. This approach can help motivate clients to learn how to manage their nutritional requirements and help the dietitian assist them.

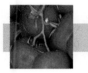

SUMMARY

The kidneys rid the body of wastes, maintain fluid, electrolyte, and acid-base balance, and secrete hormones. When they are damaged by disease or injury, the entire body is affected. Diet therapy for renal disorders can be extremely complex because of the multifaceted nature of the kidneys' functions. Untreated severe kidney disease can result in death unless dialysis or kidney transplant is undertaken.

DISCUSSION TOPICS

1. Discuss the three main tasks of the kidneys.
2. Define nephrons, and explain what they do.
3. Discuss some causes of kidney disease.
4. What is nephritis? Glomerulonephritis? Nephrosclerosis?
5. Why is diet therapy for renal disease so complex?
6. Discuss why protein is typically decreased for clients with renal disease.
7. Why are sodium and water sometimes restricted in renal disease?
8. Why is potassium sometimes restricted in renal disease? What is hyperkalemia?
9. Why is phosphorus sometimes restricted in renal disease?
10. Why might calories be restricted in renal disease?
11. What is nephrolithiasis? How is it treated?

SUGGESTED ACTIVITIES

1. Invite a registered nurse or renal dietitian to discuss renal disease with your class.
2. Invite a dialysis client to discuss her or his condition and reactions to dialysis.
3. Using outside sources, prepare a short report on the functions of the circulatory system, the liver, and the kidneys in eliminating nitrogenous waste products from the body.

REVIEW

Multiple choice. Select the *letter* that precedes the best answer.

1. The kidneys maintain the body's
   a. acid-base balance   c. fluid balance
   b. electrolyte balance d. all of these

2. The specialized part within each nephron that actually filters the blood is called the
   a. ureter   c. glomerulus
   b. filter   d. capillary bunch

3. Kidney disorders may be caused by
   a. diabetes   c. burns
   b. infections   d. all of these

4. When renal tissue has been destroyed to a point at which it can no longer filter the blood, the following occurs:
   a. nephritis   c. uremia
   b. nephrosclerosis   d. nephrolithiasis

5. The general term referring to the inflammatory diseases of the kidneys is
   a. nephritis   c. uremia
   b. nephrosclerosis   d. nephrolithiasis

6. The term referring to the hardening of renal arteries is
   a. nephritis   c. uremia
   b. nephrosclerosis   d. nephrolithiasis

7. The rare hereditary disease causing cysts to develop on the kidneys is called
   a. nephritis   c. renal stones
   b. glomerulonephritis   d. polycystic
                               kidney disease

8. The condition in which stones develop in the kidneys, ureters, or bladder is called
   a. nephritis
   b. nephrolithiasis
   c. polycystic kidney disease
   d. glomerulonephritis

9. Because its nitrogenous wastes contribute to uremia, the following nutrient may be restricted in diets of renal clients:

a. carbohydrate
c. protein
b. saturated fat
d. vitamin A

10. Kidney dialysis
    a. is a means of filtering all protein from the blood
    b. is a means of removing toxic substances from the blood
    c. always requires the client be on a low-protein diet
    d. requires the client to increase his or her sodium intake

11. Sodium and water may be restricted in the diets of renal clients because they
    a. contribute to uremia
    b. increase hypercalcemia
    c. contribute to hyperlipidemia
    d. contribute to fluid retention

12. If osteomalacia occurs in renal clients, the following nutrient may be prescribed:
    a. potassium
    c. calcium
    b. protein
    d. phosphorus

13. In a case of hyperkalemia, the following nutrient may be restricted:
    a. potassium
    c. calcium
    b. protein
    d. phosphorus

14. Fruits are an especially rich source of
    a. potassium
    c. calcium
    b. protein
    d. phosphorus

15. The vitamins renal clients may have an increased need for are
    a. the water-soluble vitamins
    b. the fat-soluble vitamins
    c. vitamins B, C, and D
    d. vitamins E and A

16. An excess of the following nutrient can compound bone loss in renal clients:
    a. phosphorus
    c. calcium
    b. carbohydrate
    d. iron

17. Purine-rich foods include
    a. meats
    b. dairy foods
    c. vegetables, except corn and lentils
    d. fruits, except cranberries, plums, and prunes

18. An example of nitrogenous waste found in the urine is
    a. ureter
    c. urea
    b. uremia
    d. all of these

CASE IN POINT

ALFRED: MANAGING DIET AFTER A KIDNEY STONE

Alfred is a third-generation Iowa farmer of Russian heritage who was proud to say he lived off the land. He raised wheat, corn, sheep, cattle, and chickens. He proudly pointed out that they used every part of the animals they slaughtered. His wife, Alice, planted a 1-acre garden each year and canned enough to provide for most of their winter fruit and vegetable needs.

Alfred had not felt well lately. He had a sharp stabbing pain in his left side and down his left leg. Sometimes it was so sharp, he would stop in his

tracks and double up. He finally got scared enough to go to the doctor. The doctor did some tests and found that Alfred had a kidney stone. Once Alfred passed the stone, the doctor was able to determine it was a uric acid stone. He told Alfred he would have to be on a low-purine diet and drink at least 10 glasses of water a day. Alfred was relieved to find out what the problem was but was not too sure about the diet aspect. Alfred had an appointment with the dietitian.

ASSESSMENT

1. What do you know about Alfred that put him at risk for kidney stones?
2. What were Alfred's symptoms?
3. How will this condition affect Alfred for the rest of his life?
4. How significant is this dietary change?

DIAGNOSIS

5. What is the cause of uric acid stones?
6. Complete the following diagnostic statement, Alfred's deficient knowledge is related to _____ .

PLAN/GOAL

7. What are reasonable, measurable goals for Alfred's change in health?

IMPLEMENTATION

8. What changes does Alfred need to make in his diet?
9. What would the consequences be if Alfred ignored the doctor's advice?
10. Could Alfred have another stone?

EVALUATION/OUTCOME CRITERIA

11. How will the doctor know if the plan is effective?

THINKING FURTHER

12. What could someone else learn from Alfred's experience?

⊚ RATE ⅛ PLATE

Alfred certainly didn't want another kidney stone, and after meeting with the dietitian, he was relieved to learn there were only a few foods that he should not eat. He told his wife his restrictions, and this is what she planned for dinner. Rate the plate.

5-oz chicken breast

Mashed potatoes made with cream and butter

Tossed salad with honey mustard dressing (2 to 4 Tbsp)

1/2 cup glazed carrots

Cherry pie

Check the Internet to familiarize yourself with low-purine diets. How did Alfred and his wife do planning this meal? Is restricting food the only way to control kidney stones?

CASE IN POINT

DONTELLE: LIVING WITH CHRONIC RENAL FAILURE

Dontelle is a 34-year-old African American male with a history of severe hypertension and noncompliance with his diet and medications. He is well known by the hospital staff for his numerous admissions due to kidney disease and chronic renal failure. Today is different. Dontelle has a gray cast to his skin, especially around his mouth and nose, and he is nauseated and has vomited a large amount of clear fluid. He is complaining of a headache and feeling as if his legs will not hold him up. Upon admission, his blood pressure is 230/120, his heart rate is 110, he has difficulty breathing, and he is slow to respond to questions. His doctor orders numerous blood tests, including a BUN, creatinine and K. His BUN is 180, his creatinine is 7, and his K is 7.

The doctor calls the dialysis on-call nurse to come in and dialyze Dontelle immediately. The doctor puts in a Quentin catheter in his jugular vein, and dialysis is initiated.

ASSESSMENT

1. What do you know about Dontelle that puts him at risk for this problem?
2. How significant is his health problem?
3. How will dialysis alter his life?

DIAGNOSIS

4. Write a diagnostic statement about what Dontelle needs to know about high blood pressure and renal failure.
5. Write a statement about the risk of excess fluid in the body.
6. Write a statement about the risk of high-potassium levels in the body.
7. Write a statement about the risk of noncompliance for renal patients.

PLAN/GOAL

8. Write a plan for Dontelle's new renal diet of 1 gram of sodium, low potassium, and 30 grams of protein.
9. What goals are important for Dontelle?

IMPLEMENTATION

10. What major topics would be important for the dietitian to discuss with Dontelle?
11. Create a day's menu for Dontelle using the dietitian's new diet. Spread the protein out throughout the day.
12. What teaching aids could the dietitian give Dontelle to help him remember his new diet?
13. How could the Web site www.mypyramid.gov help with meal planning?
14. What impact will his CRF have on his ability to be employed? What impact will it have on his physical and psychological status?

EVALUATION/OUTCOME CRITERIA

15. After discharge from the hospital, how will the physician know that Dontelle has been compliant with his diet and medications?
16. During the dialysis treatment, what is important for Dontelle to do in order to have the appropriate clearances of his blood and ultrafiltration of his fluids?

THINKING FURTHER

17. Why is it important for clients with hypertension to control it?

◎ RATE THIS PLATE

On Dontelle's plate are:

Barbecued pork ribs

Collard greens made with fatback

Potato salad

Corn bread with butter

Mixed fruit for dessert (watermelon, cantaloupe, strawberries, peaches, and grapes)

Rate the plate.

DIET AND GASTROINTESTINAL PROBLEMS

OBJECTIVES

After studying this chapter, you should be able to:

⬐ Explain the uses of diet therapy in gastrointestinal disturbances

⬐ Identify the foods allowed and disallowed in the therapeutic diets discussed

⬐ Adapt normal diets to meet the requirements of clients with these conditions

The gastrointestinal (GI) tract is where digestion and absorption of food occur. The primary organs include the mouth, esophagus, stomach, and small and large intestine. The liver, gallbladder, and pancreas are accessory organs that are also involved in these processes.

Numerous disorders of the gastrointestinal system cause countless individuals distress and consequently affect the nation's economy because they keep so many people home from work. Some problems are physiologically caused; others can be psychological in origin. It is sometimes difficult to determine the cause or causes of a GI problem. Consequently, controversy exists in some cases about proper treatment.

DISORDERS OF THE PRIMARY ORGANS

Dyspepsia

dyspepsia
gastrointestinal discomfort of vague origin

Dyspepsia, or indigestion, is a condition of discomfort in the digestive tract that can be physical or psychological in origin. Symptoms include heartburn, bloating, pain and, sometimes, regurgitation. If the cause is physical, it can be due to overeating or spicy foods, or it may be a symptom of another problem, such as appendicitis or a kidney, gallbladder, or colon disease or possibly cancer. If the problem is organic in origin, treatment of the underlying cause will be the normal procedure.

Psychological stress can affect stomach secretions and trigger dyspepsia. Treatment should include counseling to help the client:

- Find relief from the underlying stress
- Allow sufficient time to relax and enjoy meals
- Learn to improve eating habits

Esophagitis

esophagitis
inflammation of mucosal lining of the esophagus

gastroesophageal reflux (GER)
backflow of stomach contents into the esophagus

Esophagitis is caused by the irritating effect of acidic gastric reflux on the mucosa of the esophagus. Heartburn, regurgitation, and dysphagia (difficulty swallowing) are common symptoms. Acute esophagitis is caused by ingesting an irritating agent, by intubation, or by an infection. Chronic, or reflux, esophagitis is caused by recurrent **gastroesophageal reflux (GER).** This can be caused by a hiatal hernia, reduced lower esophageal sphincter (LES) pressure, abdominal pressure, recurrent vomiting, alcohol use, overweight, or smoking. Cancer of the esophagus and silent aspiration may be life-threatening for those with gastroesophageal reflux disease (GERD).

Hiatal Hernia

hiatal hernia
condition wherein part of the stomach protrudes through the diaphragm into the chest cavity

diaphragm
thin membrane or partition

Hiatal hernia is a condition in which a part of the stomach protrudes through the **diaphragm** into the thoracic cavity (Figure 20-1). The hernia prevents the food from moving normally along the digestive tract, although the food does mix somewhat with the gastric juices. Sometimes the food will move back into the esophagus, creating a burning sensation (heartburn), and sometimes food will be regurgitated into the mouth. This condition can be very uncomfortable.

Medical Nutrition Therapy. The symptoms can sometimes be alleviated by serving small, frequent meals (from a well-balanced diet) so that the amount of food in the stomach is never large. Avoid irritants to the esophagus such as carbonated beverages, citrus fruits and juices, tomato products, spicy foods, coffee, pepper, and some herbs. Some foods can cause the lower esophageal sphincter to relax, and these should be avoided. Examples are alcohol, garlic, onion, oil of peppermint and spearmint, chocolate, cream sauces, gravies, margarine, butter, and oil. If the client is obese, weight loss may be recommended to reduce pressure on the abdomen. It may also be helpful if clients

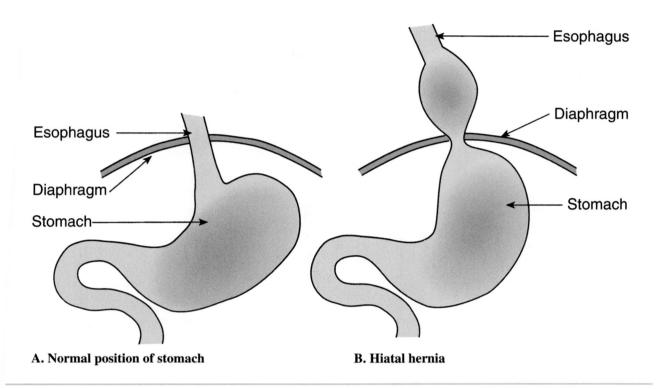

Esophagus	Esophagus
Diaphragm	Diaphragm
Stomach	Stomach

A. Normal position of stomach   **B. Hiatal hernia**

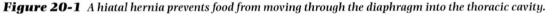

Figure 20-1 *A hiatal hernia prevents food from moving through the diaphragm into the thoracic cavity.*

avoid late-night dinners and lying down for 2 to 3 hours after eating. When they do lie down, they may be more comfortable sleeping with their heads and upper torso somewhat elevated and wearing loose-fitting clothing. If discomfort cannot be controlled, surgery may be necessary.

Peptic Ulcers

An ulcer is an erosion of the mucous membrane (Figure 20-2). **Peptic ulcers** may occur in the stomach **(gastric ulcer)** or the duodenum **(duodenal ulcer).** The specific cause of ulcers is not clear, but some physicians believe that a number of factors including genetic predisposition, abnormally high secretion of hydrochloric acid by the stomach, stress, excessive use of aspirin or ibuprofen (analgesics), cigarette smoking and, in some cases, a bacterium called *Helicobacter pylori* may contribute to their development.

    A classic symptom is gastric pain, which is sometimes described as burning, and in some cases, hemorrhage is also a symptom. The pain is typically relieved with food or antacids. A hemorrhage usually requires surgery.

    Ulcers are generally treated with drugs such as antibiotics and cimetidine. The antibiotics kill the bacteria, and cimetidine inhibits acid secretion in the stomach and thus helps to heal the ulcer. Antacids containing calcium carbonate can also be prescribed to neutralize any excess acid. Stress management may also be beneficial in the treatment of ulcers.

peptic ulcers
ulcer of the stomach or duodenum

gastric ulcer
ulcer in the stomach

duodenal ulcer
ulcer occurring in the duodenum

Helicobacter pylori
bacteria that can cause peptic ulcer

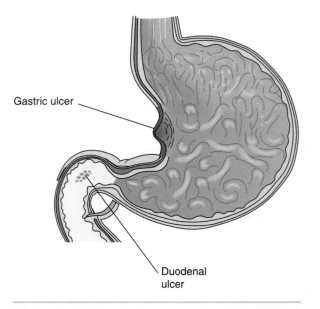

Gastric ulcer

Duodenal ulcer

Figure 20-2 *Peptic ulcers are erosion of the mucous membrane in the stomach or the duodenum.*

Sufficient low-fat protein should be provided, but not in excess because of its ability to stimulate gastric acid secretion. It is recommended that clients receive no less than 0.8 gram of protein per kilogram of body weight. However, if there has been blood loss, protein may be increased to 1 or 1.5 grams per kilogram of body weight. Vitamin and mineral supplements, especially iron if there has been hemorrhage, may be prescribed.

Although fat inhibits gastric secretions, because of the danger of atherosclerosis, the amount of fat in the diet should not be excessive. Carbohydrates have little effect on gastric acid secretion.

Spicy foods may be eaten as tolerated. Coffee, tea, or anything else that contains caffeine or that seems to cause indigestion in the client or stimulates gastric secretion should be avoided. Alcohol and aspirin irritate the mucous membrane of the stomach, and cigarette smoking decreases the secretion of the pancreas that buffers gastric acid in the duodenum. Currently, a well-balanced diet of three meals a day consisting of foods that do not irritate the client is generally recommended.

Diverticulosis/Diverticulitis

diverticulosis
intestinal disorder characterized by little pockets forming in the sides of the intestines; pockets are called diverticula

diverticulitis
inflammation of the diverticula

Diverticulosis is an intestinal disorder characterized by little pockets in the sides of the large intestine (colon) (Figure 20-3). When fecal matter collects in these pockets instead of moving on through the colon, bacteria may breed, and inflammation and pain can result, causing **diverticulitis.** If a diverticulum ruptures, surgery may be needed. This condition is thought to be caused by a diet lacking sufficient fiber. A high-fiber diet is commonly recommended for clients with diverticulosis.

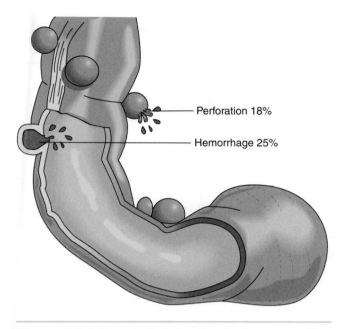

Figure 20-3 *Diverticulosis is a disorder characterized by little pockets forming in the sides of the large intestine. Rupture of the pockets may result in the need for corrective surgery.*

Along with antibiotics, diet therapy for diverticulitis may begin with a clear liquid diet, followed by a low-residue diet that allows the bowel to rest and heal. Then very gradually (over several weeks), the person progresses to a high-fiber diet. The bulk provided by the high-fiber diet increases stool volume, reduces the pressure in the colon, and shortens the time the food is in the intestine, giving bacteria less time to grow.

Inflammatory Bowel Disease

Inflammatory bowel diseases (IBDs) are chronic conditions causing inflammation in the gastrointestinal tract. The inflammation causes malabsorption that often leads to malnutrition. The acute phases of these diseases occur at irregular intervals and are followed by periods in which clients are relatively free of symptoms. Neither cause nor cure for these conditions is known.

Two examples are **ulcerative colitis** and **Crohn's disease** (Table 20-1). Ulcerative colitis causes inflammation and ulceration of the colon, the rectum, or sometimes the entire large intestine. Crohn's disease is a chronic progressive disorder that can affect both the small and large intestines. The ulcers can penetrate the entire intestinal wall, and the chronic inflammation can thicken the intestinal wall, causing obstruction.

Both conditions cause bloody diarrhea, cramps, fatigue, nausea, anorexia, malnutrition, and weight loss. Electrolytes, fluids, vitamins, and other minerals are lost in the diarrhea, and the bleeding can cause loss of iron and protein.

⊙ inflammatory bowel disease (IBD)
chronic condition causing inflammation in the gastrointestinal tract

⊙ ulcerative colitis
disease characterized by inflammation and ulceration of the colon, rectum, and sometimes entire large intestine

⊙ Crohn's disease
a chronic progressive disorder that causes inflammation, ulcers, and thickening of intestinal walls, sometimes causing obstruction

Table 20-1 *Crohn's Disease and Ulcerative Colitis*		
	CROHN'S DISEASE	**ULCERATIVE COLITIS**
Involvement	Patchy areas; can involve small and large intestines	Starts in lower colon and spreads progressively throughout colon
Tissue affected	Entire thickness of bowel	Mucosal lining of the bowel
Major complication	Malabsorption	Toxic megacolon
Long-term complications	Intestinal obstruction, fistulas, abscesses, perforations; cancer risk increases with age	Fissures, abscesses, increased risk for colorectal cancer
Surgical intervention	Usually needed at some point to repair structural damage; does not cure or limit the progress of the disease	Ileostomy performed in approximately 20% of cases to remove the colon; cures the disease
Cause	Unknown; possibly altered immune state	Unknown; possibly enteric bacterium *Escherichia coli*
Stools	3 to 4 semisoft/day; rarely bloody; steatorrhea (fat in stool), mucus	15 to 20 liquid/day; blood present; no steatorrhea (fat in stool)

Source: From *Foundations of Adult Health Nursing* (2nd ed., p. 194), by L. White, 2005, Clifton Park, NY: Thomson Delmar Learning.

⊙ **total parenteral nutrition (TPN)**
process of providing all nutrients intravenously

Treatment may involve anti-inflammatory drugs plus medical nutrition therapy. Usually a low-residue diet is required to avoid irritating the inflamed area and to avoid the danger of obstruction. When tolerated, the diet should include about 100 grams of protein, additional calories, vitamins, and minerals.

In severe cases, **total parenteral nutrition (TPN)** (a process in which nutrients are delivered directly into the superior vena cava; see Chapter 22) may be necessary for a period. As the client begins to regain health, the diet may be increasingly liberalized to suit the client's tastes while maintaining good nutrition.

((• In The Media

YOGURT, FERMENTED DRINKS GOOD FOR BOWEL DISEASE

Yogurts and fermented drinks containing "good" bacteria may not be merely a fad. These products, called probiotics, contain one or more types of bacteria from the lactobacillus family, which promote improved digestive function.

One study examined clients with inflammatory bowel disease (IBD). The two conditions categorized as IBD are ulcerative colitis and Crohn's disease, which are characterized by severe inflammation of the intestines. The probiotic (150 grams of two types of yogurt per day) were given to healthy people and clients with IBD. The results of the study showed that this probiotic got down to the large bowel and changed something within the lining of the large bowel.

(Source: Adapted from Reuters, September 29, 2001.)

Ileostomy or Colostomy

Clients with severe ulcerative colitis or Crohn's disease frequently require a surgical opening from the body surface to the intestine for the purpose of defecation. The opening that is created is called a **stoma** and is about the size of a nickel. An **ileostomy** (from the ileum to abdomen surface) is required when the entire colon, rectum, and anus must be removed. A **colostomy** (from the colon to abdomen surface) can provide entrance into the colon if the rectum and anus are removed. This can be a temporary or a permanent procedure.

Clients with ileostomies have a greater than normal need for salt and water because of excess losses. A vitamin C supplement is recommended and, in some cases, a B_{12} supplement may be needed. Eating a well-balanced individualized diet will prevent a nutritional deficiency for clients with ileostomies and colostomies.

stoma
surgically created opening in the abdominal wall

ileostomy
opening from ileum to abdomen surface

colostomy
opening from colon to abdomen surface

Celiac Disease

Celiac disease, also called **nontropical sprue** or gluten sensitivity, is a disorder characterized by malabsorption of virtually all nutrients. It is thought to be due to heredity.

Symptoms include diarrhea, weight loss, and malnutrition. Stools are usually foul-smelling, light-colored, and bulky. The cause is unknown, but it has been found that the elimination of **gluten** from the diet gives relief. Untreated, it is life-threatening because of the severe malnutrition and weight loss it can cause.

A gluten-controlled diet (Table 20-2) is used in the treatment of celiac disease. Gluten is a protein found in barley, oats, rye, and wheat. All products

nontropical sprue
a disorder of the gastrointestinal tract characterized by malabsorption; also called gluten sensitivity

gluten
protein found in grains

Table 20-2 *Sources of Gluten*			
FOOD GROUP	**FOODS THAT DO NOT CONTAIN GLUTEN**	**FOODS THAT CONTAIN GLUTEN**	**FOODS THAT MAY CONTAIN GLUTEN**
Beverage	Coffee, tea, decaffeinated coffee, carbonated beverages, chocolate drinks made with pure cocoa powder, wine, distilled liquor	Cereal beverages (e.g., Postum), malt, Ovaltine, beer, ale	Commercial chocolate milk, cocoa mixes, other beverage mixes, dietary supplements
Meat and meat substitutes	Pure meat, fish, fowl, eggs, cottage cheese, and peanut butter	Commercially breaded meats	Meatloaf and patties, cold cuts and prepared meats, stuffing, cheese foods and spreads; commercial souffles, omelets, and fondue; soy protein meat substitutes
Fat and oil	Butter, margarine, vegetable oil	Commercial gravies, white and cream sauces	Commercial salad dressing and mayonnaise, nondairy creamer

(continued)

Table 20-2 *Continued*

FOOD GROUP	FOODS THAT DO NOT CONTAIN GLUTEN	FOODS THAT CONTAIN GLUTEN	FOODS THAT MAY CONTAIN GLUTEN
Milk	Whole, low-fat, fat-free milk; buttermilk	Milk beverages that contain malt	Commercial chocolate milk
Grains and grain products	Specially prepared breads made with wheat starch, rice, potato, or soybean flour or cornmeal; pure corn or rice cereals; hominy grits; white, brown, and wild rice; quinoa; millet; amaranth; sorghum; popcorn; low-protein pasta made from wheat starch	Bread, crackers, cereal and pasta that contain wheat, oats, rye, malt, malt flavoring, graham flour, durham flour, pastry flour, bran, or wheat germ; barley; buckwheat; pretzels; communion wafers	Commercially seasoned rice and potato mixes
Vegetable	All fresh vegetables, plain commercially frozen or canned vegetables	Commercially breaded vegetables or vegetables with a cream or cheese sauce	Commercial seasoned vegetable mixes, canned baked beans
Fruit	All plain or sweetened fruits, fruit thickened with tapioca or cornstarch		Commercial pie fillings
Soup	Soup thickened with cornstarch, wheat starch, or potato, rice, or soybean flour; pure broth	Most commercial soup and soup mixes; soup that contains barley, wheat pasta; soup thickened with wheat flour or other gluten-containing grains	
Desserts	Gelatin; custard; fruit ice; specially prepared cakes, cookies, and pastries made with gluten-free flour or starch; pudding and fruit filling thickened with tapioca, cornstarch, or arrowroot flour	Commercial cakes, cookies, and pastries; commercial dessert mixes	Commercial ice cream and sherbet, puddings
Sweets			Commercial candies, especially chocolates
Miscellaneous	Monosodium glutamate, salt, pepper, pure spices and herbs, yeast, pure baking chocolate or cocoa powder, carob, flavoring extracts, artificial flavoring, cider and wine vinegar		Ketchup, prepared mustard, soy sauce, commercially prepared meat sauces and pickles, white vinegar, flavoring syrups (syrups for pancakes or ice cream)

Source: *Mayo clinic diet manual: A handbook of nutrition practices* (7th ed.), by J. K. Nelson, K. E. Moxness, C. F. Gastineau, and M. D. Jenson, 1994, St. Louis, MO: Mosby. Reprinted with permission of Mayo Foundation for Medical Education and Research.

Table 20-3 High-calories, High-Protein, Low-Residue Diet Menus

BREAKFAST	LUNCH	DINNER
Orange juice	Baked chicken	Ground beef patty
Poached egg	Rice	Mashed potato
Rice toast	Pureed green beans	Mashed acorn squash
Butter and jelly	Rolls made from wheat starch	Rice bread and butter
Coffee with milk and sugar	and butter	Applesauce with sponge cake
	Lemon chiffon pudding	made from wheat starch
	Tea with milk and sugar	Coffee with milk and sugar
SNACK	**SNACK**	**SNACK**
Eggnog, if tolerated	Sugar cookies baked with	Beef broth
	gluten-free flour	Rice cakes
	Pineapple juice	

containing these grains are disallowed. Rice and corn may be used. A reduction in the fiber content is also frequently recommended. If the client is under weight, the diet should also be high in calories, carbohydrates, and protein (Table 20-3). Fat may be restricted until bowel function is normalized. Vitamin and mineral supplements may be prescribed. Lactose intolerance sometimes develops with celiac disease.

It is not easy to avoid food products containing wheat. Breads, cereals, crackers, pasta products, desserts, gravies, white sauces, and beer contain wheat or other cereal grains with gluten. The client will have to learn to read food labels carefully and to avoid restaurant foods such as breaded meats or fish, meatloaf, creamed vegetables, and cream soups.

DISORDERS OF THE ACCESSORY ORGANS

Cirrhosis

The liver is of major importance to, and plays many roles in, metabolism. Except for a few of the fatty acids, all nutrients that are absorbed in the intestines are transported to the liver. The liver dismantles some of these nutrients, stores others, and uses some to synthesize other substances.

The liver determines where amino acids are needed and synthesizes some proteins, enzymes, and urea. It changes the simple sugars to glycogen, provides glucose to body cells, and synthesizes glucose from amino acids if needed. It converts fats to lipoproteins and synthesizes cholesterol. It stores iron, copper, zinc, and magnesium as well as the fat-soluble vitamins and B vitamins. The liver synthesizes bile and stores it in the gallbladder. It detoxifies many substances such as barbiturates and morphine.

Liver disease may be acute or chronic. Early treatment can usually lead to recovery. **Cirrhosis** is a general term referring to all types of liver disease

cirrhosis
generic term for liver disease
characterized by cell loss

characterized by cell loss. Alcohol abuse is the most common cause of cirrhosis, but it can also be caused by congenital defects, infections, or other toxic chemicals.

Although the liver does regenerate, the replacement during cirrhosis does not match the loss. In addition to the cell loss during cirrhosis, there is fatty infiltration and **fibrosis.** These developments prevent the liver from functioning normally. Blood flow through the liver is upset, and a form of hypertension, anemia, and hemorrhage in the esophagus can occur. The normal metabolic processes will also be disturbed to such a degree that, in severe cases, death may result.

The dietary treatment of cirrhosis provides at least 25 to 35 calories or more, and 0.8 to 1.0 gram of protein per kilogram of weight each day, depending on the client's condition. If hepatic coma appears imminent, the lower amount is advocated. Supplements of vitamins and minerals are usually needed. In advanced cirrhosis, 50% to 60% of the calories should be from carbohydrates.

In some forms of cirrhosis, clients cannot tolerate fat well, so it is restricted. In another form, protein may not be well tolerated, so it is restricted to 35 to 40 grams a day. Sometimes cirrhosis causes **ascites.** In such a case, sodium and fluids may be restricted. If there is bleeding in the esophagus, fiber can be restricted to prevent irritation of the tissue. Smaller feedings will be better accepted than larger ones. No alcohol is allowed.

Hepatitis

Hepatitis is an inflammation of the liver. It is caused by viruses or toxic agents such as drugs and alcohol. **Necrosis** occurs, and the liver's normal metabolic activities are constricted. Hepatitis may be acute or chronic.

Hepatitis A virus (HAV) is contracted through contaminated drinking water, food, and sewage via a fecal-oral route. Hepatitis B virus (HBV) and hepatitis C virus (HCV) are transmitted through blood, blood products, semen, and saliva. Hepatitis B and C can lead to chronic active hepatitis (CAH), which is diagnosed by liver biopsy. Chronic active hepatitis can lead to liver failure and end-stage liver disease (ESLD).

In mild cases, the cells can be replaced. In severe cases, the damage can be so extensive that the necrosis leads to liver failure and death. There can be bile **stasis** and decreased blood albumin levels. Clients experience nausea, headache, fever, fatigue, tender and enlarged liver, anorexia, and **jaundice.** Weight loss can be pronounced.

Treatment is usually bed rest, plenty of fluids, and medical nutrition therapy. The diet should provide 35 to 40 calories per kilogram of body weight. Most of the calories should be provided by carbohydrates; there should be moderate amounts of fat and, if the necrosis has not been severe, up to 70 to 80 grams of protein for cell regeneration. If the necrosis has been severe and the proteins cannot be properly metabolized, they must be limited to prevent the accumulation of ammonia in the blood. Clients may prefer frequent, small meals rather than three large ones.

Clients with liver disease require a great deal of encouragement because their anorexia and consequent feelings of general malaise can be severe. Their recovery takes patience, rest, and time.

---

fibrosis
development of tough, stringy tissue

ascites
abnormal collection of fluid in the abdomen

hepatitis
inflammation of the liver caused by viruses, drugs, or alcohol

necrosis
tissue death due to lack of blood supply

stasis
stoppage or slowing

jaundice
yellow cast of the skin and eyes

Cholecystitis and Cholelithiasis

The dual function of the gallbladder is the concentration and storage of bile. After bile is formed in the liver, the gallbladder concentrates it to several times its original strength and stores it until needed. Fat in the duodenum triggers the gallbladder to contract and release bile into the common duct for the digestion of fat in the small intestine. If this flow is hindered, there may be pain.

The precise etiology of gallbladder disease is unknown, but heredity factors may be involved. Women develop gallbladder disease more often than men do. Obesity, total parenteral nutrition (TPN), very low calorie diets for rapid weight loss, the use of estrogen, and various diseases of the small intestine are frequently associated with gallbladder disease.

Cholecystitis (inflammation) and **cholelithiasis** (gallstones) may inhibit the flow of bile and cause pain. Cholecystitis can cause changes in the gallbladder tissue, which in turn can affect the cholesterol (a constituent of bile), causing it to harden and form stones. It is also thought that chronic overindulgence in fats may contribute to gallstones because the fat stimulates the liver to produce more cholesterol for the bile, which is necessary for the digestion of fat. In addition to pain, which can be severe, there may be indigestion and vomiting, particularly after the ingestion of fatty foods.

Treatment may include medication to dissolve the stones and diet therapy. If medication does not succeed, surgery to remove the gallbladder (**cholecystectomy**) may be indicated.

Medical nutrition therapy includes abstinence during the acute phase. This is followed by a clear liquid diet and, gradually, a regular but fat-restricted diet. Amounts of fats allowed run from 40 to 45 grams a day. In chronic cases, fat may be restricted on a permanent basis. For obese clients, weight loss is recommended in addition to a fat-restricted diet. (For information on fat-restricted diets, see Chapter 18.) Clients with chronic gallbladder conditions may require the water-miscible forms of fat-soluble vitamins.

cholecystitis
inflammation of the gallbladder

cholelithiasis
gallstones

cholecystectomy
removal of the gallbladder

Pancreatitis

In addition to the hormone insulin, the pancreas produces other hormones and enzymes that are important in the digestion of protein, fats, and carbohydrates. When food reaches the duodenum, the pancreas sends its enzymes to the small intestine to aid in digestion.

Pancreatitis is an inflammation of the pancreas. It may be caused by infections, surgery, alcoholism, biliary tract (includes bile ducts and gallbladder) disease, or certain drugs. It may be acute or chronic.

Abdominal pain, nausea, and **steatorrhea** are symptoms. Malabsorption (particularly of fat-soluble vitamins) and weight loss occur and, in cases in which the islets of Langerhans are destroyed, diabetes mellitus may result.

Diet therapy is intended to reduce pancreatic secretions and bile. Just as fat stimulates the gallbladder to secrete bile, protein and hydrochloric acid stimulate the pancreas to secrete its juices and enzymes. During acute pancreatitis, the client is nourished strictly parenterally. Later, when the client can tolerate oral feedings, a liquid diet consisting mainly of carbohydrates is given because, of these three nutrients, carbohydrates have the least stimulatory effect on pancreatic secretions.

pancreatitis
inflammation of the pancreas

steatorrhea
abnormal amounts of fat in the feces

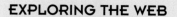

EXPLORING THE WEB

Choose one of the disorders discussed and thoroughly research on the Internet. Create a list of the signs and symptoms, the possible causes, and the treatment choices for the disorder. Identify the nutritional needs for a person with this disorder. Can the disorder(s) be controlled through proper nutrition?

As recovery progresses, small, frequent feedings of carbohydrates and protein with little fat or fiber are given. The fat is restricted because of deficiencies of pancreatic lipase. The client is gradually returned to a less-restricted diet as tolerated. Vitamin supplements may be given. Alcohol is forbidden in all cases.

RESIDUE-CONTROLLED DIETS

Fiber is that part of food that is not broken down by digestive enzymes. It is called **dietary fiber**. Most dietary fiber is found in plant foods. Some is soluble, and some is insoluble (see Chapter 4). Examples of dietary fiber in plants include the outer shells of corn kernels, strings of celery, seeds of strawberries, and the connective tissue of citrus fruits.

Residue is the solid part of feces. Residue is made up of all the undigested and unabsorbed parts of food (including fiber), connective tissue in animal foods, dead cells, and intestinal bacteria and their products. Most of this residue is composed of fiber.

Diets can be adjusted to increase or decrease fiber and residue. The specific names of these diets vary among health care facilities. The specific foods allowed, and thus the amount of fiber and residue allowed, will depend on the physician's experience and the client's condition.

The High-Fiber Diet

High-fiber diets containing 30 grams or more of dietary fiber are believed to help prevent diverticulosis, constipation, hemorrhoids, and colon cancer. They also are helpful in the treatment of diabetes mellitus (see Chapter 17) and atherosclerosis (see Chapter 18).

It is currently estimated that the normal diet in the United States contains about 11 grams of dietary fiber each day. A high-fiber diet is often 25 to 35 grams and should not exceed 50 grams a day. The recommended foods for this diet include coarse- and whole-grain breads and cereals, bran, all fruits, vegetables (especially raw), and legumes. Milk, meats, and fats do not contain fiber (Table 20-4). The diet is nutritionally adequate. High-fiber diets must be introduced gradually to prevent the formation of gas and the discomfort that accompanies it. Eight 8-ounce glasses of water also must be consumed along with the increased fiber.

dietary fiber
indigestible parts of plants; absorbs water in large intestine, helping to create soft, bulky stool; some is believed to bind cholesterol in the colon, helping to rid cholesterol from the body; some is believed to lower blood glucose levels

SUPERSIZE USA

"Baseball games are an American institution. Couldn't wait to eat the hotdogs, peanuts, and nachos and, of course, drink soda to my heart's content! There were nine innings, and then the score was tied at the end of the ninth. I ate my way through all nine and even into the extra innings. Upon leaving the ballpark, I was feeling pain in the upper-right quadrant of my abdomen and straight through to my back. I had had this pain before but never to this extent. What is wrong with me? Did I eat something specifically to cause the pain? What should I eliminate from my diet to prevent future pain?"

You may be having a gallbladder attack. All the foods that have a lot of fat—hotdogs, nachos, peanuts—can cause it. Follow a low-fat diet to prevent future pain.

Table 20-4 *Sample Menus for a High-Fiber Diet*

BREAKFAST	DINNER	LUNCH OR SUPPER
Stewed prunes	Baked pork chops	Fresh fruit cup
Bran cereal with	Baked potato	Roast beef sandwich on
milk and sugar	Fresh corn	cracked wheat bread
Whole wheat toast	Green salad with oil	Coleslaw
with marmalade	and vinegar dressing	Carrot cake
Coffee	Whole-grain bread with	Fat-free milk
	margarine	Coffee or tea
	Fresh pineapple	
	Fat-free milk	
	Tea	

SPOTLIGHT on Life Cycle

Here are some suggestions for helping older adults increase fiber in the diet:
• Eat fresh fruits and vegetables. If the older adult has difficulty chewing raw fruits and vegetables, gently steamed vegetables and soft fruits are appropriate.
• Eat some of the skins of potatoes, apples, pears, and other fruits or vegetables. The outer portion of these foods contains fiber and valuable nutrients.
• Use whole-grain breads and cereals instead of refined white bread and sugary cereals. Instead of meat, add beans (navy, lima, kidney, pinto), all of which are high in fiber and can also be a less expensive source of protein. Beans can also be used in casseroles, soups, stews, and other dishes.
• Try unbuttered air-popped popcorn or the reduced- or low-fat versions of microwave popcorn for a snack. Remind the older adult that dentures and teeth will need special attention during cleaning following a popcorn snack.
• Remember how important it is to increase the water in the diet when the fiber content is increased. At least 8 cups of liquid are needed each day.
• Keep moving; being active helps bowel regularity.

The Low-Residue Diet

The low-residue diet of 5 to 10 grams of dietary fiber a day is intended to reduce the normal work of the intestines by restricting the amount of dietary fiber and reducing food residue. Low-fiber or residue-restricted diets may be used in cases of severe diarrhea, diverticulitis, ulcerative colitis, and intestinal blockage and in preparation for and immediately after intestinal surgery.

In some facilities, these diets consist of foods that provide no more than 3 grams of fiber a day and that do not increase fecal residue (Tables 20-5 and 20-6). Some foods that do not actually leave residue in the colon are considered "low-residue" foods because they increase stool volume or provide a laxative effect. Milk and prune juice are examples. Milk increases stool volume, and prune juice acts as a laxative.

Table 20-5 *Foods to Allow and to Avoid on Low-Residue Diets*

FOODS TO ALLOW	FOODS TO AVOID
Milk, buttermilk (limited to 2 cups daily) if physician allows	Fresh or dried fruits and vegetables
Cottage cheese and some mild cheeses as flavorings in small amounts	Whole-grain breads and cereals
Butter and margarine	Nuts, seeds, legumes, coconut, and marmalade
Eggs, except fried	Tough meats
Tender chicken, fish, sweetbreads, ground beef, and ground lamb (meats must be baked, boiled, or broiled)	Rich pastries
Soup broth	Milk, unless physician allows
Cooked, mild-flavored vegetables without coarse fibers; strained fruit juices (except for prune); applesauce; canned fruits including white cherries, peaches, and pears; pureed apricots; ripe bananas	Meats and fish with tough connective tissue
Refined breads and cereals, white crackers, macaroni, spaghetti, and noodles	
Custard, sherbet, vanilla ice cream, junket and cereal puddings when considered as part of the 2-cup milk allowance and if physician allows; plain gelatin; angel food cake; sponge cake; plain cookies	
Coffee, tea, cocoa, carbonated beverage	
Salt, sugar, small amount of spices as permitted by physician	

Table 20-6 *Sample Menus for a Low-Residue Diet*

BREAKFAST	DINNER	LUNCH OR SUPPER
Strained orange juice	Chicken broth	Tomato juice
Cream of rice cereal with milk and sugar	Ground beef patty	Macaroni and cheese
White toast with margarine and jelly	Boiled potato, no skin	Green beans
Coffee with cream and sugar	Baked squash	White bread and butter
	Gelatin dessert	Lemon sherbet
	Milk	Tea with milk and sugar

CONSIDERATIONS FOR THE HEALTH CARE PROFESSIONAL

Clients with gastrointestinal problems can be frustrated and irritable. Their problems can be psychologically caused; they may fear surgery or cancer; and they may suffer nausea, pain, or both. Some will want to eat foods that are disallowed; others will refuse foods they need.

Health care professionals who show respect and understanding for their clients will have the most success in helping them learn what they should and should not eat and why.

SUMMARY

Disturbances of the gastrointestinal tract require a wide variety of therapeutic diets. Peptic ulcers are treated with drugs, and diet therapy generally involves only the avoidance of alcohol and caffeine. Diverticulosis may be treated with a high-fiber diet, whereas diverticulitis is treated with a gradual progression from clear liquid to the high-fiber diet. Ulcerative colitis may require a low-residue diet combined with high protein and high calories. Cirrhosis requires a substantial, balanced diet, with occasional restrictions of fat, protein, salt, or fluids. Diet therapy for hepatitis may include a full, well-balanced diet, although protein may be restricted, depending upon the client's condition. Cholecystitis and cholelithiasis clients require a fat-restricted diet and, in cases of overweight, a calorie-restricted diet as well. Pancreatitis diet therapy ranges from TPN to an individualized diet as tolerated.

DISCUSSION TOPICS

1. Name the accessory organs in the gastrointestinal system and explain their roles in digestion and metabolism.

2. Discuss dyspepsia. Include its probable causes and the suggested therapy for it.

3. Describe hiatal hernia. Name its symptoms and possible treatment.

4. Define ulcers. Where are they found in the gastrointestinal system, and how are they treated? What substances should not be allowed an ulcer client? Why?

5. Explain the difference between diverticulosis and diverticulitis. How are these conditions treated?

6. Discuss the high-fiber diet. For what conditions might it be used? Compare it with the low-fiber diet. Why is corn on the cob not allowed on the low-fiber diet? Name other foods that are not allowed on the low-fiber diet and tell why they would not be allowed.

7. Discuss ulcerative colitis. What is it? What causes it? How is it treated?

SUGGESTED ACTIVITIES

1. Write a report on one or more of the gastrointestinal disturbances included in this chapter and the dietary treatment of them.

2. Adapt the following menu to suit a client on a minimum-residue diet:

   Orange juice

   Fried egg

   Bacon

   Milk

   Whole wheat toast with butter and marmalade

   Coffee

3. List 10 of your favorite foods. Circle those foods that would not be allowed on a low-residue diet.

REVIEW

Multiple choice. Select the *letter* that precedes the best answer.

1. Dyspepsia
   a. may be an indication of serious gastrointestinal disturbance
   b. is always psychological in origin
   c. cannot be overcome with improved eating habits
   d. is caused by high-fiber foods

2. Hiatal hernia
   a. occurs only in the small intestine
   b. is a typical sign of colon cancer
   c. causes weight loss in all clients
   d. clients may be more comfortable with small, frequent meals

3. Peptic ulcers
   a. can occur in the stomach or the duodenum
   b. cannot be caused by stress
   c. are always treated with aspirin and a low-carbohydrate diet
   d. are usually treated with a low-protein diet

4. Protein foods may be somewhat restricted in cases of peptic ulcers because they
   a. contribute to uremia
   b. contain large amounts of vitamin C
   c. neutralize gastric acid secretions
   d. stimulate gastric acid secretions

5. Diverticulosis
   a. is the inflammation of diverticula
   b. may be initially treated with a clear-liquid diet
   c. may be prevented with a high-fiber diet
   d. occurs in the liver

6. Food residue
   a. is ultimately evacuated in the feces
   b. never leaves the stomach
   c. never leaves the intestines
   d. results from incorrect cooking methods

7. Large amounts of food residue cause
   a. a decrease in fecal matter
   b. an increase in fecal matter
   c. weight gain
   d. diverticulosis

8. The following would be recommended for the high-fiber diet:
   a. pureed pears   c. rice pudding
   b. mashed potatoes   d. bran cereal

9. The following would be allowed on a low-residue diet:
   a. fresh oranges   c. macaroni and cheese
   b. corn on the cob   d. fresh fruit cup

10. Ulcerative colitis
    a. affects the small intestine
    b. always requires parenteral feedings
    c. may be treated with a high-residue diet that is also high in calories and protein
    d. clients may be malnourished

11. The following foods would be recommended for an ulcerative colitis client, provided the client tolerates milk:
    a. fresh grapefruit
    b. chicken salad with chopped celery
    c. mashed potatoes with minced onion
    d. cream of tomato soup with crackers

12. The liver
    a. has no role in metabolism
    b. secretes insulin
    c. converts glucose to glycogen
    d. stores water-soluble vitamins

13. Cirrhosis
    a. is a liver disease characterized by cell loss
    b. is always caused by alcoholism
    c. inevitably results in death
    d. occurs only in the large intestine

14. Ascites
    a. is necessary for regeneration of liver cells
    b. is an accumulation of fluid in the abdomen
    c. requires the addition of sodium and water to the diet
    d. is caused by a shortage of iron

15. Hepatitis
    a. only occurs following exposure to HIV
    b. clients must have very low-carbohydrate diets
    c. is always fatal
    d. may be caused by viruses or toxic agents

16. Gallbladder problems may require
    a. the dietary restriction of dairy products
    b. cholecystectomy
    c. additional fat in the diet
    d. additional protein in the diet

17. Inflammation of the pancreas
    a. is called pancreatitis
    b. is asymptomatic
    c. can require a low-carbohydrate diet
    d. always signifies cancer

CASE IN POINT

GIRISH: LIVING WITH ULCERATIVE COLITIS

Girish is a 35-year-old CPA who owns his own company and in addition owns a metal shop that produces Christmas light displays and subsidizes his income. He has been used to working long hours through the tax season, which goes from January to April. Long hours include overnights and sometimes even 2 days without sleep. For his Christmas lights business, his busy season goes from October to January. He does not remember what he eats; for the most part it is fast foods—the hotter and spicier, the better. He loves Chinese and Japanese foods and has been eating sushi. Lately he has been having bouts of diarrhea, especially after Chinese dinners. His latest episode was very bad. Besides the diarrhea, he was nauseated and had cramps for two nights in a row. He was sure he had a temperature, but he felt too bad to get up and check it. On the second night that he saw blood in the toilet, he resolved to call the doctor. After 3 days of treatment in the hospital, his doctor suggested that Girish plan to follow a low-residue diet when he went home to help prevent further episodes of ulcerative colitis. The doctor requested a consult with a registered dietitian to teach Girish about his new diet.

ASSESSMENT

1. What do you know about Girish that puts him at risk for ulcerative colitis?

2. What symptoms did Girish have?

3. How will the disease alter his life?

4. How significant is this disease?

DIAGNOSIS

5. Write on diagnostic statement for Girish's potential alteration in nutrition.

6. Write a diagnosis for Girish's deficient knowledge related to the new diet.

PLAN/GOAL

7. What dietary goals are measurable and appropriate for Girish?

8. What education goals are specific and measurable for Girish?

IMPLEMENTATION

9. What major topics about ulcerative colitis does Girish need to understand to make necessary dietary changes?

10. What dietary changes does Girish need to learn to control the symptoms?

11. What foods are going to be a problem for Girish?

EVALUATION/OUTCOME CRITERIA

12. At his follow-up doctor's appointment, what is his doctor likely to ask to determine if the plan was successful?

THINKING FURTHER

13. Can ulcerative colitis be cured?

14. What medications are typically used to help manage this disease?

◎ RATE ꝨꞪꞮꞩ PLATE

Girish must follow a low-residue diet. He only needs to follow it until the irritation and inflammation have subsided. Then the diet will be liberalized to include more fiber. Girish decided to take the following for lunch. Rate the plate.

Sandwich
  2 slices whole wheat bread
  3 oz smoked ham
  1 oz Swiss cheese
  Leaf lettuce
  2 slices of tomato
1/2 cup applesauce
1/2 cup mandarin oranges
1/2 cup vanilla pudding
Soda

How did Girish do with his lunch? Is everything low residue? If not, what foods are not, and what would you change them to? Check the Internet for low-residue diets.

CASE IN POINT

IRINA: MANAGING AN ULCER THROUGH DIET

Irina was a 28-year-old Russian-born ballerina. She was the star of the traveling company from Moscow. She had dreamed of the opportunity to tour the United States. Her mother was traveling with her. Her mother was worried Irina's ulcer would act up because of the traveling, strange foods, and pressure that Irina put on herself to be perfect. Irina was also nursing an ankle injury and using ice packs and aspirin after each practice.

After rave reviews on opening night, Irina and her mother were able to relax. During the second week of the tour, Irina complained of burning pain in her chest and abdomen. She thought she was having a heart attack. Irina was in the emergency room that night. The doctor determined it was not a heart attack, as Irina had thought, but it was her ulcer bleeding again. She was admitted to the hospital. When she was discharged, the doctor prescribed famotodine (Pepcid), omeprazole (Prilosec), and a low-residue diet with no stimulants, spices, or alcohol.

ASSESSMENT

1. What put Irina at risk for her ulcer to bleed?
2. What symptoms did she have?
3. What could have been done to prevent this problem?
4. What impact did this health problem have on Irina?

DIAGNOSIS

5. Write two diagnoses for Irina's problems of diet and lack of knowledge.

PLAN/GOAL

6. What goals would be appropriate for Irina's education and nutrition?

IMPLEMENTATION

7. What does Irina need to learn about her new diet?
8. What does she need to learn about her ulcer and her new medications?
9. What challenges will she face in complying with the diet while on tour?
10. Construct a meal that Irina would be likely to find almost everywhere she travels.

11. Instead of aspirin, what can Irina use to treat her ankle injury that will not irritate her ulcer?

EVALUATION/OUTCOME CRITERIA

12. How will Irina's mother, who is supervising her health, know this plan is effective?

◎ RATE THIS PLATE

Irina will need to allow her ulcer to heal. Irina thought a low-residue diet might be difficult to follow and at the same time keep her weight down. She planned the following dinner. Rate the plate.

3 oz chicken breast

Baked potato with butter

1/2 cup broccoli

Salad with cucumber and tomatoes

Decaf iced tea

Did Irina do a good job of planning her dinner? Can she eat everything? If not, what needs to be changed? Check the Internet for low-residue diets.

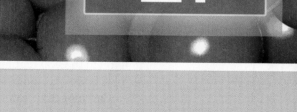

CHAPTER 21

DIET AND CANCER

KEY TERMS

cachexia
carcinogen
chemotherapy
dysphagia
endometrium
genetic predisposition
hyperglycemia
hypoalbuminemia
malignant
metastasize
neoplasia
neoplasm
oncologist
oncology
phytochemicals
resection
xerostomia

OBJECTIVES

After studying this chapter, you should be able to:

↙ Discuss how nutrition can be related to the development or the prevention of cancer

↙ State the effects of cancer on the nutritional status of the host

↙ Describe nutritional problems resulting from the medical treatment of cancer

↙ Describe nutritional therapy for cancer clients

Cancer is the second leading cause of death in the United States. It is a disease characterized by abnormal cell growth and can occur in any organ. In some way the genes lose control of cell growth, and reproduction becomes unstructured and excessive. The developing mass caused by the abnormal growth is called a tumor, or **neoplasm.** Cancer is also called **neoplasia.** Cancerous tumors are **malignant,** affecting the structure and consequently the function of organs. When cancer cells break away from their original site, move through the blood, and spread to a new site, they are said to **metastasize.** The mortality rate for cancer clients is high, but cancer does not always cause death. When it is found early in its development, prompt treatment can eradicate it. **Oncology** is the study of cancer, and a physician who specializes in cancer cases is called an **oncologist.**

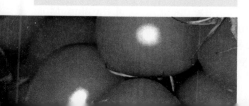

⊙ **neoplasm**
abnormal growth of new tissue

⊙ **neoplasia**
abnormal development of cells

⊙ **malignant**
life-threatening

⊙ **metastasize**
spread of cancer cells from one organ to another

⊙ **oncology**
the study of cancer

⊙ **oncologist**
doctor specializing in the study of cancer

⊙ **carcinogen**
cancer-causing substance

⊙ **genetic predisposition**
inherited tendency

THE CAUSES OF CANCER

The precise etiology of cancer is not known, but it is thought that heredity, viruses, environmental **carcinogens,** and possibly emotional stress contribute to its development. Cancer is not inherited, but some families appear to have a **genetic predisposition** for it. When such seems to be the case, environmental carcinogens should be carefully avoided and medical checkups made regularly. Environmental carcinogens include radiation (whether from X-rays, sun, or nuclear wastes), certain chemicals ingested in food or water, some chemicals that touch the skin regularly, and certain substances that are breathed in, such as tobacco smoke and asbestos.

Carcinogens are not known to cause cancer from one or even a few exposures, but after prolonged exposure. For example, skin cancer does not develop after one sunburn.

CLASSIFICATIONS OF CANCER

There are many types of cancer. A classification system was developed based on the type of cell that produced the cancer. The majority of all cancers fall under four headings: carcinomas, sarcomas, lymphomas, and leukemias.

- Carcinomas involve the epithelial cells (cells lining the body). These include the outer layer of the skin, the membranes lining the digestive tract, the bladder, the womb, and any duct or tube that goes through organs in the body.
- Sarcoma is cancer of the soft tissues of the body, such as muscle, fat, nerves, tendons, blood and lymph vessels, and any other tissues that support, surround, and protect the organs in the body. Soft-tissue sarcomas are uncommon. Sarcomas can also occur in bone rather than soft tissue and primarily in the legs.
- Lymphomas are cancer of the lymphoid tissue. This includes the lymph nodes, bone marrow, spleen, and thymus gland.
- Leukemias develop from the white blood cells and also affect the bone marrow and spleen.

The site where the cancer is located will become part of the diagnosis, such as basal cell carcinoma.

Skin Cancer

Skin cancer is becoming more prevalent. There are three types of skin cancer: basal cell, squamous cell, and melanoma. Basal cell carcinoma is the most common form of skin cancer, affecting the outer skin layer and caused by exposure to sunlight. Those at high risk have fair skin, light hair, and blue, green, or gray eyes and spend considerable leisure time in the sun. Squamous cell carcinoma affects the squamous cells that are in the upper layer of the skin. Most cases arise from chronic exposure to sunlight, but may also occur where skin has been injured—burns, scars, or long-standing sores. Melanoma is the most serious and deadliest form of skin cancer and originates in the cells that pro-

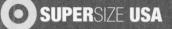

SUPERSIZE **USA**

For the last 15 years, a fast-food lunch of a double cheeseburger, large French fries, and a large soda has been your standard order. You are a meat-and-potatoes person—none of those other vegetables for you. Over the years you have gained considerable weight. How would your eating habits and the weight gain put you at risk for cancer?

High-fat diets have been associated with cancer of the prostate, colon, breast, and uterus. Excessive calories are associated with cancers of the gallbladder and endometrium. Also, you are not getting many vitamins, minerals, and phytonutrients that are protective.

duce the pigment melanin, which colors our skin, hair, and eyes. The majority of melanomas are black or brown, but some melanomas occasionally stop producing pigment and are skin colored, pink, red, or purple. If caught early, melanoma is almost 100% curable; therefore a yearly exam by a dermatologist is recommended for early diagnosis of all skin cancers.

Viral Causes of Cancer

The following viruses have been linked to cancer: Epstein Barr, hepatitis B, and herpes simplex II. Epstein Barr may cause nasopharyngeal cancer, T-cell lymphoma, Hodgkin's disease, and gastric carcinoma. The first anticancer vaccine is now available to prevent hepatitis B and its serious consequences—liver cancer. Herpes simplex II has been associated with cervical and uterine cancer. Cancer research is ongoing and continues in these and other areas.

RELATIONSHIPS OF FOOD AND CANCER

Although the relationships of food and cancer have not been proved, there appear to be associations between them—both good and bad. Certain substances in foods, for example, are thought to be carcinogenic. Nitrites in cured and smoked foods such as bacon and ham can be changed to nitrosamines (carcinogens) during cooking. Regular ingestion of these foods is associated with cancers of the stomach and esophagus. High-fat diets have been associated with cancers of the uterus, breast, prostate, and colon. The regular, excessive intake of calories is associated with cancers of the gallbladder and **endometrium.** People who smoke and drink alcohol immoderately appear to be at greater risk of cancers of the mouth, pharynx, and esophagus than those who do not.

    On the positive side, it is thought that diets high in fiber help to protect against colorectal cancer. Diets containing sufficient amounts of vitamin C–rich foods may protect against cancers of the stomach and esophagus. Diets containing sufficient carotene and vitamin A–rich foods may protect against cancers of the lung, bladder, and larynx. **Phytochemicals,** substances that occur naturally in plant foods, are thought to be anticarcinogenic agents. Examples include flavonoids, phenols, and indoles, and fruits and vegetables

○ **endometrium**
mucous membrane of the uterus

○ **phytochemicals**
substances occurring naturally in plant foods

appear to have an abundance of them. It is advisable to eat 9 or more servings of fruits and vegetables each day, including 2½ cups of vegetables and 2 cups of fruit, on a 2,000-calorie diet. Legumes such as soybeans, dried beans, and lentils contain vitamins, minerals, protein, and fiber and may protect against cancer. High intakes of soy foods are associated with a decreased risk of breast and colon cancer.

Appropriate amounts of protein foods are essential for the maintenance of a healthy immune system. An immune system that has been damaged—possibly through malnutrition—may be a contributing factor in the development of cancer. Excessive protein and fat intake, however, may be a factor in the development of cancer of the colon.

The most important principle is *moderation*. An occasional serving of bacon or buttered popcorn or wine is not likely to cause cancer, but the regular, excessive use of carcinogenic foods may contribute to cancer. Vitamins that are thought to prevent cancer should be ingested in foods that naturally contain them. Excessive intake of vitamin supplements can be harmful. For example, abnormally large amounts of vitamin A can cause bone pain and fragility, hair loss, headaches, and liver and skin problems.

EXPLORING THE WEB

Choose one particular type of cancer. Research the relationship of food to this type of cancer using the Internet. Can alterations in diet prevent, cure, or help combat this type of cancer?

(｜• In The Media

EAT BETTER, EXERCISE MORE

More than 60% of adults and 15% of children in the United States are either overweight or obese, according to the Centers for Disease Control and Prevention. Not only is obesity a major culprit in cancer development and cancer death; it's also a well-known risk factor for heart disease and diabetes. Eating a variety of vegetables, fruits, and whole grains daily, avoiding processed food and high-sugar foods, and being physically active are very important ways we can take control to reduce our risk of cancer and other chronic diseases, according to Marji McCullough with the American Cancer Society (ACS).

(Source: ACS News Center, 2003.)

THE EFFECTS OF CANCER

One of the first indications of cancer may be unexplained weight loss because the tumor cells use for their own metabolism and development the nutrients the host has taken in. The host may suffer from weakness, and anorexia may occur, which compounds the weight loss. The weight loss includes the loss of muscle tissue and **hypoalbuminemia**, and anemia may develop. The sense of taste and smell may be affected. Some foods may taste different: They may not have much taste, or everything may taste the same. Cancer clients, after chemotherapy, may experience a metallic taste when eating protein foods. Many clients complain of food tasting too sweet. Radiation to the neck and head can cause damage to the taste buds and could also affect taste and smell, causing loss of appetite and weight loss.

Cancer clients become satiated earlier than normal, possibly because of decreased digestive secretions. Insulin production may be abnormal, and **hyperglycemia** can delay the stomach's emptying and dull the appetite. Some cancers cause hypercalcemia. If this is chronic, renal stones and impaired kidney function can occur.

⊘ **hypoalbuminemia**
abnormally low amounts of protein in the blood

⊘ **hyperglycemia**
excessive amounts of sugar in the blood

The effects of cancer on the host are particularly determined by the location of a tumor. For example, an esophageal or intestinal tumor can cause blockage in the gastrointestinal tract, causing malabsorption. If the cancer is untreated, the continued anorexia and weight loss will create a state of malnutrition, which in turn can lead to **cachexia** and, ultimately, death.

THE TREATMENT OF CANCER

Medical treatment of cancer can include surgical removal, radiation, **chemotherapy,** or a combination of these methods. These treatments, unfortunately, have side effects that can further undermine the nutritional status of the client. The nutritional effects of surgery in general are discussed in Chapter 22. Cancer surgery, however, can have some additional effects. Surgery on the mouth, for example, might well affect the ability to chew or swallow. Gastric or intestinal **resection** can affect absorption and result in nutritional deficiencies. The removal of the pancreas will result in diabetes mellitus.

Radiation of the head or neck can cause a decrease in salivary secretions, which causes dry mouth (**xerostomia**) and difficulty in swallowing (**dysphagia**). This reduction in saliva also causes tooth decay and sometimes the loss of teeth. Radiation reduces the amount of absorptive tissue in the small intestine. In addition, it can cause bowel obstruction or diarrhea.

Chemotherapy reduces the ability of the small intestine to regenerate absorptive cells, and it can cause hemorrhagic colitis. Both radiation and chemotherapy depress appetite. They may cause nausea, vomiting, and diarrhea leading to fluid and electrolyte imbalances, which can lead to fluid retention. However, when the therapy is completed and the client is able to return to a well-balanced diet, these problems may disappear.

NUTRITIONAL CARE OF THE CANCER CLIENT

The nutrient and calorie needs of the cancer client are actually greater than they were before the onset of the disease. The cancer causes an increase in the metabolic rate, tissue must be rebuilt, and the nutrients lost to the cancer must be replaced. Clients who can maintain their weight or minimize its loss increase their chances of responding to treatment and, thus, their survival. Clients on high-protein and high-calorie diets tolerate the side effects of therapy and higher doses of drugs better than those who cannot eat normally. And those clients who can eat will feel better than those who cannot.

Despite their nutritional needs, however, anorexia is a major problem for cancer clients. It is particularly difficult to combat because cancer clients tend to develop strong food aversions that are thought to be caused by the effects of chemotherapy. Clients receiving chemotherapy near mealtime associate the foods at that meal with the nausea caused by the chemotherapy and often form aversions to those particular foods. These aversions result in limited acceptance of food and contribute further to the client's malnutrition. It is preferable that chemotherapy be withheld for 2 to 3 hours before and after meals. The appetite

---

cachexia
severe malnutrition and body wasting caused by chronic disease

chemotherapy
treatment of diseased tissue with chemicals

resection
reduction

xerostomia
sore, dry mouth caused by a reduction of salivary secretions; may be caused by radiation for treatment of cancer

dysphagia
difficulty swallowing

and absorption usually improve after chemotherapy, so the client can improve nutritional status between chemotherapy treatments.

Obviously, diet plans for cancer clients require special attention. The client's diet history should be taken, as usual, at the outset of hospitalization. Nutrient and calorie needs must be determined by the dietitian, and the client's diet plan should be made in consultation with the client. It is essential that favorite foods, prepared in familiar ways, be included. Nutritious food is useless if the client refuses it.

If chewing is a problem, a soft diet may be helpful. If diarrhea is a problem, a low-residue diet may help (see Chapter 20). Clients should be evaluated inconspicuously.

If the client is scheduled to undergo radiation or chemotherapy, these factors must be included in the diet planning. High-protein and high-calorie diets may be recommended. Energy demands are high because of the hypermetabolic state often caused by cancer. Calorie needs will vary from client to client, but 45 to 50 calories per kilogram of body weight may be recommended.

Carbohydrates and fat will be needed to provide this energy and spare protein for tissue building and the immune system. Clients with good nutritional status will need from 1.0 to 1.2 grams of protein per kilogram of body weight a day. Malnourished clients may need from 1.3 to 2.0 grams of protein per kilogram of body weight a day. Vitamins and minerals are essential for metabolism and tissue maintenance, and they may be supplied in supplemental form. During chemotherapy and radiation therapy, the recommendation is to eliminate vitamin A and vitamin E in supplemental form and in the diet. Intake of these vitamins may prevent cancer cells from self-destructing and work against cancer therapy. Fluids are important to help the kidneys eliminate the metabolic wastes and the toxins from drugs.

The client's food habits may require change if, before the illness, the client had avoided desserts and high-calorie foods to maintain normal weight.

Sometimes clients may be willing to eat foods that are brought from home. Some may find cold foods more appealing than hot foods. Meats may taste bitter so milk, cheese, eggs, and fish may be more appealing. If foods taste sweeter to the cancer client than to the well person, then foods with citric acid may be more acceptable.

Supplementation with high-calorie, high-protein, liquid foods between meals may be useful but should not be used if their consumption reduces the client's appetite at meals.

If the client suffers from dry mouth, salad dressings, gravies, sauces, and syrups appropriately served on foods can be helpful. Several small meals may be better tolerated than three large meals. It is preferable to serve the nutritionally richer meals early in the day because the client is less tired and may have a better appetite at that time. If nausea or pain is a continuous problem, drugs to control the problem, particularly at mealtimes, may be helpful. Although oral feedings are definitely preferred, enteral or total parenteral feedings may become necessary if cachexia is extreme. Sometimes an oral diet with a nutritional supplement may be used in conjunction with total parenteral feeding (see Chapter 22). As the client improves, calorie and nutritional content of the diet should be gradually increased.

SPOTLIGHT on Life Cycle

Children receiving chemotherapy may experience nausea and vomiting, putting their nutrition status at risk. Giving chemotherapy at bedtime may help alleviate nausea and vomiting in children. It may allow them to sleep through the emetic effects. Playing soft music, such as lullabies, or playing a recording of a caregiver singing soft songs is soothing and distracting and may alleviate symptoms of nausea and vomiting.

EXPLORING THE WEB

Search the Internet for the nutritional needs of the chemotherapy client. How do these needs change as the client progresses through therapy? Once therapy is complete, how do the client's nutritional needs change? Plan some sample menus for the chemotherapy client.

CONSIDERATIONS FOR THE HEALTH CARE PROFESSIONAL

It is important that the dietitian establish a good relationship with the client and that constant reminders to eat be avoided. The client usually understands the situation, and such comments are only depressing reminders of the cancer. When appropriate, however, it may be helpful to:

1. Explain why it is important that the client eat
2. Encourage him or her to eat foods he or she enjoys
3. Recommend that he or she avoid eating at the time of day when nausea typically occurs
4. Refrain from serving foods that give off odors that contribute to nausea

If the prognosis for the client is not good, nutritional care will not be as important as the client's feelings and immediate comfort.

SUMMARY

Cancer is a disease characterized by abnormal cell growth. It can strike any body tissue. Energy needs increase because of the hypermetabolic state and the tumor's needs for energy nutrients. At the same time, anorexia occurs in the client. It causes severe wasting, anemia, and various metabolic problems. Treatment of cancer includes surgery, radiation, and chemotherapy. Improving the client's nutritional state is difficult because of the illness and anorexia. Parenteral or enteral nutrition may be necessary.

DISCUSSION TOPICS

1. Discuss cancer, telling what it is and how it affects body functions and nutritional status.
2. Explain why cancer clients lose weight.
3. Why is the anorexia of cancer clients especially difficult to combat? What causes it? Are there any ways it can be prevented?
4. Are supplemental feedings of liquid foods useful in the nutritional rehabilitation of a cancer client? Explain.
5. Discuss enteral and parenteral nutrition in relation to cancer clients.

SUGGESTED ACTIVITIES

1. Invite an oncology nurse to speak to the class.
2. Write an essay about how you might feel if you had just been told that you had a malignant tumor.
3. Plan a day's menus for a cancer client who will eat only the following foods:

Sweetened orange juice	Soda crackers
Bananas	Milkshakes
Applesauce	Eggnog
Cooked pears	Cottage cheese
Puffed rice cereal	Cream of chicken soup
Rice pudding	Poached eggs
White toast with currant jelly	Bouillon

REVIEW

Multiple choice. Select the *letter* that precedes the best answer.

1. Cancer
   a. is characterized by reduced cell growth
   b. growth called a tumor can also be called a neoplasm
   c. inevitably causes death
   d. can metastasize only in clients 50 years and older

2. Carcinogens may include
   a. viruses
   b. certain green vegetables
   c. gluten-containing foods
   d. salmonella

3. Carcinogens
   a. cause cancer after only limited exposure
   b. include some chemical substances
   c. are never found in food or water
   d. are found only in meats and fish

4. Cancer clients
   a. seldom experience weight loss
   b. usually experience an increase in appetite
   c. seldom suffer from anorexia
   d. may suffer from cachexia

5. Radiation and chemotherapy
   a. seldom affect cancer clients' nutritional status
   b. may increase appetite
   c. have no connection to electrolyte imbalance
   d. may create food aversions

6. It is thought that cancer may be caused by
   a. frequent ingestion of smoked meats over a long period
   b. moderate use of alcohol
   c. high-fiber diets
   d. excessive use of vitamin A–rich foods

7. High-fat diets
   a. usually are harmless
   b. have been associated with breast and prostate cancer
   c. provide large amounts of fiber and vitamin C
   d. contribute to the health of the immune system

8. Phytochemicals are
   a. abundantly supplied in fruits and vegetables
   b. widely known carcinogens
   c. most prevalent in carbohydrates and fats
   d. plentifully supplied in proteins

9. High intakes of soy foods
   a. are associated with increased risk of endometrial cancer
   b. are associated with decreased risk of breast and colon cancer
   c. may increase the risk of prostate cancer
   d. are unrelated to the development of cancer

10. Cachexia
    a. is the result of continued anorexia and weight loss
    b. is inevitable in all cancer clients
    c. occurs only in clients with mouth and throat cancers
    d. does not seem to appear in untreated cancer

CASE IN POINT

GRACE: ENCOURAGING APPETITE FOLLOWING A HYSTERECTOMY

Grace has had intermittent vaginal bleeding for 3 months. At first she thought she was experiencing the first signs of menopause. After all, she was 52, and this is to be expected. She called her gynecologist just to be sure and went in for a Pap smear.

Finally, after a week, Grace's doctor called and told her she had suspicious cells on her Pap smear and he was recommending a hysterectomy. Grace had cancer of the uterus. Grace was devastated. Maybe this was why she was losing weight, something she was not trying to do. She had lost 20 pounds in the last 3 months. She had felt tired but dismissed that due to how busy she had been with her job and her quilting.

Grace had her hysterectomy and was informed that the cancer had spread throughout some of her lymph glands. She needed chemotherapy and radiation treatments.

After 5 months of treatment, Grace was continuing to lose weight. She was down 50 pounds. For her that was good since she had been 80 pounds overweight. She had no appetite, and the smell of food made her nauseated. Sometimes she could eat a banana, and other times she could eat a hamburger. But mostly she drank clear broth and ate some crackers.

ASSESSMENT

1. What do you know about Grace?
2. What barriers does she have to balance nutrition?
3. What resources does she have to overcome these barriers?
4. How important is her nutrition to her current health? How about to her future radiation treatments?

DIAGNOSIS

5. Write a diagnosis about potential alteration in nutrition.
6. Write a diagnosis about her deficient knowledge.

PLAN/GOAL

7. What is the immediate goal for Grace's nutrition?
8. What is the long-term goal?

IMPLEMENTATION

9. What does Grace need to learn?
10. List four strategies to increase what Grace eats at home.
11. How important is her nutrition to her healing?
12. What can a home health care nurse do to enhance Grace's nutrition? What can a dietitian do?

EVALUATION/OUTCOME CRITERIA

13. What can the home health nurse observe and measure as evidence of the success of the plan?

THINKING FURTHER

14. Why is it important to use nutrition to reduce your risk of cancer?

◎ RATE Ⅲ PLATE

Grace is having trouble maintaining her weight. The dietitian recommends to the physician that an antinausea medication and an appetite stimulant may be helpful. Grace is willing to try anything. She is willing to try hard to follow the dietitian's recommendations. This is the meal she planned. Rate the plate.

1/2 of a turkey sandwich on white bread with 1 tsp mayonnaise

Banana

4 oz cold supplement

Sorbet

What was the dietitian thinking when she helped Grace plan this meal? Why only half a sandwich? Will this be adequate nutritionwise?

CASE IN POINT

CHARLES: MANAGING DIET DURING CHEMOTHERAPY

Charles was a 54-year-old Asian male receiving chemotherapy for cancer. He was about to begin round four of seven rounds of chemotherapy. So far, he had experienced fear and apprehension but had little change in his weight. This pleased him. The oncologist warned Charles that it was common

that round four was "a little bit rougher" than the previous three rounds. The doctor ordered ondansetron (Zofran), an appetite stimulant, and a liquid supplement between meals. He requested a weekly assessment by a registered dietitian to help Charles maintain his weight.

ASSESSMENT

1. What has Charles's response to the chemotherapy been so far?
2. What does the doctor suspect will happen to Charles's nutrition during round four?
3. What can the dietitian assess to measure how Charles is eating?

DIAGNOSIS

4. Write a diagnostic statement describing the nutrition problems Charles could have with chemotherapy.

PLAN/GOAL

5. What is the major nutrition goal for Charles?
6. What is the rationale for aggressive proactive nutrition between rounds of chemotherapy?
7. What does Charles need to know related to the nutritional demands of ongoing chemotherapy?

IMPLEMENTATION

8. List four strategies the dietitian can use to encourage Charles to eat.
9. List three strategies that his family can use to help him eat.
10. If Charles eats only 5% to 10% of his normal food volume, what foods should be a priority? How are fluids important?
11. In preparation for round five of chemotherapy, what could Charles do to enhance his nutrition once his appetite returns?
12. How can other cancer clients undergoing chemotherapy and their families help Charles?

13. How can the Internet be of help? Check out the American Cancer Society at www.cancer.org.

EVALUATION/OUTCOME CRITERIA

14. How would the doctor evaluate the success of the diet plan?

THINKING FURTHER

15. Why is nutrition so important in the successful treatment of cancer?

◎ RATE THIS PLATE

Charles has done a good job of maintaining his weight, and his physician does not want him to backslide. Charles will be seeing the dietitian weekly for weight management and for a review of his recorded dietary intake. Can Charles continue to maintain his weight? Rate the plate.

3 oz sirloin

Mashed potatoes

Sauteed mixed vegetables

Spinach salad with dried cranberries

Light Vidalia onion salad dressing

Brownie

Clients with cancer need a lot of protein because the cancer "eats" protein. Has Charles planned enough protein, or could he have done better by adding just a few foods? What could he add to the existing menu to increase his protein intake?

DIET AND CLIENTS WITH SPECIAL NEEDS

OBJECTIVES

After studying this chapter, you should be able to:

- Describe the body's reactions to stress and relate them to nutrition
- Explain the special dietary needs of surgical and burn clients
- Discuss enteral and parenteral nutrition
- Explain the special dietary needs of clients with fever and infection
- Explain the special dietary needs of AIDS clients

Normally, the human body operates in a state of **homeostasis.** When the body experiences the trauma of surgery, severe burns, or infections, this balance is upset. The body reacts in an attempt to restore itself to homeostasis.

During its response to physical stress, the body signals the endocrine system, which activates a self-protective, **hypermetabolic** response. This increases energy output. The intensity of the response depends on the severity of the condition.

Catabolism occurs, causing the rapid breakdown of energy reserves to provide glucose and other substances necessary for the anabolic phase of wound healing and tissue maintenance. Proteins, fats, and minerals are lost in the catabolic phase just when there is an increased need for them to rebuild tissue. When the condition includes **hemorrhage** and vomiting, these losses are compounded.

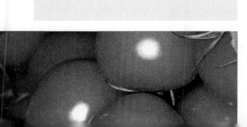

○ **homeostasis**
state of physical balance; stable condition

○ **hypermetabolic**
higher than normal rate of metabolism

○ **hemorrhage**
unusually heavy bleeding

Sufficient nutrients, fluids, and calories are required as soon as possible to replace the losses, build and repair tissue, and return the body to homeostasis. Obviously, nutrition plays an important role in the lives of clients undergoing surgery or of those who suffer from burns or infections.

THE SURGICAL CLIENT
Presurgery Nutritional Care

Surgery stresses the client regardless of whether it is elective or not. If the surgery is elective, the client's nutritional status should be evaluated before surgery; and if improvement is needed, it should be undertaken immediately. A good nutritional status before surgery enhances recovery. A nutritional assessment of the client before surgery will be helpful to the dietitian in providing nutrition that will be accepted by the client after surgery, when appetite is poor.

Improvement of nutritional status will usually mean providing extra protein, carbohydrates, vitamins, and minerals. The extra protein is needed for wound healing, tissue building, and blood regeneration. Extra carbohydrates will be converted to glycogen and stored to help provide energy after surgery, when needs are high and when clients may be unable to eat normally. The B vitamins are needed for the increased metabolism, vitamins A and C and zinc for wound healing, vitamin D for the absorption of calcium, and vitamin K for proper clotting of the blood. Iron is necessary for blood building, calcium and phosphorus for bones, and the other minerals for maintenance of acid-base, electrolyte, and fluid balance in the body.

In cases of overweight, improved nutritional status includes weight reduction before surgery whenever possible. Excess fat is a surgical hazard because the extra tissue increases the chances of infection, and fatty tissue tends to retain the anesthetic longer than other tissue.

Many physicians order their clients to be NPO (nothing by mouth) after midnight the night before surgery. Withholding food ensures that the stomach contains no food, which could be regurgitated and then **aspirated** into the lungs during surgery. If there is to be gastrointestinal surgery, a low-residue diet may be ordered for a few days before surgery (see Chapter 20). This is intended to reduce intestinal residue.

Postsurgery Nutritional Care

The postsurgery diet is intended to provide calories and nutrients in amounts sufficient to fulfill the client's increased metabolic needs and to promote healing and subsequent recovery. In general, during the 24 hours immediately following major surgery, most clients will be given intravenous solutions only. These solutions will contain water, 5% to 10% dextrose, electrolytes, vitamins, and medications as needed. The maximum calories supplied by them is about 400 to 500 calories per 24-hour period. The estimated daily calorie requirement for adults after surgery is 35 to 45 calories per kilogram of body weight. A 110-pound individual would require at least 2,000 calories a day. Obviously, until the client can take food, there will be a considerable calorie

○ **aspirated**
inhaled or suctioned

deficit each day. Body fat will be used to provide energy and to spare body protein, but the calorie intake must be increased to meet energy demands as soon as possible.

Because protein losses following surgery can be significant and because protein is especially needed then to rebuild tissue, control edema, avoid shock, resist infection, and transport fats, a high-protein diet of 80 to 100 grams a day may be recommended. In addition, extra minerals and vitamins are needed. When **peristalsis** returns, ice chips may be given; and if they are tolerated, a clear liquid diet can follow. (Peristalsis is evidenced by the presence of bowel sounds.)

Normally in postoperative cases, clients proceed from the clear-liquid diet to the regular diet. Sometimes this change is done directly and sometimes by way of the full-liquid diet, depending on the client and the type of surgery. The average client will be able to take food within 1 to 4 days after surgery. If the client cannot take food then, parenteral or enteral feeding may be necessary.

Sometimes following gastric surgery, **dumping syndrome** occurs within 15 to 30 minutes after eating. This is characterized by dizziness, weakness, cramps, vomiting, and diarrhea. It is caused by food moving too quickly from the stomach into the small intestine. It occurs secondary to an increase in insulin, in anticipation of the increase in food, which never comes.

To prevent dumping syndrome, the diet should be high in protein and fat, and carbohydrates should be restricted. Foods should contain little fiber or concentrated sugars and only limited amounts of starch. Complex carbohydrates are gradually reintroduced. Gradual reintroduction is recommended because carbohydrates leave the stomach faster than do proteins and fats. Fluids should be limited to 4 ounces at meals, or restricted completely, so as not to fill up the stomach with fluids instead of nutrients. They can be taken 30 minutes after meals. The total daily food intake may be divided and served as several small meals rather than the usual three meals in an attempt to avoid overloading the stomach. Some clients do not tolerate milk well after gastric surgery, so its inclusion in the diet will depend on the client's tolerance.

The food habits of the postoperative client should be closely observed because they will affect recovery. When the client's appetite fails to improve, the physician and the dietitian should be notified, and efforts should be made to offer nutritious foods and supplements (either in liquid or solid form) that the client will ingest. The client should be encouraged to eat and to eat slowly to avoid swallowing air, which can cause abdominal distension and pain.

THE CLIENT RECEIVING ENTERAL NUTRITION

The term **enteral nutrition** means the forms of feeding that bring nutrients directly into the digestive tract (Figure 22-1). Oral feeding is the usual method and should be used whenever possible. When clients cannot or will not take food by mouth, but their gastrointestinal tract is working, they will be given **tube feedings (TF)**. Sometimes this may be necessary because of unconsciousness, surgery, stroke, severe malnutrition, or extensive burns.

Usually, for periods that do not exceed 6 weeks, tube feeding is administered through a **nasogastric (NG) tube** inserted through the nose and into the stomach or small intestine. When the percutaneous endoscopic gastrostomy

peristalsis
muscular contractions of the intestine

dumping syndrome
nausea and diarrhea caused by food moving too quickly from the stomach to the small intestine

enteral nutrition
feeding by tube directly into the client's digestive tract

tube feeding (TF)
feeding by tube directly into the stomach or intestine or via a vein

nasogastric (NG) tube
tube leading from the nose to the stomach for tube feeding

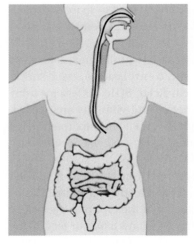

Nasogastric Route

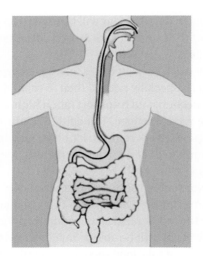

Nasoduodenal Route

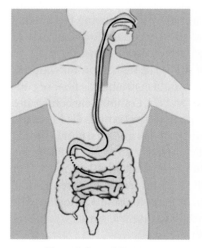

Nasojejunal Route

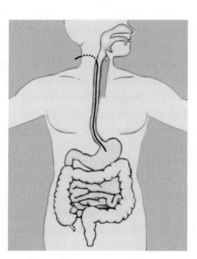

Esophagostomy Route

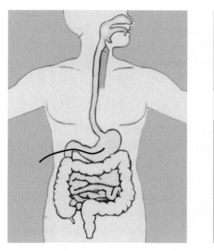

Gastrostomy Route

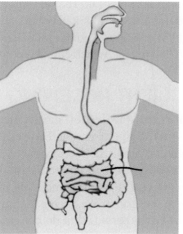

Jejunostomy Route

Figure 22-1 *Enteral feeding routes.*

(PEG) tube cannot be placed in the nose or when tube feedings will be required for more than 6 weeks, an opening called an ostomy is surgically created into the esophagus (an esophagostomy), the stomach **(gastrostomy)**, or the intestine **(jejunostomy)**.

The tubes used for these feedings are soft, flexible, and as small as they can be and still allow the feeding to pass through. Although some tubes are weighted to keep them in place in the stomach or intestine, the use of weighted tubes has not been proved to be better than unweighted.

Numerous commercial formulas are available, with varying types and amounts of nutrients. Clients who are able to digest and absorb nutrients can be given **polymeric formulas** (1–2 calories/ml) containing intact proteins, carbohydrates, and fats that require digestion. Clients who have limited ability to digest or absorb nutrients may be given **elemental** or **hydrolyzed formulas** (1.0 calories/ml) that contain the products of digestion of proteins, carbohydrates, and fats, and are lactose-free. **Modular formulas** (3.8–4.0 calories/ml) can be used as supplements to other formulas or for developing customized formulas for certain clients (such as those with extensive wound-healing needs). The use of modular formulas has been decreasing due to the development of high-protein formulas. Disease-specific formulas have been developed to be used in the acute setting and for a short period of time. Clients admitted to the hospital with renal failure, respiratory failure, or liver failure have been shown to benefit from these specialized formulas.

There are three methods for administering tube feedings: continuous, intermittent, and bolus. Intermittent can mean to only administer tube feeding at night, with solid foods eaten during the day. If there is a food-drug interaction, such as with phenytoin (Dilantin), the TF should be stopped 1 hour before and be restarted 1 hour after administration of the medication via tube.

Daily calorie needs of the client are usually divided into six servings per day (not to exceed 400 cc at a time). These feedings are given over a 15-minute time span and followed by 25 to 60 ml of water, hence the term *bolus*. This method is usually done when a client has a PEG tube, but it could also be done with an NG tube.

Usually the feedings are administered by a pump. This means the feeding is continuous during a 16- to 24-hour period. Sometimes the formula is given at half strength at a rate of from 30 to 50 ml per hour. This rate may be increased by about 25 ml every 4 hours until tolerance has been established. Once the client tolerates the half-strength formula, a full-strength formula is initiated at the appropriate rate. When clients are ready to return to oral feedings, the transfer must be done gradually.

gastrostomy
opening created by the surgeon directly into the stomach for enteral nutrition

jejunostomy
opening created by the surgeon into the intestine for enteral nutrition

polymeric formulas
commercially prepared formulas for tube feedings that contain intact proteins, carbohydrates, and fats that require digestion

elemental formulas
those formulas containing products of digestion of proteins, carbohydrates, and fats; also called hydrolyzed formulas

hydrolyzed formulas
contain products of digestion of proteins, carbohydrates, and fats; also called elemental formulas; used for clients who have difficulty digesting food

modular formulas
made by combining specific nutrients

EXPLORING THE WEB

Search the Web for information on the various types of enteral nutrition formulas discussed in the text. What are the makeups of these formulas? Are any nutrients lacking in these formulas? Is there the potential for side effects of or allergies to these formulas that clients should be aware of and monitored for?

Possible Complications with Enteral Nutrition

◔ **osmolality**

number of particles per kilogram of
solution; solutions with high osmolality
exert more pressure than do those with
fewer particles

The **osmolality** of a liquid substance means the number of particles per kilogram of solution. Solutions with more particles (high osmolality) exert more pressure than solutions with fewer particles. Solutions with high osmolality attract water from nearby fluids that contain lower osmolality. When a formula with high osmolality reaches the intestine, the body may draw fluid from the blood to dilute the formula. This process can cause weakness and diarrhea in the client. However, diarrhea should be attributed to the tube feeding only when all other causes have been ruled out. Liquid medications containing sorbitol or *Clostridium difficile* (C-dif) (the bacterium that causes dysentery) are two possible causes of diarrhea.

Aspiration can occur (some of the formula enters the lung), causing the client to develop pneumonia. The tube may become clogged, or the client may pull the tube out. The placement of the feeding tube should be checked with an X-ray to decrease the possibility of aspiration. Before beginning the tube feeding, the health care provider must administer the flush solution according to the physician's order and raise the head of the bed. If the feeding is continuous, then the head of the bed needs to remain elevated. Some facilities, to verify correct placement of the NG tube in the stomach, will check the gastric pH before each use.

Obviously, clients requiring tube feeding need a great deal of patience and understanding. They have been deprived of a basic pleasure of life—eating. They may also be uncomfortable and apprehensive.

THE CLIENT RECEIVING PARENTERAL NUTRITION

◔ **parenteral nutrition**

nutrition provided via a vein

Parenteral nutrition is the provision of nutrients intravenously. It is used if the gastrointestinal tract is not functional or if normal feeding is not adequate for the client's needs. It can be used alone or as part of a dietary plan that includes oral or tube feeding as well. When parenteral nutrition is used to provide total nutrition, it is called total parenteral nutrition (TPN) or hyperalimentation.

Nutrient solutions are prescribed by the physician and dietitian and are prepared by a pharmacist. They can be administered via a central vein or, for a period of 2 weeks or less, a **peripheral vein.** Typically, a dextrose–amino acid–fat solution is given. This solution is not combined until just before entry into the vein because the components do not form a stable solution.

◔ **peripheral vein**

a vein that is near the surface of the skin

Total parenteral nutrition that is required for an extended period is provided via a central vein. A catheter is surgically inserted, under sterile conditions, by a physician. It is inserted into a subclavian vein or the superior vena cava. The vena cava is used because the high blood flow there facilitates the quick dilution of the highly concentrated TPN solution. Dilution reduces the possibility of **phlebitis** and **thrombosis.**

◔ **phlebitis**

inflammation of a vein

◔ **thrombosis**

blockage, as a blood clot

When parenteral nutrition is no longer necessary, the client must be transferred gradually to an oral diet. Sometimes clients are given tube feeding before oral feeding as they are weaned from TPN.

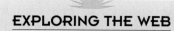

EXPLORING THE WEB

Search the Web for additional information on parenteral nutrition. What types of formulas are used for TPN? Are there nutrients lacking from this form of nutritional support? What possible side effects or allergies should the client be monitored for?

Possible Complications with Parenteral Nutrition

Infection can occur at the site of the catheter and enter the bloodstream, causing an infection of the blood called **sepsis**. Bacterial or fungal infections can develop in the solution if it is unrefrigerated for over 24 hours. Abnormal electrolyte levels may develop, as can phlebitis or blood clots. Careful monitoring of the client is essential.

sepsis
infection of the blood

THE CLIENT WITH BURNS

In cases of serious burns, the loss of skin surface leads to enormous losses of fluids, electrolytes, and proteins. Water moves from other tissues to the burn site in an effort to compensate for the loss, but this only compounds the problem. This fluid loss can reduce the blood volume and thus blood pressure, as well as urine output.

Fluids and electrolytes are replaced by intravenous therapy immediately to prevent shock. Glucose is not included in these fluids for the first 2 or 3 days after the burn, because it could cause hyperglycemia.

The hypermetabolic state after a serious burn continues until the skin is largely healed, so there is an enormous increase in energy needed for the healing process. Calorie requirements are based on weight (size) and the total burned surface, including depth of burns. Protein needs can be as high as 1.5 to 3.0 or more grams per kilogram of weight, and fat intake, 15% to 20% of nonprotein calories. A high-protein, high-calorie diet is used. There is an increased need for vitamin C and zinc for healing and B vitamins for the metabolism of the extra nutrients. Vitamin A is important for the immune system and the epithelial tissues.

Also, it is essential that severely burned clients have sufficient fluids to help the kidneys hold the unusual load of wastes in solution and to replace those lost.

If the client is able to eat, oral feedings are advisable. Liquid commercial formulas may be used at first, and solid food may be added during the second week after the burn. If the client is unable to eat, tube feedings should be started immediately. In some cases, parenteral feeding is required. The foods served should be those the client likes and is willing to eat. To determine this, a registered dietitian must perform an individualized assessment for each burn victim. The best assessment of the adequacy of the nutrients provided is wound healing.

Burn clients need a great deal of encouragement. They are in pain, worried about disfigurement, and know they face a long, costly, and painful hospital stay with the possibility of surgery.

THE CLIENT WITH INFECTION

Fever typically accompanies an infection. Fevers and infections may be acute or chronic. Fever is a hypermetabolic state in which each degree of fever on the Fahrenheit scale raises the basal metabolic rate (BMR) by 7%. If extra calories are not provided during fever, the body first uses its supply of glycogen, then its stored fat, and finally its own muscle tissue for energy.

Protein intake should be increased because of infections (sepsis). Amounts required need to be individualized. Protein is needed to replace body tissue and to produce **antibodies** to fight the infection. Minerals are needed to help build and repair body tissue and to maintain acid-base, electrolyte, and fluid balance. Extra calories are needed for the increased metabolic rate. Extra vitamins are also necessary for the increased metabolic rate and to help fight the infection causing the fever. Extra liquid is needed to replace that lost through perspiration, vomiting, or diarrhea, which often accompany infection.

Clients with fever usually have very poor appetites, but they will often accept ice water, fruit juice, and carbonated beverages. Some will accept bouillon or consommé.

Usually, the diet during fever and infection progresses from the liquid to the regular diet, with frequent, small meals recommended. It should be high in protein, calories, and vitamins. In some cases, parenteral and enteral feedings are necessary.

THE CLIENT WITH AIDS

A virus is a microscopic parasite that invades and lives in or on, and thus infects, another organism, called the host. The virus obtains nourishment from the host and duplicates itself countless times. There are many viruses that infect humans. Some, like those of the common cold, make the host only mildly ill. Others like the **human immunodeficiency virus (HIV)**, are deadly.

HIV invades the T cells, which are white blood cells that protect the body from infections. When the T cells cannot function normally, the body has no resistance to opportunistic infections. **Opportunistic infections** are caused by other microorganisms that are present but do not affect people who have healthy immune systems.

Persons infected with HIV are said to be HIV positive. HIV infection ultimately leads to **acquired immune deficiency syndrome (AIDS)**, which is incurable and fatal.

HIV can affect anyone exposed to it, regardless of age, sex, or physical condition. HIV infection cannot be cured, but it can be prevented. The virus is not transmitted through casual contact, such as shaking hands. It is transmitted via body fluids, specifically:

- Through sexual contact
- By transfusions of contaminated blood
- By use of contaminated needles during ear piercing, tattooing, acupuncture, or injection of illegal drugs
- By infected mothers to their fetuses during pregnancy or to their infants during lactation

⟳ antibodies
substances produced by the body in reaction to foreign substance; neutralize toxins from foreign bodies

⟳ human immunodeficiency virus (HIV)
a virus that weakens the body's immune system and ultimately leads to AIDS

⟳ opportunistic infections
caused by microorganisms that are present but that do not normally affect people with healthy immune systems

⟳ acquired immune deficiency syndrome (AIDS)
caused by the human immunodeficiency virus (HIV), which weakens the body's immune system, leaving it susceptible to fatal infections

Table 22-1 *Causes of Nutrient Loss in AIDS Clients*
• Anorexia • Cancer • Diarrhea • Increased metabolism due to fever • Certain medications • Malabsorption caused by cancer or diarrhea • Protein energy malnutrition

Progression from HIV Infection to AIDS

There are essentially three stages in the progress of AIDS. The first stage begins soon after exposure to HIV, when the body produces antibodies in an attempt to destroy the virus. At that time, some people may experience a few days of symptoms resembling mild flu. Others may have no symptoms. At this point and thereafter, the infected person will test positive to HIV and will be among those called HIV positive. Unless tested, the individual will feel normal and will have no idea that he or she is HIV positive for a period ranging from a few months to 10 years.

During this period, the virus is incubating. Viral cells are multiplying in the tonsils, adenoid glands, and spleen, gradually taking over the body's T cells.

Anyone suspecting that he or she has been exposed to HIV should be tested as soon as possible. An ever-growing number of medications are available that may increase the time the virus needs to multiply and, thus, may prolong the life of the host.

The second stage of HIV is known as the *ARC period. ARC* stands for AIDS-related complex. The body's immune system has by this point grown weaker, and symptoms and opportunistic infections occur. There may be fatigue, skin rashes, headache, night sweats, diarrhea, weight loss, oral lesions or thrush (candidiasis, a fungal infection of the mouth), cough, sore throat, fevers, or shortness of breath (Table 22-1).

The third and end stage of HIV infection is known as AIDS (acquired immune deficiency syndrome). It is manifested by a very low T-cell count, which makes it impossible for the body to fight off infections. Tuberculosis or **Kaposi's sarcoma** commonly develops at this point. As the T-cell count continues to diminish, other parasites invade and, ultimately, overwhelm the body, causing death.

Kaposi's sarcoma
type of cancer common to AIDS clients

The Relationship of HIV Infection and Nutrition

A healthful diet is essential for a healthy immune system, which may delay the onset of AIDS. Persons diagnosed as being HIV positive should have a baseline nutrition and diet assessment by a registered dietitian. Unhealthful eating habits can be corrected at an early stage of the disease, and future nutritional needs can be explained.

As the condition progresses, the client begins to experience the physical problems previously listed. Infections increase the metabolic rate and

Table 22-2 Causes of Anorexia among AIDS Clients	
Medications	Cause nausea, vomiting
Oral infections	Diminish saliva, alter taste, cause mouth pain
Altered taste	Changes or exaggerates flavors
Fever	Depresses appetite
Pain	Depresses appetite
Depression	Depresses appetite
Dysphagia	Makes swallowing difficult
Dementia	May cause client to forget to eat

nutrient and calorie needs and, at the same time, decrease the appetite and often the body's ability to absorb nutrients. Medications may further reduce the appetite and cause nausea. When there are oral infections, taste may change, and swallowing can become painful. Anorexia, or loss of appetite, commonly occurs (Table 22-2).

AIDS clients experience serious protein-energy malnutrition (PEM) and, thus, body wasting. This may be referred to as HIV wasting syndrome, which results in **hypoalbuminemia** and weight loss. The immune system is further damaged by insufficient amounts of protein and calories, thus hastening death.

Problems Related to Feeding AIDS Clients

Just when an AIDS client most needs a nutrient- and calorie-rich diet, he or she is most apt to refuse it. In some cases, it may be useful to discuss nutritional care with the client. When possible, medications should be given after meals to reduce the chance of nausea. Sores in the mouth or esophagus can make eating painful, and soft foods may be better tolerated than others. Taste can be affected by the disease, so spicy, highly acidic, extremely hot, or extremely cold foods may be rejected. Frequent small meals and, sometimes, liquid supplements may be helpful. Additional sugar and flavoring may increase the acceptability of liquid supplements. Because of the nausea and diarrhea, sufficient fluids are essential. If the client has difficulty swallowing or simply cannot eat, tube feeding may be imperative. If the tube causes pain or if severe diarrhea or malabsorption is present, parenteral nutrition may be necessary.

The client should be helped to eat as much as possible, especially on "good" days (Table 22-3). Clients may suffer from pain and depression, and they may worry about finances and what people think of them. These factors can further diminish their appetites, but positive discussions can help.

Neurological impairment usually occurs in varying degrees in AIDS clients and may cause confusion and dysphagia. In such cases, meal trays should be kept simple, the consistency of food modified to best suit the client, and special utensils provided if needed.

Some clients may want to try nontraditional diets, thinking they will help or even cure them. These clients need to be made aware of any potentially harmful effects from such diets. In some cases, the idea of improvement may help the client's appetite.

⊙ **hypoalbuminemia**
abnormally low amounts of protein in the blood

Table 22-3 *Methods To Improve the Appetite of an AIDS Client*
• Give medications *after* meals
• Offer soft food
• Avoid spicy, acidic, and extremely hot or cold foods
• Serve frequent, small meals
• Add sugar and flavorings to liquid supplements
• Take advantage of the "good" days and offer any food the client tolerates
• Talk with the client to help ease concerns about finances, family, and friends

Those clients who will benefit no further from either medication or nutrition can still be comforted by the health care professional or hospice nurse who shows support, understanding, and respect for them.

CONSIDERATIONS FOR THE HEALTH CARE PROFESSIONAL

Clients who fall within the categories of conditions discussed in this chapter can be a challenge for the health care professional. Surgical clients may seem to make excessive demands due to pain, uncertainty, or anxiety. Clients suffering burns may require extreme patience and the ability of the health care provider to detach emotionally. Clients with fatal infections will require extra time and attention. Clients receiving tube feedings or some medications may suffer from frequent diarrhea and require total client care.

In each of these cases, the health care professional can help herself or himself as well as the client by thinking positively and using therapeutic communication with the client and family.

SUMMARY

Surgery, burns, fevers, and infections are traumas that cause the body to respond hypermetabolically. This response creates the need for additional nutrients at the same time that the injury causes a loss of nutrients. Care must be taken to provide extra fluid, proteins, calories, vitamins, minerals, and carbohydrates as needed in these situations. When surgery is elective, nutritional status should be improved before surgery, if necessary. When food cannot be taken orally, enteral or parenteral nutrition may be used.

DISCUSSION TOPICS

1. Describe the body's reaction to trauma and how nutrition is related to it.

2. Why are extra nutrients needed during trauma?

3. When might surgery be elective?

4. In what ways might a diet history of a presurgical client be helpful?

5. Explain why a burn client needs extra protein. What happens when the extra protein is not provided?

6. Why does a surgical client need extra minerals?

7. Why must a client's stomach be empty at the time of surgery?

8. Explain why intravenous dextrose solutions are not sufficient to fulfill nutritional requirements after surgery.

9. Describe dumping syndrome, and tell how it may be alleviated.

10. Describe parenteral nutrition. What is it? How is it delivered? What are some dangers related to it?

SUGGESTED ACTIVITIES

1. Ask a certified nutrition support dietitian (CNSD) to visit the class and discuss tube feedings, telling why and when they are used and problems associated with them.

2. Invite a nurse from a local hospital to discuss burns and the nutritional challenges facing clients with burns.

3. If a class member has experienced any of the traumas discussed in this chapter, ask that person to recount it and describe her or his reactions, appetite, and recovery.

4. Role-play a situation in which a client is 5 days postsurgery and cannot eat, and the nurse is trying to convince her to eat.

REVIEW

Multiple choice. Select the *letter* that precedes the best answer.

1. Trauma
   a. can be described as injury
   b. causes a hypometabolic response in the body
   c. usually decreases the body's need for protein
   d. has no relation to nutrition

2. During trauma, there is usually
   a. reduced need for protein and minerals
   b. a hypermetabolic response in the body
   c. only minor changes in nutritional requirements
   d. a decreased need for calories

3. Wound healing, tissue building, and blood regeneration all require
   a. extra fat
   b. extra cholesterol
   c. reduced calorie intake
   d. protein

4. Intravenous solutions
   a. rarely contain vitamins
   b. usually contain cellulose
   c. are usually given after surgery
   d. provide 2,000 calories per day

5. Protein is needed to
   a. provide calories
   b. resist infection
   c. control fat metabolism during trauma
   d. kill bacteria

6. It would not be surprising for TPN to be used in the treatment of
   a. a fractured hip
   b. third-degree burns over a large part of the client's body
   c. a broken leg
   d. appendicitis

7. Dumping syndrome is characterized by
   a. migraine headache
   b. hypertension and tremors
   c. reduced clotting time
   d. dizziness and cramps

8. TPN for more than 2 weeks is given through
   a. a nasogastric tube
   b. a peripheral vein in the ankle
   c. the superior vena cava
   d. an esophagostomy

9. Severely burned clients will need
   a. to replace protein and fluids
   b. extra amounts of glucose the first 2 to 3 days after the burn
   c. reduced amounts of liquid
   d. a low-protein, low-calorie diet

10. Fever
    a. creates a need for extra calories
    b. clients have enormous appetites
    c. clients experience reduced metabolic rate
    d. clients should be kept on a low-calorie diet

CASE IN POINT

HONG-TSE: SURVIVING SEVERE BURNS

Hong-Tse is a 15-year-old boy who was helping his father in the yard during fall cleanup. They had raked leaves and trimmed bushes and picked up a lot of yard debris. To get rid of this trash they decided to burn it in a 50-gallon trash can. Jing-Li, Hong-Tse's father, got the lighter fluid and some matches to ignite the debris. No one can explain what happened next, but Hong-Tse caught on fire. In the hospital Jing-Li learned that Hong-Tse had third-degree burns over 78% of his body. Fortunately, Hong-Tse's face and neck were spared from the flames. Narcotics are controlling his pain, and he is being watched closely for hypotension, kidney failure, and electrolyte imbalances.

ASSESSMENT

1. What do you know about Hong-Tse's need for fluids?
2. What do you know about Hong-Tse's need for electrolyte balance?
3. What would help you identify Hong-Tse's health before his accident?

DIAGNOSIS

4. Write a diagnostic statement describing the problems Hong-Tse could have with his severe burns.
5. Write a diagnostic statement about the risk of infection for Hong-Tse.

PLAN/GOAL

6. What is the overall nutritional goal for Hong-Tse?

IMPLEMENTATION

7. What strategies can the dietitian use to assure proper nutritional balance for Hong-Tse?
8. If Hong-Tse would require tube feedings, what can the dietitian expect to happen? What strategies can the dietitian use to prevent side effects of tube feedings?

9. What categories of food are priorities for Hong-Tse right now?

EVALUATION/OUTCOME CRITERIA

10. What criteria could be used to evaluate the plan?

THINKING FURTHER

11. Why is nutrition so critical in the treatment of the client with burns?

◎ RATE THIS PLATE

Hong-Tse is in the burn unit of the Shriners Hospital in Ohio. He is losing a lot of fluid, and immediately upon arrival, a feeding tube was inserted for nutrition. He is receiving fluid from IVs. The physician started the following tube feeding: A 1-calorie/ml product such as Nutren 1.0 or Jevity 1.0.

Is this the best product for the client with severe burns? What nutrient would this client need for building and repairing his burns? Search the Internet for Nestle and Ross nutritional products to determine which product would be best for the client.

CASE IN POINT

KEVIN: LIVING WITH HIV

Kevin was a 32-year-old Caucasian corporate nurse. He was 6 feet tall and weighed 185 pounds. He loved what he did, training sales reps for a pharmaceutical company. He had an active social life and just enjoyed life in general. When he was diagnosed with HIV, he was devastated.

He was an only child of a widowed mother. He had grown up on a farm in a small rural town. His mother always boasted of his nursing success and her pride in him and his career. He didn't want to embarrass or hurt his mother. When he finally told her about his HIV status, she just cried and hugged him and told him she loved him.

Within months of his revelation to his mother, his T-cell counts dropped to the lowest level yet. He was having a hard time shaking his first episode of pneumonia. His mother came to take care of him. She cooked all his favorite foods, sometimes serving him four desserts for dinner. She always watched that he took his medications as prescribed.

Kevin's mother consulted with the hospital dietitian to learn how she could help her son, who now weighed about 120 pounds.

ASSESSMENT

1. What do you know about Kevin and his nutrition?
2. What barriers to good nutrition does he have?
3. What resources does he have?
4. Why would his mother talk to a dietitian?
5. How important is nutrition to health maintenance in an HIV-positive person?

DIAGNOSIS

6. Write a diagnostic statement describing the reasons Kevin was unable to remain well nourished.

PLAN/GOAL

7. What is the priority goal for Kevin?

IMPLEMENTATION

8. What strategies can the dietitian suggest?
9. What can she teach Kevin's mother about HIV and nutrition?
10. What foods are a priority during his active infection? Why is protein so important?
11. How could appetite stimulants help?
12. How could timing medications between meals help?
13. How could friends help, especially at meals? What about local AIDS network volunteers?

14. How could the information at the AIDS Treatment Network Web site, www.aidsinfonyc.org, help Kevin?

EVALUATION/OUTCOME CRITERIA

15. What criteria can his mother use to see if her plan is successful?

THINKING FURTHER

16. Why is nutrition so critical in managing AIDS?

⊙ RATE THIS PLATE

Kevin has been steadily losing weight. What could his mother plan that would be high in protein and calories? Rate the plate.

5 oz filet mignon

1 cup mashed sweet potatoes

5 stalks steamed asparagus

1/2 cup rice pudding

1 cup milk

Does this meal have all the protein that it could have? What could Kevin's mother do to increase the protein and calories when she is cooking? Are there any nutritional products that she could use to add more nutrients?

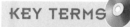

NUTRITIONAL CARE OF CLIENTS

OBJECTIVES

After studying this chapter, you should be able to:

- Describe how illness and surgery can affect the nutrition of clients

- Identify and describe three or more nutrition-related health problems that are common among elderly clients needing long-term care

- Demonstrate correct procedures for feeding a bed-bound client

- Explain the importance of adapting the family's meal to suit the client's nutritional requirements

HOSPITALIZED CLIENTS

Illness and surgery can have devastating effects on nutritional status. Fever, nausea, fear, depression, chemotherapy, and radiation can destroy appetite. Vomiting, diarrhea, chemotherapy, radiation, and some medications can reduce or prevent absorption of nutrients. In addition, food is restricted before surgery and some diagnostic tests. Ironically, this reduced nutrient and calories intake occurs just at a time when requirements are increased. Fluid may also be restricted as most clients are NPO (nothing by mouth) for 12 hours prior to surgery.

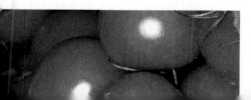

Protein Energy Malnutrition

When the increased needs for energy and protein are not met by food intake, the body must use its stores of glycogen and fat. When they have been used, the body breaks down its own tissues to provide protein for energy. It has no other "stores" of protein. Protein-energy malnutrition, commonly called PEM, can be a problem among hospitalized clients. It can delay wound healing, contribute to anemia, depress the immune system, and increase susceptibility to infections. Symptoms of PEM include weight loss and dry, pale skin. When malnutrition occurs as a result of hospitalization, it is called **iatrogenic malnutrition.**

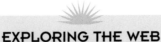

iatrogenic malnutrition
caused by treatment or diagnostic procedures

Improving the Client's Nutritional Status

The importance of improving a client's nutritional status is obvious. Formal nutritional assessments of clients should be made on a regular basis, but all members of the health care team should be alert to signs of malnutrition every day. The nurse or nursing assistant who sees the client regularly is in the best position to help the client. This person will be most familiar to the client and will hear the client's complaints about and see the reactions to the food served. She or he can bring problems to the attention of the dietitian responsible for the client's nutrition. The client may:

1. Need information about nutritional needs
2. Need a supplement
3. Want other foods

If not contraindicated by the client's health condition, it can be helpful to invite friends and relatives to bring the client some of his or her favorite foods.

EXPLORING THE WEB

Search the Web for information on nutritional status during acute or chronic illness. Why is appetite effected by illness? For what length of time is it normal to have a decreased appetite when ill? What can be done to improve appetite and maintain nutritional balance when ill?

FEEDING THE CLIENT

In the home, the family menu should serve as the basis of the client's meal whenever possible. This usually pleases the client because it makes her or him feel a part of the family. It also reduces food preparation time and costs.

Family meals are easily adapted for the client by omitting or adding certain foods or by varying the method of preparation. Suppose the client was to limit fat intake and the family menu was the following:

Fried hamburgers

Mashed potatoes with butter

Buttered peas

Tossed salad with French dressing

Ice cream with fresh strawberries

Whole milk

Broiling the hamburgers for everyone instead of frying would help limit the fat content. The client's mashed potatoes might be served with little or no butter, and the peas with only salt and pepper and perhaps a suitable spice, herb, or lemon. The client could be served the tossed salad with fat-free dressing and, for dessert, strawberries with low-fat ice cream. Fat-free milk is a simple substitute for whole milk.

Serving the Meal

When a meal is served at the bedside, the tray should be lined with a pretty cloth or paper liner. Attractive dishes that fit the tray conveniently without crowding it should be used. The food should be arranged attractively on the plate, with a colorful garnish such as a slice of fruit, parsley, or vegetable stick. The garnish must fit into the client's diet plan, however. Utensils must be arranged conveniently. Water should be served as well as another beverage (unless it is prohibited by the physician). Foods must be served at proper temperatures.

When the client is on complete bed rest, special preparations are required before the meal is served. The client should be given the opportunity to use the bedpan and to wash before the meal is served. The room can be ventilated and the bedcovers straightened. The client should be helped to a comfortable position, and any unpleasant sights should be removed before the meal is served. Pleasant conversation during the preparations can improve the client's mood considerably. Certain topics of conversation can help stimulate the client's interest in eating. The client might be told that the family is anticipating the same meal. Perhaps the recipes used will interest some clients. Appropriate remarks on the client's progress, whenever possible, are helpful.

When the meal preparations are complete, the tray should be placed so that it is easy for the client to feed herself or himself or, if necessary, convenient for someone else to do the feeding. If the client needs help, the napkin should be opened and placed, the bread spread, the meat cut, and the straw offered. The client should be encouraged to eat and be allowed sufficient time. If the meal is interrupted, the tray should be reheated and served again as soon as the interruption has resolved.

The tray should be removed and the client helped to brush her or his teeth when the meal is finished. The kinds and amounts of food refused, the time, type of diet, and client's appetite should be recorded on the client's chart after each meal. At times, the provider may request a calorie and protein count, which is an accurate report of the types and amounts of food eaten.

◎ SUPERSIZE USA

The elderly have lived through many changes in their lives. One change that might not be easily understood is the supersizing of the dishes they use. Why does a cereal bowl need to hold three or four servings? Plates, cereal-soup bowls, fruit-dessert bowls, and especially serving bowls have all been supersized. Several recent studies have shown that the larger the bowl, the larger the portion one will take. This may be why some elderly complain about "too big of a serving"; it can be overwhelming, causing them to eat very little, or not at all. Having lived through several world wars and the Great Depression, it is distressing for them to know that food will be thrown away. "That is such a waste!" Other elderly clients have adapted to the larger portions and are fighting weight gain and obesity.

Check out some antique dishes and notice the difference in sizes from those you use at home. Measuring portions, rather than eyeballing them, may be wise.

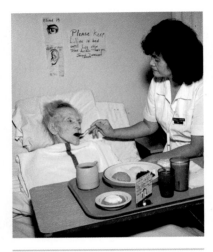

Figure 23-1 *Some clients require assistance when eating.*

EXPLORING THE WEB

Search the Web for adaptive devices that may help a client with a disability self-feed. Become familiar with the operation of these devices so that you can aid in teaching clients how to help themselves.

Feeding the Client Who Requires Assistance

If the client is unable to feed herself or himself, the person doing the feeding should sit near the side of the bed (Figure 23-1). Small amounts of food should be placed toward the back of the mouth with a slight pressure on the tongue with the spoon or fork. Clients should not be fed with a syringe. If the client is suffering from one-sided paralysis, the food and drinking straw must be placed in the nonparalyzed side of the mouth. The client must be allowed to help herself or himself as much as possible. If the client begins to choke, help her or him sit up straight. Do not give food or water while the client is choking. The client's mouth should be wiped as needed. A client diagnosed with dysphagia will require a specialized diet. Depending upon the swallowing abnormality, the client may need pureed foods with either thin or thickened (to a nectar or honey consistency) liquids. A dysphagic client should not use straws.

((In The Media

NUTRITION AND HEALTH OF THE ELDERLY

Malnutrition poses a great risk for Americans 65 and older. Malnutrition leads to frailty and allows a minor aliment to become a major one. It is estimated that 20%–60% of elderly home-bound clients are either malnourished or heading in that direction. There are many reasons why an elderly person may become malnourished, such as low income, physical changes resulting in difficulty digesting and absorbing nutrients, diminished sense of taste and smell, altered appetite, difficulty shopping for food and preparing meals, malabsorption of nutrients due to medications, isolation, depression, and being a caregiver. When the elderly make small dietary changes to take better care of themselves, they can avoid more serious problems. If the elderly have poor nutrition status and become ill with even a cold, it really sets them back for a much longer time than their well-nourished peers.

(Source: Adapted from the *New York Times*, April 2005.)

Feeding the Blind Client

Special care must be taken in serving a meal to a client who is blind. An appetizing description of the meal can help create a desire to eat. To help the client who is blind feed herself or himself, arrange the food as if the plate were the face of a clock (Figure 23-2). The meat might be put at 6 o'clock, vegetables at 9 o'clock, salad at 12, and bread at 3 o'clock. The person who regularly arranges the meal should remember to use the same pattern for all meals. People who are blind usually feel better when they can help themselves.

LONG-TERM CARE OF THE ELDERLY

Because of increasing **longevity,** the number of elderly people requiring long-term care is increasing. The changes people undergo with age that can affect their nutritional status are discussed in Chapter 15.

longevity
length of life

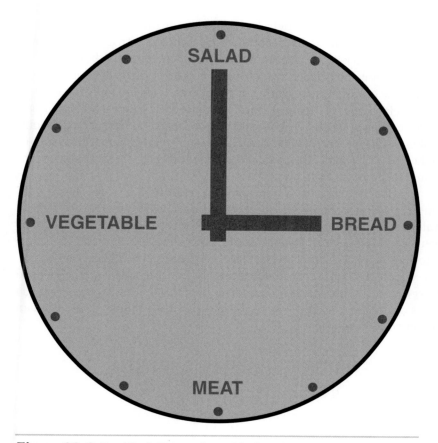

Figure 23-2 *To a blind client, a plate of food can be pictured as the face of a clock.*

Physical Problems of the Institutionalized Elderly

It is estimated that the majority of people 85 and over have at least one chronic disease such as arthritis, osteoporosis, diabetes mellitus, cardiovascular disease, or mental disorder. These conditions affect their attitudes, physical activities, appetites and, thus, nutritional status. PEM is a major concern for this population.

Anemia can develop if the client has insufficient iron intake. It can contribute to confusion and depression but may go unnoticed because one of its major symptoms, fatigue, may be simply thought to be a characteristic of old age. It is helpful to make sure there is sufficient animal protein and vitamin C (an iron enhancer) in the client's diet.

Pressure ulcers (bedsores) can develop in bedridden clients. The ulcers develop in areas where unrelieved pressure on the skin prevents the blood from bringing nutrients and oxygen and removing wastes. Healing requires treatment of the ulcer, relief of the pressure, a high-calorie diet with sufficient protein, and vitamin C and zinc supplements. Prevention is a must.

Constipation can be caused by inadequate fiber, fluid, or exercise; by medication; by reduced peristalsis; or by former abuse of laxatives. It can be relieved by increased fluid, fiber, and exercise (if possible).

pressure ulcers
bedsores

Diarrhea can be caused by lack of muscle tone in the colon. It will reduce the absorption of nutrients and can contribute to dehydration. An increase of fiber in the diet combined with supplemental vitamins and minerals may be helpful.

The sense of smell declines with age, and the appetite diminishes. A reduced sense of taste can be caused by medications, disease, mineral deficiencies, or xerostomia (dry mouth). The addition of spices, herbs, salt, and sugar (if allowed) can be helpful. Xerostomia can be caused by disease or medications. Drinking water, eating frequent small meals, and chewing sugar-free gums or candies may be helpful. The inadequate amount of saliva in these clients contributes to increased tooth decay.

Dysphagia (difficulty swallowing) can result from a stroke, closed head trauma, head or neck cancer, surgery, or Alzheimer's and other diseases. A swallow study needs to be done to determine the consistency of diet needed by clients with dysphagia. A swallow study is done by a speech therapist using a video fluoroscope. While being videotaped, the client is given liquids, semi-liquids, pureed food, and solid food to determine the consistency of the bolus (food mass) that he or she is able to swallow without aspirating. Many dysphagia clients must have thickened liquids. Dysphagia clients should always be in an upright position when eating.

CONSIDERATIONS FOR THE HEALTH CARE PROFESSIONAL

EXPLORING THE WEB

Search the Web for information relating to the nutritional status of the elderly. Why does nutritional status decline as one ages? What can be done to prevent the decline of nutritional status among the elderly? Does the American Association of Retired Persons (AARP) offer any guidelines?

The needs of bedridden clients are nearly total. They are unable to walk, use the bathroom, brush their teeth, or wash their hands without help. The feelings of helplessness they endure are considerable. In addition, they may be embarrassed by their appearance, or by needing a bedpan when only a thin curtain separates them from their roommate's guests. It is helpful to the client if the health care professional can imagine himself or herself in the place of the client.

The needs of many elderly clients in nursing homes are also total. They may be arthritic and unable to walk; some may be incontinent; others may forget their names and how to dress; they may wander off the premises unless they are constantly watched; they may need to be fed. Each remains an individual. They all need, respond to, and deserve warmth and respect from their caregivers.

SUMMARY

Illness and surgery can have devastating effects on clients' nutritional status. PEM can be a significant problem in hospitals. The health care team should work together to improve clients' nutritional status.

Once a client is at home, her or his meals should be adapted from the family's meals. This saves time and ex-

pense and allows the client to feel less of a burden and more a part of the family.

A bedridden client should be given the bedpan and then allowed to wash her or his hands before the meal. Clients should be encouraged to feed themselves. However, help should be offered if it is needed. The client who is blind can eat more easily if food is arranged in a set pattern on the plate. Pleasant conversation and cheerfulness on the part of the nurse can improve the client's appetite. The type of diet, time of meal, client's appetite, and type and amount of food eaten should all be recorded on the client's chart. Elderly clients requiring long-term care may suffer from several nutrition-related health problems that, with proper treatment, can sometimes be relieved.

DISCUSSION TOPICS

1. How do illness and surgery affect one's nutrition?

2. What is iatrogenic malnutrition? How might it develop?

3. In what ways might the nurse help improve the client's nutrition?

4. When might it be unwise to invite a client's friends and family to bring foods to the client? When might it be appropriate? Who would decide?

5. Discuss the importance of proper preparation of the client and room before the meal. What could disturb a client and affect appetite?

6. How may the appearance of the tray affect the client's appetite?

7. Why should the client be encouraged to feed herself or himself?

8. Why is it important to remove the tray as soon as the client has finished the meal?

9. How can the behavior and attitude of the attending person affect the appetite of the client?

10. Why is anemia so easily overlooked in elderly clients?

11. Discuss how a diminished sense of smell might affect one's appetite.

SUGGESTED ACTIVITIES

1. Have two students participate in the following role-playing situation. The class should evaluate and discuss the "nurse's" tact and skill in dealing with the "client."

    Mrs. Jones is a young, active woman with a family. She is recovering from viral pneumonia. Although she is allowed out of bed, she is not supposed to prepare meals or do housework until her condition improves. Dr. Malcolm has told Ms. Wilson, the nurse, that it is important for Mrs. Jones to regain her lost weight. One day, before her dinner was served, Mrs. Jones complained to Ms. Wilson. She was discouraged about her lack of energy and stated that her family needed her. Ms. Wilson noticed that Mrs. Jones had eaten very little for breakfast and lunch. What should she say to Mrs. Jones?

2. Invite a dietitian to speak to the class on nutrition and the elderly.

3. Invite a nurse who works in a nursing home to talk to the class. Ask him or her to describe how these clients are fed.

4. Visit a local nursing home in groups of two or three. Talk to some of the clients. Write a report on your visit.

REVIEW

Multiple choice. Select the *letter* that precedes the best answer.

1. Surgery
    a. reduces the number of calories normally needed
    b. has only a slight effect on appetite
    c. is always followed by TPN
    d. can temporarily devastate a client's nutritional status

2. Normal absorption of nutrients
    a. is not affected by chemotherapy
    b. is unaffected by diarrhea
    c. can be decreased after surgery
    d. is unaffected by PEM

3. When energy and protein needs are not met by food intake, the body will
    a. first use its stores of fat and second its glycogen
    b. first use its stores of glycogen and second its fat
    c. first use its stores of protein
    d. increase its metabolic rate

4. PEM
    a. can delay wound healing
    b. has no relationship to the development of anemia
    c. strengthens the immune system
    d. decreases the risk of infection

5. Surgery may
   a. reduce nutritional requirements
   b. decrease one's calorie requirement
   c. contribute to the development of PEM
   d. increase one's fat requirements

6. Favorite foods brought to hospitalized clients from home
   a. should not be allowed
   b. have no effect on the client's nutritional status
   c. should be approved by the dietitian before being given to the client
   d. are neither helpful nor harmful

7. Iatrogenic malnutrition
   a. is the inevitable result of surgery
   b. is commonly caused by low-grade fevers
   c. can be a result of hospitalization
   d. has no effect on wound healing

8. Dysphagia
   a. means memory loss
   b. is common following bone surgery
   c. can safely be ignored
   d. clients should not be in a supine position when eating

9. Anemia
   a. can result from insufficient fat intake
   b. can contribute to hyperthyroidism
   c. occurs only in males over 50
   d. can be helped by the addition of vitamin C and iron

10. Pressure ulcers
   a. occur only in the stomach
   b. can occur in the duodenum
   c. do not affect bedridden clients
   d. develop in areas where, because of pressure, blood cannot get to the tissue

CASE IN POINT

GERALD: RECOVERING FOLLOWING SURGERY

Gerald was a 30-year-old African American man who had been a paraplegic for 5 years. He lived in a house with his three brothers, who helped take care of him. John did the cooking. He made fried eggs, grits and bacon, and coffee for breakfast. Pork and potatoes with greens were a typical dinner. Gerald didn't like milk; it gave him gas.

Gerald loved to play wheelchair basketball with the neighborhood kids. He would have his boom box blasting on the side of the court and play for hours. The kids loved the attention, and Gerald loved to be outside. During the school year, Gerald took classes at the local college and tried to sell his drawings to any admirer. He felt most alive when he was just wheeling around the neighborhood in the warmer months. Gerald was no good at limiting the amount of time he was in his "chair." He was even worse at staying in bed, off his buttocks. He had a tendency to develop pressure ulcers. This time Gerald had the worst problem yet. His doctor said he had to go into the hospital for skin flap surgery to close the decubiti. He would have to stay off his back at least 3 weeks, possibly more, until the incision lines had healed. Gerald could not smoke in the hospital. The doctor was willing to let him use a nicotine patch if needed.

Initially, Gerald did well after surgery. He made the transition to regular food. Within 2 weeks, he was complaining of dry, itchy skin, and the doctor was worried about his 5-pound weight loss. The provider ordered a dietary assessment.

ASSESSMENT

1. What do you know about Gerald and his nutrition?
2. Did he eat a balanced diet?
3. What barriers were there to his healing?
4. What foods are a priority for healing?
5. How significant is nutrition to this problem?

DIAGNOSIS

6. Write at least two diagnoses that apply to Gerald's problem.

PLAN/GOAL

7. What is the priority goal for Gerald?

IMPLEMENTATION

8. What does the dietitian need to know about Gerald to help?
9. What is the dietitian likely to recommend?
10. How could vitamin supplements help?
11. Who else can help?
12. What strategies could be helpful to get Gerald to eat?
13. What could a home health nurse do?
14. What does Gerald need to do to help himself?
15. If Gerald is unable to eat enough food to maintain his weight, what alternatives does the doctor have?

EVALUATION/OUTCOME

16. What needs to happen for Gerald to avoid having a feeding tube?

THINKING FURTHER

18. How are Gerald's needs similar to those of any surgical client?
19. What are the most serious consequences if Gerald is unable to heal, even with tube feedings?

◎ RATE THIS PLATE

The dietitian met with Gerald to discuss how to incorporate more protein into his diet. Gerald is trying to teach his brother John, the cook. What do you think of the meal that Gerald has planned? Figure how much protein Gerald had planned in his meal.

6 oz sirloin steak

Baked potato with butter and cheddar cheese (1 oz)

1 cup stir-fried mixed vegetables (zucchini, yellow squash, carrots, and green beans)

Hard roll with butter

1 cup custard

CASE IN POINT

PEGGY: MAINTAINING INDEPENDENCE AT 75

When Peggy's husband died, her only daughter, Sissy, insisted that she move to a nursing home nearby. Peggy, whose family had moved to the United States from New Zealand when she was 7, was now 75 years old and did not want to move away from her only brother, Bert, and her friends. However, she reluctantly agreed to move.

When Peggy saw the assisted-living area and the tiny room she had, she cried. The food was bad, and there weren't too many people she could play cards with or have a conversation with. When her brother came to visit her, he was shocked at Peggy's appearance. She looked thin and pale. She was still in her pajamas at noon, something she never did at home. She seemed withdrawn and sullen. Bert knew he had to take her back home with him. Sissy, Peggy's daughter, agreed. Bert's wife, Molly, was a wonderful cook and enjoyed Peggy's company. Within a month, Peggy had regained some weight and was out walking every day with Molly. Peggy was alert, she was back to playing cards, and she said she felt like her old self.

Peggy was able to return to her old home after 2 months at her brother's.

When Sissy visited her mother, she had to admit that she had made a mistake. She was very happy to see her mother doing so well.

ASSESSMENT

1. What do you know about Peggy?
2. What caused the change in her health?
3. How significant was the problem?

DIAGNOSIS

4. Write two diagnoses about Peggy.

PLAN/GOAL

5. What was her brother's goal when he took Peggy out of assisted living?

IMPLEMENTATION

6. What factors contributed to her return to her old self?
7. How significant is maintaining independence in elders?
8. What are nutritional priorities for elders?

EVALUATION/OUTCOME CRITERIA

9. What had Sissy and Molly observed that deemed the plan successful?

THINKING FURTHER

10. What was the likely outcome if Peggy had not gone to stay with her brother?
11. Why is this lesson so important in the survival of elders?

◎ RATE THIS PLATE

Peggy hadn't eaten much for quite awhile due to depression. One of the meals served at the assistant-living facility was as follows. Rate the plate.

Baked chicken breast, no salt or seasoning

Mashed potatoes

Lima beans

Lemon gelatin with fruit

Vanilla pudding

We eat with our eyes first—what color is this meal? Are there any distinct flavors? Why do you think they didn't add any seasoning to the food? What would you change or add to this meal to make it more colorful and appealing?

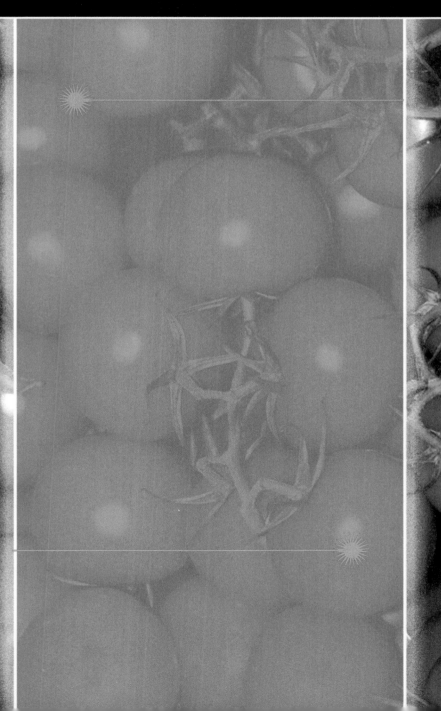

Appendices

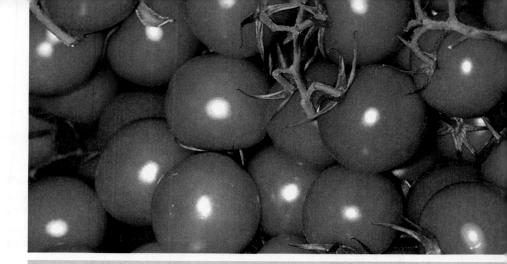

APPENDIX A

MYPYRAMID FOOD INTAKE PATTERN CALORIE LEVELS

Source: U.S. Department of Agriculture, Center for Nutrition Policy and Promotion. (2005, April). Publication CNPP-XX. Washington, DC: Author.

MyPyramid assigns Individuals to a calorie level based on their sex, age, and activity level.
The chart below identifies the calorie levels for males and females by age and activity level. Calorie levels are provided for each year of childhood, from 2 to 18 years, and for adults in 5-year increments.

	MALES				FEMALES		
Activity level	Sedentary*	Mod. active*	Active*	Activity level	Sedentary*	Mod. active*	Active*
AGE				AGE			
2	1,000	1,000	1,000	2	1,000	1,000	1,000
3	1,000	1,400	1,400	3	1,000	1,200	1,400
4	1,200	1,400	1,600	4	1,200	1,400	1,400
5	1,200	1,400	1,600	5	1,200	1,400	1,600
6	1,400	1,600	1,800	6	1,200	1,400	1,600
7	1,400	1,600	1,800	7	1,200	1,600	1,800
8	1,400	1,600	2,000	8	1,400	1,600	1,800
9	1,600	1,800	2,000	9	1,400	1,600	1,800
10	1,600	1,800	2,200	10	1,400	1,800	2,000
11	1,800	2,000	2,200	11	1,600	1,800	2,000
12	1,800	2,200	2,400	12	1,600	2,000	2,200
13	2,000	2,200	2,600	13	1,600	2,000	2,200

continued

	MALES				FEMALES		
Activity level	Sedentary*	Mod. active*	Active*	Activity level	Sedentary*	Mod. active*	Active*
AGE				**AGE**			
14	2,000	2,400	2,800	14	1,800	2,000	2,400
15	2,200	2,600	3,000	15	1,800	2,000	2,400
16	2,400	2,800	3,200	16	1,800	2,000	2,400
17	2,400	2,800	3,200	17	1,800	2,000	2,400
18	2,400	2,800	3,200	18	1,800	2,000	2,400
19–20	2,600	2,800	3,000	19–20	2,000	2,200	2,400
21–25	2,400	2,800	3,000	21–25	2,000	2,200	2,400
26–30	2,400	2,600	3,000	26–30	1,800	2,000	2,400
31–35	2,400	2,600	3,000	31–35	1,800	2,000	2,200
36–40	2,400	2,600	2,800	36–40	1,800	2,000	2,200
41–45	2,200	2,600	2,800	41–45	1,800	2,000	2,200
46–50	2,200	2,400	2,800	46–50	1,800	2,000	2,200
51–55	2,200	2,400	2,800	51–55	1,600	1,800	2,200
56–60	2,200	2,400	2,600	56–60	1,600	1,800	2,200
61–65	2,000	2,400	2,600	61–65	1,600	1,800	2,000
66–70	2,000	2,200	2,600	66–70	1,600	1,800	2,000
71–75	2,000	2,200	2,600	71–75	1,600	1,800	2,000
76 and up	2,000	2,200	2,400	76 and up	1,600	1,800	2,000

*Calorie levels are based on the estimated energy requirements (EER) and activity levels from the *Institute of Medicine Dietary Reference Intakes Macronutrients Report*, 2002.
Sedentary = less than 30 minutes a day of moderate physical activity in addition to daily activities.
Mod. Active = at least 30 minutes up to 60 minutes a day of moderate physical activity in addition to daily activities.
Active = 60 or more minutes a day of moderate physical activity in addition to daily activities.

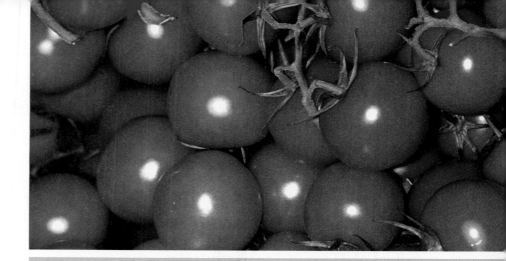

APPENDIX B

DIETARY GUIDELINES FOR AMERICANS 2005: FOOD SOURCES OF SELECTED NUTRIENTS

Reprinted from *Dietary Guidelines for Americans 2005* (6th ed.), by the U.S. Department of Health and Human Services and U.S. Department of Agriculture, 2005, Washington, DC: U.S. Government Printing Office.

Appendix B-1
Food Sources of Potassium

Food sources of potassium ranked by milligrams of potassium per standard amount, also showing calories in the standard amount. (The AI for adults is 4,700 mg/day potassium.)

Food, Standard Amount	Potassium (mg)	Calories
Sweet potato, baked, 1 potato (146 g)	694	131
Tomato paste, 1/4 cup	664	54
Beet greens, cooked, 1/2 cup	655	19
Potato, baked, flesh, 1 potato (156 g)	610	145
White beans, canned, 1/2 cup	595	153
Yogurt, plain, nonfat, 8-oz container	579	127
Tomato puree, 1/2 cup	549	48
Clams, canned, 3 oz	534	126
Yogurt, plain, low-fat, 8-oz container	531	143
Prune juice, 3/4 cup	530	136
Carrot juice, 3/4 cup	517	71
Blackstrap molasses, 1 Tbsp	498	47

Food, Standard Amount	Potassium (mg)	Calories
Halibut, cooked, 3 oz	490	119
Soybeans, green, cooked, 1/2 cup	485	127
Tuna, yellowfin, cooked, 3 oz	484	118
Lima beans, cooked, 1/2 cup	484	104
Winter squash, cooked, 1/2 cup	448	40
Soybeans, mature, cooked, 1/2 cup	443	149
Rockfish, Pacific, cooked, 3 oz	442	103
Cod, Pacific, cooked, 3 oz	439	89
Bananas, 1 medium	422	105
Spinach, cooked, 1/2 cup	419	21
Tomato juice, 3/4 cup	417	31
Tomato sauce, 1/2 cup	405	39
Peaches, dried, uncooked, 1/4 cup	398	96
Prunes, stewed, 1/2 cup	398	133
Milk, nonfat, 1 cup	382	83
Pork chop, center loin, cooked, 3 oz	382	197
Apricots, dried, uncooked, 1/4 cup	378	78
Rainbow trout, farmed, cooked, 3 oz	375	144
Pork loin, center rib (roasts), lean, roasted, 3 oz	371	190
Buttermilk, cultured, low fat, 1 cup	370	98
Cantaloupe, 1/4 medium	368	47
1%–2% milk, 1 cup	366	102–122
Honeydew melon, 1/8 medium	365	58
Lentils, cooked, 1/2 cup	365	115
Plantains, cooked, 1/2 cup slices	358	90
Kidney beans, cooked, 1/2 cup	358	112
Orange juice, 3/4 cup	355	85
Split peas, cooked, 1/2 cup	355	116
Yogurt, plain, whole milk, 8-oz container	352	138

Source: Nutrient values from Agricultural Research Service (ARS) Nutrient Database for Standard Reference, Release 17. Foods are from ARS single nutrient reports, sorted in descending order by nutrient content in terms of common household measures. Food items and weights in the single nutrient reports are adapted from those in the 2002 revision of *USDA Home and Garden Bulletin No. 72,* Nutritive Value of Foods. Mixed dishes and multiple preparations of the same food item have been omitted from this table.

Appendix B-2
Food Sources of Vitamin E

Food sources of vitamin E ranked by milligrams of vitamin E per standard amount; also calories in the standard amount. (All provide >−10% of RDA for vitamin E for adults, which is 15 mg a-tocopherol [AT]/day.)

Food, Standard Amount	AT (mg)	Calories
Fortified ready-to-eat cereals, about 1 oz	1.6–12.8	90–107
Sunflower seeds, dry roasted, 1 oz	7.4	165
Almonds, 1 oz	7.3	164
Sunflower oil, high linoleic, 1 Tbsp	5.6	120
Cottonseed oil, 1 Tbsp	4.8	120

Food, Standard Amount	AT (mg)	Calories
Safflower oil, high oleic, 1 Tbsp	4.6	120
Hazelnuts (filberts), 1 oz	4.3	178
Mixed nuts, dry roasted, 1 oz	3.1	168
Turnip greens, frozen, cooked, 1/2 cup	2.9	24
Tomato paste, 1/4 cup	2.8	54
Pine nuts, 1 oz	2.6	191
Peanut butter, 2 Tbsp	2.5	192
Tomato puree, 1/2 cup	2.5	48
Tomato sauce, 1/2 cup	2.5	39
Canola oil, 1 Tbsp	2.4	124
Wheat germ, toasted, plain, 2 Tbsp	2.3	54
Peanuts, 1 oz	2.2	166
Avocado, raw, 1/2 avocado	2.1	161
Carrot juice, canned, 3/4 cup	2.1	71
Peanut oil, 1 Tbsp	2.1	119
Corn oil, 1 Tbsp	1.9	120
Olive oil, 1 Tbsp	1.9	119
Spinach, cooked, 1/2 cup	1.9	21
Dandelion greens, cooked, 1/2 cup	1.8	18
Sardine, Atlantic, in oil, drained, 3 oz	1.7	177
Blue crab, cooked/canned, 3 oz	1.6	84
Brazil nuts, 1 oz	1.6	186
Herring, Atlantic, pickled, 3 oz	1.5	222

Source: Nutrient values from Agricultural Research Service (ARS) Nutrient Database for Standard Reference, Release 17. Foods are from ARS single nutrient reports, sorted in descending order by nutrient content in terms of common household measures. Food items and weights in the single nutrient reports are adapted from those in the 2002 revision of *USDA Home and Garden Bulletin No. 72,* Nutritive Value of Foods. Mixed dishes and multiple preparations of the same food item have been omitted from this table.

Appendix B-3
Food Sources of Iron

Food sources of iron ranked by milligrams of iron per standard amount; also calories in the standard amount. (All are > − 10% of RDA for teen and adult females, which is 18 mg/day.)

Food, Standard Amount	Iron (mg)	Calories
Clams, canned, drained, 3 oz	23.8	126
Fortified ready-to-eat cereals (various), about 1 oz	1.8–21.1	54–127
Oysters, eastern, wild, cooked, moist heat, 3 oz	10.2	116
Organ meats (liver, giblets), various, cooked, 3 oz[a]	5.2–9.9	134–235
Fortified instant cooked cereals (various), 1 packet	4.9–8.1	Varies
Soybeans, mature, cooked, 1/2 cup	4.4	149
Pumpkin and squash seed kernels, roasted, 1 oz	4.2	148
White beans, canned, 1/2 cup	3.9	153
Blackstrap molasses, 1 Tbsp	3.5	47
Lentils, cooked, 1/2 cup	3.3	115
Spinach, cooked from fresh, 1/2 cup	3.2	21

Food, Standard Amount	Iron (mg)	Calories
Beef, chuck, blade roast, lean, cooked, 3 oz	3.1	215
Beef, bottom round, lean, 0" fat, all grades, cooked, 3 oz	2.8	182
Kidney beans, cooked, 1/2 cup	2.6	112
Sardines, canned in oil, drained, 3 oz	2.5	177
Beef, rib, lean, 1/4" fat, all grades, 3 oz	2.4	195
Chickpeas, cooked, 1/2 cup	2.4	134
Duck, meat only, roasted, 3 oz	2.3	171
Lamb, shoulder, arm, lean, 1/4" fat, choice, cooked, 3 oz	2.3	237
Prune juice, 3/4 cup	2.3	136
Shrimp, canned, 3 oz	2.3	102
Cowpeas, cooked, 1/2 cup	2.2	100
Ground beef, 15% fat, cooked, 3 oz	2.2	212
Tomato puree, 1/2 cup	2.2	48
Lima beans, cooked, 1/2 cup	2.2	108
Soybeans, green, cooked, 1/2 cup	2.2	127
Navy beans, cooked, 1/2 cup	2.1	127
Refried beans, 1/2 cup	2.1	118
Beef, top sirloin, lean, 0" fat, all grades, cooked, 3 oz	2.0	156
Tomato paste, 1/4 cup	2.0	54

[a]High in cholesterol.

Source: Nutrient values from Agricultural Research Service (ARS) Nutrient Database for Standard Reference, Release 17. Foods are from ARS single nutrient reports, sorted in descending order by nutrient content in terms of common household measures. Food items and weights in the single nutrient reports are adapted from those in the 2002 revision of *USDA Home and Garden Bulletin No. 72*, Nutritive Value of Foods. Mixed dishes and multiple preparations of the same food item have been omitted from this table.

Appendix B-4
Nondairy Food Sources of Calcium

Nondairy food sources of calcium ranked by milligrams of calcium per standard amount; also calories in the standard amount. The bioavailability may vary. (The AI for adults is 1,000 mg/day.)[a]

Food, Standard Amount	Calcium (mg)	Calories
Fortified ready-to-eat cereals (various), 1 oz	236–1,043	88–106
Soy beverage, calcium fortified, 1 cup	368	98
Sardines, Atlantic, in oil, drained, 3 oz	325	177
Tofu, firm, prepared with nigari,[b] 1/2 cup	253	88
Pink salmon, canned, with bone, 3 oz	181	118
Collards, cooked from frozen, 1/2 cup	178	31
Molasses, blackstrap, 1 Tbsp	172	47
Spinach, cooked from frozen, 1/2 cup	146	30
Soybeans, green, cooked, 1/2 cup	130	127
Turnip greens, cooked from frozen, 1/2 cup	124	24
Ocean perch, Atlantic, cooked, 3 oz	116	103
Oatmeal, plain and flavored, instant, fortified, 1 packet prepared	99–110	97–157
Cowpeas, cooked, 1/2 cup	106	80
White beans, canned, 1/2 cup	96	153

Food, Standard Amount	Calcium (mg)	Calories
Kale, cooked from frozen, 1/2 cup	90	20
Okra, cooked from frozen, 1/2 cup	88	26
Soybeans, mature, cooked, 1/2 cup	88	149
Blue crab, canned, 3 oz	86	84
Beet greens, cooked from fresh, 1/2 cup	82	19
Pak-choi, Chinese cabbage, cooked from fresh, 1/2 cup	79	10
Clams, canned, 3 oz	78	126
Dandelion greens, cooked from fresh, 1/2 cup	74	17
Rainbow trout, farmed, cooked, 3 oz	73	144

[a]Both calcium content and bioavailability should be considered when selecting dietary sources of calcium. Some plant foods have calcium that is well absorbed, but the large quantity of plant foods that would be needed to provide as much calcium as in a glass of milk may be unachievable for many. Many other calcium-fortified foods are available, but the percentage of calcium that can be absorbed is unavailable for many of them.

[b]Calcium sulfate and magnesium chloride.

Source: Nutrient values from Agricultural Research Service (ARS) Nutrient Database for Standard Reference, Release 17. Foods are from ARS single nutrient reports, sorted in descending order by nutrient content in terms of common household measures. Food items and weights in the single nutrient reports are adapted from those in the 2002 revision of *USDA Home and Garden Bulletin No. 72*, Nutritive Value of Foods. Mixed dishes and multiple preparations of the same food item have been omitted from this table.

Appendix B-5
Food Sources of Calcium

Food sources of calcium ranked by milligrams of calcium per standard amount; also calories in the standard amount. (All are > − 20% of AI for adults 19–50, which is 1,000 mg/day.)

Food, Standard Amount	Calcium (mg)	Calories
Plain yogurt, nonfat (13 g protein/8 oz), 8-oz container	452	127
Romano cheese, 1.5 oz	452	165
Pasteurized process Swiss cheese, 2 oz	438	190
Plain yogurt, low fat (12 g protein/8 oz), 8-oz container	415	143
Fruit yogurt, low fat (10 g protein/8 oz), 8-oz container	345	232
Swiss cheese, 1.5 oz	336	162
Ricotta cheese, part skim, 1/2 cup	335	170
Pasteurized process American cheese food, 2 oz	323	188
Provolone cheese, 1.5 oz	321	150
Mozzarella cheese, part skim, 1.5 oz	311	129
Cheddar cheese, 1.5 oz	307	171
Fat-free (skim) milk, 1 cup	306	83
Muenster cheese, 1.5 oz	305	156
1% low-fat milk, 1 cup	290	102
Low-fat chocolate milk (1%), 1 cup	288	158
2% reduced-fat milk, 1 cup	285	122
Reduced-fat chocolate milk (2%), 1 cup	285	180
Buttermilk, low fat, 1 cup	284	98
Chocolate milk, 1 cup	280	208
Whole milk, 1 cup	276	146

Food, Standard Amount	Calcium (mg)	Calories
Yogurt, plain, whole milk (8 g protein/8 oz), 8-oz container	275	138
Ricotta cheese, whole milk, 1/2 cup	255	214
Blue cheese, 1.5 oz	225	150
Mozzarella cheese, whole milk, 1.5 oz	215	128
Feta cheese, 1.5 oz	210	113

Source: Nutrient values from Agricultural Research Service (ARS) Nutrient Database for Standard Reference, Release 17. Foods are from ARS single nutrient reports, sorted in descending order by nutrient content in terms of common household measures. Food items and weights in the single nutrient reports are adapted from those in the 2002 revision of *USDA Home and Garden Bulletin No. 72*, Nutritive Value of Foods. Mixed dishes and multiple preparations of the same food item have been omitted from this table.

Appendix B-6
Food Sources of Vitamin A

Food sources of vitamin A ranked by micrograms of retinol activity equivalents (RAE) of vitamin A per standard amount; also calories in the standard amount. (All are > −20% of RDA for adult men, which is 900 mg/day RAE.)

Food, Standard Amount	Vitamin A (μg RAE)	Calories
Organ meats (liver, giblets), various, cooked, 3 oz[a]	1,490–9,126	134–235
Carrot juice, 3/4 cup	1,692	71
Sweet potato with peel, baked, 1 medium	1,096	103
Pumpkin, canned, 1/2 cup	953	42
Carrots, cooked from fresh, 1/2 cup	671	27
Spinach, cooked from frozen, 1/2 cup	573	30
Collards, cooked from frozen, 1/2 cup	489	31
Kale, cooked from frozen, 1/2 cup	478	20
Mixed vegetables, canned, 1/2 cup	474	40
Turnip greens, cooked from frozen, 1/2 cup	441	24
Instant cooked cereals, fortified, prepared, 1 packet	285–376	75–97
Various ready-to-eat cereals, with added vitamin A, about 1 oz	180–376	100–117
Carrot, raw, 1 small	301	20
Beet greens, cooked, 1/2 cup	276	19
Winter squash, cooked, 1/2 cup	268	38
Dandelion greens, cooked, 1/2 cup	260	18
Cantaloupe, raw, 1/4 medium melon	233	46
Mustard greens, cooked, 1/2 cup	221	11
Pickled herring, 3 oz	219	222
Red sweet pepper, cooked, 1/2 cup	186	19
Chinese cabbage, cooked, 1/2 cup	180	10

[a]High in cholesterol.

Source: Nutrient values from Agricultural Research Service (ARS) Nutrient Database for Standard Reference, Release 17. Foods are from ARS single nutrient reports, sorted in descending order by nutrient content in terms of common household measures. Food items and weights in the single nutrient reports are adapted from those in the 2002 revision of *USDA Home and Garden Bulletin No. 72*, Nutritive Value of Foods. Mixed dishes and multiple preparations of the same food item have been omitted from this table.

Appendix B-7
Food Sources of Magnesium

Food sources of magnesium ranked by milligrams of magnesium per standard amount; also calories in the standard amount. (All are > − 10% of RDA for adult men, which is 420 mg/day.)

Food, Standard Amount	Magnesium (mg)	Calories
Pumpkin and squash seed kernels, roasted, 1 oz	151	148
Brazil nuts, 1 oz	107	186
Bran ready-to-eat cereal (100%), about 1 oz	103	74
Halibut, cooked, 3 oz	91	119
Quinoa, dry, 1/4 cup	89	159
Spinach, canned, 1/2 cup	81	25
Almonds, 1 oz	78	164
Spinach, cooked from fresh, 1/2 cup	78	20
Buckwheat flour, 1/4 cup	75	101
Cashews, dry roasted, 1 oz	74	163
Soybeans, mature, cooked, 1/2 cup	74	149
Pine nuts, dried, 1 oz	71	191
Mixed nuts, oil roasted, with peanuts, 1 oz	67	175
White beans, canned, 1/2 cup	67	154
Pollock, walleye, cooked, 3 oz	62	96
Black beans, cooked, 1/2 cup	60	114
Bulgur, dry, 1/4 cup	57	120
Oat bran, raw, 1/4 cup	55	58
Soybeans, green, cooked, 1/2 cup	54	127
Tuna, yellowfin, cooked, 3 oz	54	118
Artichokes (hearts), cooked, 1/2 cup	50	42
Peanuts, dry roasted, 1 oz	50	166
Lima beans, baby, cooked from frozen, 1/2 cup	50	95
Beet greens, cooked, 1/2 cup	49	19
Navy beans, cooked, 1/2 cup	48	127
Tofu, firm, prepared with nigari,[a] 1/2 cup	47	88
Okra, cooked from frozen, 1/2 cup	47	26
Soy beverage, 1 cup	47	127
Cowpeas, cooked, 1/2 cup	46	100
Hazelnuts, 1 oz	46	178
Oat bran muffin, 1 oz	45	77
Great northern beans, cooked, 1/2 cup	44	104
Oat bran, cooked, 1/2 cup	44	44
Buckwheat groats, roasted, cooked, 1/2 cup	43	78
Brown rice, cooked, 1/2 cup	42	108
Haddock, cooked, 3 oz	42	95

[a]Calcium sulfate and magnesium chloride.

Source: Nutrient values from Agricultural Research Service (ARS) Nutrient Database for Standard Reference, Release 17. Foods are from ARS single nutrient reports, sorted in descending order by nutrient content in terms of common household measures. Food items and weights in the single nutrient reports are adapted from those in the 2002 revision of *USDA Home and Garden Bulletin No. 72*, Nutritive Value of Foods. Mixed dishes and multiple preparations of the same food item have been omitted from this table.

Appendix B-8
Food Sources of Dietary Fiber

Food sources of dietary fiber ranked by grams of dietary fiber per standard amount; also calories in the standard amount. (All are $> -10\%$ of AI for adult women, which is 25 grams/day.)

Food, Standard Amount	Dietary Fiber (g)	Calories
Navy beans, cooked, 1/2 cup	9.5	128
Bran ready-to-eat cereal (100%), 1/2 cup	8.8	78
Kidney beans, canned, 1/2 cup	8.2	109
Split peas, cooked, 1/2 cup	8.1	116
Lentils, cooked, 1/2 cup	7.8	115
Black beans, cooked, 1/2 cup	7.5	114
Pinto beans, cooked, 1/2 cup	7.7	122
Lima beans, cooked, 1/2 cup	6.6	108
Artichoke, globe, cooked, 1 each	6.5	60
White beans, canned, 1/2 cup	6.3	154
Chickpeas, cooked, 1/2 cup	6.2	135
Great northern beans, cooked, 1/2 cup	6.2	105
Cowpeas, cooked, 1/2 cup	5.6	100
Soybeans, mature, cooked, 1/2 cup	5.2	149
Bran ready-to-eat cereals, various, about 1 oz	2.6–5.0	90–108
Crackers, rye wafers, plain, 2 wafers	5.0	74
Sweet potato, baked, with peel, 1 medium (146 g)	4.8	131
Asian pear, raw, 1 small	4.4	51
Green peas, cooked, 1/2 cup	4.4	67
Whole wheat English muffin, 1 each	4.4	134
Pear, raw, 1 small	4.3	81
Bulgur, cooked, 1/2 cup	4.1	76
Mixed vegetables, cooked, 1/2 cup	4.0	59
Raspberries, raw, 1/2 cup	4.0	32
Sweet potato, boiled, no peel, 1 medium (156 g)	3.9	119
Blackberries, raw, 1/2 cup	3.8	31
Potato, baked, with skin, 1 medium	3.8	161
Soybeans, green, cooked, 1/2 cup	3.8	127
Stewed prunes, 1/2 cup	3.8	133
Figs, dried, 1/4 cup	3.7	93
Dates, 1/4 cup	3.6	126
Oat bran, raw, 1/4 cup	3.6	58
Pumpkin, canned, 1/2 cup	3.6	42
Spinach, frozen, cooked, 1/2 cup	3.5	30
Shredded wheat ready-to-eat cereals, various, about 1 oz	2.8–3.4	96
Almonds, 1 oz	3.3	164
Apple with skin, raw, 1 medium	3.3	72
Brussels sprouts, frozen, cooked, 1/2 cup	3.2	33
Whole wheat spaghetti, cooked, 1/2 cup	3.1	87
Banana, 1 medium	3.1	105
Orange, raw, 1 medium	3.1	62

Food, Standard Amount	Dietary Fiber (g)	Calories
Oat bran muffin, 1 small	3.0	178
Guava, 1 medium	3.0	37
Pearled barley, cooked, 1/2 cup	3.0	97
Sauerkraut, canned, solids, and liquids, 1/2 cup	3.0	23
Tomato paste, 1/4 cup	2.9	54
Winter squash, cooked, 1/2 cup	2.9	38
Broccoli, cooked, 1/2 cup	2.8	26
Parsnips, cooked, chopped, 1/2 cup	2.8	55
Turnip greens, cooked, 1/2 cup	2.5	15
Collards, cooked, 1/2 cup	2.7	25
Okra, frozen, cooked, 1/2 cup	2.6	26
Peas, edible-podded, cooked, 1/2 cup	2.5	42

Source: ARS Nutrient Database for Standard Reference, Release 17. Foods are from single nutrient reports, which are sorted either by food description or in descending order by nutrient content in terms of common household measures. The food items and weights in these reports are adapted from those in the 2002 revision of *USDA Home and Garden Bulletin No. 72. Nutritive Value of Foods.* Mixed dishes and multiple preparations of the same food item have been omitted.

Appendix B-9
Food Sources of Vitamin C

Food sources of vitamin C ranked by milligrams of vitamin C per standard amount; also calories in the standard amount. (All provide > − 20% of RDA for adult men, which is 90 mg/day.)

Food, Standard Amount	Vitamin C (mg)	Calories
Guava, raw, 1/2 cup	188	56
Red sweet pepper, raw, 1/2 cup	142	20
Red sweet pepper, cooked, 1/2 cup	116	19
Kiwi fruit, 1 medium	70	46
Orange, raw, 1 medium	70	62
Orange juice, 3/4 cup	61–93	79–84
Green pepper, sweet, raw, 1/2 cup	60	15
Green pepper, sweet, cooked, 1/2 cup	51	19
Grapefruit juice, 3/4 cup	50–70	71–86
Vegetable juice cocktail, 3/4 cup	50	34
Strawberries, raw, 1/2 cup	49	27
Brussels sprouts, cooked, 1/2 cup	48	28
Cantaloupe, 1/4 medium	47	51
Papaya, raw, 1/4 medium	47	30
Kohlrabi, cooked, 1/2 cup	45	24
Broccoli, raw, 1/2 cup	39	15
Edible-pod peas, cooked, 1/2 cup	38	34
Broccoli, cooked, 1/2 cup	37	26
Sweet potato, canned, 1/2 cup	34	116
Tomato juice, 3/4 cup	33	31
Cauliflower, cooked, 1/2 cup	28	17

Food, Standard Amount	Vitamin C (mg)	Calories
Pineapple, raw, 1/2 cup	28	37
Kale, cooked, 1/2 cup	27	18
Mango, 1/2 cup	23	54

Source: Nutrient values from Agricultural Research Service (ARS) Nutrient Database for Standard Reference, Release 17. Foods are from ARS single nutrient reports, sorted in descending order by nutrient content in terms of common household measures. Food items and weights in the single nutrient reports are adapted from those in the 2002 revision of *USDA Home and Garden Bulletin No. 72*, Nutritive Value of Foods. Mixed dishes and multiple preparations of the same food item have been omitted from this table.

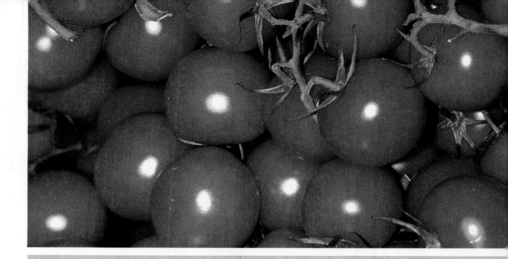

APPENDIX C

DIETARY GUIDELINES FOR AMERICANS 2005: EATING PATTERNS

Reprinted from *Dietary Guidelines for Americans 2005* (6th ed.), by the U.S. Department of Health and Human Services and U.S. Department of Agriculture, 2005, Washington, DC: U.S. Government Printing Office.

Appendix C-1
The DASH Eating Plan at 1,600-, 2,000-, 2600-, and 3,100-Calorie Levels[a]

The DASH Eating Plan is based on 1,600, 2,000, 2,600 and 3,100 calories. The number of daily servings in a food group varies depending on caloric needs (see Appendix A to determine caloric needs). This chart can aid in planning menus and food selection in restaurants and grocery stores.

Food Groups	1,600 Calories	2,000 Calories	2,600 Calories	3,100 Calories	Serving Sizes	Examples and Notes	Significance of Each Food Group to the DASH Eating Plan
Grains[b]	6 servings	7–8 servings	10–11 servings	12–13 servings	1 slice bread, 1 oz dry cereal, ½ cup cooked rice, pasta, or cereal[c]	Whole wheat bread, English muffin, pita bread, bagel, cereals, grits, oatmeal, crackers, unsalted pretzels, and popcorn	Major sources of energy and fiber
Vegetables	3–4 servings	4–5 servings	5–6 servings	6 servings	1 cup raw leafy vegetable ½ cup cooked vegetable 6 oz vegetable juice	Tomatoes, potatoes, carrots, green peas, squash, broccoli, turnip greens, collards, kale, spinach, artichokes, green beans, lima beans, sweet potatoes	Rich sources of potassium, magnesium, and fiber
Fruits	4 servings	4–5 servings	5–6 servings	6 servings	6 oz fruit juice 1 medium fruit ¼ cup dried fruit ½ cup fresh, frozen, or canned fruit	Apricots, bananas, dates, grapes, oranges, orange juice, grapefruit, grapefruit juice, mangoes, melons, peaches, pineapples, prunes, raisins, strawberries, tangerines	Important sources of potassium, magnesium, and fiber
Low-fat or fat-free dairy foods	2–3 servings	2–3 servings	3 servings	3–4 servings	8 oz milk 1 cup yogurt 1½ oz cheese	Fat-free or low-fat milk, fat-free or low-fat buttermilk, fat-free or low-fat regular or frozen yogurt, low-fat and fat-free cheese	Major sources of calcium and protein

Appendix C-1
Continued

Food Groups	1,600 Calories	2,000 Calories	2,600 Calories	3,100 Calories	Serving Sizes	Examples and Notes	Significance of Each Food Group to the DASH Eating Plan
Meat, poultry, fish	1–2 servings	2 or less servings	2 servings	2–3 servings	3 oz cooked meats, poultry, or fish	Select only lean; trim away visible fats; broil, roast, or boil instead of frying; remove skin from poultry	Rich sources of protein and magnesium
Nuts, seeds, legumes	3–4 servings/week	4–5 servings/week	1 serving	1 serving	⅓ cup or 1½ oz nuts 2 Tbsp or ½ oz seeds ½ cup cooked dry beans or peas	Almonds, filberts, mixed nuts, peanuts, walnuts, sunflower seeds, kidney beans, lentils	Rich sources of energy, magnesium, potassium, protein, and fiber
Fat and oils[d]	2 servings	2–3 servings	3 servings	4 servings	1 tsp soft margarine 1 Tbsp low-fat mayonnaise 2 Tbsp light salad dressing 1 tsp vegetable oil	Soft margarine, low-fat mayonnaise, light salad dressing, vegetable oil (such as olive, corn, canola, or safflower)	DASH has 27% of calories as fat (low in saturated fat), including fat in or added to foods
Sweets	0 servings	5 servings/week	2 servings	2 servings	1 Tbsp sugar 1 Tbsp jelly or jam ½ oz jelly beans 8 oz lemonade	Maple syrup, sugar, jelly, jam, fruit-flavored gelatin, jelly beans, hard candy, fruit punch sorbet, ices	Sweets should be low in fat

[a]NIH publication No. 03-4082; Karanja, N.M. et al., *JADA* 8:S19–27, 1999.

[b]Whole grains are recommended for most servings to meet fiber recommendations.

[c]Equals ½–1¼ cups, depending on cereal type. Check the product's nutrition facts label.

[d]Fat content changes serving counts for fats and oils: For example, 1 Tbsp of regular salad dressing equals 1 serving; 1 Tbsp of a low-fat dressing equals ½ serving; 1 Tbsp of a fat-free dressing equals 0 servings.

Appendix C-2
USDA Food Guide

The suggested amounts of food to consume from the basic food groups, subgroups, and oils to meet recommended nutrient intakes at 12 different calorie levels. Nutrient and energy contributions from each group are calculated according to the nutrient dense forms of foods in each group (e.g., lean meats and fat-free milk). The table also shows the discretionary calorie allowance that can be accommodated within each calorie level, in addition to the suggested amounts of nutrient-dense forms of foods in each group.

Daily Amount of Food from Each Group (vegetable subgroup amounts are per week)

Calorie Level	1,000	1,200	1,400	1,600	1,800	2,000	2,200	2,400	2,600	2,800	3,000	3,200
Food Group[1]	Food group amounts shown in cup (c) or ounce-equivalents (oz-eq), with number of servings (srv) in parentheses when it differs from the other units. See note for quantity equivalents for foods in each group.[2] Oils are shown in grams (g).											
Fruits	1 c (2 srv)	1 c (2 srv)	1.5 c (3 srv)	1.5 c (3 srv)	1.5 c (3 srv)	2 c (4 srv)	2 c (4 srv)	2 c (4 srv)	2 c (4 srv)	2.5 c (5 srv)	2.5 c (5 srv)	2.5 c (5 srv)
Vegetables[3]	1 c (2 srv)	1.5 c (3 srv)	1.5 c (3 srv)	2 c (4 srv)	2.5 c (5 srv)	2.5 c (5 srv)	3 c (6 srv)	3 c (6 srv)	3.5 c (7 srv)	3.5 c (7 srv)	4 c (8 srv)	4 c (8 srv)
Dark green veg.	1 c/wk	1.5 c/wk	1.5 c/wk	2 c/wk	3 c/wk	3 c/wk	3 c/wk	3 c/wk	3 c/wk	3 c/wk	3 c/wk	3 c/wk
Orange veg.	0.5 c/wk	1 c/wk	1 c/wk	1.5 c/wk	2 c/wk	2 c/wk	2 c/wk	2 c/wk	2.5 c/wk	2.5 c/wk	2.5 c/wk	2.5 c/wk
Legumes	0.5 c/wk	1 c/wk	1 c/wk	2.5 c/wk	3 c/wk	3 c/wk	3 c/wk	3 c/wk	3.5 c/wk	3.5 c/wk	3.5 c/wk	3.5 c/wk
Starchy veg.	1.5 c/wk	2.5 c/wk	2.5 c/wk	2.5 c/wk	3 c/wk	3 c/wk	6 c/wk	6 c/wk	7 c/wk	7 c/wk	9 c/wk	9 c/wk
Other veg.	3.5 c/wk	4.5 c/wk	4.5 c/wk	5.5 c/wk	6.5 c/wk	6.5 c/wk	7 c/wk	7 c/wk	8.5 c/wk	8.5 c/wk	10 c/wk	10 c/wk
Grains[4]	3 oz-eq	4 oz-eq	5 oz-eq	5 oz-eq	6 oz-eq	6 oz-eq	7 oz-eq	8 oz-eq	9 oz-eq	10 oz-eq	10 oz-eq	10 oz-eq
Whole grains	1.5	2	2.5	3	3	3	3.5	4	4.5	5	5	5
Other grains	1.5	2	2.5	2	3	3	3.5	4	4.5	5	5	5
Lean meat and beans	2 oz-eq	3 oz-eq	4 oz-eq	5 oz-eq	5 oz-eq	5.5 oz-eq	6 oz-eq	6.5 oz-eq	6.5 oz-eq	7 oz-eq	7 oz-eq	7 oz-eq
Milk	2 c	2 c	2 c	3 c	3 c	3 c	3 c	3 c	3 c	3 c	3 c	3 c
Oils[5]	15 g	17 g	17 g	22 g	24 g	27 g	29 g	31 g	34 g	36 g	44 g	51 g
Discretionary calorie allowance[6]	165	171	171	132	195	267	290	362	410	426	512	648

[1]Food items included in each group and subgroup:

Fruits	All fresh, frozen, canned, and dried fruits and fruit juices: for example, oranges and orange juice, apples and apple juice, bananas, grapes, melons, berries, raisins. In developing the food patterns, only fruits and juices with no added sugars or fats were used. *See note 6 on discretionary calories if products with added sugars or fats are consumed.*
Vegetables	In developing the food patterns, only vegetables with no added fats or sugars were used. *See note 6 on discretionary calories if products with added fats or sugars are consumed.*
▪ Dark green vegetables	All fresh, frozen, and canned dark green vegetables, cooked or raw: for example, broccoli; spinach; romaine; collard, turnip, and mustard greens.
▪ Orange vegetables	All fresh, frozen, and canned orange and deep yellow vegetables, cooked or raw: for example, carrots, sweet potatoes, winter squash, and pumpkin.
▪ Legumes (dry beans and peas)	All cooked dry beans and peas and soybean products: for example, pinto beans, kidney beans, lentils, chickpeas, tofu. (See comment under meat and beans group about counting legumes in the vegetable or the meat and beans group.)

- Starchy vegetables   All fresh, frozen, and canned starchy vegetables: for example, white potatoes, corn, green peas.

- Other vegetables   All fresh, frozen, and canned other vegetables, cooked or raw: for example, tomatoes, tomato juice, lettuce, green beans, onions.

Grains   In developing the food patterns, only grains in low-fat and low-sugar forms were used. *See note 6 on discretionary calories if products that are higher in fat and/or added sugars are consumed.*

- Whole grains   All whole-grain products and whole grains used as ingredients: for example, whole wheat and rye breads, whole-grain cereals and crackers, oatmeal, and brown rice.

- Other grains   All refined grain products and refined grains used as ingredients: for example, white breads, enriched grain cereals and crackers, enriched pasta, white rice.

Meat, poultry, fish, dry beans, eggs, and nuts (meat and beans)   All meat, poultry, fish, dry beans and peas, eggs, nuts, seeds. Most choices should be lean or low-fat. *See note 6 on discretionary calories if higher fat products are consumed.*
Dry beans and peas and soybean products are considered part of this group as well as the vegetable group, but should be counted in one group only.

Milk, yogurt, and cheese (milk)   All milks, yogurts, frozen yogurts, dairy desserts, cheeses (except cream cheese), including lactose-free and lactose-reduced products. Most choices should be fat-free or low fat. In developing the food patterns, only fat-free milk was used. *See note 6 on discretionary calories if low-fat, reduced fat, or whole milk or milk products–or milk products that contain added sugars are consumed.* Calcium-fortified soy beverages are an option for those who want a nondairy calcium source.

[2]Quantity equivalents for each food group:

Grains   The following each count as 1 ounce-equivalent (1 serving) of grains: ½ cup cooked rice, pasta, or cooked cereal; 1 ounce dry pasta or rice; 1 slice bread; 1 small muffin (1 oz); 1 cup ready-to-eat cereal flakes.

Fruits and vegetables   The following each count as 1 cup (2 servings) of fruits or vegetables: 1 cup cut up raw or cooked fruit or vegetable, 1 cup fruit or vegetable juice, 2 cups leafy salad greens.

Meat and beans   The following each count as 1 ounce-equivalent: 1 ounce lean meat, poultry, or fish; 1 egg; ¼ cup cooked dry beans or tofu; 1 Tbsp peanut butter; ½ ounce nuts or seeds.

Milk   The following each count as 1 cup (1 serving) of milk: 1 cup milk or yogurt, 1½ ounces natural cheese such as Cheddar cheese or 2 ounces processed cheese. Discretionary calories must be counted for all choices, except fat-free milk.

[3]Explanation of vegetable subgroup amounts: Vegetable subgroup amounts are shown in this table as weekly amounts, because it would be difficult for consumers to select foods from each subgroup daily. A daily amount that is one-seventh of the weekly amount listed is used in calculations of nutrient and energy levels in each pattern.

[4]Explanation of grain subgroup amounts: The whole-grain subgroup amounts shown in this table represent at least three 1-ounce servings and one-half of the total amount as whole grains for all calorie levels of 1,600 and above. This is the minimum suggested amount of whole grains to consume as part of the food patterns. More whole grains up to all of the grains recommended may be selected, with offsetting decreases in the amounts of other (enriched) grains. In patterns designed for younger children (1,000, 1,200, and 1,400 calories), one-half of the total amount of grains is shown as whole grains.

[5]Explanation of oils: Oils (including soft margarine with zero trans fat) shown in this table represent the amounts that are added to foods during processing, during cooking, or at the table. Oils and soft margarines include vegetable oils and soft vegetable oil table spreads that have no trans fats. The amounts of oils listed in this table are not considered to be part of discretionary calories because they are a major source of the vitamin E and polyunsaturated fatty acids, including the essential fatty acids, in the food pattern. In contrast, solid fats are listed separately in the discretionary calorie table (Appendix C-3) because, compared with oils, they are higher in saturated fatty acids and lower in vitamin E and polyunsaturated and monounsaturated fatty acids, including essential fatty acids. The amounts of each type of fat in the food intake pattern were based on 60% oils and/or soft margarines with no *trans* fats and 40% solid fat. The amounts in typical American diets are about 42% oils or soft margarines and about 58% solid fats.

[6]Explanation of discretionary calorie allowance: The discretionary calorie allowance is the remaining amount of calories in each food pattern after selecting the specified number of nutrient-dense forms of foods in each food group. The number of discretionary calories assumes that food items in each food group are selected in nutrient-dense forms (that is, forms that are fat-

free or low-fat and that contain no added sugars). Solid fat and sugar calories always need to be counted as discretionary calories, as in the following examples:

- The fat in low-fat, reduced-fat, or whole milk or milk products or cheese and the sugar and fat in chocolate milk, ice cream, pudding, etc.
- The fat in higher-fat meats (e.g., ground beef with more than 5% fat by weight, poultry with skin, higher-fat luncheon meats, sausages)
- The sugars added to fruits and fruit juices with added sugars or fruits canned in syrup
- The added fat or sugars in vegetables prepared with added fat or sugars
- The added fats and/or sugars in grain products containing higher levels of fats and/or sugars (e.g., sweetened cereals, higher-fat crackers, pies and other pastries, cakes, cookies)

Total discretionary calories should be limited to the amounts shown in the table at each calorie level. The number of discretionary calories is lower in the 1,600-calorie pattern than in the 1,000-, 1,200-, and 1,400-calorie patterns. These lower-calorie patterns are designed to meet the nutrient needs of children 2 to 8 years old. The nutrient goals for the 1,600 calorie pattern are set to meet the needs of adult women, which are higher and require that more calories be used in selections from the basic food groups. Additional information about discretionary calories, including an example of the division of these calories between solid fats and added sugars, is provided in Appendix C-3.

Appendix C-3
Discretionary Calorie Allowance in the USDA Food Guide

Discretionary calorie allowance is the remaining amount of calories in each calorie level after nutrient-dense forms of foods in each food group are selected. This table shows the number of discretionary calories remaining in each calorie level if nutrient-dense foods are selected. Those trying to lose weight may choose not to use discretionary calories. For those wanting to maintain their weight, discretionary calories may be used to increase the amount of food selected from each food group; to consume foods that are not in the lowest-fat form (such as 2% milk or medium-fat meat) or that contain added sugars; to add oil, fat, or sugars to foods; or to consume alcohol. The table shows an example of how these calories may be divided between solid fats and added sugars.

Discretionary calories that remain at each calorie level												
Food guide calorie level	1,000	1,200	1,400	1,600	1,800	2,000	2,200	2,400	2,600	2,800	3,000	3,200
Discretionary calories[1]	165	171	171	132	195	267	290	362	410	426	512	648
Example of division of discretionary calories: Solid fats are shown in grams (g); added sugars in grams (g) and teaspoons (tsp)												
Solid fats[2]	11g	14 g	14 g	11 g	15 g	18 g	19 g	22 g	24 g	24 g	29 g	34 g
Added sugars[3]	20 g	16 g	16 g	12 g	20 g	32 g	36 g	48 g	56 g	60 g	72 g	96 g
	(5 tsp)	(4 tsp)	(4 tsp)	(3 tsp)	(5 tsp)	(8 tsp)	(9 tsp)	(12 tsp)	(14 tsp)	(15 tsp)	(18 tsp)	(24 tsp)

[1]Discretionary calories: In developing the food guide, food items in nutrient-dense forms (that is, forms that are fat-free or low-fat and that contain no added sugars) were used. The number of discretionary calories assumes that food items in each food group are selected in nutrient-dense forms. Solid fat and sugar calories always need to be counted as discretionary calories, as in the following examples:

The fat in low-fat, reduced-fat, or whole milk or milk products or cheese and the sugar and fat in chocolate milk, ice cream, pudding, etc.

The fat in higher-fat meats (e.g., ground beef with more than 5% fat by weight, poultry with skin, higher-fat luncheon meats, sausages)

The sugars added to fruits and fruit juices with added sugars or fruits canned in syrup

The added fat or sugars in vegetables prepared with added fat or sugars

The added fats and/or sugars in grain products containing higher levels of fats and/or sugars (e.g., sweetened cereals, higher-fat crackers, pies and other pastries, cakes, cookies)

Total discretionary calories should be limited to the amounts shown in the table at each calorie level. The number of discretionary calories is lower in the 1,600-calorie pattern than in the 1,000-, 1,200-, and 1,400-calorie patterns. These lower-calorie patterns are designed to meet the nutrient needs of children 2 to 8 years old. The nutrient goals for the 1,600-calorie pattern are set to meet the needs of adult women, which are higher and require that more calories be used in selections from the basic food groups. The calories assigned to discretionary calories may be used to increase intake from the basic food groups; to select foods from these groups that are higher in fat or with added sugars; to add oils, solid fats, or sugars to foods or beverages; or to consume alcohol. See note 2 on limits for solid fats.

[2]Solid fats: Amounts of solid fats listed in the table represent about 7% to 8% of calories from saturated fat. Foods in each food group are represented in their lowest-fat forms, such as fat-free milk and skinless chicken. Solid fats shown in this table represent the amounts of fats that may be added in cooking or at the table, and fats consumed when higher-fat items are selected from the food groups (e.g., whole milk instead of fat-free milk, chicken with skin, or cookies instead of bread), without exceeding the recommended limits on saturated fat intake. Solid fats include meat and poultry fats eaten either as part of the meat or poultry product or separately; milk fat such as that in whole milk, cheese, and butter; shortenings used in baked products; and hard margarines.

Solid fats and oils are separated because their fatty acid compositions differ. Solid fats are higher in saturated fatty acids, and commonly consumed oils and soft margarines with no trans fats are higher in vitamin E and polyunsaturated and monounsaturated fatty acids, including essential fatty acids. Oils listed in Appendix C-2 are not considered to be part of the discretionary calorie allowance because they are a major source of the essential fatty acids and vitamin E in the food pattern.

The gram weights for solid fats are the amounts of these products that can be included in the pattern and are not identical to the amount of lipids in these items, because some products (margarines, butter) contain water or other ingredients, in addition to lipids.

[3]Added sugars: Added sugars are the sugars and syrups added to foods and beverages in processing or preparation, not the naturally occurring sugars in fruits or milk. The amounts of added sugars suggested in the example are NOT specific recommendations for amounts of added sugars to consume, but rather represent the amounts that can be included at each calorie level without overconsuming calories. The suggested amounts of added sugars may be helpful as part of the food guide to allow for some sweetened foods or beverages, without exceeding energy needs. This use of added sugars as a calorie balance requires two assumptions: (1) that selections are made from all food groups in accordance with the suggested amounts and (2) that additional fats are used in the amounts shown, which, together with the fats in the core food groups, represent about 27%–30% of calories from fat.

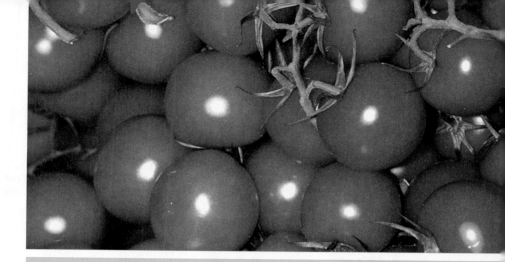

APPENDIX D

NUTRITIVE VALUE OF THE EDIBLE PART OF FOOD

Reprinted from "Nutritive value of foods" by S. E. Gebhardt and R. G. Thomas, 2002, U. S. Department of Agriculture, Agricultural Research, *Home and Garden Bulletin, 72,* 14–89.

								Fatty acids		
Food No.	Food Description	Measure of edible portion	Weight (g)	Water (%)	Calories (kcal)	Protein (g)	Total fat (g)	Satu- rated (g)	Mono- unsatu- rated (g)	Poly- unsatu- rated (g)
BEVERAGES										
	ALCOHOLIC									
	BEER									
1	REGULAR	12 FL OZ	355	92	146	1	0	0.0	0.0	0.0
2	LIGHT	12 FL OZ	354	95	99	1	0	0.0	0.0	0.0
	GIN, RUM, VODKA, WHISKEY									
3	80 PROOF	1.5 FL OZ	42	67	97	0	0	0.0	0.0	0.0
4	86 PROOF	1.5 FL OZ	42	64	105	0	0	0.0	0.0	0.0
5	90 PROOF	1.5 FL OZ	42	62	110	0	0	0.0	0.0	0.0
6	LIQUEUR, COFFEE, 53 PROOF	1.5 FL OZ	52	31	175	TR	TR	0.1	TR	0.1
	MIXED DRINKS, PREPARED FROM RECIPE									
7	DAIQUIRI	2 FL OZ	60	70	112	TR	TR	TR	TR	TR
8	PINA COLADA	4.5 FL OZ	141	65	262	1	3	1.2	0.2	0.5
	WINE									
	DESSERT									
9	DRY	3.5 FL OZ	103	80	130	TR	0	0.0	0.0	0.0
10	SWEET	3.5 FL OZ	103	73	158	TR	0	0.0	0.0	0.0
	TABLE									
11	RED	3.5 FL OZ	103	89	74	TR	0	0.0	0.0	0.0
12	WHITE	3.5 FL OZ	103	90	70	TR	0	0.0	0.0	0.0
	CARBONATED*									
13	CLUB SODA	12 FL OZ	355	100	0	0	0	0.0	0.0	0.0
14	COLA TYPE	12 FL OZ	370	89	152	0	0	0.0	0.0	0.0
	DIET, SWEETENED WITH ASPARTAME									
15	COLA	12 FL OZ	355	100	4	TR	0	0.0	0.0	0.0
16	OTHER THAN COLA OR PEPPER TYPE	12 FL OZ	355	100	0	TR	0	0.0	0.0	0.0
17	GINGER ALE	12 FL OZ	366	91	124	0	0	0.0	0.0	0.0
18	GRAPE	12 FL OZ	372	89	160	0	0	0.0	0.0	0.0
19	LEMON LIME	12 FL OZ	368	90	147	0	0	0.0	0.0	0.0
20	ORANGE	12 FL OZ	372	88	179	0	0	0.0	0.0	0.0
21	PEPPER TYPE	12 FL OZ	368	89	151	0	TR	0.3	0.0	0.0
22	ROOT BEER	12 FL OZ	370	89	152	0	0	0.0	0.0	0.0
	CHOCOLATE-FLAVORED BEVERAGE MIX									
23	POWDER	2–3 HEAPING TSP	22	1	75	1	1	0.4	0.2	TR
24	PREPARED WITH MILK	1 CUP	266	81	226	9	9	5.5	2.6	0.3
	COCOA									
	POWDER CONTAINING NONFAT DRY MILK									
25	POWDER	3 HEAPING TSP	28	2	102	3	1	0.7	0.4	TR
26	PREPARED (6 OZ WATER PLUS 1 OZ POWDER)	1 SERVING	206	86	103	3	1	0.7	0.4	TR
	POWDER CONTAINING NONFAT DRY MILK AND ASPARTAME									
27	POWDER	1/2-OZ ENVELOPE	5	3	48	4	TR	0.3	0.1	TR
28	PREPARED (6 OZ WATER PLUS 1 ENVELOPE MIX)	1 SERVING	192	92	48	4	TR	0.3	0.1	TR
	COFFEE									
29	BREWED	6 FL OZ	178	99	4	TR	0	TR	0.0	TR
30	ESPRESSO	2 FL OZ	60	98	5	TR	TR	0.1	0.0	0.1
31	INSTANT, PREPARED (1 ROUNDED TSP POWDER PLUS 6 FL OZ WATER)	6 FL OZ	179	99	4	TR	0	TR	0.0	TR

*Mineral content varies depending on water source.

Cholesterol (mg)	Carbo-hydrate (g)	Total dietary fiber (g)	Calcium (mg)	Iron (mg)	Potassium (mg)	Sodium (mg)	Vitamin A (IU)	Vitamin A (RE)	Thiamine (mg)	Ribo-flavin (mg)	Niacin (mg)	Ascorbic acid (mg)	Food No.
0	13	0.7	18	0.1	89	18	0	0	0.02	0.09	1.6	0	1
0	5	0.0	18	0.1	64	11	0	0	0.03	0.11	1.4	0	2
0	0	0.0	0	TR	1	TR	0	0	TR	TR	TR	0	3
0	TR	0.0	0	TR	1	TR	0	0	TR	TR	TR	0	4
0	0	0.0	0	TR	1	TR	0	0	TR	TR	TR	0	5
0	24	0.0	1	TR	16	4	0	0	TR	0.01	0.1	0	6
0	4	0.0	2	0.1	13	3	2	0	0.01	TR	TR	1	7
0	40	0.8	11	0.3	100	8	3	0	0.04	0.02	0.2	7	8
0	4	0.0	8	0.2	95	9	0	0	0.02	0.02	0.2	0	9
0	12	0.0	8	0.2	95	9	0	0	0.02	0.02	0.2	0	10
0	2	0.0	8	0.4	115	5	0	0	0.01	0.03	0.1	0	11
0	1	0.0	9	0.3	82	5	0	0	TR	0.01	0.1	0	12
0	0	0.0	18	TR	7	75	0	0	0.00	0.00	0.0	0	13
0	38	0.0	11	0.1	4	15	0	0	0.00	0.00	0.0	0	14
0	TR	0.0	14	0.1	0	21	0	0	0.02	0.08	0.0	0	15
0	0	0.0	14	0.1	7	21	0	0	0.00	0.00	0.0	0	16
0	32	0.0	11	0.7	4	26	0	0	0.00	0.00	0.0	0	17
0	42	0.0	11	0.3	4	56	0	0	0.00	0.00	0.0	0	18
0	38	0.0	7	0.3	4	40	0	0	0.00	0.00	0.1	0	19
0	46	0.0	19	0.2	7	45	0	0	0.00	0.00	0.0	0	20
0	38	0.0	11	0.1	4	37	0	0	0.00	0.00	0.0	0	21
0	39	0.0	19	0.2	4	48	0	0	0.00	0.00	0.0	0	22
0	20	1.3	8	0.7	128	45	4	TR	0.01	0.03	0.1	TR	23
32	31	1.3	301	0.8	497	165	311	77	0.10	0.43	0.3	2	24
1	22	0.3	92	0.3	202	143	4	1	0.03	0.16	0.2	1	25
2	22	2.5	97	0.4	202	148	4	0	0.03	0.16	0.2	TR	26
1	9	0.4	86	0.7	405	168	5	1	0.04	0.21	0.2	0	27
2	8	0.4	90	0.7	405	173	4	0	0.04	0.21	0.2	0	28
0	1	0.0	4	0.1	96	4	0	0	0.00	0.00	0.4	0	29
0	1	0.0	1	0.1	69	8	0	0	TR	0.11	3.1	TR	30
0	1	0.0	5	0.1	64	5	0	0	0.00	TR	0.5	0	31

Food No.	Food Description	Measure of edible portion	Weight (g)	Water (%)	Calories (kcal)	Protein (g)	Total fat (g)	Fatty acids Saturated (g)	Mono-unsaturated (g)	Poly-unsaturated (g)
BEVERAGES (CONTINUED)										
	FRUIT DRINKS, NONCARBONATED, CANNED OR BOTTLED, WITH ADDED ASCORBIC ACID									
32	CRANBERRY JUICE COCKTAIL	8 FL OZ	253	86	144	0	TR	TR	TR	0.1
33	FRUIT PUNCH DRINK	8 FL OZ	248	88	117	0	0	TR	TR	TR
34	GRAPE DRINK	8 FL OZ	250	88	113	0	0	TR	0.0	TR
35	PINEAPPLE GRAPEFRUIT JUICE DRINK	8 FL OZ	250	88	118	1	TR	TR	TR	0.1
36	PINEAPPLE ORANGE JUICE DRINK	8 FL OZ	250	87	125	3	0	0.0	0.0	0.0
	LEMONADE									
37	FROZEN CONCENTRATE, PREPARED	8 FL OZ	248	89	99	TR	0	TR	TR	TR
	POWDER, PREPARED WITH WATER									
38	REGULAR	8 FL OZ	266	89	112	0	0	TR	TR	TR
39	LOW CALORIE, SWEETENED WITH ASPARTAME	8 FL OZ	237	99	5	0	0	0.0	0.0	0.0
	MALTED MILK, WITH ADDED NUTRIENTS CHOCOLATE									
40	POWDER	3 HEAPING TSP	21	3	75	1	1	0.4	0.2	0.1
41	PREPARED	1 CUP	265	81	225	9	9	5.5	2.6	0.4
	NATURAL									
42	POWDER	4–5 HEAPING TSP	21	3	80	2	1	0.3	0.2	0.1
43	PREPARED	1 CUP	265	81	231	10	9	5.4	2.5	0.4
	MILK AND MILK BEVERAGES. SEE DAIRY PRODUCTS.									
44	RICE BEVERAGE, CANNED (RICE DREAM)	1 CUP	245	89	120	TR	2	0.2	1.3	0.3
	SOY MILK. SEE LEGUMES, NUTS, AND SEEDS.									
	TEA BREWED									
45	BLACK	6 FL OZ	178	100	2	0	0	TR	TR	TR
	HERB									
46	CHAMOMILE	6 FL OZ	178	100	2	0	0	TR	TR	TR
47	OTHER THAN CHAMOMILE	6 FL OZ	178	100	2	0	0	TR	TR	TR
	INSTANT, POWDER, PREPARED									
48	UNSWEETENED	8 FL OZ	237	100	2	0	0	0.0	0.0	0.0
49	SWEETENED, LEMON FLAVOR	8 FL OZ	259	91	88	TR	0	TR	TR	TR
50	SWEETENED WITH SACCHARIN, LEMON FLAVOR	8 FL OZ	237	99	5	0	0	0.0	0.0	TR
51	WATER, TAP	8 FL OZ	237	100	0	0	0	0.0	0.0	0.0
DAIRY PRODUCTS										
	BUTTER. SEE FATS AND OILS. CHEESE NATURAL									
52	BLUE	1 OZ	28	42	100	6	8	5.3	2.2	0.2
53	CAMEMBERT (3 WEDGES PER 4-OZ CONTAINER)	1 WEDGE	38	52	114	8	9	5.8	2.7	0.3
	CHEDDAR									
54	CUT PIECES	1 OZ	28	37	114	7	9	6.0	2.7	0.3
55		1 CUBIC IN.	17	37	68	4	6	3.6	1.6	0.2
56	SHREDDED	1 CUP	113	37	455	28	37	23.8	10.6	1.1

Cholesterol (mg)	Carbo-hydrate (g)	Total dietary fiber (g)	Calcium (mg)	Iron (mg)	Potassium (mg)	Sodium (mg)	Vitamin A		Thiamine (mg)	Ribo-flavin (mg)	Niacin (mg)	Ascorbic acid (mg)	Food No.
							(IU)	(RE)					
0	36	0.3	8	0.4	46	5	10	0	0.02	0.02	0.1	90	32
0	30	0.2	20	0.5	62	55	35	2	0.05	0.06	0.1	73	33
0	29	0.0	8	0.4	13	15	3	0	0.01	0.01	0.1	85	34
0	29	0.3	18	0.8	153	35	88	10	0.08	0.04	0.7	115	35
0	30	0.3	13	0.7	115	8	1,328	133	0.08	0.05	0.5	56	36
0	26	0.2	7	0.4	37	7	52	5	0.01	0.05	TR	10	37
0	29	0.0	29	0.1	3	19	0	0	0.00	TR	0.0	34	38
0	1	0.0	50	0.1	0	7	0	0	0.00	0.00	0.0	6	39
1	18	0.2	93	3.6	251	125	2,751	824	0.64	0.86	10.7	32	40
34	29	0.3	384	3.8	620	244	3,058	901	0.73	1.26	10.9	34	41
4	17	0.1	79	3.5	203	85	2,222	668	0.62	0.75	10.2	27	42
34	28	0.0	371	3.6	572	204	2,531	742	0.71	1.14	10.4	29	43
0	25	0.0	20	0.2	69	86	5	0	0.08	0.01	1.9	1	44
0	1	0.0	0	TR	66	5	0	0	0.00	0.02	0.0	0	45
0	TR	0.0	4	0.1	16	2	36	4	0.02	0.01	0.0	0	46
0	TR	0.0	4	0.1	16	2	0	0	0.02	0.01	0.0	0	47
0	TR	0.0	5	TR	47	7	0	0	0.00	TR	0.1	0	48
0	22	0.0	5	0.1	49	8	0	0	0.00	0.05	0.1	0	49
0	1	0.0	5	0.1	40	24	0	0	0.00	0.01	0.1	0	50
0	0	0.0	5	TR	0	7	0	0	0.00	0.00	0.0	0	51
21	1	0.0	150	0.1	73	396	204	65	0.01	0.11	0.3	0	52
27	TR	0.0	147	0.1	71	320	351	96	0.01	0.19	0.2	0	53
30	TR	0.0	204	0.2	28	176	300	79	0.01	0.11	TR	0	54
18	TR	0.0	123	0.1	17	105	180	47	TR	0.06	TR	0	55
119	1	0.0	815	0.8	111	701	1,197	314	0.03	0.42	0.1	0	56

Food No.	Food Description	Measure of edible portion	Weight (g)	Water (%)	Calories (kcal)	Protein (g)	Total fat (g)	Fatty acids Saturated (g)	Mono-unsaturated (g)	Poly-unsaturated (g)
DAIRY PRODUCTS (CONTINUED)										
	CHEESE (CONTINUED)									
	NATURAL (CONTINUED)									
	COTTAGE									
	CREAMED (4% FAT)									
57	LARGE CURD	1 CUP	225	79	233	28	10	6.4	2.9	0.3
58	SMALL CURD	1 CUP	210	79	217	26	9	6.0	2.7	0.3
59	WITH FRUIT	1 CUP	226	72	279	22	8	4.9	2.2	0.2
60	LOW FAT (2%)	1 CUP	226	79	203	31	4	2.8	1.2	0.1
61	LOW FAT (1%)	1 CUP	226	82	164	28	2	1.5	0.7	0.1
62	UNCREAMED (DRY CURD, LESS THAN 1/2% FAT)	1 CUP	145	80	123	25	1	0.4	0.2	TR
	CREAM									
63	REGULAR	1 OZ	28	54	99	2	10	6.2	2.8	0.4
64		1 TBSP	15	54	51	1	5	3.2	1.4	0.2
65	LOW FAT	1 TBSP	15	64	35	2	3	1.7	0.7	0.1
66	FAT FREE	1 TBSP	16	76	15	2	TR	0.1	0.1	TR
67	FETA	1 OZ	28	55	75	4	6	4.2	1.3	0.2
68	LOW FAT, CHEDDAR OR COLBY	1 OZ	28	63	49	7	2	1.2	0.6	0.1
	MOZZARELLA, MADE WITH									
69	WHOLE MILK	1 OZ	28	54	80	6	6	3.7	1.9	0.2
70	PART SKIM MILK (LOW MOISTURE)	1 OZ	28	49	79	8	5	3.1	1.4	0.1
71	MUENSTER	1 OZ	28	42	104	7	9	5.4	2.5	0.2
72	NEUFCHATEL	1 OZ	28	62	74	3	7	4.2	1.9	0.2
73	PARMESAN, GRATED	1 CUP	100	18	456	42	30	19.1	8.7	0.7
74		1 TBSP	5	18	23	2	2	1.0	0.4	TR
75		1 OZ	28	18	129	12	9	5.4	2.5	0.2
76	PROVOLONE	1 OZ	28	41	100	7	8	4.8	2.1	0.2
	RICOTTA, MADE WITH									
77	WHOLE MILK	1 CUP	246	72	428	28	32	20.4	8.9	0.9
78	PART SKIM MILK	1 CUP	246	74	340	28	19	12.1	5.7	0.6
79	SWISS	1 OZ	28	37	107	8	8	5.0	2.1	0.3
	PASTEURIZED PROCESS CHEESE									
	AMERICAN									
80	REGULAR	1 OZ	28	39	106	6	9	5.6	2.5	0.3
81	FAT FREE	1 SLICE	21	57	31	5	TR	0.1	TR	TR
82	SWISS	1 OZ	28	42	95	7	7	4.5	2.0	0.2
83	PASTEURIZED PROCESS CHEESE FOOD, AMERICAN	1 OZ	28	43	93	6	7	4.4	2.0	0.2
84	PASTEURIZED PROCESS CHEESE SPREAD, AMERICAN	1 OZ	28	48	82	5	6	3.8	1.8	0.2
	CREAM, SWEET									
85	HALF AND HALF (CREAM AND MILK)	1 CUP	242	81	315	7	28	17.3	8.0	1.0
86		1 TBSP	15	81	20	TR	2	1.1	0.5	0.1
87	LIGHT, COFFEE, OR TABLE	1 CUP	240	74	469	6	46	28.8	13.4	1.7
88		1 TBSP	15	74	29	TR	3	1.8	0.8	0.1
	WHIPPING, UNWHIPPED (VOLUME ABOUT DOUBLE WHEN WHIPPED)									
89	LIGHT	1 CUP	239	64	699	5	74	46.2	21.7	2.1
90		1 TBSP	15	64	44	TR	5	2.9	1.4	0.1
91	HEAVY	1 CUP	238	58	821	5	88	54.8	25.4	3.3
92		1 TBSP	15	58	52	TR	6	3.5	1.6	0.2

Cholesterol (mg)	Carbo-hydrate (g)	Total dietary fiber (g)	Calcium (mg)	Iron (mg)	Potassium (mg)	Sodium (mg)	Vitamin A (IU)	Vitamin A (RE)	Thiamine (mg)	Ribo-flavin (mg)	Niacin (mg)	Ascorbic acid (mg)	Food No.
34	6	0.0	135	0.3	190	911	367	108	0.05	0.37	0.3	0	57
31	6	0.0	126	0.3	177	850	342	101	0.04	0.34	0.3	0	58
25	30	0.0	108	0.2	151	915	278	81	0.04	0.29	0.2	0	59
19	8	0.0	155	0.4	217	918	158	45	0.05	0.42	0.3	0	60
10	6	0.0	138	0.3	193	918	84	25	0.05	0.37	0.3	0	61
10	3	0.0	46	0.3	47	19	44	12	0.04	0.21	0.2	0	62
31	1	0.0	23	0.3	34	84	405	108	TR	0.06	TR	0	63
16	TR	0.0	12	0.2	17	43	207	55	TR	0.03	TR	0	64
8	1	0.0	17	0.3	25	44	108	33	TR	0.04	TR	0	65
1	1	0.0	29	TR	25	85	145	44	0.01	0.03	TR	0	66
25	1	0.0	140	0.2	18	316	127	36	0.04	0.24	0.3	0	67
6	1	0.0	118	0.1	19	174	66	18	TR	0.06	TR	0	68
22	1	0.0	147	0.1	19	106	225	68	TR	0.07	TR	0	69
15	1	0.0	207	0.1	27	150	199	54	0.01	0.10	TR	0	70
27	TR	0.0	203	0.1	38	178	318	90	TR	0.09	TR	0	71
22	1	0.0	21	0.1	32	113	321	85	TR	0.06	TR	0	72
79	4	0.0	1,376	1.0	107	1,862	701	173	0.05	0.39	0.3	0	73
4	TR	0.0	69	TR	5	93	35	9	TR	0.02	TR	0	74
22	1	0.0	390	0.3	30	528	199	49	0.01	0.11	0.1	0	75
20	1	0.0	214	0.1	39	248	231	75	0.01	0.09	TR	0	76
124	7	0.0	509	0.9	257	207	1,205	330	0.03	0.48	0.3	0	77
76	13	0.0	669	1.1	308	307	1,063	278	0.05	0.46	0.2	0	78
26	1	0.0	272	TR	31	74	240	72	0.01	0.10	TR	0	79
27	TR	0.0	174	0.1	46	406	343	82	0.01	0.10	TR	0	80
2	3	0.0	145	0.1	60	321	308	92	0.01	0.10	TR	0	81
24	1	0.0	219	0.2	61	388	229	65	TR	0.08	TR	0	82
18	2	0.0	163	0.2	79	337	259	62	0.01	0.13	TR	0	83
16	2	0.0	159	0.1	69	381	223	54	0.01	0.12	TR	0	84
89	10	0.0	254	0.2	314	98	1,050	259	0.08	0.36	0.2	2	85
6	1	0.0	16	TR	19	6	65	16	0.01	0.02	TR	TR	86
159	9	0.0	231	0.1	292	95	1,519	437	0.08	0.36	0.1	2	87
10	1	0.0	14	TR	18	6	95	27	TR	0.02	TR	TR	88
265	7	0.0	166	0.1	231	82	2,694	705	0.06	0.30	0.1	1	89
17	TR	0.0	10	TR	15	5	169	44	TR	0.02	TR	TR	90
326	7	0.0	154	0.1	179	89	3,499	1,002	0.05	0.26	0.1	1	91
21	TR	0.0	10	TR	11	6	221	63	TR	0.02	TR	TR	92

Food No.	Food Description	Measure of edible portion	Weight (g)	Water (%)	Calories (kcal)	Protein (g)	Total fat (g)	Fatty acids Saturated (g)	Fatty acids Monounsaturated (g)	Fatty acids Polyunsaturated (g)
DAIRY PRODUCTS (CONTINUED)										
93	WHIPPED TOPPING (PRESSURIZED)	1 CUP	60	61	154	2	13	8.3	3.9	0.5
94		1 TBSP	3	61	8	TR	1	0.4	0.2	TR
	CREAM, SOUR									
95	REGULAR	1 CUP	230	71	493	7	48.0	30.0	13.9	1.8
96		1 TBSP	12	71	26	TR	3	1.6	0.7	0.1
97	REDUCED FAT	1 TBSP	15	80	20	TR	2	1.1	0.5	0.1
98	FAT FREE	1 TBSP	16	81	12	TR	0	0.0	0.0	0.0
	CREAM PRODUCT, IMITATION (MADE WITH VEGETABLE FAT)									
	SWEET									
	CREAMER									
99	LIQUID (FROZEN)	1 TBSP	15	77	20	TR	1	0.3	1.1	TR
100	POWDERED	1 TSP	2	2	11	TR	1	0.7	TR	TR
	WHIPPED TOPPING									
101	FROZEN	1 CUP	75	50	239	1	19	16.3	1.2	0.4
102		1 TBSP	4	50	13	TR	1	0.9	0.1	TR
103	POWDERED, PREPARED WITH WHOLE MILK	1 CUP	80	67	151	3	10	8.5	0.7	0.2
104		1 TBSP	4	67	8	TR	TR	0.4	TR	TR
105	PRESSURIZED	1 CUP	70	60	184	1	16	13.0	2.0	1.3
106		1 TBSP	4	60	11	TR	1	0.8	0.1	TR
107	SOUR DRESSING (FILLED CREAM TYPE, NONBUTTERFAT)	1 CUP	235	75	417	8	39	31.2	4.6	1.1
108		1 TBSP	12	75	21	TR	2	1.6	0.2	0.1
	FROZEN DESSERT									
	FROZEN YOGURT, SOFT SERVE									
109	CHOCOLATE	1/2 CUP	72	64	115	3	4	2.6	1.3	0.2
110	VANILLA	1/2 CUP	72	65	114	3	4	2.5	1.1	0.2
	ICE CREAM									
	REGULAR									
111	CHOCOLATE	1/2 CUP	66	56	143	3	7	4.5	2.1	0.3
112	VANILLA	1/2 CUP	66	61	133	2	7	4.5	2.1	0.3
113	LIGHT (50% REDUCED FAT), VANILLA	1/2 CUP	66	68	92	3	3	1.7	0.8	0.1
114	PREMIUM LOW FAT, CHOCOLATE	1/2 CUP	72	61	113	3	2	1.0	0.6	0.1
115	RICH, VANILLA	1/2 CUP	74	57	178	3	12	7.4	3.4	0.4
116	SOFT SERVE, FRENCH VANILLA.	1/2 CUP	86	60	185	4	11	6.4	3.0	0.4
117	SHERBET, ORANGE	1/2 CUP	74	66	102	1	1	0.9	0.4	0.1
	MILK									
	FLUID, NO MILK SOLIDS ADDED									
118	WHOLE (3.3% FAT)	1 CUP	244	88	150	8	8	5.1	2.4	0.3
119	REDUCED FAT (2%)	1 CUP	244	89	121	8	5	2.9	1.4	0.2
120	LOW FAT (1%)	1 CUP	244	90	102	8	3	1.6	0.7	0.1
121	NONFAT (SKIM)	1 CUP	245	91	86	8	TR	0.3	0.1	TR
122	BUTTERMILK	1 CUP	245	90	99	8	2	1.3	0.6	0.1
	CANNED									
123	CONDENSED, SWEETENED	1 CUP	306	27	982	24	27	16.8	7.4	1.0
	EVAPORATED									
124	WHOLE MILK	1 CUP	252	74	339	17	19	11.6	5.9	0.6
125	SKIM MILK	1 CUP	256	79	199	19	1	0.3	0.2	TR
	DRIED									
126	BUTTERMILK	1 CUP	120	3	464	41	7	4.3	2.0	0.3

*The vitamin A values listed for imitation sweet cream produts are mostly from beta-carotene added for coloring.

Cholesterol (mg)	Carbo-hydrate (g)	Total dietary fiber (g)	Calcium (mg)	Iron (mg)	Potassium (mg)	Sodium (mg)	Vitamin A (IU)	Vitamin A (RE)	Thiamine (mg)	Ribo-flavin (mg)	Niacin (mg)	Ascorbic acid (mg)	Food No.
46	7	0.0	61	TR	88	78	506	124	0.02	0.04	TR	0	93
2	TR	0.0	3	TR	4	4	25	6	TR	TR	TR	0	94
102	10	0.0	268	0.1	331	123	1,817	449	0.08	0.34	0.2	2	95
5	1	0.0	14	TR	17	6	95	23	TR	0.02	TR	TR	96
6	1	0.0	16	TR	19	6	68	17	0.01	0.02	TR	TR	97
1	2	0.0	20	0.0	21	23	100	13	0.01	0.02	TR	0	98
0	2	0.0	1	TR	29	12	13*	1*	0.00	0.00	0.0	0	99
0	1	0.0	TR	TR	16	4	4	TR	0.00	TR	0.0	0	100
0	17	0.0	5	0.1	14	19	646*	65*	0.00	0.00	0.0	0	101
0	1	0.0	TR	TR	1	1	34*	3*	0.00	0.00	0.0	0	102
8	13	0.0	72	TR	121	53	289*	39*	0.02	0.09	TR	1	103
TR	1	0.0	4	TR	6	3	14*	2*	TR	TR	TR	TR	104
0	11	0.0	4	TR	13	43	331*	33*	0.00	0.00	0.0	0	105
0	1	0.0	TR	TR	1	2	19*	2*	0.00	0.00	0.0	0	106
13	11	0.0	266	0.1	380	113	24	5	0.09	0.38	0.2	2	107
1	1	0.0	14	TR	19	6	1	TR	TR	0.02	TR	TR	108
4	18	1.6	106	0.9	188	71	115	31	0.03	0.15	0.2	TR	109
1	17	0.0	103	0.2	152	63	153	41	0.03	0.16	0.2	1	110
22	19	0.8	72	0.6	164	50	275	79	0.03	0.13	0.1	TR	111
29	16	0.0	84	0.1	131	53	270	77	0.03	0.16	0.1	TR	112
9	15	0.0	92	0.1	139	56	109	31	0.04	0.17	0.1	1	113
7	22	0.7	107	0.4	179	50	163	47	0.02	0.13	0.1	1	114
45	17	0.0	87	TR	118	41	476	136	0.03	0.12	0.1	1	115
78	19	0.0	113	0.2	152	52	464	132	0.04	0.16	0.1	1	116
4	22	0.0	40	0.1	71	34	56	10	0.02	0.06	TR	2	117
33	11	0.0	291	0.1	370	120	307	76	0.09	0.40	0.2	2	118
18	12	0.0	297	0.1	377	122	500	139	0.10	0.40	0.2	2	119
10	12	0.0	300	0.1	381	123	500	144	0.10	0.41	0.2	2	120
4	12	0.0	302	0.1	406	126	500	149	0.09	0.34	0.2	2	121
9	12	0.0	285	0.1	371	257	81	20	0.08	0.38	0.1	2	122
104	166	0.0	868	0.6	1,136	389	1,004	248	0.28	1.27	0.6	8	123
74	25	0.0	657	0.5	764	267	612	136	0.12	0.80	0.5	5	124
9	29	0.0	741	0.7	849	294	1,004	300	0.12	0.79	0.4	3	125
83	59	0.0	1,421	0.4	1,910	621	262	65	0.47	1.89	1.1	7	126

Food No.	Food Description	Measure of edible portion	Weight (g)	Water (%)	Calories (kcal)	Protein (g)	Total fat (g)	Fatty acids		
								Satu-rated (g)	Mono-unsatu-rated (g)	Poly-unsatu-rated (g)
DAIRY PRODUCTS (CONTINUED)										
127	NONFAT, INSTANT, WITH ADDED VITAMIN A	1 CUP	68	4	244	24	TR	0.3	0.1	TR
	MILK BEVERAGE									
	CHOCOLATE MILK (COMMERCIAL)									
128	WHOLE	1 CUP	250	82	208	8	8	5.3	2.5	0.3
129	REDUCED FAT (2%)	1 CUP	250	84	179	8	5	3.1	1.5	0.2
130	LOW FAT (1%)	1 CUP	250	85	158	8	3	1.5	0.8	0.1
131	EGGNOG (COMMERCIAL)	1 CUP	254	74	342	10	19	11.3	5.7	0.9
	MILK SHAKE, THICK									
132	CHOCOLATE	10.6 FL OZ	300	72	356	9	8	5.0	2.3	0.3
133	VANILLA	11 FL OZ	313	74	350	12	9	5.9	2.7	0.4
	SHERBET. SEE DAIRY PRODUCTS, FROZEN DESSERT									
	YOGURT									
	WITH ADDED MILK SOLIDS									
	MADE WITH LOW FAT MILK									
134	FRUIT FLAVORED	8-OZ CONTAINER	227	74	231	10	2	1.6	0.7	0.1
135	PLAIN	8-OZ CONTAINER	227	85	144	12	4	2.3	1.0	0.1
	MADE WITH NONFAT MILK									
136	FRUIT FLAVORED	8-OZ CONTAINER	227	75	213	10	TR	0.3	0.1	TR
137	PLAIN	8-OZ CONTAINER	227	85	127	13	TR	0.3	0.1	TR
	WITHOUT ADDED MILK SOLIDS									
138	MADE WITH WHOLE MILK, PLAIN	8-OZ CONTAINER	227	88	139	8	7	4.8	2.0	0.2
139	MADE WITH NON-FAT MILK, LOW-CALORIE SWEETENER, VANILLA OR LEMON FLAVOR	8-OZ CONTAINER	227	87	98	9	TR	0.3	0.1	TR
EGGS										
	EGG									
	RAW									
140	WHOLE	1 MEDIUM	44	75	66	5	4	1.4	1.7	0.6
141		1 LARGE	50	75	75	6	5	1.6	1.9	0.7
142		1 EXTRA LARGE	58	75	86	7	6	1.8	2.2	0.8
143	WHITE	1 LARGE	33	88	17	4	0	0.0	0.0	0.0
144	YOLK	1 LARGE	17	49	59	3	5	1.6	1.9	0.7
	COOKED, WHOLE									
145	FRIED, IN MARGARINE, WITH SALT	1 LARGE	46	69	92	6	7	1.9	2.7	1.3
146	HARD COOKED, SHELL REMOVED	1 LARGE	50	75	78	6	5	1.6	2.0	0.7
147		1 CUP, CHOPPED	136	75	211	17	14	4.4	5.5	1.9
148	POACHED, WITH SALT	1 LARGE	50	75	75	6	5	1.5	1.9	0.7
149	SCRAMBLED, IN MARGARINE, WITH WHOLE MILK, SALT	1 LARGE	61	73	101	7	7	2.2	2.9	1.3
150	EGG SUBSTITUTE, LIQUID	1/4 CUP	63	83	53	8	2	0.4	0.6	1.0
FATS AND OILS										
	BUTTER (4 STICKS PER LB)									
151	SALTED	1 STICK	113	16	813	1	92	57.3	26.6	3.4
152		1 TBSP	14	16	102	TR	12	7.2	3.3	0.4
153		1 TSP	5	16	36	TR	4	2.5	1.2	0.2
154	UNSALTED	1 STICK	113	18	813	1	92	57.3	26.6	3.4

Cholesterol (mg)	Carbo-hydrate (g)	Total dietary fiber (g)	Calcium (mg)	Iron (mg)	Potassium (mg)	Sodium (mg)	Vitamin A (IU)	Vitamin A (RE)	Thiamine (mg)	Ribo-flavin (mg)	Niacin (mg)	Ascorbic acid (mg)	Food No.
12	35	0.0	837	0.2	1,160	373	1,612	483	0.28	1.19	0.6	4	127
31	26	2.0	280	0.6	417	149	303	73	0.09	0.41	0.3	2	128
17	26	1.3	284	0.6	422	151	500	143	0.09	0.41	0.3	2	129
7	26	1.3	287	0.6	426	152	500	148	0.10	0.42	0.3	2	130
149	34	0.0	330	0.5	420	138	894	203	0.09	0.48	0.3	4	131
32	63	0.9	396	0.9	672	333	258	63	0.14	0.67	0.4	0	132
37	56	0.0	457	0.3	572	299	357	88	0.09	0.61	0.5	0	133
10	43	0.0	345	0.2	442	133	104	25	0.08	0.40	0.2	1	134
14	16	0.0	415	0.2	531	159	150	36	0.10	0.49	0.3	2	135
5	43	0.0	345	0.2	440	132	16	5	0.09	0.41	0.2	2	136
4	17	0.0	452	0.2	579	174	16	5	0.11	0.53	0.3	2	137
29	11	0.0	274	0.1	351	105	279	68	0.07	0.32	0.2	1	138
5	17	0.0	325	0.3	402	134	0	0	0.08	0.37	0.2	2	139
187	1	0.0	22	0.6	53	55	279	84	0.03	0.22	TR	0	140
213	1	0.0	25	0.7	61	63	318	96	0.03	0.25	TR	0	141
247	1	0.0	28	0.8	70	73	368	111	0.04	0.29	TR	0	142
0	TR	0.0	2	TR	48	55	0	0	TR	0.15	TR	0	143
213	TR	0.0	23	0.6	16	7	323	97	0.03	0.11	TR	0	144
211	1	0.0	25	0.7	61	162	394	114	0.03	0.24	TR	0	145
212	1	0.0	25	0.6	63	62	280	84	0.03	0.26	TR	0	146
577	2	0.0	68	1.6	171	169	762	228	0.09	0.70	0.1	0	147
212	1	0.0	25	0.7	60	140	316	95	0.02	0.22	TR	0	148
215	1	0.0	43	0.7	84	171	416	119	0.03	0.27	TR	TR	149
1	TR	0.0	33	1.3	208	112	1,361	136	0.07	0.19	0.1	0	150
248	TR	0.0	27	0.2	29	937	3,468	855	0.01	0.04	TR	0	151
31	TR	0.0	3	TR	4	117	434	107	TR	TR	TR	0	152
11	TR	0.0	1	TR	1	41	153	38	TR	TR	TR	0	153
248	TR	0.0	27	0.2	29	12	3,468	855	0.01	0.04	TR	0	154

Food No.	Food Description	Measure of edible portion	Weight (g)	Water (%)	Calories (kcal)	Protein (g)	Total fat (g)	Fatty acids Satu- rated (g)	Mono- unsatu- rated (g)	Poly- unsatu- rated (g)
FATS AND OILS (CONTINUED)										
155	LARD	1 CUP	205	0	1,849	0	205	80.4	92.5	23.0
156		1 TBSP	13	0	115	0	13	5.0	5.8	1.4
	MARGARINE, VITAMIN A–FORTIFIED, SALT ADDED									
	REGULAR (ABOUT 80% FAT)									
157	HARD (4 STICKS PER LB)	1 STICK	113	16	815	1	91	17.9	40.6	28.8
158		1 TBSP	14	16	101	TR	11	2.2	5.0	3.6
159		1 TSP	5	16	34	TR	4	0.7	1.7	1.2
160	SOFT	1 CUP	227	16	1,626	2	183	31.3	64.7	78.5
161		1 TSP	5	16	34	TR	4	0.6	1.3	1.6
	SPREAD (ABOUT 60% FAT)									
162	HARD (4 STICKS PER LB)	1 STICK	115	37	621	1	70	16.2	29.9	20.8
163		1 TBSP	14	37	76	TR	9	2.0	3.6	2.5
164		1 TSP	5	37	26	TR	3	0.7	1.2	0.9
165	SOFT	1 CUP	229	37	1,236	1	139	29.3	72.1	31.6
166		1 TSP	5	37	26	TR	3	0.6	1.5	0.7
167	SPREAD (ABOUT 40% FAT)	1 CUP	232	58	801	1	90	17.9	36.4	32.0
168		1 TSP	5	58	17	TR	2	0.4	0.8	0.7
169	MARGARINE BUTTER BLEND	1 STICK	113	16	811	1	91	32.1	37.0	18.0
170		1 TBSP	14	16	102	TR	11	4.0	4.7	2.3
	OILS, SALAD OR COOKING									
171	CANOLA	1 CUP	218	0	1,927	0	218	15.5	128.4	64.5
172		1 TBSP	14	0	124	0	14	1.0	8.2	4.1
173	CORN	1 CUP	218	0	1,927	0	218	27.7	52.8	128.0
174		1 TBSP	14	0	120	0	14	1.7	3.3	8.0
175	OLIVE	1 CUP	216	0	1,909	0	216	29.2	159.2	18.1
176		1 TBSP	14	0	119	0	14	1.8	9.9	1.1
177	PEANUT	1 CUP	216	0	1,909	0	216	36.5	99.8	69.1
178		1 TBSP	14	0	119	0	14	2.3	6.2	4.3
179	SAFFLOWER, HIGH OLEIC	1 CUP	218	0	1,927	0	218	13.5	162.7	31.3
180		1 TBSP	14	0	120	0	14	0.8	10.2	2.0
181	SESAME	1 CUP	218	0	1,927	0	218	31.0	86.5	90.9
182		1 TBSP	14	0	120	0	14	1.9	5.4	5.7
183	SOYBEAN, HYDROGENATED	1 CUP	218	0	1,927	0	218	32.5	93.7	82.0
184		1 TBSP	14	0	120	0	14	2.0	5.8	5.1
185	SOYBEAN, HYDROGENATED AND COTTONSEED OIL BLEND	1 CUP	218	0	1,927	0	218	39.2	64.3	104.9
186		1 TBSP	14	0	120	0	14	2.4	4.0	6.5
187	SUNFLOWER	1 CUP	218	0	1,927	0	218	22.5	42.5	143.2
188		1 TBSP	14	0	120	0	14	1.4	2.7	8.9
	SALAD DRESSINGS									
	COMMERCIAL									
	BLUE CHEESE									
189	REGULAR	1 TBSP	15	32	77	1	8	1.5	1.9	4.3
190	LOW CALORIE	1 TBSP	15	80	15	1	1	0.4	0.3	0.4
	CAESAR									
191	REGULAR	1 TBSP	15	34	78	TR	8	1.3	2.0	4.8
192	LOW CALORIE	1 TBSP	15	73	17	TR	1	0.1	0.2	0.4
	FRENCH									
193	REGULAR	1 TBSP	16	38	67	TR	6	1.5	1.2	3.4
194	LOW CALORIE	1 TBSP	16	69	22	TR	1	0.1	0.2	0.6

Cholesterol (mg)	Carbo-hydrate (g)	Total dietary fiber (g)	Calcium (mg)	Iron (mg)	Potassium (mg)	Sodium (mg)	Vitamin A (IU)	(RE)	Thiamine (mg)	Ribo-flavin (mg)	Niacin (mg)	Ascorbic acid (mg)	Food No.
195	0	0.0	TR	0.0	TR	TR	0	0	0.00	0.00	0.0	0	155
12	0	0.0	TR	0.0	TR	TR	0	0	0.00	0.00	0.0	0	156
0	1	0.0	34	0.1	48	1,070	4,050	906	0.01	0.04	TR	TR	157
0	TR	0.0	4	TR	6	132	500	112	TR	0.01	TR	TR	158
0	TR	0.0	1	TR	2	44	168	38	TR	TR	TR	TR	159
0	1	0.0	60	0.0	86	2,449	8,106	1,814	0.02	0.07	TR	TR	160
0	TR	0.0	1	0.0	2	51	168	38	TR	TR	TR	TR	161
0	0	0.0	24	0.0	34	1,143	4,107	919	0.01	0.03	TR	TR	162
0	0	0.0	3	0.0	4	139	500	112	TR	TR	TR	TR	163
0	0	0.0	1	0.0	1	48	171	38	TR	TR	TR	TR	164
0	0	0.0	48	0.0	68	2,276	8,178	1,830	0.02	0.06	TR	TR	165
0	0	0.0	1	0.0	1	48	171	38	TR	TR	TR	TR	166
0	1	0.0	41	0.0	59	2,226	8,285	1,854	0.01	0.05	TR	TR	167
0	TR	0.0	1	0.0	1	46	171	38	TR	TR	TR	TR	168
99	1	0.0	32	0.1	41	1,014	4,035	903	0.01	0.04	TR	TR	169
12	TR	0.0	4	TR	5	127	507	113	TR	TR	TR	TR	170
0	0	0.0	0	0.0	0	0	0	0	0.00	0.00	0.0	0	171
0	0	0.0	0	0.0	0	0	0	0	0.00	0.00	0.0	0	172
0	0	0.0	0	0.0	0	0	0	0	0.00	0.00	0.0	0	173
0	0	0.0	0	0.0	0	0	0	0	0.00	0.00	0.0	0	174
0	0	0.0	TR	0.8	0	TR	0	0	0.00	0.00	0.0	0	175
0	0	0.0	TR	0.1	0	TR	0	0	0.00	0.00	0.0	0	176
0	0	0.0	TR	0.1	TR	TR	0	0	0.00	0.00	0.0	0	177
0	0	0.0	TR	TR	TR	TR	0	0	0.00	0.00	0.0	0	178
0	0	0.0	0	0.0	0	0	0	0	0.00	0.00	0.0	0	179
0	0	0.0	0	0.0	0	0	0	0	0.00	0.00	0.0	0	180
0	0	0.0	0	0.0	0	0	0	0	0.00	0.00	0.0	0	181
0	0	0.0	0	0.0	0	0	0	0	0.00	0.00	0.0	0	182
0	0	0.0	0	0.0	0	0	0	0	0.00	0.00	0.0	0	183
0	0	0.0	0	0.0	0	0	0	0	0.00	0.00	0.0	0	184
0	0	0.0	0	0.0	0	0	0	0	0.00	0.00	0.0	0	185
0	0	0.0	0	0.0	0	0	0	0	0.00	0.00	0.0	0	186
0	0	0.0	0	0.0	0	0	0	0	0.00	0.00	0.0	0	187
0	0	0.0	0	0.0	0	0	0	0	0.00	0.00	0.0	0	188
3	1	0.0	12	TR	6	167	32	10	TR	0.02	TR	TR	189
TR	TR	0.0	14	0.1	1	184	2	TR	TR	0.02	TR	TR	190
TR	TR	TR	4	TR	4	158	3	TR	TR	TR	TR	0	191
TR	3	TR	4	TR	4	162	3	TR	TR	TR	TR	0	192
0	3	0.0	2	0.1	12	214	203	20	TR	TR	TR	0	193
0	4	0.0	2	0.1	13	128	212	21	0.00	0.00	0.0	0	194

Food No.	Food Description	Measure of edible portion	Weight (g)	Water (%)	Calories (kcal)	Protein (g)	Total fat (g)	Fatty acids Saturated (g)	Mono-unsaturated (g)	Poly-unsaturated (g)
FATS AND OILS (CONTINUED)										
	ITALIAN									
195	REGULAR	1 TBSP	15	38	69	TR	7	1.0	1.6	4.1
196	LOW CALORIE	1 TBSP	15	82	16	TR	1	0.2	0.3	0.9
	MAYONNAISE									
197	REGULAR	1 TBSP	14	15	99	TR	11	1.6	3.1	5.7
198	LIGHT, CHOLESTEROL FREE	1 TBSP	15	56	49	TR	5	0.7	1.1	2.8
199	FAT FREE	1 TBSP	16	84	12	0	TR	0.1	0.1	0.2
	RUSSIAN									
200	REGULAR	1 TBSP	15	35	76	TR	8	1.1	1.8	4.5
201	LOW CALORIE	1 TBSP	16	65	23	TR	1	0.1	0.1	0.4
	THOUSAND ISLAND									
202	REGULAR	1 TBSP	16	46	59	TR	6	0.9	1.3	3.1
203	LOW CALORIE	1 TBSP	15	69	24	TR	2	0.2	0.4	0.9
	PREPARED FROM HOME RECIPE									
204	COOKED, MADE WITH MARGARINE	1 TBSP	16	69	25	1	2	0.5	0.6	0.3
205	FRENCH	1 TBSP	14	24	88	TR	10	1.8	2.9	4.7
206	VINEGAR AND OIL	1 TBSP	16	47	70	0	8	1.4	2.3	3.8
207	SHORTENING (HYDROGENATED SOYBEAN AND COTTON-SEED OILS)	1 CUP	205	0	1,812	0	205	51.3	91.2	53.5
208		1 TBSP	13	0	113	0	13	3.2	5.7	3.3
FISH AND SHELLFISH										
209	CATFISH, BREADED, FRIED	3 OZ	85	59	195	15	11	2.8	4.8	2.8
	CLAM									
210	RAW, MEAT ONLY	3 OZ	85	82	63	11	1	0.1	0.1	0.2
211		1 MEDIUM	15	82	11	2	TR	TR	TR	TR
212	BREADED, FRIED	3/4 CUP	115	29	451	13	26	6.6	11.4	6.8
213	CANNED, DRAINED SOLIDS	3 OZ	85	64	126	22	2	0.2	0.1	0.5
214		1 CUP	160	64	237	41	3	0.3	0.3	0.9
	COD									
215	BAKED OR BROILED	3 OZ	85	76	89	20	1	0.1	0.1	0.3
216		1 FILLET	90	76	95	21	1	0.1	0.1	0.3
217	CANNED, SOLIDS AND LIQUID	3 OZ	85	76	89	19	1	0.1	0.1	0.2
	CRAB									
	ALASKA KING									
218	STEAMED	1 LEG	134	78	130	26	2	0.2	0.2	0.7
219		3 OZ	85	78	82	16	1	0.1	0.2	0.5
220	IMITATION, FROM SURIMI	3 OZ	85	74	87	10	1	0.2	0.2	0.6
	BLUE									
221	STEAMED	3 OZ	85	77	87	17	2	0.2	0.2	0.6
222	CANNED CRABMEAT	1 CUP	135	76	134	28	2	0.3	0.3	0.6
223	CRAB CAKE, WITH EGG, ONION, FRIED IN MARGARINE	1 CAKE	60	71	93	12	5	0.9	1.7	1.4
224	FISH FILLET, BATTERED OR BREADED, FRIED	1 FILLET	91	54	211	13	11	2.6	2.3	5.7
225	FISH STICK AND PORTION, BREADED, FROZEN, REHEATED	1 STICK (4″ × 1″ × 1/2″)	28	46	76	4	3	0.9	1.4	0.9
226		1 PORTION (4″ × 2″ × 1/2″)	57	46	155	9	7	1.8	2.9	1.8
227	FLOUNDER OR SOLE, BAKED OR BROILED	3 OZ	85	73	99	21	1	0.3	0.2	0.5
228		1 FILLET	127	73	149	31	2	0.5	0.3	0.8

Cholesterol (mg)	Carbo-hydrate (g)	Total dietary fiber (g)	Calcium (mg)	Iron (mg)	Potassium (mg)	Sodium (mg)	Vitamin A (IU)	Vitamin A (RE)	Thiamine (mg)	Ribo-flavin (mg)	Niacin (mg)	Ascorbic acid (mg)	Food No.
0	1	0.0	1	TR	2	116	11	4	TR	TR	TR	0	195
1	1	TR	TR	TR	2	118	0	0	0.00	0.00	0.0	0	196
8	TR	0.0	2	0.1	5	78	39	12	0.00	0.00	TR	0	197
0	1	0.0	0	0.0	10	107	18	2	0.00	0.00	0.0	0	198
0	2	0.6	0	0.0	15	190	0	0	0.00	0.00	0.0	0	199
3	2	0.0	3	0.1	24	133	106	32	0.01	0.01	0.1	1	200
1	4	TR	3	0.1	26	141	9	3	TR	TR	TR	1	201
4	2	0.0	2	0.1	18	109	50	15	TR	TR	TR	0	202
2	2	0.2	2	0.1	17	153	49	15	TR	TR	TR	0	203
9	2	0.0	13	0.1	19	117	66	20	0.01	0.02	TR	TR	204
0	TR	0.0	1	TR	3	92	72	22	TR	TR	TR	TR	205
0	TR	0.0	0	0.0	1	TR	0	0	0.00	0.00	0.0	0	206
0	0	0.0	0	0.0	0	0	0	0	0.00	0.00	0.0	0	207
0	0	0.0	0	0.0	0	0	0	0	0.00	0.00	0.0	0	208
69	7	0.6	37	1.2	289	238	24	7	0.06	0.11	1.9	0	209
29	2	0.0	39	11.9	267	48	255	77	0.07	0.18	1.5	11	210
5	TR	0.0	7	2.0	46	8	44	13	0.01	0.03	0.3	2	211
87	39	0.3	21	3.0	266	834	122	37	0.21	0.26	2.9	0	212
57	4	0.0	78	23.8	534	95	485	145	0.13	0.36	2.9	19	213
107	8	0.0	147	44.7	1,005	179	912	274	0.24	0.68	5.4	35	214
40	0	0.0	8	0.3	439	77	27	9	0.02	0.04	2.1	3	215
42	0	0.0	8	0.3	465	82	29	9	0.02	0.05	2.2	3	216
47	0	0.0	18	0.4	449	185	39	12	0.07	0.07	2.1	1	217
71	0	0.0	79	1.0	351	1,436	39	12	0.07	0.07	1.8	10	218
45	0	0.0	50	0.6	223	911	25	8	0.05	0.05	1.1	6	219
17	9	0.0	11	0.3	77	715	56	17	0.03	0.02	0.2	0	220
85	0	0.0	88	0.8	275	237	5	2	0.09	0.04	2.8	3	221
120	0	0.0	136	1.1	505	450	7	3	0.11	0.11	1.8	4	222
90	TR	0.0	63	0.6	194	198	151	49	0.05	0.05	1.7	2	223
31	15	0.5	16	1.9	291	484	35	11	0.10	0.10	1.9	0	224
31	7	0.0	6	0.2	73	163	30	9	0.04	0.05	0.6	0	225
64	14	0.0	11	0.4	149	332	60	18	0.07	0.10	1.2	0	226
58	0	0.0	15	0.3	292	89	32	9	0.07	0.10	1.9	0	227
86	0	0.0	23	0.4	437	133	48	14	0.10	0.14	2.8	0	228

Food No.	Food Description	Measure of edible portion	Weight (g)	Water (%)	Calories (kcal)	Protein (g)	Total fat (g)	Fatty acids Satu-rated (g)	Mono-unsatu-rated (g)	Poly-unsatu-rated (g)
FISH AND SHELLFISH (CONTINUED)										
229	HADDOCK, BAKED OR BROILED	3 OZ	85	74	95	21	1	0.1	0.1	0.3
230		1 FILLET	150	74	168	36	1	0.3	0.2	0.5
231	HALIBUT, BAKED OR BROILED	3 OZ	85	72	119	23	2	0.4	0.8	0.8
232		1/2 FILLET	159	72	223	42	5	0.7	1.5	1.5
233	HERRING, PICKLED	3 OZ	85	55	223	12	15	2.0	10.2	1.4
234	LOBSTER, STEAMED	3 OZ	85	76	83	17	1	0.1	0.1	0.1
235	OCEAN PERCH, BAKED OR BROILED	3 OZ	85	73	103	20	2	0.3	0.7	0.5
236		1 FILLET	50	73	61	12	1	0.2	0.4	0.3
	OYSTER									
237	RAW, MEAT ONLY	1 CUP	248	85	169	17	6	1.9	0.8	2.4
238		6 MEDIUM	84	85	57	6	2	0.6	0.3	0.8
239	BREADED, FRIED	3 OZ	85	65	167	7	11	2.7	4.0	2.8
240	POLLOCK, BAKED OR BROILED	3 OZ	85	74	96	20	1	0.2	0.1	0.4
241		1 FILLET	60	74	68	14	1	0.1	0.1	0.3
242	ROCKFISH, BAKED OR BROILED	3 OZ	85	73	103	20	2	0.4	0.4	0.5
243		1 FILLET	149	73	180	36	3	0.7	0.7	0.9
244	ROUGHY, ORANGE, BAKED OR BROILED	3 OZ	85	69	76	16	1	TR	0.5	TR
	SALMON									
245	BAKED OR BROILED (RED)	3 OZ	85	62	184	23	9	1.6	4.5	2.0
246		1/2 FILLET	155	62	335	42	17	3.0	8.2	3.7
247	CANNED (PINK), SOLIDS AND LIQUID (INCLUDES BONES)	3 OZ	85	69	118	17	5	1.3	1.5	1.7
248	SMOKED (CHINOOK)	3 OZ	85	72	99	16	4	0.8	1.7	0.8
249	SARDINE, ATLANTIC, CANNED IN OIL, DRAINED SOLIDS (INCLUDES BONES)	3 OZ	85	60	177	21	10	1.3	3.3	4.4
	SCALLOP, COOKED									
250	BREADED, FRIED	6 LARGE	93	58	200	17	10	2.5	4.2	2.7
251	STEAMED	3 OZ	85	73	95	20	1	0.1	0.1	0.4
	SHRIMP									
252	BREADED, FRIED	3 OZ	85	53	206	18	10	1.8	3.2	4.3
253		6 LARGE	45	53	109	10	6	0.9	1.7	2.3
254	CANNED, DRAINED SOLIDS	3 OZ	85	73	102	20	2	0.3	0.2	0.6
255	SWORDFISH, BAKED OR BROILED	3 OZ	85	69	132	22	4	1.2	1.7	1.0
256		1 PIECE	106	69	164	27	5	1.5	2.1	1.3
257	TROUT, BAKED OR BROILED	3 OZ	85	68	144	21	6	1.8	1.8	2.0
258		1 FILLET	71	68	120	17	5	1.5	1.5	1.7
	TUNA									
259	BAKED OR BROILED	3 OZ	85	63	118	25	1	0.3	0.2	0.3
	CANNED, DRAINED SOLIDS									
260	OIL PACK, CHUNK LIGHT	3 OZ	85	60	168	25	7	1.3	2.5	2.5
261	WATER PACK, CHUNK LIGHT	3 OZ	85	75	99	22	1	0.2	0.1	0.3
262	WATER PACK, SOLID WHITE	3 OZ	85	73	109	20	3	0.7	0.7	0.9
263	TUNA SALAD: LIGHT TUNA IN OIL, PICKLE RELISH, MAYO-TYPE SALAD DRESSING	1 CUP	205	63	383	33	19	3.2	5.9	8.5
FRUITS AND FRUIT JUICES										
	APPLES									
	RAW									
264	UNPEELED, 2 3/4" DIA (ABOUT 3 PER LB)	1 APPLE	138	84	81	TR	TR	0.1	TR	0.1

Cholesterol (mg)	Carbo-hydrate (g)	Total dietary fiber (g)	Calcium (mg)	Iron (mg)	Potassium (mg)	Sodium (mg)	Vitamin A (IU)	Vitamin A (RE)	Thiamine (mg)	Ribo-flavin (mg)	Niacin (mg)	Ascorbic acid (mg)	Food No.
63	0	0.0	36	1.1	339	74	54	16	0.03	0.04	3.9	0	229
111	0	0.0	63	2.0	599	131	95	29	0.06	0.07	6.9	0	230
35	0	0.0	51	0.9	490	59	152	46	0.06	0.08	6.1	0	231
65	0	0.0	95	1.7	916	110	285	86	0.11	0.14	11.3	0	232
11	8	0.0	65	1.0	59	740	732	219	0.03	0.12	2.8	0	233
61	1	0.0	52	0.3	299	323	74	22	0.01	0.06	0.9	0	234
46	0	0.0	116	1.0	298	82	39	12	0.11	0.11	2.1	1	235
27	0	0.0	69	0.6	175	48	23	7	0.07	0.07	1.2	TR	236
131	10	0.0	112	16.5	387	523	248	74	0.25	0.24	3.4	9	237
45	3	0.0	38	5.6	131	177	84	25	0.08	0.08	1.2	3	238
69	10	0.2	53	5.9	207	354	257	77	0.13	0.17	1.4	3	239
82	0	0.0	5	0.2	329	99	65	20	0.06	0.06	1.4	0	240
58	0	0.0	4	0.2	232	70	46	14	0.04	0.05	1.0	0	241
37	0	0.0	10	0.5	442	65	186	56	0.04	0.07	3.3	0	242
66	0	0.0	18	0.8	775	115	326	98	0.07	0.13	5.8	0	243
22	0	0.0	32	0.2	327	69	69	20	0.10	0.16	3.1	0	244
74	0	0.0	6	0.5	319	56	178	54	0.18	0.15	5.7	0	245
135	0	0.0	11	0.9	581	102	324	98	0.33	0.27	10.3	0	246
47	0	0.0	181	0.7	277	471	47	14	0.02	0.16	5.6	0	247
20	0	0.0	9	0.7	149	666	75	22	0.02	0.09	4.0	0	248
121	0	0.0	325	2.5	337	429	190	57	0.07	0.19	4.5	0	249
57	9	0.2	39	0.8	310	432	70	20	0.04	0.10	1.4	2	250
45	3	0.0	98	2.6	405	225	85	26	0.09	0.05	1.1	0	251
150	10	0.3	57	1.1	191	292	161	48	0.11	0.12	2.6	1	252
80	5	0.2	30	0.6	101	155	85	25	0.06	0.06	1.4	1	253
147	1	0.0	50	2.3	179	144	51	15	0.02	0.03	2.3	2	254
43	0	0.0	5	0.9	314	98	116	35	0.04	0.10	10.0	1	255
53	0	0.0	6	1.1	391	122	145	43	0.05	0.12	12.5	1	256
58	0	0.0	73	0.3	375	36	244	73	0.20	0.07	7.5	3	257
48	0	0.0	61	0.2	313	30	204	61	0.17	0.06	6.2	2	258
49	0	0.0	18	0.8	484	40	58	17	0.43	0.05	10.1	1	259
15	0	0.0	11	1.2	176	301	66	20	0.03	0.10	10.5	0	260
26	0	0.0	9	1.3	201	287	48	14	0.03	0.06	11.3	0	261
36	0	0.0	12	0.8	201	320	16	5	0.01	0.04	4.9	0	262
27	19	0.0	35	2.1	365	824	199	55	0.06	0.14	13.7	5	263
0	21	3.7	10	0.2	159	0	73	7	0.02	0.02	0.1	8	264

Food No.	Food Description	Measure of edible portion	Weight (g)	Water (%)	Calories (kcal)	Protein (g)	Total fat (g)	Fatty acids Satu-rated (g)	Mono-unsatu-rated (g)	Poly-unsatu-rated (g)
FRUITS AND FRUIT JUICES (CONTINUED)										
265	PEELED, SLICED	1 CUP	110	84	63	TR	TR	0.1	TR	0.1
266	DRIED (SODIUM BISULFITE USED TO PRESERVE COLOR)	5 RINGS	32	32	78	TR	TR	TR	TR	TR
267	APPLE JUICE, BOTTLED OR CANNED	1 CUP	248	88	117	TR	TR	TR	TR	0.1
268	APPLE PIE FILLING, CANNED	1/8 OF 21-OZ CAN	74	73	75	TR	TR	TR	0.0	TR
	APPLESAUCE, CANNED									
269	SWEETENED	1 CUP	255	80	194	TR	TR	0.1	TR	0.1
270	UNSWEETENED	1 CUP	244	88	105	TR	TR	TR	TR	TR
	APRICOTS									
271	RAW, WITHOUT PITS (ABOUT 12 PER LB WITH PITS)	1 APRICOT	35	86	17	TR	TR	TR	0.1	TR
	CANNED, HALVES, FRUIT AND LIQUID									
272	HEAVY SYRUP PACK	1 CUP	258	78	214	1	TR	TR	0.1	TR
273	JUICE PACK	1 CUP	244	87	117	2	TR	TR	TR	TR
274	DRIED, SULFURED	10 HALVES	35	31	83	1	TR	TR	0.1	TR
275	APRICOT NECTAR, CANNED, WITH ADDED ASCORBIC ACID	1 CUP	251	85	141	1	TR	TR	0.1	TR
	ASIAN PEAR, RAW									
276	2 1/4″ HIGH × 2 1/2″ DIA	1 PEAR	122	88	51	1	TR	TR	0.1	0.1
277	3 3/8″ HIGH × 3″ DIA	1 PEAR	275	88	116	1	1	TR	0.1	0.2
	AVOCADOS, RAW, WITHOUT SKIN AND SEED									
278	CALIFORNIA (ABOUT 1/5 WHOLE)	1 OZ	28	73	50	1	5	0.7	3.2	0.6
279	FLORIDA (ABOUT 1/10 WHOLE)	1 OZ	28	80	32	TR	3	0.5	1.4	0.4
	BANANAS, RAW									
280	WHOLE, MEDIUM (7″ TO 7 7/8″ LONG)	1 BANANA	118	74	109	1	1	0.2	TR	0.1
281	SLICED	1 CUP	150	74	138	2	1	0.3	0.1	0.1
282	BLACKBERRIES, RAW	1 CUP	144	86	75	1	1	TR	0.1	0.3
	BLUEBERRIES									
283	RAW	1 CUP	145	85	81	1	1	TR	0.1	0.2
284	FROZEN, SWEETENED, THAWED	1 CUP	230	77	186	1	TR	TR	TR	0.1
	CANTALOUPE. SEE MELONS.									
	CARAMBOLA (STARFRUIT), RAW									
285	WHOLE (3 5/8″ LONG)	1 FRUIT	91	91	30	TR	TR	TR	TR	0.2
286	SLICED	1 CUP	108	91	36	1	TR	TR	TR	0.2
	CHERRIES									
287	SOUR, RED, PITTED, CANNED, WATER PACK	1 CUP	244	90	88	2	TR	0.1	0.1	0.1
288	SWEET, RAW, WITHOUT PITS AND STEMS	10 CHERRIES	68	81	49	1	1	0.1	0.2	0.2
289	CHERRY PIE FILLING, CANNED	1/5 OF 21-OZ CAN	74	71	85	TR	TR	TR	TR	TR
290	CRANBERRIES, DRIED, SWEETENED	1/4 CUP	28	12	92	TR	TR	TR	TR	0.1
291	CRANBERRY SAUCE, SWEETENED, CANNED (ABOUT 8 SLICES PER CAN)	1 SLICE	57	61	86	TR	TR	TR	TR	TR
	DATES, WITHOUT PITS									
292	WHOLE	5 DATES	42	23	116	1	TR	0.1	0.1	TR
293	CHOPPED	1 CUP	178	23	490	4	1	0.3	0.3	0.1
294	FIGS, DRIED	2 FIGS	38	28	97	1	TR	0.1	0.1	0.2
	FRUIT COCKTAIL, CANNED, FRUIT AND LIQUID									

Cholesterol (mg)	Carbo-hydrate (g)	Total dietary fiber (g)	Calcium (mg)	Iron (mg)	Potassium (mg)	Sodium (mg)	Vitamin A		Thiamine (mg)	Ribo-flavin (mg)	Niacin (mg)	Ascorbic acid (mg)	Food No.
							(IU)	(RE)					
0	16	2.1	4	0.1	124	0	48	4	0.02	0.01	0.1	4	265
0	21	2.8	4	0.4	144	28	0	0	0.00	0.05	0.3	1	266
0	29	0.2	17	0.9	295	7	2	0	0.05	0.04	0.2	2	267
0	19	0.7	3	0.2	33	33	10	1	0.01	0.01	TR	1	268
0	51	3.1	10	0.9	156	8	28	3	0.03	0.07	0.5	4	269
0	28	2.9	7	0.3	183	5	71	7	0.03	0.06	0.5	3	270
0	4	0.8	5	0.2	104	TR	914	91	0.01	0.01	0.2	4	271
0	55	4.1	23	0.8	361	10	3,173	317	0.05	0.06	1.0	8	272
0	30	3.9	29	0.7	403	10	4,126	412	0.04	0.05	0.8	12	273
0	22	3.2	16	1.6	482	4	2,534	253	TR	0.05	1.0	1	274
0	36	1.5	18	1.0	286	8	3,303	331	0.02	0.04	0.7	137	275
0	13	4.4	5	0.0	148	0	0	0	0.01	0.01	0.3	5	276
0	29	9.9	11	0.0	333	0	0	0	0.02	0.03	0.6	10	277
0	2	1.4	3	0.3	180	3	174	17	0.03	0.03	0.5	2	278
0	3	1.5	3	0.2	138	1	174	17	0.03	0.03	0.5	2	279
0	28	2.8	7	0.4	467	1	96	9	0.05	0.12	0.6	11	280
0	35	3.6	9	0.5	594	2	122	12	0.07	0.15	0.8	14	281
0	18	7.6	46	0.8	282	0	238	23	0.04	0.06	0.6	30	282
0	20	3.9	9	0.2	129	9	145	15	0.07	0.07	0.5	19	283
0	50	4.8	14	0.9	138	2	101	9	0.05	0.12	0.6	2	284
0	7	2.5	4	0.2	148	2	449	45	0.03	0.02	0.4	19	285
0	8	2.9	4	0.3	176	2	532	53	0.03	0.03	0.4	23	286
0	22	2.7	27	3.3	239	17	1,840	183	0.04	0.10	0.4	5	287
0	11	1.6	10	0.3	152	0	146	14	0.03	0.04	0.3	5	288
0	21	0.4	8	0.2	78	13	152	16	0.02	0.01	0.1	3	289
0	24	2.5	5	0.1	24	1	0	0	0.01	0.03	TR	TR	290
0	22	0.6	2	0.1	15	17	11	1	0.01	0.01	0.1	1	291
0	31	3.2	13	0.5	274	1	21	2	0.04	0.04	0.9	0	292
0	131	13.4	57	2.0	1,161	5	89	9	0.16	0.18	3.9	0	293
0	25	4.6	55	0.8	271	4	51	5	0.03	0.03	0.3	TR	294

Food No.	Food Description	Measure of edible portion	Weight (g)	Water (%)	Calories (kcal)	Protein (g)	Total fat (g)	Fatty acids Satu-rated (g)	Fatty acids Mono-unsatu-rated (g)	Fatty acids Poly-unsatu-rated (g)
FRUITS AND FRUIT JUICES (CONTINUED)										
295	HEAVY SYRUP PACK	1 CUP	248	80	181	1	TR	TR	TR	0.1
296	JUICE PACK	1 CUP	237	87	109	1	TR	TR	TR	TR
	GRAPEFRUIT									
	RAW, WITHOUT PEEL, MEMBRANE AND SEEDS (3 3/4″ DIA)									
297	PINK OR RED	1/2 GRAPEFRUIT	123	91	37	1	TR	TR	TR	TR
298	WHITE	1/2 GRAPEFRUIT	118	90	39	1	TR	TR	TR	TR
299	CANNED, SECTIONS WITH LIGHT SYRUP	1 CUP	254	84	152	1	TR	TR	TR	0.1
	GRAPEFRUIT JUICE									
	RAW									
300	PINK	1 CUP	247	90	96	1	TR	TR	TR	0.1
301	WHITE	1 CUP	247	90	96	1	TR	TR	TR	0.1
	CANNED									
302	UNSWEETENED	1 CUP	247	90	94	1	TR	TR	TR	0.1
303	SWEETENED	1 CUP	250	87	115	1	TR	TR	TR	0.1
	FROZEN CONCENTRATE, UNSWEETENED									
304	UNDILUTED	6-FL-OZ CAN	207	62	302	4	1	0.1	0.1	0.2
305	DILUTED WITH 3 PARTS WATER BY VOLUME	1 CUP	247	89	101	1	TR	TR	TR	0.1
306	GRAPES, SEEDLESS, RAW	10 GRAPES	50	81	36	TR	TR	0.1	TR	0.1
307		1 CUP	160	81	114	1	1	0.3	TR	0.3
	GRAPE JUICE									
308	CANNED OR BOTTLED	1 CUP	253	84	154	1	TR	0.1	TR	0.1
	FROZEN CONCENTRATE, SWEETENED, WITH ADDED VITAMIN C									
309	UNDILUTED	6-FL-OZ CAN	216	54	387	1	1	0.2	TR	0.2
310	DILUTED WITH 3 PARTS WATER BY VOLUME	1 CUP	250	87	128	TR	TR	0.1	TR	0.1
311	KIWI FRUIT, RAW, WITHOUT SKIN (ABOUT 5 PER LB WITH SKIN)	1 MEDIUM	76	83	46	1	TR	TR	TR	0.2
312	LEMONS, RAW, WITHOUT PEEL (2 1/8″ DIA WITH PEEL)	1 LEMON	58	89	17	1	TR	TR	TR	0.1
	LEMON JUICE									
313	RAW (FROM 2 1/8″ -DIA LEMON)	JUICE OF 1 LEMON	47	91	12	TR	0	0.0	0.0	0.0
314	CANNED OR BOTTLED, UNSWEETENED	1 CUP	244	92	51	1	1	0.1	TR	0.2
315		1 TBSP	15	92	3	TR	TR	TR	TR	TR
	LIME JUICE									
316	RAW (FROM 2″-DIA LIME)	JUICE OF 1 LIME	38	90	10	TR	TR	TR	TR	TR
317	CANNED, UNSWEETENED	1 CUP	246	93	52	1	1	0.1	0.1	0.2
318		1 TBSP	15	93	3	TR	TR	TR	TR	TR
	MANGOS, RAW, WITHOUT SKIN AND SEED (ABOUT 1 1/2 PER LB WITH SKIN AND SEED)									
319	WHOLE	1 MANGO	207	82	135	1	1	0.1	0.2	0.1
320	SLICED	1 CUP	165	82	107	1	TR	0.1	0.2	0.1
	MELONS, RAW, WITHOUT RIND AND CAVITY CONTENTS									

*Sodium benzoate and sodium bisulfite added as preservatives.

Cholesterol (mg)	Carbo-hydrate (g)	Total dietary fiber (g)	Calcium (mg)	Iron (mg)	Potassium (mg)	Sodium (mg)	Vitamin A (IU)	Vitamin A (RE)	Thiamine (mg)	Ribo-flavin (mg)	Niacin (mg)	Ascorbic acid (mg)	Food No.
0	47	2.5	15	0.7	218	15	508	50	0.04	0.05	0.9	5	295
0	28	2.4	19	0.5	225	9	723	73	0.03	0.04	1.0	6	296
0	9	1.4	14	0.1	159	0	319	32	0.04	0.02	0.2	47	297
0	10	1.3	14	0.1	175	0	12	1	0.04	0.02	0.3	39	298
0	39	1.0	36	1.0	328	5	0	0	0.10	0.05	0.6	54	299
0	23	0.2	22	0.5	400	2	1,087	109	0.10	0.05	0.5	94	300
0	23	0.2	22	0.5	400	2	25	2	0.10	0.05	0.5	94	301
0	22	0.2	17	0.5	378	2	17	2	0.10	0.05	0.6	72	302
0	28	0.3	20	0.9	405	5	0	0	0.10	0.06	0.8	67	303
0	72	0.8	56	1.0	1,002	6	64	6	0.30	0.16	1.6	248	304
0	24	0.2	20	0.3	336	2	22	2	0.10	0.05	0.5	83	305
0	9	0.5	6	0.1	93	1	37	4	0.05	0.03	0.2	5	306
0	28	1.6	18	0.4	296	3	117	11	0.15	0.09	0.5	17	307
0	38	0.3	23	0.6	334	8	20	3	0.07	0.09	0.7	TR	308
0	96	0.6	28	0.8	160	15	58	6	0.11	0.20	0.9	179	309
0	32	0.3	10	0.3	53	5	20	3	0.04	0.07	0.3	60	310
0	11	2.6	20	0.3	252	4	133	14	0.02	0.04	0.4	74	311
0	5	1.6	15	0.3	80	1	17	2	0.02	0.01	0.1	31	312
0	4	0.2	3	TR	58	TR	9	1	0.01	TR	TR	22	313
0	16	1.0	27	0.3	249	51*	37	5	0.10	0.02	0.5	61	314
0	1	0.1	2	TR	16	3*	2	TR	0.01	TR	TR	4	315
0	3	0.2	3	TR	41	TR	4	TR	0.01	TR	TR	11	316
0	16	1.0	30	0.6	185	39*	39	5	0.08	0.01	0.4	16	317
0	1	0.1	2	TR	11	2*	2	TR	TR	TR	TR	1	318
0	35	3.7	21	0.3	323	4	8,061	805	0.12	0.12	1.2	57	319
0	28	3.0	17	0.2	257	3	6,425	642	0.10	0.09	1.0	46	320

Food No.	Food Description	Measure of edible portion	Weight (g)	Water (%)	Calories (kcal)	Protein (g)	Total fat (g)	Fatty acids Saturated (g)	Fatty acids Mono-unsaturated (g)	Fatty acids Poly-unsaturated (g)
FRUITS AND FRUIT JUICES (CONTINUED)										
	CANTALOUPE (5″ DIA)									
321	WEDGE	1/8 MELON	69	90	24	1	TR	TR	TR	0.1
322	CUBES	1 CUP	160	90	56	1	TR	0.1	TR	0.2
	HONEYDEW (6″–7″ DIA)									
323	WEDGE	1/8 MELON	160	90	56	1	TR	TR	TR	0.1
324	DICED (ABOUT 20 PIECES PER CUP)	1 CUP	170	90	60	1	TR	TR	TR	0.1
325	MIXED FRUIT, FROZEN, SWEETENED, THAWED (PEACH, CHERRY, RASPBERRY, GRAPE, ANDBOYSENBERRY)	1 CUP	250	74	245	4	TR	0.1	0.1	0.2
326	NECTARINES, RAW (2 1/2″ DIA)	1 NECTARINE	136	86	67	1	1	0.1	0.2	0.3
	ORANGES, RAW									
327	WHOLE, WITHOUT PEEL AND SEEDS (2 5/8″ DIA)	1 ORANGE	131	87	62	1	TR	TR	TR	TR
328	SECTIONS WITHOUT MEMBRANES	1 CUP	180	87	85	2	TR	TR	TR	TR
	ORANGE JUICE									
329	RAW, ALL VARIETIES	1 CUP	248	88	112	2	TR	0.1	0.1	0.1
330		JUICE FROM 1 ORANGE	86	88	39	1	TR	TR	TR	TR
331	CANNED, UNSWEETENED	1 CUP	249	89	105	1	TR	TR	0.1	0.1
332	CHILLED (REFRIGERATOR CASE)	1 CUP	249	88	110	2	1	0.1	0.1	0.2
	FROZEN CONCENTRATE									
333	UNDILUTED	6-FL-OZ CAN	213	58	339	5	TR	0.1	0.1	0.1
334	DILUTED WITH 3 PARTS WATER BY VOLUME	1 CUP	249	88	112	2	TR	TR	TR	TR
	PAPAYAS, RAW									
335	1/2″ CUBES	1 CUP	140	89	55	1	TR	0.1	0.1	TR
336	WHOLE (5 1/8″ LONG × 3″ DIA)	1 PAPAYA	304	89	119	2	TR	0.1	0.1	0.1
	PEACHES									
	RAW									
337	WHOLE, 2 1/2″ DIA, PITTED (ABOUT 4 PER LB)	1 PEACH	98	88	42	1	TR	TR	TR	TR
338	SLICED	1 CUP	170	88	73	1	TR	TR	0.1	0.1
	CANNED, FRUIT AND LIQUID									
339	HEAVY SYRUP PACK	1 CUP	262	79	194	1	TR	TR	0.1	0.1
340		1 HALF	98	79	73	TR	TR	TR	TR	TR
341	JUICE PACK	1 CUP	248	87	109	2	TR	TR	TR	TR
342		1 HALF	98	87	43	1	TR	TR	TR	TR
343	DRIED, SULFURED	3 HALVES	39	32	93	1	TR	TR	0.1	0.1
344	FROZEN, SLICED, SWEETENED, WITH ADDED ASCORBIC ACID, THAWED	1 CUP	250	75	235	2	TR	TR	0.1	0.2
	PEARS									
345	RAW, WITH SKIN, CORED, 2 1/2″ DIA	1 PEAR	166	84	98	1	1	TR	0.1	0.2
	CANNED, FRUIT AND LIQUID									
346	HEAVY SYRUP PACK	1 CUP	266	80	197	1	TR	TR	0.1	0.1
347		1 HALF	76	80	56	TR	TR	TR	TR	TR
348	JUICE PACK	.1 CUP	248	86	124	1	TR	TR	TR	TR
349		1 HALF	76	86	38	TR	TR	TR	TR	TR
	PINEAPPLE									
350	RAW, DICED	1 CUP	155	87	76	1	1	TR	0.1	0.2

Cholesterol (mg)	Carbo-hydrate (g)	Total dietary fiber (g)	Calcium (mg)	Iron (mg)	Potassium (mg)	Sodium (mg)	Vitamin A (IU)	(RE)	Thiamine (mg)	Ribo-flavin (mg)	Niacin (mg)	Ascorbic acid (mg)	Food No.
0	6	0.6	8	0.1	213	6	2,225	222	0.02	0.01	0.4	29	321
0	13	1.3	18	0.3	494	14	5,158	515	0.06	0.03	0.9	68	322
0	15	1.0	10	0.1	434	16	64	6	0.12	0.03	1.0	40	323
0	16	1.0	10	0.1	461	17	68	7	0.13	0.03	1.0	42	324
0	61	4.8	18	0.7	328	8	805	80	0.04	0.09	1.0	188	325
0	16	2.2	7	0.2	288	0	1,001	101	0.02	0.06	1.3	7	326
0	15	3.1	52	0.1	237	0	269	28	0.11	0.05	0.4	70	327
0	21	4.3	72	0.2	326	0	369	38	0.16	0.07	0.5	96	328
0	26	0.5	27	0.5	496	2	496	50	0.22	0.07	1.0	124	329
0	9	0.2	9	0.2	172	1	172	17	0.08	0.03	0.3	43	330
0	25	0.5	20	1.1	436	5	436	45	0.15	0.07	0.8	86	331
0	25	0.5	25	0.4	473	2	194	20	0.28	0.05	0.7	82	332
0	81	1.7	68	0.7	1,436	6	588	60	0.60	0.14	1.5	294	333
0	27	0.5	22	0.2	473	2	194	20	0.20	0.04	0.5	97	334
0	14	2.5	34	0.1	360	4	398	39	0.04	0.04	0.5	87	335
0	30	5.5	73	0.3	781	9	863	85	0.08	0.10	1.0	188	336
0	11	2.0	5	0.1	193	0	524	53	0.02	0.04	1.0	6	337
0	19	3.4	9	0.2	335	0	910	92	0.03	0.07	1.7	11	338
0	52	3.4	8	0.7	241	16	870	86	0.03	0.06	1.6	7	339
0	20	1.3	3	0.3	90	6	325	32	0.01	0.02	0.6	3	340
0	29	3.2	15	0.7	317	10	945	94	0.02	0.04	1.4	9	341
0	11	1.3	6	0.3	125	4	373	37	0.01	0.02	0.6	4	342
0	24	3.2	11	1.6	388	3	844	84	TR	0.08	1.7	2	343
0	60	4.5	8	0.9	325	15	710	70	0.03	0.09	1.6	236	344
0	25	4.0	18	0.4	208	0	33	3	0.03	0.07	0.2	7	345
0	51	4.3	13	0.6	173	13	0	0	0.03	0.06	0.6	3	346
0	15	1.2	4	0.2	49	4	0	0	0.01	0.02	0.2	1	347
0	32	4.0	22	0.7	238	10	15	2	0.03	0.03	0.5	4	348
0	10	1.2	7	0.2	73	3	5	1	0.01	0.01	0.2	1	349
0	19	1.9	11	0.6	175	2	36	3	0.14	0.06	0.7	24	350

Food No.	Food Description	Measure of edible portion	Weight (g)	Water (%)	Calories (kcal)	Protein (g)	Total fat (g)	Fatty acids		
								Satu-rated (g)	Mono-unsatu-rated (g)	Poly-unsatu-rated (g)
FRUITS AND FRUIT JUICES (CONTINUED)										
	CANNED, FRUIT AND LIQUID									
	HEAVY SYRUP PACK									
351	CRUSHED, SLICED, OR CHUNKS	1 CUP	254	79	198	1	TR	TR	TR	0.1
352	SLICES (3" DIA)	1 SLICE	49	79	38	TR	TR	TR	TR	TR
	JUICE PACK									
353	CRUSHED, SLICED, OR CHUNKS	1 CUP	249	84	149	1	TR	TR	TR	0.1
354	SLICE (3" DIA)	1 SLICE	47	84	28	TR	TR	TR	TR	TR
355	PINEAPPLE JUICE, UNSWEETENED, CANNED	1 CUP	250	86	140	1	TR	TR	TR	0.1
	PLANTAIN, WITHOUT PEEL									
356	RAW	1 MEDIUM	179	65	218	2	1	0.3	0.1	0.1
357	COOKED, SLICES	1 CUP	154	67	179	1	TR	0.1	TR	0.1
	PLUMS									
358	RAW (2 1/8" DIA)	1 PLUM	66	85	36	1	TR	TR	0.3	0.1
	CANNED, PURPLE, FRUIT AND LIQUID									
359	HEAVY SYRUP PACK	1 CUP	258	76	230	1	TR	TR	0.2	0.1
360		1 PLUM	46	76	41	TR	TR	TR	TR	TR
361	JUICE PACK	1 CUP	252	84	146	1	TR	TR	TR	TR
362		1 PLUM	46	84	27	TR	TR	TR	TR	TR
	PRUNES, DRIED, PITTED									
363	UNCOOKED	5 PRUNES	42	32	100	1	TR	TR	0.1	TR
364	STEWED, UNSWEETENED,									
	FRUIT AND LIQUID	1 CUP	248	70	265	3	1	TR	0.4	0.1
365	PRUNE JUICE, CANNED OR BOTTLED	1 CUP	256	81	182	2	TR	TR	0.1	TR
	RAISINS, SEEDLESS									
366	CUP, NOT PACKED	1 CUP	145	15	435	5	1	0.2	TR	0.2
367	PACKET, 1/2 OZ (1 1/2 TBSP)	1 PACKET	14	15	42	TR	TR	TR	TR	TR
	RASPBERRIES									
368	RAW	1 CUP	123	87	60	1	1	TR	0.1	0.4
369	FROZEN, SWEETENED, THAWED	1 CUP	250	73	258	2	TR	TR	TR	0.2
370	RHUBARB, FROZEN, COOKED, WITH SUGAR	1 CUP	240	68	278	1	TR	TR	TR	0.1
	STRAWBERRIES									
	RAW, CAPPED									
371	LARGE (1 1/8" DIA)	1 STRAWBERRY	18	92	5	TR	TR	TR	TR	TR
372	MEDIUM (1 1/4" DIA)	1 STRAWBERRY	12	92	4	TR	TR	TR	TR	TR
373	SLICED	1 CUP	166	92	50	1	1	TR	0.1	0.3
374	FROZEN, SWEETENED,									
	SLICED, THAWED	1 CUP	255	73	245	1	TR	TR	TR	0.2
	TANGERINES									
375	RAW, WITHOUT PEEL AND SEEDS									
	(2 3/8" DIA)	1 TANGERINE	84	88	37	1	TR	TR	TR	TR
376	CANNED (MANDARIN ORANGES),									
	LIGHT SYRUP, FRUIT AND LIQUID	1 CUP	252	83	154	1	TR	TR	TR	0.1
377	TANGERINE JUICE, CANNED, SWEETENED	1 CUP	249	87	125	1	TR	TR	TR	0.1
	WATERMELON, RAW (15" LONG × 7 1/2" DIA)									
378	WEDGE (ABOUT 1/16 OF MELON)	1 WEDGE	286	92	92	2	1	0.1	0.3	0.4
379	DICED	1 CUP	152	92	49	1	1	0.1	0.2	0.2
GRAIN PRODUCTS										
	BAGELS, ENRICHED									
380	PLAIN	3 1/2" BAGEL	71	33	195	7	1	0.2	0.1	0.5
381		4" BAGEL	89	33	245	9	1	0.2	0.1	0.6

Cholesterol (mg)	Carbo-hydrate (g)	Total dietary fiber (g)	Calcium (mg)	Iron (mg)	Potassium (mg)	Sodium (mg)	Vitamin A (IU)	Vitamin A (RE)	Thiamine (mg)	Ribo-flavin (mg)	Niacin (mg)	Ascorbic acid (mg)	Food No.
0	51	2.0	36	1.0	264	3	36	3	0.23	0.06	0.7	19	351
0	10	0.4	7	0.2	51	TR	7	TR	0.04	0.01	0.1	4	352
0	39	2.0	35	0.7	304	2	95	10	0.24	0.05	0.7	24	353
0	7	0.4	7	0.1	57	TR	18	2	0.04	0.01	0.1	4	354
0	34	0.5	43	0.7	335	3	13	0	0.14	0.06	0.6	27	355
0	57	4.1	5	1.1	893	7	2,017	202	0.09	0.10	1.2	33	356
0	48	3.5	3	0.9	716	8	1,400	140	0.07	0.08	1.2	17	357
0	9	1.0	3	0.1	114	0	213	21	0.03	0.06	0.3	6	358
0	60	2.6	23	2.2	235	49	668	67	0.04	0.10	0.8	1	359
0	11	0.5	4	0.4	42	9	119	12	0.01	0.02	0.1	TR	360
0	38	2.5	25	0.9	388	3	2,543	255	0.06	0.15	1.2	7	361
0	7	0.5	5	0.2	71	TR	464	46	0.01	0.03	0.2	1	362
0	26	3.0	21	1.0	313	2	835	84	0.03	0.07	0.8	1	363
0	70	16.4	57	2.8	828	5	759	77	0.06	0.25	1.8	7	364
0	45	2.6	31	3.0	707	10	8	0	0.04	0.18	2.0	10	365
0	115	5.8	71	3.0	1,089	17	12	1	0.23	0.13	1.2	5	366
0	11	0.6	7	0.3	105	2	1	TR	0.02	0.01	0.1	TR	367
0	14	8.4	27	0.7	187	0	160	16	0.04	0.11	1.1	31	368
0	65	11.0	38	1.6	285	3	150	15	0.05	0.11	0.6	41	369
0	75	4.8	348	0.5	230	2	166	17	0.04	0.06	0.5	8	370
0	1	0.4	3	0.1	30	TR	5	1	TR	0.01	TR	10	371
0	1	0.3	2	TR	20	TR	3	TR	TR	0.01	TR	7	372
0	12	3.8	23	0.6	276	2	45	5	0.03	0.11	0.4	94	373
0	66	4.8	28	1.5	250	8	61	5	0.04	0.13	1.0	106	374
0	9	1.9	12	0.1	132	1	773	77	0.09	0.02	0.1	26	375
0	41	1.8	18	0.9	197	15	2,117	212	0.13	0.11	1.1	50	376
0	30	0.5	45	0.5	443	2	1,046	105	0.15	0.05	0.2	55	377
0	21	1.4	23	0.5	332	6	1,047	106	0.23	0.06	0.6	27	378
0	11	0.8	12	0.3	176	3	556	56	0.12	0.03	0.3	15	379
0	38	1.6	53	2.5	72	379	0	0	0.38	0.22	3.2	0	380
0	48	2.0	66	3.2	90	475	0	0	0.48	0.28	4.1	0	381

Food No.	Food Description	Measure of edible portion	Weight (g)	Water (%)	Calories (kcal)	Protein (g)	Total fat (g)	Fatty acids Satu-rated (g)	Fatty acids Mono-unsatu-rated (g)	Fatty acids Poly-unsatu-rated (g)
GRAIN PRODUCTS (CONTINUED)										
382	CINNAMON RAISIN	3 1/2" BAGEL	71	32	195	7	1	0.2	0.1	0.5
383		4" BAGEL	89	32	244	9	2	0.2	0.2	0.6
384	EGG	3 1/2" BAGEL	71	33	197	8	1	0.3	0.3	0.5
385		4" BAGEL	89	33	247	9	2	0.4	0.4	0.6
386	BANANA BREAD, PREPARED FROM RECIPE, WITH MARGARINE	1 SLICE	60	29	196	3	6	1.3	2.7	1.9
	BARLEY, PEARLED									
387	UNCOOKED	1 CUP	200	10	704	20	2	0.5	0.3	1.1
388	COOKED	1 CUP	157	69	193	4	1	0.1	0.1	0.3
	BISCUITS, PLAIN OR BUTTERMILK, ENRICHED									
389	PREPARED FROM RECIPE, WITH 2% MILK	2 1/2" BISCUIT	60	29	212	4	10	2.6	4.2	2.5
390		4" BISCUIT	101	29	358	7	16	4.4	7.0	4.2
	REFRIGERATED DOUGH, BAKED									
391	REGULAR	2 1/2" BISCUIT	27	28	93	2	4	1.0	2.2	0.5
392	LOWER FAT	2 1/4" BISCUIT	21	28	63	2	1	0.3	0.6	0.2
	BREADS, ENRICHED									
393	CRACKED WHEAT	1 SLICE	25	36	65	2	1	0.2	0.5	0.2
394	EGG BREAD (CHALLAH)	1/2" SLICE	40	35	115	4	2	0.6	0.9	0.4
395	FRENCH OR VIENNA (INCLUDES SOURDOUGH)	1/2 SLICE	25	34	69	2	1	0.2	0.3	0.2
396	INDIAN FRY (NAVAJO) BREAD	5" BREAD	90	27	296	6	9	2.1	3.6	2.3
397		10 1/2" BREAD	160	27	526	11	15	3.7	6.4	4.1
398	ITALIAN	1 SLICE	20	36	54	2	1	0.2	0.2	0.3
	MIXED GRAIN									
399	UNTOASTED	1 SLICE	26	38	65	3	1	0.2	0.4	0.2
400	TOASTED	1 SLICE	24	32	65	3	1	0.2	0.4	0.2
	OATMEAL									
401	UNTOASTED	1 SLICE	27	37	73	2	1	0.2	0.4	0.5
402	TOASTED	1 SLICE	25	31	73	2	1	0.2	0.4	0.5
403	PITA	4 PITA	28	32	77	3	TR	TR	TR	0.1
404		6 1/2" PITA	60	32	165	5	1	0.1	0.1	0.3
	PUMPERNICKEL									
405	UNTOASTED	1 SLICE	32	38	80	3	1	0.1	0.3	0.4
406	TOASTED	1 SLICE	29	32	80	3	1	0.1	0.3	0.4
	RAISIN									
407	UNTOASTED	1 SLICE	26	34	71	2	1	0.3	0.6	0.2
408	TOASTED	1 SLICE	24	28	71	2	1	0.3	0.6	0.2
	RYE									
409	UNTOASTED	1 SLICE	32	37	83	3	1	0.2	0.4	0.3
410	TOASTED	1 SLICE	24	31	68	2	1	0.2	0.3	0.2
411	RYE, REDUCED CALORIE	1 SLICE	23	46	47	2	1	0.1	0.2	0.2
	WHEAT									
412	UNTOASTED	1 SLICE	25	37	65	2	1	0.2	0.4	0.2
413	TOASTED	1 SLICE	23	32	65	2	1	0.2	0.4	0.2
414	WHEAT, REDUCED CALORIE	1 SLICE	23	43	46	2	1	0.1	0.1	0.2
	WHITE									
415	UNTOASTED	1 SLICE	25	37	67	2	1	0.1	0.2	0.5
416	TOASTED	1 SLICE	22	30	64	2	1	0.1	0.2	0.5
417	SOFT CRUMBS	1 CUP	45	37	120	4	2	0.2	0.3	0.9
418	WHITE, REDUCED CALORIE	1 SLICE	23	43	48	2	1	0.1	0.2	0.1

Cholesterol (mg)	Carbo-hydrate (g)	Total dietary fiber (g)	Calcium (mg)	Iron (mg)	Potassium (mg)	Sodium (mg)	Vitamin A (IU)	Vitamin A (RE)	Thiamine (mg)	Ribo-flavin (mg)	Niacin (mg)	Ascorbic acid (mg)	Food No.
0	39	1.6	13	2.7	105	229	52	0	0.27	0.20	2.2	TR	382
0	49	2.0	17	3.4	132	287	65	0	0.34	0.25	2.7	1	383
17	38	1.6	9	2.8	48	359	77	23	0.38	0.17	2.4	TR	384
21	47	2.0	12	3.5	61	449	97	29	0.48	0.21	3.1	1	385
26	33	0.7	13	0.8	80	181	278	72	0.10	0.12	0.9	1	386
0	155	31.2	58	5.0	560	18	44	4	0.38	0.23	9.2	0	387
0	44	6.0	17	2.1	146	5	11	2	0.13	0.10	3.2	0	388
2	27	0.9	141	1.7	73	348	49	14	0.21	0.19	1.8	TR	389
3	45	1.5	237	2.9	122	586	83	23	0.36	0.31	3.0	TR	390
0	13	0.4	5	0.7	42	325	0	0	0.09	0.06	0.8	0	391
0	12	0.4	4	0.6	39	305	0	0	0.09	0.05	0.7	0	392
0	12	1.4	11	0.7	44	135	0	0	0.09	0.06	0.9	0	393
20	19	0.9	37	1.2	46	197	30	9	0.18	0.17	1.9	0	394
0	13	0.8	19	0.6	28	152	0	0	0.13	0.08	1.2	0	395
0	48	1.6	210	3.2	67	626	0	0	0.39	0.27	3.3	0	396
0	85	2.9	373	5.8	118	1,112	0	0	0.69	0.49	5.8	0	397
0	10	0.5	16	0.6	22	117	0	0	0.09	0.06	0.9	0	398
0	12	1.7	24	0.9	53	127	0	0	0.11	0.09	1.1	TR	399
0	12	1.6	24	0.9	53	127	0	0	0.08	0.08	1.0	TR	400
0	13	1.1	18	0.7	38	162	4	1	0.11	0.06	0.8	0	401
0	13	1.1	18	0.7	39	163	4	1	0.09	0.06	0.8	TR	402
0	16	0.6	24	0.7	34	150	0	0	0.17	0.09	1.3	0	403
0	33	1.3	52	1.6	72	322	0	0	0.36	0.20	2.8	0	404
0	15	2.1	22	0.9	67	215	0	0	0.10	0.10	1.0	0	405
0	15	2.1	21	0.9	66	214	0	0	0.08	0.09	0.9	0	406
0	14	1.1	17	0.8	59	101	0	0	0.09	0.10	0.9	TR	407
0	14	1.1	17	0.8	59	102	TR	0	0.07	0.09	0.8	TR	408
0	15	1.9	23	0.9	53	211	2	TR	0.14	0.11	1.2	TR	409
0	13	1.5	19	0.7	44	174	1	0	0.09	0.08	0.9	TR	410
0	9	2.8	17	0.7	23	93	1	0	0.08	0.06	0.6	TR	411
0	12	1.1	26	0.8	50	133	0	0	0.10	0.07	1.0	0	412
0	12	1.2	26	0.8	50	132	0	0	0.08	0.06	0.9	0	413
0	10	2.8	18	0.7	28	118	0	0	0.10	0.07	0.9	TR	414
TR	12	0.6	27	0.8	30	135	0	0	0.12	0.09	1.0	0	415
TR	12	0.6	26	0.7	29	130	0	0	0.09	0.07	0.9	0	416
TR	22	1.0	49	1.4	54	242	0	0	0.21	0.15	1.8	0	417
0	10	2.2	22	0.7	17	104	1	TR	0.09	0.07	0.8	TR	418

Food No.	Food Description	Measure of edible portion	Weight (g)	Water (%)	Calories (kcal)	Protein (g)	Total fat (g)	Fatty acids Saturated (g)	Fatty acids Mono-unsaturated (g)	Fatty acids Poly-unsaturated (g)
GRAIN PRODUCTS (CONTINUED)										
	BREAD, WHOLE WHEAT									
419	UNTOASTED	1 SLICE	28	38	69	3	1	0.3	0.5	0.3
420	TOASTED	1 SLICE	25	30	69	3	1	0.3	0.5	0.3
	BREAD CRUMBS, DRY, GRATED									
421	PLAIN, ENRICHED	1 CUP	108	6	427	14	6	1.3	2.6	1.2
422		1 OZ	28	6	112	4	2	0.3	0.7	0.3
423	SEASONED, UNENRICHED	1 CUP	120	6	440	17	3	0.9	1.2	0.8
	BREAD CRUMBS, SOFT. SEE WHITE BREAD.									
424	BREAD STUFFING, PREPARED FROM DRY MIX	1/2 CUP	100	65	178	3	9	1.7	3.8	2.6
425	BREAKFAST BAR, CEREAL CRUST WITH FRUIT FILLING, FAT FREE	1 BAR	37	14	121	2	TR	TR	TR	0.1
	BREAKFAST CEREALS									
	HOT TYPE, COOKED									
	CORN (HOMINY) GRITS									
	REGULAR OR QUICK, ENRICHED									
426	WHITE	1 CUP	242	85	145	3	TR	0.1	0.1	0.2
427	YELLOW	1 CUP	242	85	145	3	TR	0.1	0.1	0.2
428	INSTANT, PLAIN	1 PACKET	137	82	89	2	TR	TR	TR	0.1
	CREAM OF WHEAT									
429	REGULAR	1 CUP	251	87	133	4	1	0.1	0.1	0.3
430	QUICK	1 CUP	239	87	129	4	TR	0.1	0.1	0.3
431	MIX'N EAT, PLAIN	1 PACKET	142	82	102	3	TR	TR	TR	0.2
432	MALT O MEAL	1 CUP	240	88	122	4	TR	0.1	0.1	TR
	OATMEAL									
433	REGULAR, QUICK OR INSTANT, PLAIN, NONFORTIFIED	1 CUP	234	85	145	6	2	0.4	0.7	0.9
434	INSTANT, FORTIFIED, PLAIN	1 PACKET	177	86	104	4	2	0.3	0.6	0.7
	QUAKER INSTANT									
435	APPLES AND CINNAMON	1 PACKET	149	79	125	3	1	0.3	0.5	0.6
436	MAPLE AND BROWN SUGAR	1 PACKET	155	75	153	4	2	0.4	0.6	0.7
437	WHEATENA	1 CUP	243	85	136	5	1	0.2	0.2	0.6
	READY TO EAT									
438	ALL BRAN	1/2 CUP	30	3	79	4	1	0.2	0.2	0.5
439	APPLE CINNAMON CHEERIOS	3/4 CUP	30	3	118	2	2	0.3	0.6	0.2
440	APPLE JACKS	1 CUP	30	3	116	1	TR	0.1	0.1	0.2
441	BASIC 4	1 CUP	55	7	201	4	3	0.4	1.0	1.1
442	BERRY BERRY KIX	3/4 CUP	30	2	120	1	1	0.2	0.5	0.1
443	CAP'N CRUNCH	3/4 CUP	27	2	107	1	1	0.4	0.3	0.2
444	CAP'N CRUNCH'S CRUNCHBERRIES	3/4 CUP	26	2	104	1	1	0.3	0.3	0.2
445	CAP'N CRUNCH'S PEANUT BUTTER CRUNCH	3/4 CUP	27	2	112	2	2	0.5	0.8	0.5
446	CHEERIOS	1 CUP	30	3	110	3	2	0.4	0.6	0.2
	CHEX									
447	CORN	1 CUP	30	3	113	2	TR	0.1	0.1	0.2
448	HONEY NUT	3/4 CUP	30	2	117	2	1	0.1	0.4	0.2
449	MULTI BRAN	1 CUP	49	3	165	4	1	0.2	0.3	0.5
450	RICE	1 1/4 CUP	31	3	117	2	TR	TR	TR	TR
451	WHEAT	1 CUP	30	3	104	3	1	0.1	0.1	0.3
452	CINNAMON LIFE	1 CUP	50	4	190	4	2	0.3	0.6	0.8

Cholesterol (mg)	Carbo-hydrate (g)	Total dietary fiber (g)	Calcium (mg)	Iron (mg)	Potassium (mg)	Sodium (mg)	Vitamin A (IU)	Vitamin A (RE)	Thiamine (mg)	Ribo-flavin (mg)	Niacin (mg)	Ascorbic acid (mg)	Food No.
0	13	1.9	20	0.9	71	148	0	0	0.10	0.06	1.1	0	419
0	13	1.9	20	0.9	71	148	0	0	0.08	0.05	1.0	0	420
0	78	2.6	245	6.6	239	931	1	0	0.83	0.47	7.4	0	421
0	21	0.7	64	1.7	63	244	TR	0	0.22	0.12	1.9	0	422
1	84	5.0	119	3.8	324	3,180	16	4	0.19	0.20	3.3	TR	423
0	22	2.9	32	1.1	74	543	313	81	0.14	0.11	1.5	0	424
TR	28	0.8	49	4.5	92	203	1,249	125	1.01	0.42	5.0	1	425
0	31	0.5	0	1.5	53	0	0	0	0.24	0.15	2.0	0	426
0	31	0.5	0	1.5	53	0	145	15	0.24	0.15	2.0	0	427
0	21	1.2	8	8.2	38	289	0	0	0.15	0.08	1.4	0	428
0	28	1.8	50	10.3	43	3	0	0	0.25	0.00	1.5	0	429
0	27	1.2	50	10.3	45	139	0	0	0.24	0.00	1.4	0	430
0	21	0.4	20	8.1	38	241	1,252	376	0.43	0.28	5.0	0	431
0	26	1.0	5	9.6	31	2	0	0	0.48	0.24	5.8	0	432
0	25	4.0	19	1.6	131	2	37	5	0.26	0.05	0.3	0	433
0	18	3.0	163	6.3	99	285	1,510	453	0.53	0.28	5.5	0	434
0	26	2.5	104	3.9	106	121	1,019	305	0.30	0.35	4.1	TR	435
0	31	2.6	105	3.9	112	234	1,008	302	0.30	0.34	4.0	0	436
0	29	6.6	10	1.4	187	5	0	0	0.02	0.05	1.3	0	437
0	23	9.7	106	4.5	342	61	750	225	0.39	0.42	5.0	15	438
0	25	1.6	35	4.5	60	150	750	225	0.38	0.43	5.0	15	439
0	27	0.6	3	4.5	32	134	750	225	0.39	0.42	5.0	15	440
0	42	3.4	310	4.5	162	323	1,250	375	0.37	0.42	5.0	15	441
0	26	0.2	66	4.5	24	185	750	225	0.38	0.43	5.0	15	442
0	23	0.9	5	4.5	35	208	36	4	0.38	0.42	5.0	0	443
0	22	0.6	7	4.5	37	190	33	5	0.37	0.42	5.0	TR	444
0	22	0.8	3	4.5	62	204	37	4	0.38	0.42	5.0	0	445
0	23	2.6	55	8.1	89	284	1,250	375	0.38	0.43	5.0	15	446
0	26	0.5	100	9.0	32	289	0	0	0.38	0.00	5.0	6	447
0	26	0.4	102	9.0	27	224	0	0	0.38	0.44	5.0	6	448
0	41	6.4	95	13.7	191	325	0	0	0.32	0.00	4.4	5	449
0	27	0.3	104	9.0	36	291	0	0	0.38	0.02	5.0	6	450
0	24	3.3	60	9.0	116	269	0	0	0.23	0.04	3.0	4	451
0	40	3.0	135	7.5	113	220	16	2	0.63	0.71	8.4	TR	452

Food No.	Food Description	Measure of edible portion	Weight (g)	Water (%)	Calories (kcal)	Protein (g)	Total fat (g)	Fatty acids		
								Satu-rated (g)	Mono-unsatu-rated (g)	Poly-unsatu-rated (g)
GRAIN PRODUCTS (CONTINUED)										
453	CINNAMON TOAST CRUNCH	3/4 CUP	30	2	124	2	3	0.5	0.9	0.5
454	COCOA KRISPIES	3/4 CUP	31	2	120	2	1	0.6	0.1	0.1
455	COCOA PUFFS	1 CUP	30	2	119	1	1	0.2	0.3	TR
	CORN FLAKES									
456	GENERAL MILLS, TOTAL	1 1/3 CUP	30	3	112	2	TR	0.2	0.1	TR
457	KELLOGG'S	1 CUP	28	3	102	2	TR	0.1	TR	0.1
458	CORN POPS	1 CUP	31	3	118	1	TR	0.1	0.1	TR
459	CRISPIX	1 CUP	29	3	108	2	TR	0.1	0.1	0.1
460	COMPLETE WHEAT BRAN FLAKES	3/4 CUP	29	4	95	3	1	0.1	0.1	0.4
461	FROOT LOOPS	1 CUP	30	2	117	1	1	0.4	0.2	0.3
462	FROSTED FLAKES	3/4 CUP	31	3	119	1	TR	0.1	TR	0.1
	FROSTED MINI WHEATS									
463	REGULAR	1 CUP	51	5	173	5	1	0.2	0.1	0.6
464	BITE SIZE	1 CUP	55	5	187	5	1	0.2	0.2	0.6
465	GOLDEN GRAHAMS	3/4 CUP	30	3	116	2	1	0.2	0.3	0.2
466	HONEY FROSTED WHEATIES	3/4 CUP	30	3	110	2	TR	0.1	TR	TR
467	HONEY NUT CHEERIOS	1 CUP	30	2	115	3	1	0.2	0.5	0.2
468	HONEY NUT CLUSTERS	1 CUP	55	3	213	5	3	0.4	1.8	0.4
469	KIX	1 1/3 CUP	30	2	114	2	1	0.2	0.1	TR
470	LIFE	3/4 CUP	32	4	121	3	1	0.2	0.4	0.6
471	LUCKY CHARMS	1 CUP	30	2	116	2	1	0.2	0.4	0.2
472	NATURE VALLEY GRANOLA	3/4 CUP	55	4	248	6	10	1.3	6.5	1.9
	100% NATURAL CEREAL									
473	WITH OATS, HONEY, AND RAISINS	1/2 CUP	51	4	218	5	7	3.2	3.2	0.8
474	WITH RAISINS, LOW FAT	1/2 CUP	50	4	195	4	3	0.8	1.3	0.5
475	PRODUCT 19	1 CUP	30	3	110	3	TR	TR	0.2	0.2
476	PUFFED RICE	1 CUP	14	3	56	1	TR	TR	TR	TR
477	PUFFED WHEAT	1 CUP	12	3	44	2	TR	TR	TR	TR
	RAISIN BRAN									
478	GENERAL MILLS, TOTAL	1 CUP	55	9	178	4	1	0.2	0.2	0.2
479	KELLOGG'S	1 CUP	61	8	186	6	1	0.0	0.2	0.8
480	RAISIN NUT BRAN	1 CUP	55	5	209	5	4	0.7	1.9	0.5
481	REESE'S PEANUT BUTTER PUFFS	3/4 CUP	30	2	129	3	3	0.6	1.4	0.6
482	RICE KRISPIES	1 1/4 CUP	33	3	124	2	TR	0.1	0.1	0.2
483	RICE KRISPIES TREATS CEREAL	3/4 CUP	30	4	120	1	2	0.4	1.0	0.2
484	SHREDDED WHEAT	2 BISCUITS	46	4	156	5	1	0.1	NA	NA
485	SMACKS	3/4 CUP	27	3	103	2	1	0.3	0.1	0.2
486	SPECIAL K	1 CUP	31	3	115	6	TR	0.0	0.0	0.2
487	QUAKER TOASTED OATMEAL, HONEY NUT	1 CUP	49	3	191	5	3	0.5	1.2	0.7
488	TOTAL, WHOLE GRAIN	3/4 CUP	30	3	105	3	1	0.2	0.1	0.1
489	TRIX	1 CUP	30	2	122	1	2	0.4	0.9	0.3
490	WHEATIES	1 CUP	30	3	110	3	1	0.2	0.2	0.2
	BROWNIES, WITHOUT ICING COMMERCIALLY PREPARED									
491	REGULAR, LARGE (2 3/4″ SQ × 7/8″)	1 BROWNIE	56	14	227	3	9	2.4	5.0	1.3

Cholesterol (mg)	Carbo-hydrate (g)	Total dietary fiber (g)	Calcium (mg)	Iron (mg)	Potassium (mg)	Sodium (mg)	Vitamin A (IU)	Vitamin A (RE)	Thiamine (mg)	Ribo-flavin (mg)	Niacin (mg)	Ascorbic acid (mg)	Food No.
0	24	1.5	42	4.5	44	210	750	225	0.38	0.43	5.0	15	453
0	27	0.4	4	1.8	60	210	750	225	0.37	0.43	5.0	15	454
0	27	0.2	33	4.5	52	181	0	0	0.38	0.43	5.0	15	455
0	26	0.8	237	18.0	34	203	1,250	375	1.50	1.70	20.1	60	456
0	24	0.8	1	8.7	25	298	700	210	0.36	0.39	4.7	14	457
0	28	0.4	2	1.9	23	123	775	233	0.40	0.43	5.2	16	458
0	25	0.6	3	1.8	35	240	750	225	0.38	0.44	5.0	15	459
0	23	4.6	14	8.1	175	226	1,208	363	0.38	0.44	5.0	15	460
0	26	0.6	3	4.2	32	141	703	211	0.39	0.42	5.0	14	461
0	28	0.6	1	4.5	20	200	750	225	0.37	0.43	5.0	15	462
0	42	5.5	18	14.3	170	2	0	0	0.36	0.41	5.0	0	463
0	45	5.9	0	15.4	186	2	0	0	0.33	0.39	4.7	0	464
0	26	0.9	14	4.5	53	275	750	225	0.38	0.43	5.0	15	465
0	26	1.5	8	4.5	56	211	750	225	0.38	0.43	5.0	15	466
0	24	1.6	20	4.5	85	259	750	225	0.38	0.43	5.0	15	467
0	43	4.2	72	4.5	171	239	0	0	0.37	0.42	5.0	9	468
0	26	0.8	44	8.1	41	263	1,250	375	0.38	0.43	5.0	15	469
0	25	2.0	98	9.0	79	174	12	1	0.40	0.45	5.3	0	470
0	25	1.2	32	4.5	54	203	750	225	0.38	0.43	5.0	15	471
0	36	3.5	41	1.7	183	89	0	0	0.17	0.06	0.6	0	472
1	36	3.7	39	1.7	214	11	4	1	0.14	0.09	0.8	TR	473
1	40	3.0	30	1.3	169	129	9	1	0.15	0.06	0.9	TR	474
0	25	1.0	3	18.0	41	216	750	225	1.50	1.71	20.0	60	475
0	13	0.2	1	4.4	16	TR	0	0	0.36	0.25	4.9	0	476
0	10	0.5	3	3.8	42	TR	0	0	0.31	0.22	4.2	0	477
0	43	5.0	238	18.0	287	240	1,250	375	1.50	1.70	20.0	0	478
0	47	8.2	35	5.0	437	354	832	250	0.43	0.49	5.6	0	479
0	41	5.1	74	4.5	218	246	0	0	0.37	0.42	5.0	0	480
0	23	0.4	21	4.5	62	177	750	225	0.38	0.43	5.0	15	481
0	29	0.4	3	2.0	42	354	825	248	0.43	0.46	5.5	17	482
0	26	0.3	2	1.8	19	190	750	225	0.39	0.42	5.0	15	483
0	38	5.3	20	1.4	196	3	0	NA	0.12	0.05	2.6	0	484
0	24	0.9	3	1.8	42	51	750	225	0.38	0.43	5.0	15	485
0	22	1.0	5	8.7	55	250	750	225	0.53	0.59	7.0	15	486
TR	39	3.3	27	4.5	185	166	500	150	0.37	0.42	5.0	6	487
0	24	2.6	258	18.0	97	199	1,250	375	1.50	1.70	20.1	60	488
0	26	0.7	32	4.5	18	197	750	225	0.38	0.43	5.0	15	489
0	24	2.1	55	8.1	104	222	750	225	0.38	0.43	5.0	15	490
10	36	1.2	16	1.3	83	175	39	3	0.14	0.12	1.0	0	491

Food No.	Food Description	Measure of edible portion	Weight (g)	Water (%)	Calories (kcal)	Protein (g)	Total fat (g)	Fatty acids Satu-rated (g)	Mono-unsatu-rated (g)	Poly-unsatu-rated (g)
GRAIN PRODUCTS (CONTINUED)										
492	FAT FREE, 2″ SQ	1 BROWNIE	28	12	89	1	TR	0.2	0.1	TR
493	PREPARED FROM DRY MIX, REDUCED CALORIE, 2″ SQ	1 BROWNIE	22	13	84	1	2	1.1	1.0	0.2
494	BUCKWHEAT FLOUR, WHOLE GROAT	1 CUP	120	11	402	15	4	0.8	1.1	1.1
495	BUCKWHEAT GROATS, ROASTED (KASHA), COOKED	1 CUP	168	76	155	6	1	0.2	0.3	0.3
	BULGUR									
496	UNCOOKED	1 CUP	140	9	479	17	2	0.3	0.2	0.8
497	COOKED	1 CUP	182	78	151	6	TR	0.1	0.1	0.2
	CAKES, PREPARED FROM DRY MIX									
498	ANGELFOOD (1/12 OF 10″ DIA)	1 PIECE	50	33	129	3	TR	TR	TR	0.1
499	YELLOW, LIGHT, WITH WATER, EGG WHITES, NO FROSTING (1/12 OF 9″ DIA)	1 PIECE	69	37	181	3	2	1.1	0.9	0.2
	CAKES, PREPARED FROM RECIPE									
500	CHOCOLATE, WITHOUT FROSTING (1/12 OF 9″ DIA)	1 PIECE	95	24	340	5	14	5.2	5.7	2.6
501	GINGERBREAD (1/9 OF 8″ SQUARE)	1 PIECE	74	28	263	3	12	3.1	5.3	3.1
502	PINEAPPLE UPSIDE DOWN (1/9 OF 8″ SQUARE)	1 PIECE	115	32	367	4	14	3.4	6.0	3.8
503	SHORTCAKE, BISCUIT TYPE (ABOUT 3″ DIA)	1 SHORTCAKE	65	28	225	4	9	2.5	3.9	2.4
504	SPONGE (1/12 OF 16-OZ CAKE)	1 PIECE	63	29	187	5	3	0.8	1.0	0.4
	WHITE									
505	WITH COCONUT FROSTING (1/12 OF 9″ DIA)	1 PIECE	112	21	399	5	12	4.4	4.1	2.4
506	WITHOUT FROSTING (1/12 OF 9″ DIA)	1 PIECE	74	23	264	4	9	2.4	3.9	2.3
	CAKES, COMMERCIALLY PREPARED									
507	ANGELFOOD (1/12 OF 12-OZ CAKE)	1 PIECE	28	33	72	2	TR	TR	TR	0.1
508	BOSTON CREAM (1/6 OF PIE)	1 PIECE	92	45	232	2	8	2.2	4.2	0.9
509	CHOCOLATE WITH CHOCOLATE FROSTING (1/8 OF 18-OZ CAKE)	1 PIECE	64	23	235	3	10	3.1	5.6	1.2
510	COFFEECAKE, CRUMB (1/9 OF 20-OZ CAKE)	1 PIECE	63	22	263	4	15	3.7	8.2	2.0
511	FRUITCAKE	1 PIECE	43	25	139	1	4	0.5	1.8	1.4
	POUND									
512	BUTTER (1/12 OF 12-OZ CAKE)	1 PIECE	28	25	109	2	6	3.2	1.7	0.3
513	FAT FREE (3 1/4″ × 2 3/4″ × 5/8″ SLICE)	1 SLICE	28	31	79	2	TR	0.1	TR	0.1
	SNACK CAKES									
514	CHOCOLATE, CREAM FILLED, WITH FROSTING	1 CUPCAKE	50	20	188	2	7	1.4	2.8	2.6
515	CHOCOLATE, WITH FROSTING, LOW FAT	1 CUPCAKE	43	23	131	2	2	0.5	0.8	0.2
516	SPONGE, CREAM FILLED	1 CAKE	43	20	155	1	5	1.1	1.7	1.4
517	SPONGE, INDIVIDUAL SHORTCAKE	1 SHORTCAKE	30	30	87	2	1	0.2	0.3	0.1
	YELLOW									
518	WITH CHOCOLATE FROSTING	1 PIECE	64	22	243	2	11	3.0	6.1	1.4
519	WITH VANILLA FROSTING	1 PIECE	64	22	239	2	9	1.5	3.9	3.3
520	CHEESECAKE (1/6 OF 17-OZ CAKE)	1 PIECE	80	46	257	4	18	7.9	6.9	1.3
521	CHEESE FLAVOR PUFFS OR TWISTS	1 OZ	28	2	157	2	10	1.9	5.7	1.3
522	CHEX MIX	1 OZ (ABOUT 2/3 CUP)	28	4	120	3	5	1.6	NA	NA
	COOKIES									
523	BUTTER, COMMERCIALLY PREPARED CHOCOLATE CHIP, MEDIUM (2 1/4″–2 1/2″ DIA)	1 COOKIE	5	5	23	TR	1	0.6	0.3	TR

Cholesterol (mg)	Carbo-hydrate (g)	Total dietary fiber (g)	Calcium (mg)	Iron (mg)	Potassium (mg)	Sodium (mg)	Vitamin A (IU)	Vitamin A (RE)	Thiamine (mg)	Ribo-flavin (mg)	Niacin (mg)	Ascorbic acid (mg)	Food No.
0	22	1.0	17	0.7	89	90	1	TR	0.03	0.04	0.3	TR	492
0	16	0.8	3	0.3	69	21	0	0	0.02	0.03	0.2	0	493
0	85	12.0	49	4.9	692	13	0	0	0.50	0.23	7.4	0	494
0	33	4.5	12	1.3	148	7	0	0	0.07	0.07	1.6	0	495
0	106	25.6	49	3.4	574	24	0	0	0.32	0.16	7.2	0	496
0	34	8.2	18	1.7	124	9	0	0	0.10	0.05	1.8	0	497
0	29	0.1	42	0.1	68	255	0	0	0.05	0.10	0.1	0	498
0	37	0.6	69	0.6	41	279	6	1	0.06	0.12	0.6	0	499
55	51	1.5	57	1.5	133	299	133	38	0.13	0.20	1.1	TR	500
24	36	0.7	53	2.1	325	242	36	10	0.14	0.12	1.3	TR	501
25	58	0.9	138	1.7	129	367	291	75	0.18	0.18	1.4	1	502
2	32	0.8	133	1.7	69	329	47	12	0.20	0.18	1.7	TR	503
107	36	0.4	26	1.0	89	144	163	49	0.10	0.19	0.8	0	504
1	71	1.1	101	1.3	111	318	43	12	0.14	0.21	1.2	TR	505
1	42	0.6	96	1.1	70	242	41	12	0.14	0.18	1.1	TR	506
0	16	0.4	39	0.1	26	210	0	0	0.03	0.14	0.2	0	507
34	39	1.3	21	0.3	36	132	74	21	0.38	0.25	0.2	TR	508
27	35	1.8	28	1.4	128	214	54	16	0.02	0.09	0.4	TR	509
20	29	1.3	34	1.2	77	221	70	21	0.13	0.14	1.1	TR	510
2	26	1.6	14	0.9	66	116	9	2	0.02	0.04	0.3	TR	511
62	14	0.1	10	0.4	33	111	170	44	0.04	0.06	0.4	0	512
0	17	0.3	12	0.6	31	95	27	8	0.04	0.08	0.2	0	513
9	30	0.4	37	1.7	61	213	9	3	0.11	0.15	1.2	0	514
0	29	1.8	15	0.7	96	178	0	0	0.02	0.06	0.3	0	515
7	27	0.2	19	0.5	37	155	7	2	0.07	0.06	0.5	TR	516
31	18	0.2	21	0.8	30	73	46	14	0.07	0.08	0.6	0	517
35	35	1.2	24	1.3	114	216	70	21	0.08	0.10	0.8	0	518
35	38	0.2	40	0.7	34	220	40	12	0.06	0.04	0.3	0	519
44	20	0.3	41	0.5	72	166	438	117	0.02	0.15	0.2	TR	520
1	15	0.3	16	0.7	47	298	75	10	0.07	0.10	0.9	TR	521
0	18	1.6	10	7.0	76	288	41	4	0.44	0.14	4.8	13	522
6	3	TR	1	0.1	6	18	34	8	0.02	0.02	0.2	0	523

Food No.	Food Description	Measure of edible portion	Weight (g)	Water (%)	Calories (kcal)	Protein (g)	Total fat (g)	Fatty acids Satu- rated (g)	Mono- unsatu- rated (g)	Poly- unsatu- rated (g)
GRAIN PRODUCTS (CONTINUED)										
	COMMERCIALLY PREPARED									
524	REGULAR	1 COOKIE	10	4	48	1	2	0.7	1.2	0.2
525	REDUCED FAT	1 COOKIE	10	4	45	1	2	0.4	0.6	0.5
526	FROM REFRIGERATED DOUGH (SPOONED FROM ROLL)	1 COOKIE	26	3	128	1	6	2.0	2.9	0.6
527	PREPARED FROM RECIPE, WITH MARGARINE	1 COOKIE	16	6	78	1	5	1.3	1.7	1.3
528	DEVIL'S FOOD, COMMERCIALLY PREPARED, FAT FREE	1 COOKIE	16	18	49	1	TR	0.1	TR	TR
529	FIG BAR	1 COOKIE	16	17	56	1	1	0.2	0.5	0.4
	MOLASSES									
530	MEDIUM	1 COOKIE	15	6	65	1	2	0.5	1.1	0.3
531	LARGE (3 1/2"–4" DIA)	1 COOKIE	32	6	138	2	4	1.0	2.3	0.6
	OATMEAL									
	COMMERCIALLY PREPARED, WITH OR WITHOUT RAISINS									
532	REGULAR, LARGE	1 COOKIE	25	6	113	2	5	1.1	2.5	0.6
533	SOFT TYPE	1 COOKIE	15	11	61	1	2	0.5	1.2	0.3
534	FAT FREE	1 COOKIE	11	13	36	1	TR	TR	TR	0.1
535	PREPARED FROM RECIPE, WITH RAISINS (2 5/8" DIA)	1 COOKIE	15	6	65	1	2	0.5	1.0	0.8
	PEANUT BUTTER									
536	COMMERCIALLY PREPARED	1 COOKIE	15	6	72	1	4	0.7	1.9	0.8
537	PREPARED FROM RECIPE, WITH MARGARINE (3" DIA)	1 COOKIE	20	6	95	2	5	0.9	2.2	1.4
	SANDWICH TYPE, WITH CREAM FILLING									
538	CHOCOLATE COOKIE	1 COOKIE	10	2	47	TR	2	0.4	0.9	0.7
	VANILLA COOKIE									
539	OVAL	1 COOKIE	15	2	72	1	3	0.4	1.3	1.1
540	ROUND	1 COOKIE	10	2	48	TR	2	0.3	0.8	0.8
	SHORTBREAD, COMMERCIALLY PREPARED									
541	PLAIN (1 5/8" SQ)	1 COOKIE	8	4	40	TR	2	0.5	1.1	0.3
	PECAN									
542	REGULAR (2" DIA)	1 COOKIE	14	3	76	1	5	1.1	2.6	0.6
543	REDUCED FAT	1 COOKIE	16	5	73	1	3	0.6	1.6	0.4
	SUGAR									
544	COMMERCIALLY PREPARED	1 COOKIE	15	5	72	1	3	0.8	1.8	0.4
545	FROM REFRIGERATED DOUGH	1 COOKIE	15	5	73	1	3	0.9	2.0	0.4
546	PREPARED FROM RECIPE, WITH MARGARINE (3" DIA)	1 COOKIE	14	9	66	1	3	0.7	1.4	1.0
547	VANILLA WAFER, LOWER FAT, MEDIUM SIZE	1 COOKIE	4	5	18	TR	1	0.2	0.3	0.2
	CORN CHIPS									
548	PLAIN	1 OZ	28	1	153	2	9	1.3	2.7	4.7
549	BARBECUE FLAVOR	1 OZ	28	1	148	2	9	1.3	2.7	4.6
	CORNBREAD									
550	PREPARED FROM MIX, PIECE 3 3/4" × 2 1/2" × 3/4"	1 PIECE	60	32	188	4	6	1.6	3.1	0.7
551	PREPARED FROM RECIPE, WITH 2% MILK, PIECE 2 1/2" SQ × 1 1/2"	1 PIECE	65	39	173	4	5	1.0	1.2	2.1
	CORNMEAL, YELLOW, DRY FORM									
552	WHOLE GRAIN	1 CUP	122	10	442	10	4	0.6	1.2	2.0

Cholesterol (mg)	Carbo-hydrate (g)	Total dietary fiber (g)	Calcium (mg)	Iron (mg)	Potassium (mg)	Sodium (mg)	Vitamin A (IU)	Vitamin A (RE)	Thiamine (mg)	Ribo-flavin (mg)	Niacin (mg)	Ascorbic acid (mg)	Food No.
0	7	0.3	3	0.3	14	32	TR	0	0.02	0.03	0.3	0	524
0	7	0.4	2	0.3	12	38	TR	0	0.03	0.03	0.3	0	525
7	18	0.4	7	0.7	52	60	15	4	0.04	0.05	0.5	0	526
5	9	0.4	6	0.4	36	58	102	26	0.03	0.03	0.2	TR	527
0	12	0.3	5	0.4	18	28	TR	NA	0.01	0.03	0.2	TR	528
0	11	0.7	10	0.5	33	56	5	1	0.03	0.03	0.3	TR	529
0	11	0.1	11	1.0	52	69	0	0	0.05	0.04	0.5	0	530
0	24	0.3	24	2.1	111	147	0	0	0.11	0.08	1.0	0	531
0	17	0.7	9	0.6	36	96	5	1	0.07	0.06	0.6	TR	532
1	10	0.4	14	0.4	20	52	5	1	0.03	0.03	0.3	TR	533
0	9	0.8	4	0.2	23	33	0	0	0.02	0.03	0.1	0	534
5	10	0.5	15	0.4	36	81	96	25	0.04	0.02	0.2	TR	535
TR	9	0.3	5	0.4	25	62	1	TR	0.03	0.03	0.6	0	536
6	12	0.4	8	0.4	46	104	120	31	0.04	0.04	0.7	TR	537
0	7	0.3	3	0.4	18	60	TR	0	0.01	0.02	0.2	0	538
0	11	0.2	4	0.3	14	52	0	0	0.04	0.04	0.4	0	539
0	7	0.2	3	0.2	9	35	0	0	0.03	0.02	0.3	0	540
2	5	0.1	3	0.2	8	36	7	1	0.03	0.03	0.3	0	541
5	8	0.3	4	0.3	10	39	TR	TR	0.04	0.03	0.3	0	542
0	11	0.2	8	0.5	15	55	1	TR	0.05	0.03	0.4	TR	543
8	10	0.1	3	0.3	9	54	14	4	0.03	0.03	0.4	TR	544
5	10	0.1	14	0.3	24	70	6	2	0.03	0.02	0.4	0	545
4	8	0.2	10	0.3	11	69	135	35	0.04	0.04	0.3	TR	546
2	3	0.1	2	0.1	4	12	1	TR	0.01	0.01	0.1	0	547
0	16	1.4	36	0.4	40	179	27	3	0.01	0.04	0.3	0	548
0	16	1.5	37	0.4	67	216	173	17	0.02	0.06	0.5	TR	549
37	29	1.4	44	1.1	77	467	123	26	0.15	0.16	1.2	TR	550
26	28	1.9	162	1.6	96	428	180	35	0.19	0.19	1.5	TR	551
0	94	8.9	7	4.2	350	43	572	57	0.47	0.25	4.4	0	552

Food No.	Food Description	Measure of edible portion	Weight (g)	Water (%)	Calories (kcal)	Protein (g)	Total fat (g)	Fatty acids		
								Satu-rated (g)	Mono-unsatu-rated (g)	Poly-unsatu-rated (g)
GRAIN PRODUCTS (CONTINUED)										
553	DEGERMED, ENRICHED	1 CUP	138	12	505	12	2	0.3	0.6	1.0
554	SELF-RISING, DEGERMED, ENRICHED	1 CUP	138	10	490	12	2	0.3	0.6	1.0
555	CORNSTARCH	1 TBSP	8	8	30	TR	TR	TR	TR	TR
	COUSCOUS									
556	UNCOOKED	1 CUP	173	9	650	22	1	0.2	0.2	0.4
557	COOKED	1 CUP	157	73	176	6	TR	TR	TR	0.1
	CRACKERS									
558	CHEESE, 1" SQ	10 CRACKERS	10	3	50	1	3	0.9	1.2	0.2
	GRAHAM, PLAIN									
559	2 1/2" SQ	2 SQUARES	14	4	59	1	1	0.2	0.6	0.5
560	CRUSHED	1 CUP	84	4	355	6	8	1.3	3.4	3.2
561	MELBA TOAST, PLAIN	4 PIECES	20	5	78	2	1	0.1	0.2	0.3
562	RYE WAFER, WHOLE GRAIN, PLAIN	1 WAFER	11	5	37	1	TR	TR	TR	TR
	SALTINE									
563	SQUARE	4 CRACKERS	12	4	52	1	1	0.4	0.8	0.2
564	OYSTER TYPE	1 CUP	45	4	195	4	5	1.3	2.9	0.8
	SANDWICH TYPE									
565	WHEAT WITH CHEESE	1 SANDWICH	7	4	33	1	1	0.4	0.8	0.2
566	CHEESE WITH PEANUT BUTTER	1 SANDWICH	7	4	34	1	2	0.4	0.8	0.3
	STANDARD SNACK TYPE									
567	BITE SIZE	1 CUP	62	4	311	5	16	2.3	6.6	5.9
568	ROUND	4 CRACKERS	12	4	60	1	3	0.5	1.3	1.1
569	WHEAT, THIN SQUARE	4 CRACKERS	8	3	38	1	2	0.4	0.9	0.2
570	WHOLE WHEAT	4 CRACKERS	16	3	71	1	3	0.5	0.9	1.1
571	CROISSANT, BUTTER	1 CROISSANT	57	23	231	5	12	6.6	3.1	0.6
572	CROUTONS, SEASONED	1 CUP	40	4	186	4	7	2.1	3.8	0.9
	DANISH PASTRY, ENRICHED									
573	CHEESE FILLED	1 DANISH	71	31	266	6	16	4.8	8.0	1.8
574	FRUIT FILLED	1 DANISH	71	27	263	4	13	3.5	7.1	1.7
	DOUGHNUTS									
575	CAKE TYPE	1 HOLE	14	21	59	1	3	0.5	1.3	1.1
576		1 MEDIUM	47	21	198	2	11	1.7	4.4	3.7
577	YEAST LEAVENED, GLAZED	1 HOLE	13	25	52	1	3	0.8	1.7	0.4
578		1 MEDIUM	60	25	242	4	14	3.5	7.7	1.7
579	ECLAIR, PREPARED FROM RECIPE, 5" × 2" × 1 3/4"	1 ECLAIR	100	52	262	6	16	4.1	6.5	3.9
	ENGLISH MUFFIN, PLAIN, ENRICHED									
580	UNTOASTED	1 MUFFIN	57	42	134	4	1	0.1	0.2	0.5
581	TOASTED	1 MUFFIN	52	37	133	4	1	0.1	0.2	0.5
	FRENCH TOAST									
582	PREPARED FROM RECIPE, WITH 2% MILK, FRIED IN MARGARINE	1 SLICE	65	55	149	5	7	1.8	2.9	1.7
583	FROZEN, READY TO HEAT	1 SLICE	59	53	126	4	4	0.9	1.2	0.7
	GRANOLA BAR									
584	HARD, PLAIN	1 BAR	28	4	134	3	6	0.7	1.2	3.4
	SOFT, UNCOATED									
585	CHOCOLATE CHIP	1 BAR	28	5	119	2	5	2.9	1.0	0.6
586	RAISIN	1 BAR	28	6	127	2	5	2.7	0.8	0.9
587	SOFT, CHOCOLATE-COATED, PEANUT BUTTER	1 BAR	28	3	144	3	9	4.8	1.9	0.5
588	MACARONI (ELBOWS), ENRICHED, COOKED	1 CUP	140	66	197	7	1	0.1	0.1	0.4

Cholesterol (mg)	Carbo-hydrate (g)	Total dietary fiber (g)	Calcium (mg)	Iron (mg)	Potassium (mg)	Sodium (mg)	Vitamin A (IU)	Vitamin A (RE)	Thiamine (mg)	Ribo-flavin (mg)	Niacin (mg)	Ascorbic acid (mg)	Food No.
0	107	10.2	7	5.7	224	4	570	57	0.99	0.56	6.9	0	553
0	103	9.8	483	6.5	235	1,860	570	57	0.94	0.53	6.3	0	554
0	7	0.1	TR	TR	TR	1	0	0	0.00	0.00	0.0	0	555
0	134	8.7	42	1.9	287	17	0	0	0.28	0.13	6.0	0	556
0	36	2.2	13	0.6	91	8	0	0	0.10	0.04	1.5	0	557
1	6	0.2	15	0.5	15	100	16	3	0.06	0.04	0.5	0	558
0	11	0.4	3	0.5	19	85	0	0	0.03	0.04	0.6	0	559
0	65	2.4	20	3.1	113	508	0	0	0.19	0.26	3.5	0	560
0	15	1.3	19	0.7	40	166	0	0	0.08	0.05	0.8	0	561
0	9	2.5	4	0.7	54	87	1	0	0.05	0.03	0.2	TR	562
0	9	0.4	14	0.6	15	156	0	0	0.07	0.06	0.6	0	563
0	32	1.4	54	2.4	58	586	0	0	0.25	0.21	2.4	0	564
TR	4	0.1	18	0.2	30	98	5	1	0.03	0.05	0.3	TR	565
TR	4	0.2	6	0.2	17	69	22	2	0.03	0.02	0.5	TR	566
0	38	1.0	74	2.2	82	525	0	0	0.25	0.21	2.5	0	567
0	7	0.2	14	0.4	16	102	0	0	0.05	0.04	0.5	0	568
0	5	0.4	4	0.4	15	64	0	0	0.04	0.03	0.4	0	569
0	11	1.7	8	0.5	48	105	0	0	0.03	0.02	0.7	0	570
38	26	1.5	21	1.2	67	424	424	106	0.22	0.14	1.2	TR	571
3	25	2.0	38	1.1	72	495	16	4	0.20	0.17	1.9	0	572
11	26	0.7	25	1.1	70	320	104	32	0.13	0.18	1.4	TR	573
81	34	1.3	33	1.3	59	251	53	16	0.19	0.16	1.4	3	574
5	7	0.2	6	0.3	18	76	8	2	0.03	0.03	0.3	TR	575
17	23	0.7	21	0.9	60	257	27	8	0.10	0.11	0.9	TR	576
1	6	0.2	6	0.3	14	44	2	1	0.05	0.03	0.4	TR	577
4	27	0.7	26	1.2	65	205	8	2	0.22	0.13	1.7	TR	578
127	24	0.6	63	1.2	117	337	718	191	0.12	0.27	0.8	TR	579
0	26	1.5	99	1.4	75	264	0	0	0.25	0.16	2.2	0	580
0	26	1.5	98	1.4	74	262	0	0	0.20	0.14	2.0	TR	581
75	16	0.7	65	1.1	87	311	315	86	0.13	0.21	1.1	TR	582
48	19	0.7	63	1.3	79	292	110	32	0.16	0.22	1.6	TR	583
0	18	1.5	17	0.8	95	83	43	4	0.07	0.03	0.4	TR	584
TR	20	1.4	26	0.7	96	77	12	1	0.06	0.04	0.3	0	585
TR	19	1.2	29	0.7	103	80	0	0	0.07	0.05	0.3	0	586
3	15	0.8	31	0.4	96	55	37	10	0.03	0.06	0.9	TR	587
0	40	1.8	10	2.0	43	1	0	0	0.29	0.14	2.3	0	588

Food No.	Food Description	Measure of edible portion	Weight (g)	Water (%)	Calories (kcal)	Protein (g)	Total fat (g)	Fatty acids		
								Satu-rated (g)	Mono-unsatu-rated (g)	Poly-unsatu-rated (g)
GRAIN PRODUCTS (CONTINUED)										
589	MATZO, PLAIN	1 MATZO	28	4	112	3	TR	0.1	TR	0.2
	MUFFINS									
	BLUEBERRY									
590	COMMERCIALLY PREPARED (2 3/4″ DIA × 2″)	1 MUFFIN	57	38	158	3	4	0.8	1.1	1.4
591	PREPARED FROM MIX (2 1/4″ DIA × 1 3/4″)	1 MUFFIN	50	36	150	3	4	0.7	1.8	1.5
592	PREPARED FROM RECIPE, WITH 2% MILK	1 MUFFIN	57	40	162	4	6	1.2	1.5	3.1
593	BRAN WITH RAISINS, TOASTER TYPE, TOASTED	1 MUFFIN	34	27	106	2	3	0.5	0.8	1.7
	CORN									
594	COMMERCIALLY PREPARED (2 1/2″ DIA × 2 1/4″)	1 MUFFIN	57	33	174	3	5	0.8	1.2	1.8
595	PREPARED FROM MIX (2 1/4″ DIA × 1 1/2″)	1 MUFFIN	50	31	161	4	5	1.4	2.6	0.6
596	OAT BRAN, COMMERCIALLY PREPARED (2 1/2″ DIA × 2 1/4″)	1 MUFFIN	57	35	154	4	4	0.6	1.0	2.4
597	NOODLES, CHOW MEIN, CANNED	1 CUP	45	1	237	4	14	2.0	3.5	7.8
	NOODLES (EGG NOODLES), ENRICHED, COOKED									
598	REGULAR	1 CUP	160	69	213	8	2	0.5	0.7	0.7
599	SPINACH	1 CUP	160	69	211	8	3	0.6	0.8	0.6
600	NUTRI GRAIN CEREAL BAR, FRUIT FILLED	1 BAR	37	15	136	2	3	0.6	1.9	0.3
	OAT BRAN									
601	UNCOOKED	1 CUP	94	7	231	16	7	1.2	2.2	2.6
602	COOKED	1 CUP	219	84	88	7	2	0.4	0.6	0.7
603	ORIENTAL SNACK MIX	1 OZ (ABOUT 1/4 CUP)	28	3	156	5	7	1.1	2.8	3.0
	PANCAKES, PLAIN (4″ DIA)									
604	FROZEN, READY TO HEAT	1 PANCAKE	36	45	82	2	1	0.3	0.4	0.3
605	PREPARED FROM COMPLETE MIX	1 PANCAKE	38	53	74	2	1	0.2	0.3	0.3
606	PREPARED FROM INCOMPLETE MIX, WITH 2% MILK, EGG, AND OIL	1 PANCAKE	38	53	83	3	3	0.8	0.8	1.1
	PIE CRUST, BAKED									
	STANDARD TYPE									
607	FROM RECIPE	1 PIE SHELL	180	10	949	12	62	15.5	27.3	16.4
608	FROM FROZEN	1 PIE SHELL	126	11	648	6	41	13.3	19.8	5.1
609	GRAHAM CRACKER	1 PIE SHELL	239	4	1,181	10	60	12.4	27.2	16.5
	PIES									
	COMMERCIALLY PREPARED (1/6 OF 8″ DIA)									
610	APPLE	1 PIECE	117	52	277	2	13	4.4	5.1	2.6
611	BLUEBERRY	1 PIECE	117	53	271	2	12	2.0	5.0	4.1
612	CHERRY	1 PIECE	117	46	304	2	13	3.0	6.8	2.4
613	CHOCOLATE CREAM	1 PIECE	113	44	344	3	22	5.6	12.6	2.7
614	COCONUT CUSTARD	1 PIECE	104	49	270	6	14	6.1	5.7	1.2
615	LEMON MERINGUE	1 PIECE	113	42	303	2	10	2.0	3.0	4.1
616	PECAN	1 PIECE	113	19	452	5	21	4.0	12.1	3.6
617	PUMPKIN	1 PIECE	109	58	229	4	10	1.9	4.4	3.4
	PREPARED FROM RECIPE (1/8 OF 9″ DIA)									
618	APPLE	1 PIECE	155	47	411	4	19	4.7	8.4	5.2
619	BLUEBERRY	1 PIECE	147	51	360	4	17	4.3	7.5	4.5
620	CHERRY	1 PIECE	180	46	486	5	22	5.4	9.6	5.8
621	LEMON MERINGUE	1 PIECE	127	43	362	5	16	4.0	7.1	4.2

Cholesterol (mg)	Carbo-hydrate (g)	Total dietary fiber (g)	Calcium (mg)	Iron (mg)	Potassium (mg)	Sodium (mg)	Vitamin A (IU)	(RE)	Thiamine (mg)	Ribo-flavin (mg)	Niacin (mg)	Ascorbic acid (mg)	Food No.
0	24	0.9	4	0.9	32	1	0	0	0.11	0.08	1.1	0	589
17	27	1.5	32	0.9	70	255	19	5	0.08	0.07	0.6	1	590
23	24	0.6	13	0.6	39	219	39	11	0.07	0.16	1.1	1	591
21	23	1.1	108	1.3	70	251	80	22	0.16	0.16	1.3	1	592
3	19	2.8	13	1.0	60	179	58	16	0.07	0.10	0.8	0	593
15	29	1.9	42	1.6	39	297	119	21	0.16	0.19	1.2	0	594
31	25	1.2	38	1.0	66	398	105	23	0.12	0.14	1.1	TR	595
0	28	2.6	36	2.4	289	224	0	0	0.15	0.05	0.2	0	596
0	26	1.8	9	2.1	54	198	38	4	0.26	0.19	2.7	0	597
53	40	1.8	19	2.5	45	11	32	10	0.30	0.13	2.4	0	598
53	39	3.7	30	1.7	59	19	165	22	0.39	0.20	2.4	0	599
0	27	0.8	15	1.8	73	110	750	227	0.37	0.41	5.0	0	600
0	62	14.5	55	5.1	532	4	0	0	1.10	0.21	0.9	0	601
0	25	5.7	22	1.9	201	2	0	0	0.35	0.07	0.3	0	602
0	15	3.7	15	0.7	93	117	1	0	0.09	0.04	0.9	TR	603
3	16	0.6	22	1.3	26	183	36	10	0.14	0.17	1.4	TR	604
5	14	0.5	48	0.6	67	239	12	3	0.08	0.08	0.7	TR	605
27	11	0.7	82	0.5	76	192	95	27	0.08	0.12	0.5	TR	606
0	86	3.0	18	5.2	121	976	0	0	0.70	0.50	6.0	0	607
0	62	1.3	26	2.8	139	815	0	0	0.35	0.48	3.1	0	608
0	156	3.6	50	5.2	210	1,365	1,876	483	0.25	0.42	5.1	0	609
0	40	1.9	13	0.5	76	311	145	35	0.03	0.03	0.3	4	610
0	41	1.2	9	0.4	59	380	164	40	0.01	0.04	0.4	3	611
0	47	0.9	14	0.6	95	288	329	63	0.03	0.03	0.2	1	612
6	38	2.3	41	1.2	144	154	0	0	0.04	0.12	0.8	0	613
36	31	1.9	84	0.8	182	348	114	28	0.09	0.15	0.4	1	614
51	53	1.4	63	0.7	101	165	198	59	0.07	0.24	0.7	4	615
36	65	4.0	19	1.2	84	479	198	53	0.10	0.14	0.3	1	616
22	30	2.9	65	0.9	168	307	3,743	405	0.06	0.17	0.2	1	617
0	58	3.6	11	1.7	122	327	90	19	0.23	0.17	1.9	3	618
0	49	3.6	10	1.8	74	272	62	6	0.22	0.19	1.8	1	619
0	69	3.5	18	3.3	139	344	736	86	0.27	0.23	2.3	2	620
67	50	0.7	15	1.3	83	307	203	56	0.15	0.20	1.2	4	621

Food No.	Food Description	Measure of edible portion	Weight (g)	Water (%)	Calories (kcal)	Protein (g)	Total fat (g)	Fatty acids Satu-rated (g)	Mono-unsatu-rated (g)	Poly-unsatu-rated (g)
GRAIN PRODUCTS (CONTINUED)										
622	PECAN	1 PIECE	122	20	503	6	27	4.9	13.6	7.0
623	PUMPKIN	1 PIECE	155	59	316	7	14	4.9	5.7	2.8
624	FRIED, CHERRY	1 PIE	128	38	404	4	21	3.1	9.5	6.9
	POPCORN									
625	AIR POPPED, UNSALTED	1 CUP	8	4	31	1	TR	TR	0.1	0.2
626	OIL POPPED, SALTED	1 CUP	11	3	55	1	3	0.5	0.9	1.5
	CARAMEL-COATED									
627	WITH PEANUTS	1 CUP	42	3	168	3	3	0.4	1.1	1.4
628	WITHOUT PEANUTS	1 CUP	35	3	152	1	5	1.3	1.0	1.6
629	CHEESE FLAVOR	1 CUP	11	3	58	1	4	0.7	1.1	1.7
630	POPCORN CAKE	1 CAKE	10	5	38	1	TR	TR	0.1	0.1
	PRETZELS, MADE WITH ENRICHED FLOUR									
631	STICK, 2 1/4″ LONG	10 PRETZELS	3	3	11	TR	TR	TR	TR	TR
632	TWISTED, REGULAR	10 PRETZELS	60	3	229	5	2	0.5	0.8	0.7
633	TWISTED, DUTCH, 2 3/4″ × 2 5/8″	1 PRETZEL	16	3	61	1	1	0.1	0.2	0.2
	RICE									
634	BROWN, LONG GRAIN, COOKED	1 CUP	195	73	216	5	2	0.4	0.6	0.6
	WHITE, LONG GRAIN, ENRICHED									
	REGULAR									
635	RAW	1 CUP	185	12	675	13	1	0.3	0.4	0.3
636	COOKED	1 CUP	158	68	205	4	TR	0.1	0.1	0.1
637	INSTANT, PREPARED	1 CUP	165	76	162	3	TR	0.1	0.1	0.1
	PARBOILED									
638	RAW	1 CUP	185	10	686	13	1	0.3	0.3	0.3
639	COOKED	1 CUP	175	72	200	4	TR	0.1	0.1	0.1
640	WILD, COOKED	1 CUP	164	74	166	7	1	0.1	0.1	0.3
641	RICE CAKE, BROWN RICE, PLAIN	1 CAKE	9	6	35	1	TR	0.1	0.1	0.1
642	RICE KRISPIES TREAT SQUARES	1 BAR	22	6	91	1	2	0.3	0.6	1.1
	ROLLS									
643	DINNER	1 ROLL	28	32	84	2	2	0.5	1.0	0.3
644	HAMBURGER OR HOTDOG	1 ROLL	43	34	123	4	2	0.5	0.4	1.1
645	HARD, KAISER	1 ROLL	57	31	167	6	2	0.3	0.6	1.0
	SPAGHETTI, COOKED									
646	ENRICHED	1 CUP	140	66	197	7	1	0.1	0.1	0.4
647	WHOLE WHEAT	1 CUP	140	67	174	7	1	0.1	0.1	0.3
	SWEET ROLLS, CINNAMON									
648	COMMERCIAL, WITH RAISINS	1 ROLL	60	25	223	4	10	1.8	2.9	4.5
649	REFRIGERATED DOUGH, BAKED, WITH FROSTING	1 ROLL	30	23	109	2	4	1.0	2.2	0.5
650	TACO SHELL, BAKED	1 MEDIUM	13	6	62	1	3	0.4	1.2	1.1
651	TAPIOCA, PEARL, DRY	1 CUP	152	11	544	TR	TR	TR	TR	TR
	TOASTER PASTRIES									
652	BROWN SUGAR CINNAMON	1 PASTRY	50	11	206	3	7	1.8	4.0	0.9
653	CHOCOLATE WITH FROSTING	1 PASTRY	52	13	201	3	5	1.0	2.7	1.1
654	FRUIT FILLED	1 PASTRY	52	12	204	2	5	0.8	2.2	2.0
655	LOW FAT	1 PASTRY	52	12	193	2	3	0.7	1.7	0.5
	TORTILLA CHIPS									
	PLAIN									
656	REGULAR	1 OZ	28	2	142	2	7	1.4	4.4	1.0
657	LOW FAT, BAKED	10 CHIPS	14	2	54	2	1	0.1	0.2	0.4
	NACHO FLAVOR									
658	REGULAR	1 OZ	28	2	141	2	7	1.4	4.3	1.0
659	LIGHT, REDUCED FAT	1 OZ	28	1	126	2	4	0.8	2.5	0.6

Cholesterol (mg)	Carbo- hydrate (g)	Total dietary fiber (g)	Calcium (mg)	Iron (mg)	Potassium (mg)	Sodium (mg)	Vitamin A (IU)	Vitamin A (RE)	Thiamine (mg)	Ribo- flavin (mg)	Niacin (mg)	Ascorbic acid (mg)	Food No.
106	64	2.2	39	1.8	162	320	410	109	0.23	0.22	1.0	TR	622
65	41	2.9	146	2.0	288	349	11,833	1,212	0.14	0.31	1.2	3	623
0	55	3.3	28	1.6	83	479	220	22	0.18	0.14	1.8	2	624
0	6	1.2	1	0.2	24	TR	16	2	0.02	0.02	0.2	0	625
0	6	1.1	1	0.3	25	97	17	2	0.01	0.01	0.2	TR	626
0	34	1.6	28	1.6	149	124	27	3	0.02	0.05	0.8	0	627
2	28	1.8	15	0.6	38	73	18	4	0.02	0.02	0.8	0	628
1	6	1.1	12	0.2	29	98	27	5	0.01	0.03	0.2	TR	629
0	8	0.3	1	0.2	33	29	7	1	0.01	0.02	0.6	0	630
0	2	0.1	1	0.1	4	51	0	0	0.01	0.02	0.2	0	631
0	48	1.9	22	2.6	88	1,029	0	0	0.28	0.37	3.2	0	632
0	13	0.5	6	0.7	23	274	0	0	0.07	0.10	0.8	0	633
0	45	3.5	20	0.8	84	10	0	0	0.19	0.05	3.0	0	634
0	148	2.4	52	8.0	213	9	0	0	1.07	0.09	7.8	0	635
0	45	0.6	16	1.9	55	2	0	0	0.26	0.02	2.3	0	636
0	35	1.0	13	1.0	7	5	0	0	0.12	0.08	1.5	0	637
0	151	3.1	111	6.6	222	9	0	0	1.10	0.13	6.7	0	638
0	43	0.7	33	2.0	65	5	0	0	0.44	0.03	2.5	0	639
0	35	3.0	5	1.0	166	5	0	0	0.09	0.14	2.1	0	640
0	7	0.4	1	0.1	26	29	4	TR	0.01	0.01	0.7	0	641
0	18	0.1	1	0.5	9	77	200	60	0.15	0.18	2.0	0	642
TR	14	0.8	33	0.9	37	146	0	0	0.14	0.09	1.1	TR	643
0	22	1.2	60	1.4	61	241	0	0	0.21	0.13	1.7	TR	644
0	30	1.3	54	1.9	62	310	0	0	0.27	0.19	2.4	0	645
0	40	2.4	10	2.0	43	1	0	0	0.29	0.14	2.3	0	646
0	37	6.3	21	1.5	62	4	0	0	0.15	0.06	1.0	0	647
40	31	1.4	43	1.0	67	230	129	38	0.19	0.16	1.4	1	648
0	17	0.6	10	0.8	19	250	1	0	0.12	0.07	1.1	TR	649
0	8	1.0	21	0.3	24	49	0	0	0.03	0.01	0.2	0	650
0	135	1.4	30	2.4	17	2	0	0	0.01	0.00	0.0	0	651
0	34	0.5	17	2.0	57	212	493	112	0.19	0.29	2.3	TR	652
0	37	0.6	20	1.8	82	203	500	NA	0.16	0.16	2.0	0	653
0	37	1.1	14	1.8	58	218	501	2	0.15	0.19	2.0	TR	654
0	40	0.8	23	1.8	34	131	494	49	0.15	0.29	2.0	2	655
0	18	1.8	44	0.4	56	150	56	6	0.02	0.05	0.4	0	656
0	11	0.7	22	0.2	37	57	52	6	0.03	0.04	0.1	TR	657
1	18	1.5	42	0.4	61	201	105	12	0.04	0.05	0.4	1	658
1	20	1.4	45	0.5	77	284	108	12	0.06	0.08	0.1	TR	659

Food No.	Food Description	Measure of edible portion	Weight (g)	Water (%)	Calories (kcal)	Protein (g)	Total fat (g)	Fatty acids		
								Saturated (g)	Mono-unsaturated (g)	Poly-unsaturated (g)
GRAIN PRODUCTS (CONTINUED)										
	TORTILLAS, READY TO COOK (ABOUT 6″ DIA)									
660	CORN	1 TORTILLA	26	44	58	1	1	0.1	0.2	0.3
661	FLOUR	1 TORTILLA	32	27	104	3	2	0.6	1.2	0.3
	WAFFLES, PLAIN									
662	PREPARED FROM RECIPE, 7″ DIA	1 WAFFLE	75	42	218	6	11	2.1	2.6	5.1
663	FROZEN, TOASTED, 4″ DIA	1 WAFFLE	33	42	87	2	3	0.5	1.1	0.9
664	LOW FAT, 4″ DIA	1 WAFFLE	35	43	83	2	1	0.3	0.4	0.4
	WHEAT FLOURS									
	ALL PURPOSE, ENRICHED									
665	SIFTED, SPOONED	1 CUP	115	12	419	12	1	0.2	0.1	0.5
666	UNSIFTED, SPOONED	1 CUP	125	12	455	13	1	0.2	0.1	0.5
667	BREAD, ENRICHED	1 CUP	137	13	495	16	2	0.3	0.2	1.0
668	CAKE OR PASTRY FLOUR, ENRICHED, UNSIFTED, SPOONED	1 CUP	137	13	496	11	1	0.2	0.1	0.5
669	SELF-RISING, ENRICHED, UNSIFTED, SPOONED	1 CUP	125	11	443	12	1	0.2	0.1	0.5
670	WHOLE WHEAT, FROM HARD WHEATS, STIRRED, SPOONED	1 CUP	120	10	407	16	2	0.4	0.3	0.9
671	WHEAT GERM, TOASTED, PLAIN	1 TBSP	7	6	27	2	1	0.1	0.1	0.5
LEGUMES, NUTS, AND SEEDS										
	ALMONDS, SHELLED									
672	SLICED	1 CUP	95	5	549	20	48	3.7	30.5	11.6
673	WHOLE	1 OZ (24 NUTS)	28	5	164	6	14	1.1	9.1	3.5
	BEANS, DRY									
	COOKED									
674	BLACK	1 CUP	172	66	227	15	1	0.2	0.1	0.4
675	GREAT NORTHERN	1 CUP	177	69	209	15	1	0.2	TR	0.3
676	KIDNEY, RED	1 CUP	177	67	225	15	1	0.1	0.1	0.5
677	LIMA, LARGE	1 CUP	188	70	216	15	1	0.2	0.1	0.3
678	PEA (NAVY)	1 CUP	182	63	258	16	1	0.3	0.1	0.4
679	PINTO	1 CUP	171	64	234	14	1	0.2	0.2	0.3
	CANNED, SOLIDS AND LIQUID									
	BAKED BEANS									
680	PLAIN OR VEGETARIAN	1 CUP	254	73	236	12	1	0.3	0.1	0.5
681	WITH FRANKFURTERS	1 CUP	259	69	368	17	17	6.1	7.3	2.2
682	WITH PORK IN TOMATO SAUCE	1 CUP	253	73	248	13	3	1.0	1.1	0.3
683	WITH PORK IN SWEET SAUCE	1 CUP	253	71	281	13	4	1.4	1.6	0.5
684	KIDNEY, RED	1 CUP	256	77	218	13	1	0.1	0.1	0.5
685	LIMA, LARGE	1 CUP	241	77	190	12	TR	0.1	TR	0.2
686	WHITE	1 CUP	262	70	307	19	1	0.2	0.1	0.3
	BLACK-EYED PEAS, DRY									
687	COOKED	1 CUP	172	70	200	13	1	0.2	0.1	0.4
688	CANNED, SOLIDS AND LIQUID	1 CUP	240	80	185	11	1	0.3	0.1	0.6
689	BRAZIL NUTS, SHELLED	1 OZ (6–8 NUTS)	28	3	186	4	19	4.6	6.5	6.8
690	CAROB FLOUR	1 CUP	103	4	229	5	1	0.1	0.2	0.2
	CASHEWS, SALTED									
691	DRY ROASTED	1 OZ	28	2	163	4	13	2.6	7.7	2.2
692	OIL ROASTED	1 CUP	130	4	749	21	63	12.4	36.9	10.6
693		1 OZ (18 NUTS)	28	4	163	5	14	2.7	8.1	2.3
694	CHESTNUTS, EUROPEAN, ROASTED, SHELLED	1 CUP	143	40	350	5	3	0.6	1.1	1.2
	CHICKPEAS, DRY									

Cholesterol (mg)	Carbo-hydrate (g)	Total dietary fiber (g)	Calcium (mg)	Iron (mg)	Potassium (mg)	Sodium (mg)	Vitamin A (IU)	Vitamin A (RE)	Thiamine (mg)	Ribo-flavin (mg)	Niacin (mg)	Ascorbic acid (mg)	Food No.
0	12	1.4	46	0.4	40	42	0	0	0.03	0.02	0.4	0	660
0	18	1.1	40	1.1	42	153	0	0	0.17	0.09	1.1	0	661
52	25	0.7	191	1.7	119	383	171	49	0.20	0.26	1.6	TR	662
8	13	0.8	77	1.5	42	260	400	120	0.13	0.16	1.5	0	663
9	15	0.4	20	1.9	50	155	506	NA	0.31	0.26	2.6	0	664
0	88	3.1	17	5.3	123	2	0	0	0.90	0.57	6.8	0	665
0	95	3.4	19	5.8	134	3	0	0	0.98	0.62	7.4	0	666
0	99	3.3	21	6.0	137	3	0	0	1.11	0.70	10.3	0	667
0	107	2.3	19	10.0	144	3	0	0	1.22	0.59	9.3	0	668
0	93	3.4	423	5.8	155	1,588	0	0	0.84	0.52	7.3	0	669
0	87	14.6	41	4.7	486	6	0	0	0.54	0.26	7.6	0	670
0	3	0.9	3	0.6	66	TR	0	0	0.12	0.06	0.4	TR	671
0	19	11.2	236	4.1	692	1	10	1	0.23	0.77	3.7	0	672
0	6	3.3	70	1.2	206	TR	3	TR	0.07	0.23	1.1	0	673
0	41	15.0	46	3.6	611	2	10	2	0.42	0.10	0.9	0	674
0	37	12.4	120	3.8	692	4	2	0	0.28	0.10	1.2	2	675
0	40	13.1	50	5.2	713	4	0	0	0.28	0.10	1.0	2	676
0	39	13.2	32	4.5	955	4	0	0	0.30	0.10	0.8	0	677
0	48	11.6	127	4.5	670	2	4	0	0.37	0.11	1.0	2	678
0	44	14.7	82	4.5	800	3	3	0	0.32	0.16	0.7	4	679
0	52	12.7	127	0.7	752	1,008	434	43	0.39	0.15	1.1	8	680
16	40	17.9	124	4.5	609	1,114	399	39	0.15	0.15	2.3	6	681
18	49	12.1	142	8.3	759	1,113	314	30	0.13	0.12	1.3	8	682
18	53	13.2	154	4.2	673	850	288	28	0.12	0.15	0.9	8	683
0	40	16.4	61	3.2	658	873	0	0	0.27	0.23	1.2	3	684
0	36	11.6	51	4.4	530	810	0	0	0.13	0.08	0.6	0	685
0	57	12.6	191	7.8	1,189	13	0	0	0.25	0.10	0.3	0	686
0	36	11.2	41	4.3	478	7	26	3	0.35	0.09	0.9	1	687
0	33	7.9	48	2.3	413	718	31	2	0.18	0.18	0.8	6	688
0	4	1.5	50	1.0	170	1	0	0	0.28	0.03	0.5	TR	689
0	92	41.0	358	3.0	852	36	14	1	0.05	0.47	2.0	TR	690
0	9	0.9	13	1.7	160	181	0	0	0.06	0.06	0.4	0	691
0	37	4.9	53	5.3	689	814	0	0	0.55	0.23	2.3	0	692
0	8	1.1	12	1.2	150	177	0	0	0.12	0.05	0.5	0	693
0	76	7.3	41	1.3	847	3	34	3	0.35	0.25	1.9	37	694

Food No.	Food Description	Measure of edible portion	Weight (g)	Water (%)	Calories (kcal)	Protein (g)	Total fat (g)	Fatty acids		
								Satu-rated (g)	Mono-unsatu-rated (g)	Poly-unsatu-rated (g)
LEGUMES, NUTS, AND SEEDS (CONTINUED)										
695	COOKED	1 CUP	164	60	269	15	4	0.4	1.0	1.9
696	CANNED, SOLIDS AND LIQUID	1 CUP	240	70	286	12	3	0.3	0.6	1.2
	COCONUT									
	RAW									
697	PIECE, ABOUT 2″ × 2″ × 1/2″	1 PIECE	45	47	159	1	15	13.4	0.6	0.2
698	SHREDDED, NOT PACKED	1 CUP	80	47	283	3	27	23.8	1.1	0.3
699	DRIED, SWEETENED, SHREDDED	1 CUP	93	13	466	3	33	29.3	1.4	0.4
700	HAZELNUTS (FILBERTS), CHOPPED	1 CUP	115	5	722	17	70	5.1	52.5	9.1
701		1 OZ	28	5	178	4	17	1.3	12.9	2.2
702	HUMMUS, COMMERCIAL	1 TBSP	14	67	23	1	1	0.2	0.6	0.5
703	LENTILS, DRY, COOKED	1 CUP	198	70	230	18	1	0.1	0.1	0.3
704	MACADAMIA NUTS, DRY ROASTED, SALTED	1 CUP	134	2	959	10	102	16.0	79.4	2.0
705		1 OZ (10–12 NUTS)	28	2	203	2	22	3.4	16.8	0.4
	MIXED NUTS, WITH PEANUTS, SALTED									
706	DRY ROASTED	1 OZ	28	2	168	5	15	2.0	8.9	3.1
707	OIL ROASTED	1 OZ	28	2	175	5	16	2.5	9.0	3.8
	PEANUTS									
	DRY ROASTED									
708	SALTED	1 OZ (ABOUT 28)	28	2	166	7	14	2.0	7.0	4.4
709	UNSALTED	1 CUP	146	2	854	35	73	10.1	36.0	22.9
710		1 OZ (ABOUT 28)	28	2	166	7	14	2	7.0	4.4
711	OIL ROASTED, SALTED	1 CUP	144	2	837	38	71	9.9	35.2	22.4
712		1 OZ	28	2	165	7	14	1.9	6.9	4.4
	PEANUT BUTTER									
	REGULAR									
713	SMOOTH STYLE	1 TBSP	16	1	95	4	8	1.7	3.9	2.2
714	CHUNK STYLE	1 TBSP	16	1	94	4	8	1.5	3.8	2.3
715	REDUCED FAT, SMOOTH	1 TBSP	18	1	94	5	6	1.3	2.9	1.8
716	PEAS, SPLIT, DRY, COOKED	1 CUP	196	69	231	16	1	0.1	0.2	0.3
717	PECANS, HALVES	1 CUP	108	4	746	10	78	6.7	44.0	23.3
718		1 OZ (20 HALVES)	28	4	196	3	20	1.8	11.6	6.1
719	PINE NUTS (PIGNOLIA), SHELLED	1 OZ	28	7	160	7	14	2.2	5.4	6.1
720		1 TBSP	9	7	49	2	4	0.7	1.6	1.8
721	PISTACHIO NUTS, DRY ROASTED, WITH SALT, SHELLED	1 OZ (47 NUTS)	28	2	161	6	13	1.6	6.8	3.9
722	PUMPKIN AND SQUASH KERNELS, ROASTED, WITH SALT	1 OZ (142 SEEDS)	28	7	148	9	12	2.3	3.7	5.4
723	REFRIED BEANS, CANNED	1 CUP	252	76	237	14	3	1.2	1.4	0.4
724	SESAME SEEDS	1 TBSP	8	5	47	2	4	0.6	1.7	1.9
725	SOYBEANS, DRY, COOKED	1 CUP	172	63	298	29	15	2.2	3.4	8.7
	SOY PRODUCTS									
726	MISO	1 CUP	275	41	567	32	17	2.4	3.7	9.4
727	SOY MILK	1 CUP	245	93	81	7	5	0.5	0.8	2.0
	TOFU									
728	FIRM	1/4 BLOCK	81	84	62	7	4	0.5	0.8	2.0
729	SOFT, PIECE 2 1/2″ × 2 3/4″ × 1″	1 PIECE	120	87	73	8	4	0.6	1.0	2.5
730	SUNFLOWER SEED KERNELS, DRY ROASTED, WITH SALT	1/4 CUP	32	1	186	6	16	1.7	3.0	10.5

Cholesterol (mg)	Carbo-hydrate (g)	Total dietary fiber (g)	Calcium (mg)	Iron (mg)	Potassium (mg)	Sodium (mg)	Vitamin A (IU)	(RE)	Thiamine (mg)	Ribo-flavin (mg)	Niacin (mg)	Ascorbic acid (mg)	Food No.
0	45	12.5	80	4.7	477	11	44	5	0.19	0.10	0.9	2	695
0	54	10.6	77	3.2	413	718	58	5	0.07	0.08	0.3	9	696
0	7	4.1	6	1.1	160	9	0	0	0.03	0.01	0.2	1	697
0	12	7.2	11	1.9	285	16	0	0	0.05	0.02	0.4	3	698
0	44	4.2	14	1.8	313	244	0	0	0.03	0.02	0.4	1	699
0	19	11.2	131	5.4	782	0	46	5	0.74	0.13	2.1	7	700
0	5	2.7	32	1.3	193	0	11	1	0.18	0.03	0.5	2	701
0	2	0.8	5	0.3	32	53	4	TR	0.03	0.01	0.1	0	702
0	40	15.6	38	6.6	731	4	16	2	0.33	0.14	2.1	3	703
0	17	10.7	94	3.6	486	355	0	0	0.95	0.12	3.0	1	704
0	4	2.3	20	0.8	103	75	0	0	0.20	0.02	0.6	TR	705
0	7	2.6	20	1.0	169	190	4	TR	0.06	0.06	1.3	TR	706
0	6	2.6	31	0.9	165	185	5	1	0.14	0.06	1.4	TR	707
0	6	2.3	15	0.6	187	230	0	0	0.12	0.03	3.8	0	708
0	31	11.7	79	3.3	961	9	0	0	0.64	0.14	19.7	0	709
0	6	2.3	15	0.6	187	2	0	0	0.12	0.03	3.8	0	710
0	27	13.2	127	2.6	982	624	0	0	0.36	0.16	20.6	0	711
0	5	2.6	25	0.5	193	123	0	0	0.07	0.03	4.0	0	712
0	3	0.9	6	0.3	107	75	0	0	0.01	0.02	2.1	0	713
0	3	1.1	7	0.3	120	78	0	0	0.02	0.02	2.2	0	714
0	6	0.9	6	0.3	120	97	0	0	0.05	0.01	2.6	0	715
0	41	16.3	27	2.5	710	4	14	2	0.37	0.11	1.7	1	716
0	15	10.4	76	2.7	443	0	83	9	0.71	0.14	1.3	1	717
0	4	2.7	20	0.7	116	0	22	2	0.19	0.04	0.3	TR	718
0	4	1.3	7	2.6	170	1	8	1	0.23	0.05	1.0	1	719
0	1	0.4	2	0.8	52	TR	2	TR	0.07	0.02	0.3	TR	720
0	8	2.9	31	1.2	293	121	151	15	0.24	0.04	0.4	1	721
0	4	1.1	12	4.2	229	163	108	11	0.06	0.09	0.5	1	722
20	39	13.4	88	4.2	673	753	0	0	0.07	0.04	0.8	15	723
0	1	0.9	10	0.6	33	3	5	1	0.06	0.01	0.4	0	724
0	17	10.3	175	8.8	886	2	15	2	0.27	0.49	0.7	3	725
0	77	14.9	182	7.5	451	10,029	239	25	0.27	0.69	2.4	0	726
0	4	3.2	10	1.4	345	29	78	7	0.39	0.17	0.4	0	727
0	2	0.3	131	1.2	143	6	6	1	0.08	0.08	TR	TR	728
0	2	0.2	133	1.3	144	10	8	1	0.06	0.04	0.6	TR	729
0	8	2.9	22	1.2	272	250	0	0	0.03	0.08	2.3	TR	730

Food No.	Food Description	Measure of edible portion	Weight (g)	Water (%)	Calories (kcal)	Protein (g)	Total fat (g)	Fatty acids Saturated (g)	Fatty acids Monounsaturated (g)	Fatty acids Polyunsaturated (g)
LEGUMES, NUTS, AND SEEDS (CONTINUED)										
731		1 OZ	28	1	165	5	14	1.5	2.7	9.3
732	TAHINI	1 TBSP	15	3	89	3	8	1.1	3.0	3.5
733	WALNUTS, ENGLISH	1 CUP, CHOPPED	120	4	785	18	78	7.4	10.7	56.6
734		1 OZ (14 HALVES)	28	4	185	4	18	1.7	2.5	13.4
MEAT AND MEAT PRODUCTS										
	BEEF, COOKED									
	CUTS BRAISED, SIMMERED, OR									
	POT ROASTED									
	RELATIVELY FAT, SUCH AS CHUCK BLADE,									
	PIECE, 2 1/2″ × 2 1/2″ × 3/4″									
735	LEAN AND FAT	3 OZ	85	47	293	23	22	8.7	9.4	0.8
736	LEAN ONLY	3 OZ	85	55	213	26	11	4.3	4.8	0.4
	RELATIVELY LEAN, SUCH AS BOTTOM ROUND,									
	PIECE, 4 1/8″ × 2 1/4″ × 1/2″									
737	LEAN AND FAT	3 OZ	85	52	234	24	14	5.4	6.2	0.5
738	LEAN ONLY	3 OZ	85	58	178	27	7	2.4	3.1	0.3
	GROUND BEEF, BROILED									
739	83% LEAN	3 OZ	85	57	218	22	14	5.5	6.1	0.5
740	79% LEAN	3 OZ	85	56	231	21	16	6.2	6.9	0.6
741	73% LEAN	3 OZ	85	54	246	20	18	6.9	7.7	0.7
742	LIVER, FRIED, SLICE, 6 1/2″ × 2 3/8″ × 3/8″	3 OZ	85	56	184	23	7	2.3	1.4	1.5
	ROAST, OVEN COOKED, NO LIQUID ADDED									
	RELATIVELY FAT, SUCH AS RIB, 2 PIECES,									
	4 1/8″ × 2 1/4″ × 1/4″									
743	LEAN AND FAT	3 OZ	85	47	304	19	25	9.9	10.6	0.9
744	LEAN ONLY	3 OZ	85	59	195	23	11	4.2	4.5	0.3
	RELATIVELY LEAN, SUCH AS EYE OF ROUND,									
	2 PIECES, 2 1/2″ × 2 1/2″ × 3/8″									
745	LEAN AND FAT	3 OZ	85	59	195	23	11	4.2	4.7	0.4
746	LEAN ONLY	3 OZ	85	65	143	25	4	1.5	1.8	0.1
	STEAK, SIRLOIN, BROILED, PIECE,									
	2 1/2″ × 2 1/2″ × 3/4″									
747	LEAN AND FAT	3 OZ	85	57	219	24	13	5.2	5.6	0.5
748	LEAN ONLY	3 OZ	85	62	166	26	6	2.4	2.6	0.2
749	BEEF, CANNED, CORNED	3 OZ	85	58	213	23	13	5.3	5.1	0.5
750	BEEF, DRIED, CHIPPED	1 OZ	28	57	47	8	1	0.5	0.5	0.1
	LAMB, COOKED									
	CHOPS									
	ARM, BRAISED									
751	LEAN AND FAT	3 OZ	85	44	294	26	20	8.4	8.7	1.5
752	LEAN ONLY	3 OZ	85	49	237	30	12	4.3	5.2	0.8
	LOIN, BROILED									
753	LEAN AND FAT	3 OZ	85	52	269	21	20	8.4	8.2	1.4
754	LEAN ONLY	3 OZ	85	61	184	25	8	3.0	3.6	0.5
	LEG, ROASTED, 2 PIECES, 4 1/8″ × 2 1/4″ × 1/4″									
755	LEAN AND FAT	3 OZ	85	57	219	22	14	5.9	5.9	1.0
756	LEAN ONLY	3 OZ	85	64	162	24	7	2.3	2.9	0.4
	RIB, ROASTED, 3 PIECES, 2 1/2″ × 2 1/2″ × 1/4″									
757	LEAN AND FAT	3 OZ	85	48	305	18	25	10.9	10.6	1.8
758	LEAN ONLY	3 OZ	85	60	197	22	11	4.0	5.0	0.7

Cholesterol (mg)	Carbo-hydrate (g)	Total dietary fiber (g)	Calcium (mg)	Iron (mg)	Potassium (mg)	Sodium (mg)	Vitamin A (IU)	(RE)	Thiamine (mg)	Ribo-flavin (mg)	Niacin (mg)	Ascorbic acid (mg)	Food No.
0	7	2.6	20	1.1	241	221	0	0	0.03	0.07	2.0	TR	731
0	3	1.4	64	1.3	62	17	10	1	0.18	0.07	0.8	0	732
0	16	8.0	125	3.5	529	2	49	5	0.41	0.18	2.3	2	733
0	4	1.9	29	0.8	125	1	12	1	0.10	0.04	0.5	TR	734
88	0	0.0	11	2.6	196	54	0	0	0.06	0.20	2.1	0	735
90	0	0.0	11	3.1	224	60	0	0	0.07	0.24	2.3	0	736
82	0	0.0	5	2.7	240	43	0	0	0.06	0.20	3.2	0	737
82	0	0.0	4	2.9	262	43	0	0	0.06	0.22	3.5	0	738
71	0	0.0	6	2.0	266	60	0	0	0.05	0.23	4.2	0	739
74	0	0.0	9	1.8	256	65	0	0	0.04	0.18	4.4	0	740
77	0	0.0	9	2.1	248	71	0	0	0.03	0.16	4.9	0	741
410	7	0.0	9	5.3	309	90	30,689	9,120	0.18	3.52	12.3	20	742
71	0	0.0	9	2.0	256	54	0	0	0.06	0.14	2.9	0	743
68	0	0.0	9	2.4	318	61	0	0	0.07	0.18	3.5	0	744
61	0	0.0	5	1.6	308	50	0	0	0.07	0.14	3.0	0	745
59	0	0.0	4	1.7	336	53	0	0	0.08	0.14	3.2	0	746
77	0	0.0	9	2.6	311	54	0	0	0.09	0.23	3.3	0	747
76	0	0.0	9	2.9	343	56	0	0	0.11	0.25	3.6	0	748
73	0	0.0	10	1.8	116	855	0	0	0.02	0.12	2.1	0	749
12	TR	0.0	2	1.3	126	984	0	0	0.02	0.06	1.5	0	750
102	0	0.0	21	2.0	260	61	0	0	0.06	0.21	5.7	0	751
103	0	0.0	22	2.3	287	65	0	0	0.06	0.23	5.4	0	752
85	0	0.0	17	1.5	278	65	0	0	0.09	0.21	6.0	0	753
81	0	0.0	16	1.7	320	71	0	0	0.09	0.24	5.8	0	754
79	0	0.0	9	1.7	266	56	0	0	0.09	0.23	5.6	0	755
76	0	0.0	7	1.8	287	58	0	0	0.09	0.25	5.4	0	756
82	0	0.0	19	1.4	230	62	0	0	0.08	0.18	5.7	0	757
75	0	0.0	18	1.5	268	69	0	0	0.08	0.20	5.2	0	758

Food No.	Food Description	Measure of edible portion	Weight (g)	Water (%)	Calories (kcal)	Protein (g)	Total fat (g)	Fatty acids Saturated (g)	Mono-unsaturated (g)	Poly-unsaturated (g)
MEAT AND MEAT PRODUCTS (CONTINUED)										
	PORK, CURED, COOKED									
	BACON									
759	REGULAR	3 MEDIUM SLICES	19	13	109	6	9	3.3	4.5	1.1
760	CANADIAN STYLE (6 SLICES PER 6-OZ PKG)	2 SLICES	47	62	86	11	4	1.3	1.9	0.4
	HAM, LIGHT CURE, ROASTED, 2 PIECES, 4 1/8″ × 2 1/4″ × 1/4″									
761	LEAN AND FAT	3 OZ	85	58	207	18	14	5.1	6.7	1.5
762	LEAN ONLY	3 OZ	85	66	133	21	5	1.6	2.2	0.5
763	HAM, CANNED, ROASTED, 2 PIECES, 4 1/8″ × 21/4″ × 1/4″	3 OZ	85	67	142	18	7	2.4	3.5	0.8
	PORK, FRESH, COOKED									
	CHOP, LOIN (CUT 3 PER LB WITH BONE)									
	BROILED									
764	LEAN AND FAT	3 OZ	85	58	204	24	11	4.1	5.0	0.8
765	LEAN ONLY	3 OZ	85	61	172	26	7	2.5	3.1	0.5
	PAN FRIED									
766	LEAN AND FAT	3 OZ	85	53	235	25	14	5.1	6.0	1.6
767	LEAN ONLY	3 OZ	85	57	197	27	9	3.1	3.8	1.1
	HAM (LEG), ROASTED, PIECE, 2 1/2″ × 2 1/2″ × 3/4″									
768	LEAN AND FAT	3 OZ	85	55	232	23	15	5.5	6.7	1.4
769	LEAN ONLY	3 OZ	85	61	179	25	8	2.8	3.8	0.7
	RIB ROAST, PIECE, 2 1/2″ × 2 1/2″ × 3/4″									
770	LEAN AND FAT	3 OZ	85	56	217	23	13	5.0	5.9	1.1
771	LEAN ONLY	3 OZ	85	59	190	24	9	3.7	4.5	0.7
	RIBS, LEAN AND FAT, COOKED									
772	BACKRIBS, ROASTED	3 OZ	85	45	315	21	25	9.3	11.4	2.0
773	COUNTRY STYLE, BRAISED	3 OZ	85	54	252	20	18	6.8	7.9	1.6
774	SPARERIBS, BRAISED	3 OZ	85	40	337	25	26	9.5	11.5	2.3
	SHOULDER CUT, BRAISED, 3 PIECES, 2 1/2″ × 2 1/2″ × 1/4″									
775	LEAN AND FAT	3 OZ	85	48	280	24	20	7.2	8.8	1.9
776	LEAN ONLY	3 OZ	85	54	211	27	10	3.5	4.9	1.0
	SAUSAGES AND LUNCHEON MEATS									
777	BOLOGNA, BEEF AND PORK (8 SLICES PER 8-OZ PKG)	2 SLICES	57	54	180	7	16	6.1	7.6	1.4
778	BRAUNSCHWEIGER (6 SLICES PER 6-OZ PKG)	2 SLICES	57	48	205	8	18	6.2	8.5	2.1
779	BROWN AND SERVE, COOKED, LINK, 4″ × 7/8″ RAW	2 LINKS	26	45	103	4	9	3.4	4.5	1.0
	CANNED, MINCED LUNCHEON MEAT									
780	PORK, HAM, AND CHICKEN, REDUCED SODIUM (7 SLICES PER 7-OZ CAN)	2 SLICES	57	56	172	7	15	5.1	7.1	1.5
781	PORK WITH HAM (12 SLICES PER 12-OZ CAN)	2 SLICES	57	52	188	8	17	5.7	7.7	1.2
782	PORK AND CHICKEN (12 SLICES PER 12-OZ CAN)	2 SLICES	57	64	117	9	8	2.7	3.8	0.8
783	CHOPPED HAM (8 SLICES PER 6-OZ PKG)	2 SLICES	21	64	48	4	4	1.2	1.7	0.4
	COOKED HAM (8 SLICES PER 8-OZ PKG)									
784	REGULAR	2 SLICES	57	65	104	10	6	1.9	2.8	0.7
785	EXTRA LEAN	2 SLICES	57	71	75	11	3	0.9	1.3	0.3
	FRANKFURTER (10 PER 1-LB PKG), HEATED									

Cholesterol (mg)	Carbo-hydrate (g)	Total dietary fiber (g)	Calcium (mg)	Iron (mg)	Potassium (mg)	Sodium (mg)	Vitamin A (IU)	(RE)	Thiamine (mg)	Ribo-flavin (mg)	Niacin (mg)	Ascorbic acid (mg)	Food No.
16	TR	0.0	2	0.3	92	303	0	0	0.13	0.05	1.4	0	759
27	1	0.0	5	0.4	181	719	0	0	0.38	0.09	3.2	0	760
53	0	0.0	6	0.7	243	1,009	0	0	0.51	0.19	3.8	0	761
47	0	0.0	6	0.8	269	1,128	0	0	0.58	0.22	4.3	0	762
35	TR	0.0	6	0.9	298	908	0	0	0.82	0.21	4.3	0	763
70	0	0.0	28	0.7	304	49	8	3	0.91	0.24	4.5	TR	764
70	0	0.0	26	0.7	319	51	7	2	0.98	0.26	4.7	TR	765
78	0	0.0	23	0.8	361	68	7	2	0.97	0.26	4.8	1	766
78	0	0.0	20	0.8	382	73	7	2	1.06	0.28	5.1	1	767
80	0	0.0	12	0.9	299	51	9	3	0.54	0.27	3.9	TR	768
80	0	0.0	6	1.0	317	54	8	3	0.59	0.30	4.2	TR	769
62	0	0.0	24	0.8	358	39	5	2	0.62	0.26	5.2	TR	770
60	0	0.0	22	0.8	371	40	5	2	0.64	0.27	5.5	TR	771
100	0	0.0	38	1.2	268	86	8	3	0.36	0.17	3.0	TR	772
74	0	0.0	25	1.0	279	50	7	2	0.43	0.22	3.3	1	773
103	0	0.0	40	1.6	272	79	9	3	0.35	0.32	4.7	0	774
93	0	0.0	15	1.4	314	75	8	3	0.46	0.26	4.4	TR	775
97	0	0.0	7	1.7	344	87	7	2	0.51	0.31	5.0	TR	776
31	2	0.0	7	0.9	103	581	0	0	0.10	0.08	1.5	0	777
89	2	0.0	5	5.3	113	652	8,009	2,405	0.14	0.87	4.8	0	778
18	1	0.0	3	0.3	49	209	0	0	0.09	0.04	0.9	0	779
43	1	0.0	0	0.4	321	539	0	0	0.15	0.10	1.8	18	780
40	1	0.0	0	0.4	233	758	0	0	0.18	0.10	2.0	0	781
43	1	0.0	0	0.7	352	539	0	0	0.10	0.12	2.0	18	782
11	0	0.0	1	0.2	67	288	0	0	0.13	0.04	0.8	0	783
32	2	0.0	4	0.6	189	751	0	0	0.49	0.14	3.0	0	784
27	1	0.0	4	0.4	200	815	0	0	0.53	0.13	2.8	0	785

Food No.	Food Description	Measure of edible portion	Weight (g)	Water (%)	Calories (kcal)	Protein (g)	Total fat (g)	Fatty acids Satu-rated (g)	Mono-unsatu-rated (g)	Poly-unsatu-rated (g)
MEAT AND MEAT PRODUCTS (CONTINUED)										
786	BEEF AND PORK	1 FRANK	45	54	144	5	13	4.8	6.2	1.2
787	BEEF	1 FRANK	45	55	142	5	13	5.4	6.1	0.6
	PORK SAUSAGE, FRESH, COOKED									
788	LINK (4″ × 7/8″ RAW)	2 LINKS	26	45	96	5	8	2.8	3.6	1.0
789	PATTY (3 7/8″ × 1/4″ RAW)	1 PATTY	27	45	100	5	8	2.9	3.8	1.0
	SALAMI, BEEF AND PORK									
790	COOKED TYPE (8 SLICES PER 8-OZ PKG)	2 SLICES	57	60	143	8	11	4.6	5.2	1.2
791	DRY TYPE, SLICE, 3 1/8″ × 1/16″	2 SLICES	20	35	84	5	7	2.4	3.4	0.6
792	SANDWICH SPREAD (PORK, BEEF)	1 TBSP	15	60	35	1	3	0.9	1.1	0.4
793	VIENNA SAUSAGE (7 PER 4-OZ CAN)	1 SAUSAGE	16	60	45	2	4	1.5	2.0	0.3
	VEAL, LEAN AND FAT, COOKED									
794	CUTLET, BRAISED, 4 1/8″ × 2 1/4″ × 1/2″	3 OZ	85	55	179	31	5	2.2	2.0	0.4
795	RIB, ROASTED, 2 PIECES, 4 1/8″ × 2 1/4″ × 1/4″	3 OZ	85	60	194	20	12	4.6	4.6	0.8
MIXED DISHES AND FAST FOODS										
	MIXED DISHES									
796	BEEF MACARONI, FROZEN, HEALTHY CHOICE	1 PACKAGE	240	78	211	14	2	0.7	1.2	0.3
797	BEEF STEW, CANNED	1 CUP	232	82	218	11	12	5.2	5.5	0.5
798	CHICKEN POT PIE, FROZEN	1 SMALL PIE	217	60	484	13	29	9.7	12.5	4.5
799	CHILI CON CARNE WITH BEANS, CANNED	1 CUP	222	74	255	20	8	2.1	2.2	1.4
800	MACARONI AND CHEESE, CANNED, MADE WITH CORN OIL	1 CUP	252	82	199	8	6	3.0	NA	1.3
801	MEATLESS BURGER CRUMBLES, MORNINGSTAR FARMS	1 CUP	110	60	231	22	13	3.3	4.6	4.9
802	MEATLESS BURGER PATTY, FROZEN, MORNINGSTAR FARMS	1 PATTY	85	71	91	14	1	0.1	0.3	0.2
803	PASTA WITH MEATBALLS IN TOMATO SAUCE, CANNED	1 CUP	252	78	260	11	10	4.0	4.2	0.6
804	SPAGHETTI BOLOGNESE (MEAT SAUCE), FROZEN, HEALTHY CHOICE	1 PACKAGE	283	78	255	14	3	1.0	0.9	0.9
805	SPAGHETTI IN TOMATO SAUCE WITH CHEESE, CANNED	1 CUP	252	80	192	6	2	0.7	0.3	0.3
806	SPINACH SOUFFLE, HOME-PREPARED	1 CUP	136	74	219	11	18	7.1	6.8	3.1
807	TORTELLINI, PASTA WITH CHEESE FILLING, FROZEN	3/4 CUP (YIELDS 1 CUP COOKED)	81	31	249	11	6	2.9	1.7	0.4
	FAST FOODS									
	BREAKFAST ITEMS									
808	BISCUIT WITH EGG AND SAUSAGE	1 BISCUIT	180	43	581	19	39	15.0	16.4	4.4
809	CROISSANT WITH EGG, CHEESE, BACON	1 CROISSANT	129	44	413	16	28	15.4	9.2	1.8
	DANISH PASTRY									
810	CHEESE FILLED	1 PASTRY	91	34	353	6	25	5.1	15.6	2.4
811	FRUIT FILLED	1 PASTRY	94	29	335	5	16	3.3	10.1	1.6
812	ENGLISH MUFFIN WITH EGG, CHEESE, CANADIAN BACON	1 MUFFIN	137	57	289	17	13	4.7	4.7	1.6
813	FRENCH TOAST WITH BUTTER	2 SLICES	135	51	356	10	19	7.7	7.1	2.4
814	FRENCH TOAST STICKS	5 STICKS	141	30	513	8	29	4.7	12.6	9.9
815	HASHED BROWN POTATOES	1/2 CUP	72	60	151	2	9	4.3	3.9	0.5
816	PANCAKES WITH BUTTER, SYRUP	2 PANCAKES	232	50	520	8	14	5.9	5.3	2.0

Cholesterol (mg)	Carbo-hydrate (g)	Total dietary fiber (g)	Calcium (mg)	Iron (mg)	Potassium (mg)	Sodium (mg)	Vitamin A (IU)	Vitamin A (RE)	Thiamine (mg)	Ribo-flavin (mg)	Niacin (mg)	Ascorbic acid (mg)	Food No.
23	1	0.0	5	0.5	75	504	0	0	0.09	0.05	1.2	0	786
27	1	0.0	9	0.6	75	462	0	0	0.02	0.05	1.1	0	787
22	TR	0.0	8	0.3	94	336	0	0	0.19	0.07	1.2	1	788
22	TR	0.0	9	0.3	97	349	0	0	0.20	0.07	1.2	1	789
37	1	0.0	7	1.5	113	607	0	0	0.14	0.21	2.0	0	790
16	1	0.0	2	0.3	76	372	0	0	0.12	0.06	1.0	0	791
6	2	TR	2	0.1	17	152	13	1	0.03	0.02	0.3	0	792
8	TR	0.0	2	0.1	16	152	0	0	0.01	0.02	0.3	0	793
114	0	0.0	7	1.1	326	57	0	0	0.05	0.30	9.0	0	794
94	0	0.0	9	0.8	251	78	0	0	0.04	0.23	5.9	0	795
14	33	4.6	46	2.7	365	444	514	50	0.28	0.16	3.1	58	796
37	16	3.5	28	1.6	404	947	3,860	494	0.17	0.14	2.9	10	797
41	43	1.7	33	2.1	256	857	2,285	343	0.25	0.36	4.1	2	798
24	24	8.2	67	3.3	608	1,032	884	93	0.15	0.15	2.1	1	799
8	29	3.0	113	2.0	123	1,058	713	NA	0.28	0.25	2.5	0	800
0	7	5.1	79	6.4	178	476	0	0	9.92	0.35	3.0	0	801
0	8	4.3	87	2.9	434	383	0	0	0.26	0.55	4.1	0	802
20	31	6.8	28	2.3	416	1,053	920	93	0.19	0.16	3.3	8	803
17	43	5.1	51	3.5	408	473	492	48	0.35	3.77	0.5	15	804
8	39	7.8	40	2.8	305	963	932	58	0.35	0.28	4.5	10	805
184	3	NA	230	1.3	201	763	3,461	675	0.09	0.30	0.5	3	806
34	38	1.5	123	1.2	72	279	50	13	0.25	0.25	2.2	0	807
302	41	0.9	155	4.0	320	1,141	635	164	0.50	0.45	3.6	0	808
215	24	NA	151	2.2	201	889	472	120	0.35	0.34	2.2	2	809
20	29	NA	70	1.8	116	319	155	43	0.26	0.21	2.5	3	810
19	45	NA	22	1.4	110	333	86	24	0.29	0.21	1.8	2	811
234	27	1.5	151	2.4	199	729	586	156	0.49	0.45	3.3	2	812
116	36	NA	73	1.9	177	513	473	146	0.58	0.50	3.9	TR	813
75	58	2.7	78	3.0	127	499	45	13	0.23	0.25	3.0	0	814
9	16	NA	7	0.5	267	290	18	3	0.08	0.01	1.1	5	815
58	91	NA	128	2.6	251	1,104	281	70	0.39	0.56	3.4	3	816

Food No.	Food Description	Measure of edible portion	Weight (g)	Water (%)	Calories (kcal)	Protein (g)	Total fat (g)	Fatty acids Satu-rated (g)	Mono-unsatu-rated (g)	Poly-unsatu-rated (g)
MIXED DISHES AND FAST FOODS (CONTINUED)										
	BURRITO									
817	WITH BEANS AND CHEESE	1 BURRITO	93	54	189	8	6	3.4	1.2	0.9
818	WITH BEANS AND MEAT	1 BURRITO	116	52	255	11	9	4.2	3.5	0.6
	CHEESEBURGER									
	REGULAR SIZE, WITH CONDIMENTS									
819	DOUBLE PATTY WITH MAYO-TYPE DRESSING, VEGETABLES	1 SANDWICH	166	51	417	21	21	8.7	7.8	2.7
820	SINGLE PATTY	1 SANDWICH	113	48	295	16	14	6.3	5.3	1.1
	REGULAR SIZE, PLAIN									
821	DOUBLE PATTY	1 SANDWICH	155	42	457	28	28	13.0	11.0	1.9
822	DOUBLE PATTY WITH 3-PIECE BUN	1 SANDWICH	160	43	461	22	22	9.5	8.3	1.8
823	SINGLE PATTY	1 SANDWICH	102	37	319	15	15	6.5	5.8	1.5
	LARGE, WITH CONDIMENTS									
824	SINGLE PATTY WITH MAYO-TYPE DRESSING, VEGETABLES	1 SANDWICH	219	53	563	28	33	15.0	12.6	2.0
825	SINGLE PATTY WITH BACON	1 SANDWICH	195	44	608	32	37	16.2	14.5	2.7
826	CHICKEN FILLET (BREADED AND FRIED) SANDWICH, PLAIN	1 SANDWICH	182	47	515	24	29	8.5	10.4	8.4
	CHICKEN, FRIED. SEE POULTRY AND POULTRY PRODUCTS.									
827	CHICKEN PIECES, BONELESS, BREADED AND FRIED, PLAIN	6 PIECES	106	47	319	18	21	4.7	10.5	4.6
828	CHILI CON CARNE	1 CUP	253	77	256	25	8	3.4	3.4	0.5
829	CHIMICHANGA WITH BEEF	1 CHIMICHANGA	174	51	425	20	20	8.5	8.1	1.1
830	COLESLAW	3/4 CUP	99	74	147	1	11	1.6	2.4	6.4
	DESSERTS									
831	ICE MILK, SOFT, VANILLA, IN CONE	1 CONE	103	65	164	4	6	3.5	1.8	0.4
832	PIE, FRIED, WITH FRUIT FILLING (5″ X 3 3/4″)	1 PIE	128	38	404	4	21	3.1	9.5	6.9
833	SUNDAE, HOT FUDGE	1 SUNDAE	158	60	284	6	9	5.0	2.3	0.8
834	ENCHILADA WITH CHEESE	1 ENCHILADA	163	63	319	10	19	10.6	6.3	0.8
835	FISH SANDWICH, WITH TARTAR SAUCE AND CHEESE	1 SANDWICH	183	45	523	21	29	8.1	8.9	9.4
836	FRENCH FRIES	1 SMALL	85	35	291	4	16	3.3	9.0	2.7
837		1 MEDIUM	134	35	458	6	25	5.2	14.3	4.2
838		1 LARGE	169	35	578	7	31	6.5	18.0	5.3
839	FRIJOLES (REFRIED BEANS, CHILI SAUCE, CHEESE)	1 CUP	167	69	225	11	8	4.1	2.6	0.7
	HAMBURGER									
	REGULAR SIZE, WITH CONDIMENTS									
840	DOUBLE PATTY	1 SANDWICH	215	51	576	32	32	12.0	14.1	2.8
841	SINGLE PATTY	1 SANDWICH	106	45	272	12	10	3.6	3.4	1.0
	LARGE, WITH CONDIMENTS, MAYO-TYPE DRESSING, AND VEGETABLES									
842	DOUBLE PATTY	1 SANDWICH	226	54	540	34	27	10.5	10.3	2.8
843	SINGLE PATTY	1 SANDWICH	218	56	512	26	27	10.4	11.4	2.2
	HOT DOG									
844	PLAIN	1 SANDWICH	98	54	242	10	15	5.1	6.9	1.7
845	WITH CHILI	1 SANDWICH	114	48	296	14	13	4.9	6.6	1.2
846	WITH CORN FLOUR COATING (CORNDOG)	1 CORNDOG	175	47	460	17	19	5.2	9.1	3.5
847	HUSH PUPPIES	5 PIECES	78	32	257	5	12	2.7	7.8	0.4

Cholesterol (mg)	Carbo-hydrate (g)	Total dietary fiber (g)	Calcium (mg)	Iron (mg)	Potassium (mg)	Sodium (mg)	Vitamin A (IU)	Vitamin A (RE)	Thiamine (mg)	Ribo-flavin (mg)	Niacin (mg)	Ascorbic acid (mg)	Food No.
14	27	NA	107	1.1	248	583	625	119	0.11	0.35	1.8	1	817
24	33	NA	53	2.5	329	670	319	32	0.27	0.42	2.7	1	818
60	35	NA	171	3.4	335	1,051	398	65	0.35	0.28	8.1	2	819
37	27	NA	111	2.4	223	616	462	94	0.25	0.23	3.7	2	820
110	22	NA	233	3.4	308	636	332	79	0.25	0.37	6.0	0	821
80	44	NA	224	3.7	285	891	277	66	0.34	0.38	6.0	0	822
50	32	NA	141	2.4	164	500	153	37	0.40	0.40	3.7	0	823
88	38	NA	206	4.7	445	1,108	613	129	0.39	0.46	7.4	8	824
111	37	NA	162	4.7	332	1,043	406	80	0.31	0.41	6.6	2	825
60	39	NA	60	4.7	353	957	100	31	0.33	0.24	6.8	9	826
61	15	0.0	14	0.9	305	513	0	0	0.12	0.16	7.5	0	827
134	22	NA	68	5.2	691	1,007	1,662	167	0.13	1.14	2.5	2	828
9	43	NA	63	4.5	586	910	146	16	0.49	0.64	5.8	5	829
5	13	NA	34	0.7	177	267	338	50	0.04	0.03	0.1	8	830
28	24	0.1	153	0.2	169	92	211	52	0.05	0.26	0.3	1	831
0	55	3.3	28	1.6	83	479	35	4	0.18	0.14	1.8	2	832
21	48	0.0	207	0.6	395	182	221	57	0.06	0.30	1.1	2	833
44	29	NA	324	1.3	240	784	1,161	186	0.08	0.42	1.9	1	834
68	48	NA	185	3.5	353	939	432	97	0.46	0.42	4.2	3	835
0	34	3.0	12	0.7	586	168	0	0	0.07	0.03	2.4	10	836
0	53	4.7	19	1.0	923	265	0	0	0.11	0.05	3.8	16	837
0	67	5.9	24	1.3	1,164	335	0	0	0.14	0.07	4.8	20	838
37	29	NA	189	2.2	605	882	456	70	0.13	0.33	1.5	2	839
103	39	NA	92	5.5	527	742	54	4	0.34	0.41	6.7	1	840
30	34	2.3	126	2.7	251	534	74	10	0.29	0.24	3.9	2	841
122	40	NA	102	5.9	570	791	102	11	0.36	0.38	7.6	1	842
87	40	NA	96	4.9	480	824	312	33	0.41	0.37	7.3	3	843
44	18	NA	24	2.3	143	670	0	0	0.24	0.27	3.6	TR	844
51	31	NA	19	3.3	166	480	58	6	0.22	0.40	3.7	3	845
79	56	NA	102	6.2	263	973	207	37	0.28	0.70	4.2	0	846
135	35	NA	69	1.4	188	965	94	27	0.00	0.02	2.0	0	847

Food No.	Food Description	Measure of edible portion	Weight (g)	Water (%)	Calories (kcal)	Protein (g)	Total fat (g)	Fatty acids Satu- rated (g)	Fatty acids Mono- unsatu- rated (g)	Fatty acids Poly- unsatu- rated (g)
MIXED DISHES AND FAST FOODS (CONTINUED)										
848	MASHED POTATOES	1/3 CUP	80	79	66	2	1	0.4	0.3	0.2
849	NACHOS, WITH CHEESE SAUCE	6–8 NACHOS	113	40	346	9	19	7.8	8.0	2.2
850	ONION RINGS, BREADED AND FRIED	8–9 RINGS	83	37	276	4	16	7.0	6.7	0.7
	PIZZA (SLICE = 1/8 OF 12″ PIZZA)									
851	CHEESE	1 SLICE	63	48	140	8	3	1.5	1.0	0.5
852	MEAT AND VEGETABLES	1 SLICE	79	48	184	13	5	1.5	2.5	0.9
853	PEPPERONI	1 SLICE	71	47	181	10	7	2.2	3.1	1.2
854	ROAST BEEF SANDWICH, PLAIN	1 SANDWICH	139	49	346	22	14	3.6	6.8	1.7
855	SALAD, TOSSED, WITH CHICKEN, NO DRESSING	1 1/2 CUPS	218	87	105	17	2	0.6	0.7	0.6
856	SALAD, TOSSED, WITH EGG, CHEESE, NO DRESSING	1 1/2 CUPS	217	90	102	9	6	3.0	1.8	0.5
	SHAKE									
857	CHOCOLATE	16 FL OZ	333	72	423	11	12	7.7	3.6	0.5
858	VANILLA	16 FL OZ	333	75	370	12	10	6.2	2.9	0.4
859	SHRIMP, BREADED AND FRIED	6–8 SHRIMP	164	48	454	19	25	5.4	17.4	0.6
	SUBMARINE SANDWICH (6″ LONG), WITH OIL AND VINEGAR									
860	COLD CUTS (WITH LETTUCE, CHEESE, SALAMI, HAM, TOMATO, ONION)	1 SANDWICH	228	58	456	22	19	6.8	8.2	2.3
861	ROAST BEEF (WITH TOMATO, LETTUCE, MAYO)	1 SANDWICH	216	59	410	29	13	7.1	1.8	2.6
862	TUNA SALAD (WITH MAYO, LETTUCE)	1 SANDWICH	256	54	584	30	28	5.3	13.4	7.3
863	TACO, BEEF	1 SMALL	171	58	369	21	21	11.4	6.6	1.0
864		1 LARGE	263	58	568	32	32	17.5	10.1	1.5
865	TACO SALAD (WITH GROUND BEEF, CHEESE, TACO SHELL)	1 1/2 CUPS	198	72	279	13	15	6.8	5.2	1.7
	TOSTADA (WITH CHEESE, TOMATO, LETTUCE)									
866	WITH BEANS AND BEEF	1 TOSTADA	225	70	333	16	17	11.5	3.5	0.6
867	WITH GUACAMOLE	1 TOSTADA	131	73	181	6	12	5.0	4.3	1.5
POULTRY AND POULTRY PRODUCTS										
	CHICKEN									
	FRIED IN VEGETABLE SHORTENING, MEAT WITH SKIN									
	BATTER DIPPED									
868	BREAST, 1/2 BREAST (5.6 OZ WITH BONES)	1/2 BREAST	140	52	364	35	18	4.9	7.6	4.3
869	DRUMSTICK (3.4 OZ WITH BONES)	1 DRUMSTICK	72	53	193	16	11	3.0	4.6	2.7
870	THIGH	1 THIGH	86	52	238	19	14	3.8	5.8	3.4
871	WING	1 WING	49	46	159	10	11	2.9	4.4	2.5
	FLOUR-COATED									
872	BREAST, 1/2 BREAST (4.2 OZ WITH BONES)	1/2 BREAST	98	57	218	31	9	2.4	3.4	1.9
873	DRUMSTICK (2.6 OZ WITH BONES)	1 DRUMSTICK	49	57	120	13	7	1.8	2.7	1.6
	FRIED, MEAT ONLY									
874	DARK MEAT	3 OZ	85	56	203	25	10	2.7	3.7	2.4
875	LIGHT MEAT	3 OZ	85	60	163	28	5	1.3	1.7	1.1
	ROASTED, MEAT ONLY									
876	BREAST, 1/2 BREAST (4.2 OZ WITH BONE AND SKIN)	1/2 BREAST	86	65	142	27	3	0.9	1.1	0.7
877	DRUMSTICK (2.9 OZ WITH BONE AND SKIN)	1 DRUMSTICK	44	67	76	12	2	0.7	0.8	0.6

Cholesterol (mg)	Carbo-hydrate (g)	Total dietary fiber (g)	Calcium (mg)	Iron (mg)	Potassium (mg)	Sodium (mg)	Vitamin A (IU)	Vitamin A (RE)	Thiamine (mg)	Ribo-flavin (mg)	Niacin (mg)	Ascorbic acid (mg)	Food No.
2	13	NA	17	0.4	235	182	33	8	0.07	0.04	1.0	TR	848
18	36	NA	272	1.3	172	816	559	92	0.19	0.37	1.5	1	849
14	31	NA	73	0.8	129	430	8	1	0.08	0.10	0.9	1	850
9	21	NA	117	0.6	110	336	382	74	0.18	0.16	2.5	1	851
21	21	NA	101	1.5	179	382	524	101	0.21	0.17	2.0	2	852
14	20	NA	65	0.9	153	267	282	55	0.13	0.23	3.0	2	853
51	33	NA	54	4.2	316	792	210	21	0.38	0.31	5.9	2	854
72	4	NA	37	1.1	447	209	935	96	0.11	0.13	5.9	17	855
98	5	NA	100	0.7	371	119	822	115	0.09	0.17	1.0	10	856
43	68	2.7	376	1.0	666	323	310	77	0.19	0.82	0.5	1	857
37	60	1.3	406	0.3	579	273	433	107	0.15	0.61	0.6	3	858
200	40	NA	84	3.0	184	1,446	120	36	0.21	0.90	0.0	0	859
36	51	NA	189	2.5	394	1,651	424	80	1.00	0.80	5.5	12	860
73	44	NA	41	2.8	330	845	413	50	0.41	0.41	6.0	6	861
49	55	NA	74	2.6	335	1,293	187	41	0.46	0.33	11.3	4	862
56	27	NA	221	2.4	474	802	855	147	0.15	0.44	3.2	2	863
87	41	NA	339	3.7	729	1,233	1,315	226	0.24	0.68	4.9	3	864
44	24	NA	192	2.3	416	762	588	77	0.10	0.36	2.5	4	865
74	30	NA	189	2.5	491	871	1,276	173	0.09	0.50	2.9	4	866
20	16	NA	212	0.8	326	401	879	109	0.07	0.29	1.0	2	867
119	13	0.4	28	1.8	281	385	94	28	0.16	0.20	14.7	0	868
62	6	0.2	12	1.0	134	194	62	19	0.08	0.15	3.7	0	869
80	8	0.3	15	1.2	165	248	82	25	0.10	0.20	4.9	0	870
39	5	0.1	10	0.6	68	157	55	17	0.05	0.07	2.6	0	871
87	2	0.1	16	1.2	254	74	49	15	0.08	0.13	13.5	0	872
44	1	TR	6	0.7	112	44	41	12	0.04	0.11	3.0	0	873
82	2	0.0	15	1.3	215	82	67	20	0.08	0.21	6.0	0	874
77	TR	0.0	14	1.0	224	69	26	8	0.06	0.11	11.4	0	875
73	0	0.0	13	0.9	220	64	18	5	0.06	0.10	11.8	0	876
41	0	0.0	5	0.6	108	42	26	8	0.03	0.10	2.7	0	877

Food No.	Food Description	Measure of edible portion	Weight (g)	Water (%)	Calories (kcal)	Protein (g)	Total fat (g)	Fatty acids Satu- rated (g)	Mono- unsatu- rated (g)	Poly- unsatu- rated (g)
POULTRY AND POULTRY PRODUCTS (CONTINUED)										
878	THIGH	1 THIGH	52	63	109	13	6	1.6	2.2	1.3
879	STEWED, MEAT ONLY, LIGHT AND DARK MEAT, CHOPPED OR DICED	1 CUP	140	56	332	43	17	4.3	5.7	4.0
880	CHICKEN GIBLETS, SIMMERED, CHOPPED	1 CUP	145	68	228	37	7	2.2	1.7	1.6
881	CHICKEN LIVER, SIMMERED	1 LIVER	20	68	31	5	1	0.4	0.3	0.2
882	CHICKEN NECK, MEAT ONLY, SIMMERED	1 NECK	18	67	32	4	1	0.4	0.5	0.4
883	DUCK, ROASTED, FLESH ONLY	1/2 DUCK	221	64	444	52	25	9.2	8.2	3.2
	TURKEY									
	ROASTED, MEAT ONLY									
884	DARK MEAT	3 OZ	85	63	159	24	6	2.1	1.4	1.8
885	LIGHT MEAT	3 OZ	85	66	133	25	3	0.9	0.5	0.7
886	LIGHT AND DARK MEAT, CHOPPED OR DICED	1 CUP	140	65	238	41	7	2.3	1.4	2.0
	GROUND, COOKED									
887	PATTY, FROM 4 OZ RAW	1 PATTY	82	59	193	22	11	2.8	4.0	2.6
888	CRUMBLED	1 CUP	127	59	298	35	17	4.3	6.2	4.1
889	TURKEY GIBLETS, SIMMERED, CHOPPED	1 CUP	145	65	242	39	7	2.2	1.7	1.7
890	TURKEY NECK, MEAT ONLY, SIMMERED	1 NECK	152	65	274	41	11	3.7	2.5	3.3
	POULTRY FOOD PRODUCTS									
	CHICKEN									
891	CANNED, BONELESS	5 OZ	142	69	234	31	11	3.1	4.5	2.5
892	FRANKFURTER (10 PER 1-LB PKG)	1 FRANK	45	58	116	6	9	2.5	3.8	1.8
893	ROLL, LIGHT MEAT (6 SLICES PER 6-OZ PKG)	2 SLICES	57	69	90	11	4	1.1	1.7	0.9
	TURKEY									
894	GRAVY AND TURKEY, FROZEN	5-OZ PACKAGE	142	85	95	8	4	1.2	1.4	0.7
895	PATTIES, BREADED OR BATTERED, FRIED (2.25 OZ)	1 PATTY	64	50	181	9	12	3.0	4.8	3.0
896	ROAST, BONELESS, FROZEN, SEASONED, LIGHT AND DARK MEAT, COOKED	3 OZ	85	68	132	18	5	1.6	1.0	1.4
SOUPS, SAUCES, AND GRAVIES										
	SOUPS									
	CANNED, CONDENSED									
	PREPARED WITH EQUAL VOLUME OF WHOLE MILK									
897	CLAM CHOWDER, NEW ENGLAND	1 CUP	248	85	164	9	7	3.0	2.3	1.1
898	CREAM OF CHICKEN	1 CUP	248	85	191	7	11	4.6	4.5	1.6
899	CREAM OF MUSHROOM	1 CUP	248	85	203	6	14	5.1	3.0	4.6
900	TOMATO	1 CUP	248	85	161	6	6	2.9	1.6	1.1
	PREPARED WITH EQUAL VOLUME OF WATER									
901	BEAN WITH PORK	1 CUP	253	84	172	8	6	1.5	2.2	1.8
902	BEEF BROTH, BOUILLON, CONSOMME	1 CUP	241	96	29	5	0	0.0	0.0	0.0
903	BEEF NOODLE	1 CUP	244	92	83	5	3	1.1	1.2	0.5
904	CHICKEN NOODLE	1 CUP	241	92	75	4	2	0.7	1.1	0.6
905	CHICKEN AND RICE	1 CUP	241	94	60	4	2	0.5	0.9	0.4
906	CLAM CHOWDER, MANHATTAN	1 CUP	244	92	78	2	2	0.4	0.4	1.3
907	CREAM OF CHICKEN	1 CUP	244	91	117	3	7	2.1	3.3	1.5
908	CREAM OF MUSHROOM	1 CUP	244	90	129	2	9	2.4	1.7	4.2
909	MINESTRONE	1 CUP	241	91	82	4	3	0.6	0.7	1.1
910	PEA, GREEN	1 CUP	250	83	165	9	3	1.4	1.0	0.4
911	TOMATO	1 CUP	244	90	85	2	2	0.4	0.4	1.0

Cholesterol (mg)	Carbo-hydrate (g)	Total dietary fiber (g)	Calcium (mg)	Iron (mg)	Potassium (mg)	Sodium (mg)	Vitamin A (IU)	Vitamin A (RE)	Thiamine (mg)	Ribo-flavin (mg)	Niacin (mg)	Ascorbic acid (mg)	Food No.
49	0	0.0	6	0.7	124	46	34	10	0.04	0.12	3.4	0	878
116	0	0.0	18	2.0	283	109	157	46	0.16	0.39	9.0	0	879
570	1	0.0	17	9.3	229	84	10,775	3,232	0.13	1.38	5.9	12	880
126	TR	0.0	3	1.7	28	10	3,275	983	0.03	0.35	0.9	3	881
14	0	0.0	8	0.5	25	12	22	6	0.01	0.05	0.7	0	882
197	0	0.0	27	6.0	557	144	170	51	0.57	1.04	11.3	0	883
72	0	0.0	27	2.0	247	67	0	0	0.05	0.21	3.1	0	884
59	0	0.0	16	1.1	259	54	0	0	0.05	0.11	5.8	0	885
106	0	0.0	35	2.5	417	98	0	0	0.09	0.25	7.6	0	886
84	0	0.0	21	1.6	221	88	0	0	0.04	0.14	4.0	0	887
130	0	0.0	32	2.5	343	136	0	0	0.07	0.21	6.1	0	888
606	3	0.0	19	9.7	290	86	8,752	2,603	0.07	1.31	6.5	2	889
185	0	0.0	56	3.5	226	85	0	0	0.05	0.29	2.6	0	890
88	0	0.0	20	2.2	196	714	166	48	0.02	0.18	9.0	3	891
45	3	0.0	43	0.9	38	617	59	17	0.03	0.05	1.4	0	892
28	1	0.0	24	0.5	129	331	46	14	0.04	0.07	3.0	0	893
26	7	0.0	20	1.3	87	787	60	18	0.03	0.18	2.6	0	894
40	10	0.3	9	1.4	176	512	24	7	0.06	0.12	1.5	0	895
45	3	0.0	4	1.4	253	578	0	0	0.04	0.14	5.3	0	896
22	17	1.5	186	1.5	300	992	164	40	0.07	0.24	1.0	3	897
27	15	0.2	181	0.7	273	1,047	714	94	0.07	0.26	0.9	1	898
20	15	0.5	179	0.6	270	918	154	37	0.08	0.28	0.9	2	899
17	22	2.7	159	1.8	449	744	848	109	0.13	0.25	1.5	68	900
3	23	8.6	81	2.0	402	951	888	89	0.09	0.03	0.6	2	901
0	2	0.0	10	0.5	154	636	0	0	0.02	0.03	0.7	1	902
5	9	0.7	15	1.1	100	952	630	63	0.07	0.06	1.1	TR	903
7	9	0.7	17	0.8	55	1,106	711	72	0.05	0.06	1.4	TR	904
7	7	0.7	17	0.7	101	815	660	65	0.02	0.02	1.1	TR	905
2	12	1.5	27	1.6	188	578	964	98	0.03	0.04	0.8	4	906
10	9	0.2	34	0.6	88	986	561	56	0.03	0.06	0.8	TR	907
2	9	0.5	46	0.5	100	881	0	0	0.05	0.09	0.7	1	908
2	11	1.0	34	0.9	313	911	2,338	234	0.05	0.04	0.9	1	909
0	27	2.8	28	2.0	190	918	203	20	0.11	0.07	1.2	2	910
0	17	0.5	12	1.8	264	695	688	68	0.09	0.05	1.4	66	911

Food No.	Food Description	Measure of edible portion	Weight (g)	Water (%)	Calories (kcal)	Protein (g)	Total fat (g)	Fatty acids Satu-rated (g)	Mono-unsatu-rated (g)	Poly-unsatu-rated (g)
SOUPS, SAUCES, AND GRAVIES (CONTINUED)										
912	VEGETABLE BEEF	1 CUP	244	92	78	6	2	0.9	0.8	0.1
913	VEGETARIAN VEGETABLE	1 CUP	241	92	72	2	2	0.3	0.8	0.7
	CANNED, READY TO SERVE, CHUNKY									
914	BEAN WITH HAM	1 CUP	243	79	231	13	9	3.3	3.8	0.9
915	CHICKEN NOODLE	1 CUP	240	84	175	13	6	1.4	2.7	1.5
916	CHICKEN AND VEGETABLE	1 CUP	240	83	166	12	5	1.4	2.2	1.0
917	VEGETABLE	1 CUP	240	88	122	4	4	0.6	1.6	1.4
	CANNED, READY TO SERVE, LOW FAT, REDUCED SODIUM									
918	CHICKEN BROTH	1 CUP	240	97	17	3	0	0.0	0.0	0.0
919	CHICKEN NOODLE	1 CUP	237	92	76	6	2	0.4	0.6	0.4
920	CHICKEN AND RICE	1 CUP	241	88	116	7	3	0.9	1.3	0.7
921	CHICKEN AND RICE WITH VEGETABLES	1 CUP	239	91	88	6	1	0.4	0.5	0.5
922	CLAM CHOWDER, NEW ENGLAND	1 CUP	244	89	117	5	2	0.5	0.7	0.4
923	LENTIL	1 CUP	242	88	126	8	2	0.3	0.8	0.2
924	MINESTRONE	1 CUP	241	87	123	5	3	0.4	0.9	1.0
925	VEGETABLE	1 CUP	238	91	81	4	1	0.3	0.4	0.3
	DEHYDRATED									
	UNPREPARED									
926	BEEF BOUILLON	1 PACKET	6	3	14	1	1	0.3	0.2	TR
927	ONION	1 PACKET	39	4	115	5	2	0.5	1.4	0.3
	PREPARED WITH WATER									
928	CHICKEN NOODLE	1 CUP	252	94	58	2	1	0.3	0.5	0.4
929	ONION	1 CUP	246	96	27	1	1	0.1	0.3	0.1
	HOME PREPARED, STOCK									
930	BEEF	1 CUP	240	96	31	5	TR	0.1	0.1	TR
931	CHICKEN	1 CUP	240	92	86	6	3	0.8	1.4	0.5
932	FISH	1 CUP	233	97	40	5	2	0.5	0.5	0.3
	SAUCES									
	HOME RECIPE									
933	CHEESE	1 CUP	243	67	479	25	36	19.5	11.5	3.4
934	WHITE, MEDIUM, MADE WITH WHOLE MILK	1 CUP	250	75	368	10	27	7.1	11.1	7.2
	READY TO SERVE									
935	BARBECUE	1 TBSP	16	81	12	TR	TR	TR	0.1	0.1
936	CHEESE	1/4 CUP	63	71	110	4	8	3.8	2.4	1.6
937	HOISIN	1 TBSP	16	44	35	1	1	0.1	0.2	0.3
938	NACHO CHEESE	1/4 CUP	63	70	119	5	10	4.2	3.1	2.1
939	PEPPER OR HOT	1 TSP	5	90	1	TR	TR	TR	TR	TR
940	SALSA	1 TBSP	16	90	4	TR	TR	TR	TR	TR
941	SOY	1 TBSP	16	69	9	1	TR	TR	TR	TR
942	SPAGHETTI/MARINARA/PASTA	1 CUP	250	87	143	4	5	0.7	2.2	1.8
943	TERIYAKI	1 TBSP	18	68	15	1	0	0.0	0.0	0.0
944	TOMATO CHILI	1/4 CUP	68	68	71	2	TR	TR	TR	0.1
945	WORCESTERSHIRE	1 TBSP	17	70	11	0	0	0.0	0.0	0.0
	GRAVIES, CANNED									
946	BEEF	1/4 CUP	58	87	31	2	1	0.7	0.6	TR
947	CHICKEN	1/4 CUP	60	85	47	1	3	0.8	1.5	0.9
948	COUNTRY SAUSAGE	1/4 CUP	62	75	96	3	8	2.0	2.9	2.2
949	MUSHROOM	1/4 CUP	60	89	30	1	2	0.2	0.7	0.6
950	TURKEY	1/4 CUP	60	89	31	2	1	0.4	0.5	0.3

Cholesterol (mg)	Carbo-hydrate (g)	Total dietary fiber (g)	Calcium (mg)	Iron (mg)	Potassium (mg)	Sodium (mg)	Vitamin A (IU)	Vitamin A (RE)	Thiamine (mg)	Ribo-flavin (mg)	Niacin (mg)	Ascorbic acid (mg)	Food No.
5	10	0.5	17	1.1	173	791	1,891	190	0.04	0.05	1.0	2	912
0	12	0.5	22	1.1	210	822	3,005	301	0.05	0.05	0.9	1	913
22	27	11.2	78	3.2	425	972	3,951	396	0.15	0.15	1.7	4	914
19	17	3.8	24	1.4	108	850	1,222	122	0.07	0.17	4.3	0	915
17	19	NA	26	1.5	367	1,068	5,990	600	0.04	0.17	3.3	6	916
0	19	1.2	55	1.6	396	1,010	5,878	588	0.07	0.06	1.2	6	917
0	1	0.0	19	0.6	204	554	0	0	TR	0.03	1.6	1	918
19	9	1.2	19	1.1	209	460	920	95	0.11	0.11	3.4	1	919
14	14	0.7	22	1.0	422	482	2,010	202	0.05	0.13	5.0	2	920
17	12	0.7	24	1.2	275	459	1,644	165	0.12	0.07	2.6	1	921
5	20	1.2	17	0.9	283	529	244	59	0.05	0.09	0.9	5	922
0	20	5.6	41	2.7	336	443	951	94	0.11	0.09	0.7	1	923
0	20	1.2	39	1.7	306	470	1,357	135	0.15	0.08	1.0	1	924
5	13	1.4	31	1.5	290	466	3,196	319	0.08	0.07	1.8	1	925
1	1	0.0	4	0.1	27	1,019	3	TR	TR	0.01	0.3	0	926
2	21	4.1	55	0.6	260	3,493	8	1	0.11	0.24	2.0	1	927
10	9	0.3	5	0.5	33	578	15	5	0.20	0.08	1.1	0	928
0	5	1.0	12	0.1	64	849	2	0	0.03	0.06	0.5	TR	929
0	3	0.0	19	0.6	444	475	0	0	0.08	0.22	2.1	0	930
7	8	0.0	7	0.5	252	343	0	0	0.08	0.20	3.8	TR	931
2	0	0.0	7	TR	336	363	0	0	0.08	0.18	2.8	TR	932
92	13	0.2	756	0.9	345	1,198	1,473	389	0.11	0.59	0.5	1	933
18	23	0.5	295	0.8	390	885	1,383	138	0.17	0.46	1.0	2	934
0	2	0.2	3	0.1	28	130	139	14	TR	TR	0.1	1	935
18	4	0.3	116	0.1	19	522	199	40	TR	0.07	TR	TR	936
TR	7	0.4	5	0.2	19	258	2	TR	TR	0.03	0.2	TR	937
20	3	0.5	118	0.2	20	492	128	32	TR	0.08	TR	TR	938
0	TR	0.1	TR	TR	7	124	14	1	TR	TR	TR	4	939
0	1	0.3	5	0.2	34	69	96	10	0.01	0.01	0.1	2	940
0	1	0.1	3	0.3	64	871	0	0	0.01	0.03	0.4	0	941
0	21	4.0	55	1.8	738	1,030	938	95	0.14	0.10	2.7	20	942
0	3	TR	5	0.3	41	690	0	0	0.01	0.01	0.2	0	943
0	17	4.0	14	0.5	252	910	462	46	0.06	0.05	1.1	11	944
0	3	0.0	18	0.9	136	167	18	2	0.01	0.02	0.1	2	945
2	3	0.2	3	0.4	47	325	0	0	0.02	0.02	0.4	0	946
1	3	0.2	12	0.3	65	346	221	67	0.01	0.03	0.3	0	947
13	4	0.4	4	0.3	48	236	0	0	0.10	0.04	0.7	TR	948
0	3	0.2	4	0.4	64	342	0	0	0.02	0.04	0.4	0	949
1	3	0.2	2	0.4	65	346	0	0	0.01	0.05	0.8	0	950

SUGARS AND SWEETS

Food No.	Food Description	Measure of edible portion	Weight (g)	Water (%)	Calories (kcal)	Protein (g)	Total fat (g)	Fatty acids Saturated (g)	Fatty acids Mono-unsaturated (g)	Fatty acids Poly-unsaturated (g)
	CANDY									
951	BUTTERFINGER (NESTLE)	1 FUN SIZE BAR	7	2	34	1	1	0.7	0.4	0.2
	CARAMEL									
952	PLAIN	1 PIECE	10	9	39	TR	1	0.7	0.1	TR
953	CHOCOLATE-FLAVORED ROLL	1 PIECE	7	7	25	TR	TR	TR	0.1	0.1
954	CAROB	1 OZ	28	2	153	2	9	8.2	0.1	0.1
	CHOCOLATE, MILK									
955	PLAIN	1 BAR (1.55 OZ)	44	1	226	3	14	8.1	4.4	0.5
956	WITH ALMONDS	1 BAR (1.45 OZ)	41	2	216	4	14	7.0	5.5	0.9
957	WITH PEANUTS, MR. GOODBAR (HERSHEY)	1 BAR (1.75 OZ)	49	1	267	5	17	7.3	5.7	2.4
958	WITH RICE CEREAL, NESTLE CRUNCH	1 BAR (1.55 OZ)	44	1	230	3	12	6.7	3.8	0.4
	CHOCOLATE CHIPS									
959	MILK	1 CUP	168	1	862	12	52	31.0	16.7	1.8
960	SEMISWEET	1 CUP	168	1	805	7	50	29.8	16.7	1.6
961	WHITE	1 CUP	170	1	916	10	55	33.0	15.5	1.7
962	CHOCOLATE COATED PEANUTS	10 PIECES	40	2	208	5	13	5.8	5.2	1.7
963	CHOCOLATE COATED RAISINS	10 PIECES	10	11	39	TR	1	0.9	0.5	0.1
964	FRUIT LEATHER, PIECES	1 OZ	28	12	97	TR	2	0.3	0.9	0.8
965	FRUIT LEATHER, ROLLS	1 LARGE	21	11	74	TR	1	0.1	0.3	0.1
966	FUDGE, PREPARED FROM RECIPE	1 SMALL	14	11	49	TR	TR	0.1	0.2	0.1
	CHOCOLATE									
967	PLAIN	1 PIECE	17	10	65	TR	1	0.9	0.4	0.1
968	WITH NUTS	1 PIECE	19	7	81	1	3	1.1	0.8	1.0
	VANILLA									
969	PLAIN	1 PIECE	16	11	59	TR	1	0.5	0.2	TR
970	WITH NUTS	1 PIECE	15	8	62	TR	2	0.6	0.5	0.8
	GUMDROPS/GUMMY CANDIES									
971	GUMDROPS (3/4" DIA)	1 CUP	182	1	703	0	0	0.0	0.0	0.0
972		1 MEDIUM	4	1	16	0	0	0.0	0.0	0.0
973	GUMMY BEARS	10 BEARS	22	1	85	0	0	0.0	0.0	0.0
974	GUMMY WORMS	10 WORMS	74	1	286	0	0	0.0	0.0	0.0
975	HARD CANDY	1 PIECE	6	1	24	0	TR	0.0	0.0	0.0
976		1 SMALL PIECE	3	1	12	0	TR	0.0	0.0	0.0
977	JELLY BEANS	10 LARGE	28	6	104	0	TR	TR	0.1	TR
978		10 SMALL	11	6	40	0	TR	TR	TR	TR
979	KIT KAT (HERSHEY)	1 BAR (1.5 OZ)	42	2	216	3	11	6.8	3.1	0.3
	MARSHMALLOWS									
980	MINIATURE	1 CUP	50	16	159	1	TR	TR	TR	TR
981	REGULAR	1 REGULAR	7	16	23	TR	TR	TR	TR	TR
	M&M'S (M&M MARS)									
982	PEANUT	1/4 CUP	43	2	222	4	11	4.4	4.7	1.8
983		10 PIECES	20	2	103	2	5	2.1	2.2	0.8
984	PLAIN	1/4 CUP	52	2	256	2	11	6.8	3.6	0.3
985		10 PIECES	7	2	34	TR	1	0.9	0.5	TR
986	MILKY WAY (M&M MARS)	1 FUN SIZE BAR	18	6	76	1	3	1.4	1.1	0.1
987		1 BAR (2.15 OZ)	61	6	258	3	10	4.8	3.7	0.4
988	REESE'S PEANUT BUTTER CUP (HERSHEY)	1 MINIATURE CUP	7	2	38	1	2	0.8	0.9	0.4

Cholesterol (mg)	Carbo-hydrate (g)	Total dietary fiber (g)	Calcium (mg)	Iron (mg)	Potassium (mg)	Sodium (mg)	Vitamin A (IU)	(RE)	Thiamine (mg)	Ribo-flavin (mg)	Niacin (mg)	Ascorbic acid (mg)	Food No.
TR	5	0.2	2	0.1	27	14	0	0	0.01	TR	0.2	0	951
1	8	0.1	14	TR	22	25	3	1	TR	0.02	TR	TR	952
0	6	TR	2	TR	7	6	1	TR	TR	0.01	TR	TR	953
1	16	1.1	86	0.4	179	30	7	2	0.03	0.05	0.3	TR	954
10	26	1.5	84	0.6	169	36	81	24	0.03	0.13	0.1	TR	955
8	22	2.5	92	0.7	182	30	30	6	0.02	0.18	0.3	TR	956
4	25	1.7	53	0.6	219	73	70	18	0.08	0.12	1.6	TR	957
6	29	1.1	74	0.2	151	59	30	9	0.15	0.25	1.7	TR	958
37	99	5.7	321	2.3	647	138	311	92	0.13	0.51	0.5	1	959
0	106	9.9	54	5.3	613	18	35	3	0.09	0.15	0.7	0	960
36	101	0.0	338	0.4	486	153	60	2	0.11	0.48	1.3	1	961
4	20	1.9	42	0.5	201	16	0	0	0.05	0.07	1.7	0	962
TR	7	0.4	9	0.2	51	4	4	1	0.01	0.02	TR	TR	963
0	22	1.0	5	0.2	46	114	33	3	0.01	0.03	TR	16	964
0	18	0.8	7	0.2	62	13	24	3	0.01	TR	TR	1	965
0	12	0.5	4	0.1	41	9	16	2	0.01	TR	TR	1	966
2	14	0.1	7	0.1	18	11	32	8	TR	0.01	TR	TR	967
3	14	0.2	10	0.1	30	11	38	9	0.01	0.02	TR	TR	968
3	13	0.0	6	TR	8	11	33	8	TR	0.01	TR	TR	969
2	11	0.1	7	0.1	17	9	30	7	0.01	0.01	TR	TR	970
0	180	0.0	5	0.7	9	80	0	0	0.00	TR	TR	0	971
0	4	0.0	TR	TR	TR	2	0	0	0.00	TR	TR	0	972
0	22	0.0	1	0.1	1	10	0	0	0.00	TR	TR	0	973
0	73	0.0	2	0.3	4	33	0	0	0.00	TR	TR	0	974
0	6	0.0	TR	TR	TR	2	0	0	TR	TR	TR	0	975
0	3	0.0	TR	TR	TR	1	0	0	TR	TR	TR	0	976
0	26	0.0	1	0.3	10	7	0	0	0.00	0.00	0.0	0	977
0	10	0.0	TR	0.1	4	3	0	0	0.00	0.00	0.0	0	978
3	27	0.8	69	0.4	122	32	68	20	0.07	0.23	1.1	TR	979
0	41	0.1	2	0.1	3	24	1	0	TR	TR	TR	0	980
0	6	TR	TR	TR	TR	3	TR	0	TR	TR	TR	0	981
4	26	1.5	43	0.5	149	21	40	10	0.04	0.07	1.6	TR	982
2	12	0.7	20	0.2	69	10	19	5	0.02	0.03	0.7	TR	983
7	37	1.3	55	0.6	138	32	106	28	0.03	0.11	0.1	TR	984
1	5	0.2	7	0.1	19	4	14	4	TR	0.01	TR	TR	985
3	13	0.3	23	0.1	43	43	19	6	0.01	0.04	0.1	TR	986
9	44	1.0	79	0.5	147	146	66	20	0.02	0.14	0.2	1	987
TR	4	0.2	5	0.1	25	22	5	1	0.02	0.01	0.3	TR	988

Food No.	Food Description	Measure of edible portion	Weight (g)	Water (%)	Calories (kcal)	Protein (g)	Total fat (g)	Fatty acids		
								Satu-rated (g)	Mono-unsatu-rated (g)	Poly-unsatu-rated (g)
SUGARS AND SWEETS (CONTINUED)										
989		1 PACKAGE (CONTAINS 2)	45	2	243	5	14	5.0	5.9	2.5
990	SNICKERS BAR (M&M MARS)	1 FUN SIZE BAR	15	5	72	1	4	1.3	1.6	0.7
991		1 KING SIZE BAR (4 OZ)	113	5	541	9	28	10.2	11.8	5.6
992		1 BAR (2 OZ)	57	5	273	5	14	5.1	6.0	2.8
993	SPECIAL DARK SWEETCHOCOLATE (HERSHEY)	1 MINIATURE	8	1	46	TR	3	1.7	0.9	0.1
994	STARBURST FRUIT CHEWS (M&M MARS)	1 PIECE	5	7	20	TR	TR	0.1	0.2	0.2
995		1 PACKAGE (2.07 OZ)	59	7	234	TR	5	0.7	2.1	1.8
	FROSTING, READY TO EAT									
996	CHOCOLATE	1/12 PACKAGE	38	17	151	TR	7	2.1	3.4	0.8
997	VANILLA	1/12 PACKAGE	38	13	159	TR	6	1.9	3.3	0.9
	FROZEN DESSERTS (NONDAIRY)									
998	FRUIT AND JUICE BAR	1 BAR (2.5 FL OZ)	77	78	63	1	TR	0.0	0.0	TR
999	ICE POP	1 BAR (2 FL OZ)	59	80	42	0	0	0.0	0.0	0.0
1000	ITALIAN ICES	1/2 CUP	116	86	61	TR	TR	0.0	0.0	0.0
1001	FRUIT BUTTER, APPLE	1 TBSP	17	56	29	TR	0	0.0	0.0	0.0
	GELATIN DESSERT, PREPARED WITH GELATIN DESSERT POWDER AND WATER									
1002	REGULAR	1/2 CUP	135	85	80	2	0	0.0	0.0	0.0
1003	REDUCED CALORIE (WITH ASPARTAME)	1/2 CUP	117	98	8	1	0	0.0	0.0	0.0
1004	HONEY, STRAINED OR EXTRACTED	1 TBSP	21	17	64	TR	0	0.0	0.0	0.0
1005		1 CUP	339	17	1,031	1	0	0.0	0.0	0.0
1006	JAMS AND PRESERVES	1 TBSP	20	30	56	TR	TR	TR	TR	0.0
1007		1 PACKET (0.5 OZ)	14	30	39	TR	TR	TR	TR	0.0
1008	JELLIES	1 TBSP	19	29	54	TR	TR	TR	TR	TR
1009		1 PACKET (0.5 OZ)	14	29	40	TR	TR	TR	TR	TR
	PUDDINGS PREPARED WITH DRY MIX AND 2% MILK CHOCOLATE									
1010	INSTANT	1/2 CUP	147	75	150	5	3	1.6	0.9	0.2
1011	REGULAR (COOKED)	1/2 CUP	142	74	151	5	3	1.8	0.8	0.1
	VANILLA									
1012	INSTANT	1/2 CUP	142	75	148	4	2	1.4	0.7	0.1
1013	REGULAR (COOKED)	1/2 CUP	140	76	141	4	2	1.5	0.7	0.1
	READY TO EAT REGULAR									
1014	CHOCOLATE	4 OZ	113	69	150	3	5	0.8	1.9	1.6
1015	RICE	4 OZ	113	68	184	2	8	1.3	3.6	3.2
1016	TAPIOCA	4 OZ	113	74	134	2	4	0.7	1.8	1.5
1017	VANILLA	4 OZ	113	71	147	3	4	0.6	1.7	1.5
	FAT FREE									
1018	CHOCOLATE	4 OZ	113	76	107	3	TR	0.3	0.1	TR
1019	TAPIOCA	4 OZ	113	77	98	2	TR	0.1	TR	TR
1020	VANILLA	4 OZ	113	76	105	2	TR	0.1	TR	TR

Cholesterol (mg)	Carbo-hydrate (g)	Total dietary fiber (g)	Calcium (mg)	Iron (mg)	Potassium (mg)	Sodium (mg)	Vitamin A (IU)	Vitamin A (RE)	Thiamine (mg)	Ribo-flavin (mg)	Niacin (mg)	Ascorbic acid (mg)	Food No.
2	25	1.4	35	0.5	158	143	33	9	0.11	0.08	2.1	TR	989
2	9	0.4	14	0.1	49	40	23	6	0.01	0.02	0.6	TR	990
15	67	2.8	106	0.9	366	301	172	44	0.11	0.17	4.7	1	991
7	34	1.4	54	0.4	185	152	87	22	0.06	0.09	2.4	TR	992
TR	5	0.4	2	0.2	25	1	3	TR	TR	0.01	TR	0	993
0	4	0.0	TR	TR	TR	3	0	0	TR	TR	TR	3	994
0	50	0.0	2	0.1	1	33	0	0	TR	TR	TR	31	995
0	24	0.2	3	0.5	74	70	249	75	TR	0.01	TR	0	996
0	26	TR	1	TR	14	34	283	86	0.00	TR	TR	0	997
0	16	0.0	4	0.1	41	3	22	2	0.01	0.01	0.1	7	998
0	11	0.0	0	0.0	2	7	0	0	0.00	0.00	0.0	0	999
0	16	0.0	1	0.1	7	5	194	0	0.01	0.01	0.8	1	1000
0	7	0.3	2	0.1	15	1	20	2	TR	TR	TR	TR	1001
0	19	0.0	3	TR	1	57	0	0	0.00	TR	TR	0	1002
0	1	0.0	2	TR	0	56	0	0	0.00	TR	TR	0	1003
0	17	TR	1	0.1	11	1	0	0	0.00	0.01	TR	TR	1004
0	279	0.7	20	1.4	176	14	0	0	0.00	0.13	0.4	2	1005
0	14	0.2	4	0.1	15	6	2	TR	0.00	TR	TR	2	1006
0	10	0.2	3	0.1	11	4	2	TR	0.00	TR	TR	1	1007
0	13	0.2	2	TR	12	5	3	TR	TR	TR	TR	TR	1008
0	10	0.1	1	TR	9	4	2	TR	TR	TR	TR	TR	1009
9	28	0.6	153	0.4	247	417	253	56	0.05	0.21	0.1	1	1010
10	28	0.4	160	0.5	240	149	253	68	0.05	0.21	0.2	1	1011
9	28	0.0	146	0.1	185	406	241	64	0.05	0.20	0.1	1	1012
10	26	0.0	153	0.1	193	224	252	70	0.04	0.20	0.1	1	1013
3	26	1.1	102	0.6	203	146	41	12	0.03	0.18	0.4	2	1014
1	25	0.1	59	0.3	68	96	129	40	0.02	0.08	0.2	1	1015
1	22	0.1	95	0.3	110	180	0	0	0.02	0.11	0.4	1	1016
8	25	0.1	99	0.1	128	153	24	7	0.02	0.16	0.3	0	1017
2	23	0.9	89	0.6	235	192	174	52	0.02	0.12	0.1	TR	1018
1	23	0.1	76	0.2	99	251	121	36	0.02	0.09	0.1	TR	1019
1	24	0.1	86	TR	123	241	174	52	0.02	0.10	0.1	TR	1020

Food No.	Food Description	Measure of edible portion	Weight (g)	Water (%)	Calories (kcal)	Protein (g)	Total fat (g)	Fatty acids Satu-rated (g)	Fatty acids Mono-unsatu-rated (g)	Fatty acids Poly-unsatu-rated (g)
SUGARS AND SWEETS (CONTINUED)										
	SUGAR									
	BROWN									
1021	PACKED	1 CUP	220	2	827	0	0	0.0	0.0	0.0
1022	UNPACKED	1 CUP	145	2	545	0	0	0.0	0.0	0.0
1023		1 TBSP	9	2	34	0	0	0.0	0.0	0.0
	WHITE									
1024	GRANULATED	1 PACKET	6	0	23	0	0	0.0	0.0	0.0
1025		1 TSP	4	0	16	0	0	0.0	0.0	0.0
1026		1 CUP	200	0	774	0	0	0.0	0.0	0.0
1027	POWDERED, UNSIFTED	1 TBSP	8	TR	31	0	TR	TR	TR	TR
1028		1 CUP	120	TR	467	0	TR	TR	TR	0.1
	SYRUP									
	CHOCOLATE-FLAVORED SYRUP OR TOPPING									
1029	THIN TYPE	1 TBSP	19	31	53	TR	TR	0.1	0.1	TR
1030	FUDGE TYPE	1 TBSP	19	22	67	1	2	0.8	0.7	0.1
1031	CORN, LIGHT	1 TBSP	20	23	56	0	0	0.0	0.0	0.0
1032	MAPLE	1 TBSP	20	32	52	0	TR	TR	TR	TR
1033	MOLASSES, BLACKSTRAP	1 TBSP	20	29	47	0	0	0.0	0.0	0.0
1034		1 CUP	328	29	771	0	0	0.0	0.0	0.0
	TABLE BLEND, PANCAKE									
1035	REGULAR	1 TBSP	20	24	57	0	0	0.0	0.0	0.0
1036	REDUCED CALORIE	1 TBSP	15	55	25	0	0	0.0	0.0	0.0
VEGETABLES AND VEGETABLE PRODUCTS										
1037	ALFALFA SPROUTS, RAW	1 CUP	33	91	10	1	TR	TR	TR	0.1
1038	ARTICHOKES, GLOBE OR FRENCH, COOKED, DRAINED	1 CUP	168	84	84	6	TR	0.1	TR	0.1
1039		1 MEDIUM	120	84	60	4	TR	TR	TR	0.1
	ASPARAGUS, GREEN									
	COOKED, DRAINED									
1040	FROM RAW	1 CUP	180	92	43	5	1	0.1	TR	0.2
1041		4 SPEARS	60	92	14	2	TR	TR	TR	0.1
1042	FROM FROZEN	1 CUP	180	91	50	5	1	0.2	TR	0.3
1043		4 SPEARS	60	91	17	2	TR	0.1	TR	0.1
1044	CANNED, SPEARS, ABOUT 5″ LONG, DRAINED	1 CUP	242	94	46	5	2	0.4	0.1	0.7
1045		4 SPEARS	72	94	14	2	TR	0.1	TR	0.2
1046	BAMBOO SHOOTS, CANNED, DRAINED	1 CUP	131	94	25	2	1	0.1	TR	0.2
	BEANS									
	LIMA, IMMATURE SEEDS, FROZEN, COOKED, DRAINED									
1047	FORD HOOKS	1 CUP	170	74	170	10	1	0.1	TR	0.3
1048	BABY LIMAS	1 CUP	180	72	189	12	1	0.1	TR	0.3
	SNAP, CUT									
	COOKED, DRAINED									
	FROM RAW									
1049	GREEN	1 CUP	125	89	44	2	TR	0.1	TR	0.2
1050	YELLOW	1 CUP	125	89	44	2	TR	0.1	TR	0.2
	FROM FROZEN									
1051	GREEN	1 CUP	135	91	38	2	TR	0.1	TR	0.1
1052	YELLOW	1 CUP	135	91	38	2	TR	0.1	TR	0.1
	CANNED, DRAINED									

Cholesterol (mg)	Carbo-hydrate (g)	Total dietary fiber (g)	Calcium (mg)	Iron (mg)	Potassium (mg)	Sodium (mg)	Vitamin A (IU)	(RE)	Thiamine (mg)	Ribo-flavin (mg)	Niacin (mg)	Ascorbic acid (mg)	Food No.
0	214	0.0	187	4.2	761	86	0	0	0.02	0.02	0.2	0	1021
0	141	0.0	123	2.8	502	57	0	0	0.01	0.01	0.1	0	1022
0	9	0.0	8	0.2	31	4	0	0	TR	TR	TR	0	1023
0	6	0.0	TR	TR	TR	TR	0	0	0.00	TR	0.0	0	1024
0	4	0.0	TR	TR	TR	TR	0	0	0.00	TR	0.0	0	1025
0	200	0.0	2	0.1	4	2	0	0	0.00	0.04	0.0	0	1026
0	8	0.0	TR	TR	TR	TR	0	0	0.00	0.00	0.0	0	1027
0	119	0.0	1	0.1	2	1	0	0	0.00	0.00	0.0	0	1028
0	12	0.3	3	0.4	43	14	6	1	TR	0.01	0.1	TR	1029
TR	12	0.5	15	0.2	69	66	3	1	0.01	0.04	0.1	TR	1030
0	15	0.0	1	TR	1	24	0	0	TR	TR	TR	0	1031
0	13	0.0	13	0.2	41	2	0	0	TR	TR	TR	0	1032
0	12	0.0	172	3.5	498	11	0	0	0.01	0.01	0.2	0	1033
0	199	0.0	2,821	57.4	8,174	180	0	0	0.11	0.17	3.5	0	1034
0	15	0.0	TR	TR	TR	17	0	0	TR	TR	TR	0	1035
0	7	0.0	TR	TR	TR	30	0	0	TR	TR	TR	0	1036
0	1	0.8	11	0.3	26	2	51	5	0.03	0.04	0.2	3	1037
0	19	9.1	76	2.2	595	160	297	30	0.11	0.11	1.7	17	1038
0	13	6.5	54	1.5	425	114	212	22	0.08	0.08	1.2	12	1039
0	8	2.9	36	1.3	288	20	970	97	0.22	0.23	1.9	19	1040
0	3	1.0	12	0.4	96	7	323	32	0.07	0.08	0.6	6	1041
0	9	2.9	41	1.2	392	7	1,472	148	0.12	0.19	1.9	44	1042
0	3	1.0	14	0.4	131	2	491	49	0.04	0.06	0.6	15	1043
0	6	3.9	39	4.4	416	695	1,285	128	0.15	0.24	2.3	45	1044
0	2	1.2	12	1.3	124	207	382	38	0.04	0.07	0.7	13	1045
0	4	1.8	10	0.4	105	9	10	1	0.03	0.03	0.2	1	1046
0	32	9.9	37	2.3	694	90	323	32	0.13	0.10	1.8	22	1047
0	35	10.8	50	3.5	740	52	301	31	0.13	0.10	1.4	10	1048
0	10	4.0	58	1.6	374	4	833	84	0.09	0.12	0.8	12	1049
0	10	4.1	58	1.6	374	4	101	10	0.09	0.12	0.8	12	1050
0	9	4.1	66	1.2	170	12	541	54	0.05	0.12	0.5	6	1051
0	9	4.1	66	1.2	170	12	151	15	0.05	0.12	0.5	6	1052

Food No.	Food Description	Measure of edible portion	Weight (g)	Water (%)	Calories (kcal)	Protein (g)	Total fat (g)	Fatty acids		
								Satu- rated (g)	Mono- unsatu- rated (g)	Poly- unsatu- rated (g)
VEGETABLES AND VEGETABLE PRODUCTS (CONTINUED)										
1053	GREEN	1 CUP	135	93	27	2	TR	TR	TR	0.1
1054	YELLOW	1 CUP	135	93	27	2	TR	TR	TR	0.1
	BEANS, DRY. SEE LEGUMES.									
	BEAN SPROUTS (MUNG)									
1055	RAW	1 CUP	104	90	31	3	TR	TR	TR	0.1
1056	COOKED, DRAINED	1 CUP	124	93	26	3	TR	TR	TR	TR
	BEETS									
	COOKED, DRAINED									
1057	SLICES	1 CUP	170	87	75	3	TR	TR	0.1	0.1
1058	WHOLE BEET, 2″ DIA	1 BEET	50	87	22	1	TR	TR	TR	TR
	CANNED, DRAINED									
1059	SLICES	1 CUP	170	91	53	2	TR	TR	TR	0.1
1060	WHOLE BEET	1 BEET	24	91	7	TR	TR	TR	TR	TR
1061	BEET GREENS, LEAVES AND STEMS, COOKED, DRAINED, 1″ PIECES	1 CUP	144	89	39	4	TR	TR	0.1	0.1
	BLACK-EYED PEAS, IMMATURE SEEDS, COOKED, DRAINED									
1062	FROM RAW	1 CUP	165	75	160	5	1	0.2	0.1	0.3
1063	FROM FROZEN	1 CUP	170	66	224	14	1	0.3	0.1	0.5
	BROCCOLI									
	RAW									
1064	CHOPPED OR DICED	1 CUP	88	91	25	3	TR	TR	TR	0.1
1065	SPEAR, ABOUT 5″ LONG	1 SPEAR	31	91	9	1	TR	TR	TR	0.1
1066	FLOWER CLUSTER	1 FLOWERET	11	91	3	TR	TR	TR	TR	TR
	COOKED, DRAINED									
	FROM RAW									
1067	CHOPPED	1 CUP	156	91	44	5	1	0.1	TR	0.3
1068	SPEAR, ABOUT 5″ LONG	1 SPEAR	37	91	10	1	TR	TR	TR	0.1
1069	FROM FROZEN, CHOPPED	1 CUP	184	91	52	6	TR	TR	TR	0.1
	BRUSSELS SPROUTS, COOKED, DRAINED									
1070	FROM RAW	1 CUP	156	87	61	4	1	0.2	0.1	0.4
1071	FROM FROZEN	1 CUP	155	87	65	6	1	0.1	TR	0.3
	CABBAGE, COMMON VARIETIES, SHREDDED									
1072	RAW	1 CUP	70	92	18	1	TR	TR	TR	0.1
1073	COOKED, DRAINED	1 CUP	150	94	33	2	1	0.1	TR	0.3
	CABBAGE, CHINESE, SHREDDED, COOKED, DRAINED									
1074	PAK CHOI OR BOK CHOY	1 CUP	170	96	20	3	TR	TR	TR	0.1
1075	PE TSAI	1 CUP	119	95	17	2	TR	TR	TR	0.1
1076	CABBAGE, RED, RAW, SHREDDED	1 CUP	70	92	19	1	TR	TR	TR	0.1
1077	CABBAGE, SAVOY, RAW, SHREDDED	1 CUP	70	91	19	1	TR	TR	TR	TR
1078	CARROT JUICE, CANNED	1 CUP	236	89	94	2	TR	0.1	TR	0.2
	CARROTS									
	RAW									
1079	WHOLE, 7 1/2″ LONG	1 CARROT	72	88	31	1	TR	TR	TR	0.1
1080	GRATED	1 CUP	110	88	47	1	TR	TR	TR	0.1
1081	BABY	1 MEDIUM	10	90	4	TR	TR	TR	TR	TR
	COOKED, SLICED, DRAINED									
1082	FROM RAW	1 CUP	156	87	70	2	TR	0.1	TR	0.1
1083	FROM FROZEN	1 CUP	146	90	53	2	TR	TR	TR	0.1
1084	CANNED, SLICED, DRAINED	1 CUP	146	93	37	1	TR	0.1	TR	0.1

Cholesterol (mg)	Carbo-hydrate (g)	Total dietary fiber (g)	Calcium (mg)	Iron (mg)	Potassium (mg)	Sodium (mg)	Vitamin A (IU)	Vitamin A (RE)	Thiamine (mg)	Ribo-flavin (mg)	Niacin (mg)	Ascorbic acid (mg)	Food No.
0	6	2.6	35	1.2	147	354	471	47	0.02	0.08	0.3	6	1053
0	6	1.8	35	1.2	147	339	142	15	0.02	0.08	0.3	6	1054
0	6	1.9	14	0.9	155	6	22	2	0.09	0.13	0.8	14	1055
0	5	1.5	15	0.8	125	12	17	1	0.06	0.13	1.0	14	1056
0	17	3.4	27	1.3	519	131	60	7	0.05	0.07	0.6	6	1057
0	5	1.0	8	0.4	153	39	18	2	0.01	0.02	0.2	2	1058
0	12	2.9	26	3.1	252	330	19	2	0.02	0.07	0.3	7	1059
0	2	0.4	4	0.4	36	47	3	TR	TR	0.01	TR	1	1060
0	8	4.2	164	2.7	1,309	347	7,344	734	0.17	0.42	0.7	36	1061
0	34	8.3	211	1.8	690	7	1,305	130	0.17	0.24	2.3	4	1062
0	40	10.9	39	3.6	638	9	128	14	0.44	0.11	1.2	4	1063
0	5	2.6	42	0.8	286	24	1,357	136	0.06	0.10	0.6	82	1064
0	2	0.9	15	0.3	101	8	478	48	0.02	0.04	0.2	29	1065
0	1	0.3	5	0.1	36	3	330	33	0.01	0.01	0.1	10	1066
0	8	4.5	72	1.3	456	41	2,165	217	0.09	0.18	0.9	116	1067
0	2	1.1	17	0.3	108	10	514	51	0.02	0.04	0.2	28	1068
0	10	5.5	94	1.1	331	44	3,481	348	0.10	0.15	0.8	74	1069
0	14	4.1	56	1.9	495	33	1,122	112	0.17	0.12	0.9	97	1070
0	13	6.4	37	1.1	504	36	913	91	0.16	0.18	0.8	71	1071
0	4	1.6	33	0.4	172	13	93	9	0.04	0.03	0.2	23	1072
0	7	3.5	47	0.3	146	12	198	20	0.09	0.08	0.4	30	1073
0	3	2.7	158	1.8	631	58	4,366	437	0.05	0.11	0.7	44	1074
0	3	3.2	38	0.4	268	11	1,151	115	0.05	0.05	0.6	19	1075
0	4	1.4	36	0.3	144	8	28	3	0.04	0.02	0.2	40	1076
0	4	2.2	25	0.3	161	20	700	70	0.05	0.02	0.2	22	1077
0	22	1.9	57	1.1	689	68	25,833	2,584	0.22	0.13	0.9	20	1078
0	7	2.2	19	0.4	233	25	20,253	2,025	0.07	0.04	0.7	7	1079
0	11	3.3	30	0.6	355	39	30,942	3,094	0.11	0.06	1.0	10	1080
0	1	0.2	2	0.1	28	4	1,501	150	TR	0.01	0.1	1	1081
0	16	5.1	48	1.0	354	103	38,304	3,830	0.05	0.09	0.8	4	1082
0	12	5.1	41	0.7	231	86	25,845	2,584	0.04	0.05	0.6	4	1083
0	8	2.2	37	0.9	261	353	20,110	2,010	0.03	0.04	0.8	4	1084

Food No.	Food Description	Measure of edible portion	Weight (g)	Water (%)	Calories (kcal)	Protein (g)	Total fat (g)	Fatty acids		
								Satu-rated (g)	Mono-unsatu-rated (g)	Poly-unsatu-rated (g)
	VEGETABLES AND VEGETABLE PRODUCTS (CONTINUED)									
	CAULIFLOWER									
1085	RAW	1 FLOWERET	13	92	3	TR	TR	TR	TR	TR
1086		1 CUP	100	92	25	2	TR	TR	TR	0.1
	COOKED, DRAINED, 1″ PIECES									
1087	FROM RAW	1 CUP	124	93	29	2	1	0.1	TR	0.3
1088		3 FLOWERETS	54	93	12	1	TR	TR	TR	0.1
1089	FROM FROZEN	1 CUP	180	94	34	3	TR	0.1	TR	0.2
	CELERY									
	RAW									
1090	STALK, 7 1/2″ TO 8″ LONG	1 STALK	40	95	6	TR	TR	TR	TR	TR
1091	PIECES, DICED	1 CUP	120	95	19	1	TR	TR	TR	0.1
	COOKED, DRAINED									
1092	STALK, MEDIUM	1 STALK	38	94	7	TR	TR	TR	TR	TR
1093	PIECES, DICED	1 CUP	150	94	27	1	TR	0.1	TR	0.1
1094	CHIVES, RAW, CHOPPED	1 TBSP	3	91	1	TR	TR	TR	TR	TR
1095	CILANTRO, RAW	1 TSP	2	92	TR	TR	TR	TR	TR	TR
1096	COLESLAW, HOME PREPARED	1 CUP	120	82	83	2	3	0.5	0.8	1.6
	COLLARDS, COOKED, DRAINED, CHOPPED									
1097	FROM RAW	1 CUP	190	92	49	4	1	0.1	TR	0.3
1098	FROM FROZEN	1 CUP	170	88	61	5	1	0.1	TR	0.4
	CORN, SWEET, YELLOW									
	COOKED, DRAINED									
1099	FROM RAW, KERNELS ON COB	1 EAR	77	70	83	3	1	0.2	0.3	0.5
	FROM FROZEN									
1100	KERNELS ON COB	1 EAR	63	73	59	2	TR	0.1	0.1	0.2
1101	KERNELS	1 CUP	164	77	131	5	1	0.1	0.2	0.3
	CANNED									
1102	CREAM STYLE	1 CUP	256	79	184	4	1	0.2	0.3	0.5
1103	WHOLE KERNEL, VACUUM PACK	1 CUP	210	77	166	5	1	0.2	0.3	0.5
1104	CORN, SWEET, WHITE, COOKED, DRAINED	1 EAR	77	70	83	3	1	0.2	0.3	0.5
	CUCUMBER									
	PEELED									
1105	SLICED	1 CUP	119	96	14	1	TR	TR	TR	0.1
1106	WHOLE, 8 1/4″ LONG	1 LARGE	280	96	34	2	TR	0.1	TR	0.2
	UNPEELED									
1107	SLICED	1 CUP	104	96	14	1	TR	TR	TR	0.1
1108	WHOLE, 8 1/4″ LONG	1 LARGE	301	96	39	2	TR	0.1	TR	0.2
1109	DANDELION GREENS, COOKED, DRAINED	1 CUP	105	90	35	2	1	0.2	TR	0.3
1110	DILL WEED, RAW	5 SPRIGS	1	86	TR	TR	Total	TR	TR	TR
1111	EGGPLANT, COOKED, DRAINED	1 CUP	99	92	28	1	TR	TR	TR	0.1
1112	ENDIVE, CURLY (INCLUDING SCAROLE), RAW, SMALL PIECES	1 CUP	50	94	9	1	TR	TR	TR	TR
1113	GARLIC, RAW	1 CLOVE	3	59	4	TR	TR	TR	TR	TR
1114	HEARTS OF PALM, CANNED	1 PIECE	33	90	9	1	TR	TR	TR	0.1
1115	JERUSALEM ARTICHOKE, RAW, SLICED	1 CUP	150	78	114	3	TR	0.0	TR	TR
	KALE, COOKED, DRAINED, CHOPPED									
1116	FROM RAW	1 CUP	130	91	36	2	1	0.1	TR	0.3
1117	FROM FROZEN	1 CUP	130	91	39	4	1	0.1	TR	0.3
1118	KOHLRABI, COOKED, DRAINED, SLICES	1 CUP	165	90	48	3	TR	TR	TR	0.1
1119	LEEKS, BULB AND LOWER LEAF PORTION, CHOPPED OR DICED, COOKED, DRAINED	1 CUP	104	94	32	1	TR	TR	TR	0.1

*White varieties contain only a trace amount of vitamin A; other nutrients are the same.

Cholesterol (mg)	Carbo-hydrate (g)	Total dietary fiber (g)	Calcium (mg)	Iron (mg)	Potassium (mg)	Sodium (mg)	Vitamin A		Thiamine (mg)	Ribo-flavin (mg)	Niacin (mg)	Ascorbic acid (mg)	Food No.
							(IU)	(RE)					
0	1	0.3	3	0.1	39	4	2	TR	0.01	0.01	0.1	6	1085
0	5	2.5	22	0.4	303	30	19	2	0.06	0.06	0.5	46	1086
0	5	3.3	20	0.4	176	19	21	2	0.05	0.06	0.5	55	1087
0	2	1.5	9	0.2	77	8	9	1	0.02	0.03	0.2	24	1088
0	7	4.9	31	0.7	250	32	40	4	0.07	0.10	0.6	56	1089
0	1	0.7	16	0.2	115	35	54	5	0.02	0.02	0.1	3	1090
0	4	2.0	48	0.5	344	104	161	16	0.06	0.05	0.4	8	1091
0	2	0.6	16	0.2	108	35	50	5	0.02	0.02	0.1	2	1092
0	6	2.4	63	0.6	426	137	198	20	0.06	0.07	0.5	9	1093
0	TR	0.1	3	TR	9	TR	131	13	TR	TR	TR	2	1094
0	TR	TR	1	TR	8	1	98	10	TR	TR	TR	1	1095
10	15	1.8	54	0.7	217	28	762	98	0.08	0.07	0.3	39	1096
0	9	5.3	226	0.9	494	17	5,945	595	0.08	0.20	1.1	35	1097
0	12	4.8	357	1.9	427	85	10,168	1,017	0.08	0.20	1.1	45	1098
0	19	2.2	2	0.5	192	13	167	17	0.17	0.06	1.2	5	1099
0	14	1.8	2	0.4	158	3	133*	13*	0.11	0.04	1.0	3	1100
0	32	3.9	7	0.6	241	8	361*	36*	0.14	0.12	2.1	5	1101
0	46	3.1	8	1.0	343	730	248*	26*	0.06	0.14	2.5	12	1102
0	41	4.2	11	0.9	391	571	506*	50*	0.09	0.15	2.5	17	1103
0	19	2.1	2	0.5	192	13	0	0	0.17	0.06	1.2	5	1104
0	3	0.8	17	0.2	176	2	88	8	0.02	0.01	0.1	3	1105
0	7	2.0	39	0.4	414	6	207	20	0.06	0.03	0.3	8	1106
0	3	0.8	15	0.3	150	2	224	22	0.02	0.02	0.2	6	1107
0	8	2.4	42	0.8	433	6	647	63	0.07	0.07	0.7	16	1108
0	7	3.0	147	1.9	244	46	12,285	1,229	0.14	0.18	0.5	19	1109
0	TR	TR	2	0.1	7	1	77	8	TR	TR	TR	1	1110
0	7	2.5	6	0.3	246	3	63	6	0.08	0.02	0.6	1	1111
0	2	1.6	26	0.4	157	11	1,025	103	0.04	0.04	0.2	3	1112
0	1	0.1	5	0.1	12	1	0	0	0.01	TR	TR	1	1113
0	2	0.8	19	1.0	58	141	0	0	TR	0.02	0.1	3	1114
0	26	2.4	21	5.1	644	6	30	3	0.30	0.09	2.0	6	1115
0	7	2.6	94	1.2	296	30	9,620	962	0.07	0.09	0.7	53	1116
0	7	2.6	179	1.2	417	20	8,260	826	0.06	0.15	0.9	33	1117
0	11	1.8	41	0.7	561	35	58	7	0.07	0.03	0.6	89	1118
0	8	1.0	31	1.1	90	10	48	5	0.03	0.02	0.2	4	1119

Food No.	Food Description	Measure of edible portion	Weight (g)	Water (%)	Calories (kcal)	Protein (g)	Total fat (g)	Saturated (g)	Mono-unsaturated (g)	Poly-unsaturated (g)
	VEGETABLES AND VEGETABLE PRODUCTS (CONTINUED)									
	LETTUCE, RAW									
	BUTTERHEAD, AS BOSTON TYPES									
1120	LEAF	1 MEDIUM LEAF	8	96	1	TR	TR	TR	TR	TR
1121	HEAD, 5" DIA	1 HEAD	163	96	21	2	TR	TR	TR	0.2
	CRISPHEAD, AS ICEBERG									
1122	LEAF	1 MEDIUM	8	96	1	TR	TR	TR	TR	TR
1123	HEAD, 6" DIA	1 HEAD	539	96	65	5	1	0.1	TR	0.5
1124	PIECES, SHREDDED OR CHOPPED	1 CUP	55	96	7	1	TR	TR	TR	0.1
	LOOSELEAF									
1125	LEAF	1 LEAF	10	94	2	TR	TR	TR	TR	TR
1126	PIECES, SHREDDED	1 CUP	56	94	10	1	TR	TR	TR	0.1
	ROMAINE OR COS									
1127	INNERLEAF	1 LEAF	10	95	1	TR	TR	TR	TR	TR
1128	PIECES, SHREDDED	1 CUP	56	95	8	1	TR	TR	TR	0.1
	MUSHROOMS									
1129	RAW, PIECES OR SLICES	1 CUP	70	92	18	2	TR	TR	TR	0.1
1130	COOKED, DRAINED, PIECES	1 CUP	156	91	42	3	1	0.1	TR	0.3
1131	CANNED, DRAINED, PIECES	1 CUP	156	91	37	3	TR	0.1	TR	0.2
	MUSHROOMS, SHIITAKE									
1132	COOKED PIECES	1 CUP	145	83	80	2	TR	0.1	0.1	TR
1133	DRIED	1 MUSHROOM	4	10	11	TR	TR	TR	TR	TR
1134	MUSTARD GREENS, COOKED, DRAINED	1 CUP	140	94	21	3	TR	TR	0.2	0.1
	OKRA, SLICED, COOKED, DRAINED									
1135	FROM RAW	1 CUP	160	90	51	3	TR	0.1	TR	0.1
1136	FROM FROZEN	1 CUP	184	91	52	4	1	0.1	0.1	0.1
	ONIONS									
	RAW									
1137	CHOPPED	1 CUP	160	90	61	2	TR	TR	TR	0.1
1138	WHOLE, MEDIUM, 2 1/2" DIA	1 WHOLE	110	90	42	1	TR	TR	TR	0.1
1139	SLICE, 1/8" THICK	1 SLICE	14	90	5	TR	TR	TR	TR	TR
1140	COOKED (WHOLE OR SLICED), DRAINED	1 CUP	210	88	92	3	TR	0.1	0.1	0.2
1141		1 MEDIUM	94	88	41	1	TR	TR	TR	0.1
1142	DEHYDRATED FLAKES	1 TBSP	5	4	17	TR	TR	TR	TR	TR
	ONIONS, SPRING, RAW, TOP AND BULB									
1143	CHOPPED	1 CUP	100	90	32	2	TR	TR	TR	0.1
1144	WHOLE, MEDIUM, 4 1/8" LONG	1 WHOLE	15	90	5	TR	TR	TR	TR	TR
1145	ONION RINGS, 2–3" DIA, BREADED, PAR FRIED, FROZEN, OVEN HEATED	10 RINGS	60	29	244	3	16	5.2	6.5	3.1
1146	PARSLEY, RAW	10 SPRIGS	10	88	4	TR	TR	TR	TR	TR
1147	PARSNIPS, SLICED, COOKED, DRAINED	1 CUP	156	78	126	2	TR	0.1	0.2	0.1
	PEAS, EDIBLE POD, COOKED, DRAINED									
1148	FROM RAW	1 CUP	160	89	67	5	TR	0.1	TR	0.2
1149	FROM FROZEN	1 CUP	160	87	83	6	1	0.1	0.1	0.3
	PEAS, GREEN									
1150	CANNED, DRAINED	1 CUP	170	82	117	8	1	0.1	0.1	0.3
1151	FROZEN, BOILED, DRAINED	1 CUP	160	80	125	8	TR	0.1	TR	0.2
	PEPPERS									
	HOT CHILI, RAW									
1152	GREEN	1 PEPPER	45	88	18	1	TR	TR	TR	TR
1153	RED	1 PEPPER	45	88	18	1	TR	TR	TR	TR

Cholesterol (mg)	Carbo-hydrate (g)	Total dietary fiber (g)	Calcium (mg)	Iron (mg)	Potassium (mg)	Sodium (mg)	Vitamin A (IU)	(RE)	Thiamine (mg)	Ribo-flavin (mg)	Niacin (mg)	Ascorbic acid (mg)	Food No.
0	TR	0.1	2	TR	19	TR	73	7	TR	TR	TR	1	1120
0	4	1.6	52	0.5	419	8	1,581	158	0.10	0.10	0.5	13	1121
0	TR	0.1	2	TR	13	1	26	3	TR	TR	TR	TR	1122
0	11	7.5	102	2.7	852	49	1,779	178	0.25	0.16	1.0	21	1123
0	1	0.8	10	0.3	87	5	182	18	0.03	0.02	0.1	2	1124
0	TR	0.2	7	0.1	26	1	190	19	0.01	0.01	TR	2	1125
0	2	1.1	38	0.8	148	5	1,064	106	0.03	0.04	0.2	10	1126
0	TR	0.2	4	0.1	29	1	260	26	0.01	0.01	0.1	2	1127
0	1	1.0	20	0.6	162	4	1,456	146	0.06	0.06	0.3	13	1128
0	3	0.8	4	0.7	259	3	0	0	0.06	0.30	2.8	2	1129
0	8	3.4	9	2.7	555	3	0	0	0.11	0.47	7.0	6	1130
0	8	3.7	17	1.2	201	663	0	0	0.13	0.03	2.5	0	1131
0	21	3.0	4	0.6	170	6	0	0	0.05	0.25	2.2	TR	1132
0	3	0.4	TR	0.1	55	TR	0	0	0.01	0.05	0.5	TR	1133
0	3	2.8	104	1.0	283	22	4,243	424	0.06	0.09	0.6	35	1134
0	12	4.0	101	0.7	515	8	920	93	0.21	0.09	1.4	26	1135
0	11	5.2	177	1.2	431	6	946	94	0.18	0.23	1.4	22	1136
0	14	2.9	32	0.4	251	5	0	0	0.07	0.03	0.2	10	1137
0	9	2.0	22	0.2	173	3	0	0	0.05	0.02	0.2	7	1138
0	1	0.3	3	TR	22	TR	0	0	0.01	TR	TR	1	1139
0	21	2.9	46	0.5	349	6	0	0	0.09	0.05	0.3	11	1140
0	10	1.3	21	0.2	156	3	0	0	0.04	0.02	0.2	5	1141
0	4	0.5	13	0.1	81	1	0	0	0.03	0.01	TR	4	1142
0	7	2.6	72	1.5	276	16	385	39	0.06	0.08	0.5	19	1143
0	1	0.4	11	0.2	41	2	58	6	0.01	0.01	0.1	3	1144
0	23	0.8	19	1.0	77	225	135	14	0.17	0.08	2.2	1	1145
0	1	0.3	14	0.6	55	6	520	52	0.01	0.01	0.1	13	1146
0	30	6.2	58	0.9	573	16	0	0	0.13	0.08	1.1	20	1147
0	11	4.5	67	3.2	384	6	210	21	0.20	0.12	0.9	77	1148
0	14	5.0	94	3.8	347	8	267	27	0.10	0.19	0.9	35	1149
0	21	7.0	34	1.6	294	428	1,306	131	0.21	0.13	1.2	16	1150
0	23	8.8	38	2.5	269	139	1,069	107	0.45	0.16	2.4	16	1151
0	4	0.7	8	0.5	153	3	347	35	0.04	0.04	0.4	109	1152
0	4	0.7	8	0.5	153	3	4,838	484	0.04	0.04	0.4	109	1153

Food No.	Food Description	Measure of edible portion	Weight (g)	Water (%)	Calories (kcal)	Protein (g)	Total fat (g)	Fatty acids		
								Satu-rated (g)	Mono-unsatu-rated (g)	Poly-unsatu-rated (g)
VEGETABLES AND VEGETABLE PRODUCTS (CONTINUED)										
1154	JALAPENO, CANNED, SLICED, SOLIDS AND LIQUIDS	1/4 CUP	26	89	7	TR	TR	TR	TR	0.1
	SWEET (2 3/4″ LONG, 2 1/2″ DIA)									
	RAW									
	GREEN									
1155	CHOPPED	1 CUP	149	92	40	1	TR	TR	TR	0.2
1156	RING (1/4″ THICK)	1 RING	10	92	3	TR	TR	TR	TR	TR
1157	WHOLE (2 3/4″ × 2 1/2″)	1 PEPPER	119	92	32	1	TR	TR	TR	0.1
	RED									
1158	CHOPPED	1 CUP	149	92	40	1	TR	TR	TR	0.2
1159	WHOLE (2 3/4″ × 2 1/2″)	1 PEPPER	119	92	32	1	TR	TR	TR	0.1
	COOKED, DRAINED, CHOPPED									
1160	GREEN	1 CUP	136	92	38	1	TR	TR	TR	0.1
1161	RED	1 CUP	136	92	38	1	TR	TR	TR	0.1
1162	PIMENTO, CANNED	1 TBSP	12	93	3	TR	TR	TR	TR	TR
	POTATOES									
	BAKED (2 1/3″ × 3 1/4″)									
1163	WITH SKIN	1 POTATO	202	71	220	5	TR	0.1	TR	0.1
1164	FLESH ONLY	1 POTATO	156	75	145	3	TR	TR	TR	0.1
1165	SKIN ONLY	1 SKIN	58	47	115	2	TR	TR	TR	TR
	BOILED (2 1/2″ DIA)									
1166	PEELED AFTER BOILING	1 POTATO	136	77	118	3	TR	TR	TR	0.1
1167	PEELED BEFORE BOILING	1 POTATO	135	77	116	2	TR	TR	TR	0.1
1168		1 CUP	156	77	134	3	TR	TR	TR	0.1
	POTATO PRODUCTS, PREPARED									
	AU GRATIN									
1169	FROM DRY MIX, WITH WHOLE MILK, BUTTER	1 CUP	245	79	228	6	10	6.3	2.9	0.3
1170	FROM HOME RECIPE, WITH BUTTER	1 CUP	245	74	323	12	19	11.6	5.3	0.7
1171	FRENCH FRIED, FROZEN, OVEN HEATED	10 STRIPS	50	57	100	2	4	0.6	2.4	0.4
	HASHED BROWN									
1172	FROM FROZEN (ABOUT 3″ × 1 1/2″ × 1/2″)	1 PATTY	29	56	63	1	3	1.3	1.5	0.4
1173	FROM HOME RECIPE	1 CUP	156	62	326	4	22	8.5	9.7	2.5
	MASHED									
1174	FROM DEHYDRATED FLAKES (WITHOUT MILK); WHOLE MILK, BUTTER, AND SALT ADDED	1 CUP	210	76	237	4	12	7.2	3.3	0.5
	FROM HOME RECIPE									
1175	WITH WHOLE MILK	1 CUP	210	78	162	4	1	0.7	0.3	0.1
1176	WITH WHOLE MILK AND MARGARINE	1 CUP	210	76	223	4	9	2.2	3.7	2.5
1177	POTATO PANCAKES, HOME PREPARED	1 PANCAKE	76	47	207	5	12	2.3	3.5	5.0
1178	POTATO PUFFS, FROM FROZEN	10 PUFFS	79	53	175	3	8	4.0	3.4	0.6
1179	POTATO SALAD, HOME PREPARED	1 CUP	250	76	358	7	21	3.6	6.2	9.3
	SCALLOPED									
1180	FROM DRY MIX, WITH WHOLE MILK, BUTTER	1 CUP	245	79	228	5	11	6.5	3.0	0.5
1181	FROM HOME RECIPE, WITH BUTTER	1 CUP	245	81	211	7	9	5.5	2.5	0.4
	PUMPKIN									
1182	COOKED, MASHED	1 CUP	245	94	49	2	TR	0.1	TR	TR
1183	CANNED	1 CUP	245	90	83	3	1	0.4	0.1	TR
1184	RADISHES, RAW (3/4″ TO 1″ DIA)	1 RADISH	5	95	1	TR	TR	TR	TR	TR
1185	RUTABAGAS, COOKED, DRAINED, CUBES	1 CUP	170	89	66	2	TR	TR	TR	0.2
1186	SAUERKRAUT, CANNED, SOLIDS AND LIQUID	1 CUP	236	93	45	2	TR	0.1	TR	0.1

Cholesterol (mg)	Carbo-hydrate (g)	Total dietary fiber (g)	Calcium (mg)	Iron (mg)	Potassium (mg)	Sodium (mg)	Vitamin A (IU)	Vitamin A (RE)	Thiamine (mg)	Ribo-flavin (mg)	Niacin (mg)	Ascorbic acid (mg)	Food No.
0	1	0.7	6	0.5	50	434	442	44	0.01	0.01	0.1	3	1154
0	10	2.7	13	0.7	264	3	942	94	0.10	0.04	0.8	133	1155
0	1	0.2	1	TR	18	TR	63	6	0.01	TR	0.1	9	1156
0	8	2.1	11	0.5	211	2	752	75	0.08	0.04	0.6	106	1157
0	10	3.0	13	0.7	264	3	8,493	849	0.10	0.04	0.8	283	1158
0	8	2.4	11	0.5	211	2	6,783	678	0.08	0.04	0.6	226	1159
0	9	1.6	12	0.6	226	3	805	80	0.08	0.04	0.6	101	1160
0	9	1.6	12	0.6	226	3	5,114	511	0.08	0.04	0.6	233	1161
0	1	0.2	1	0.2	19	2	319	32	TR	0.01	0.1	10	1162
0	51	4.8	20	2.7	844	16	0	0	0.22	0.07	3.3	26	1163
0	34	2.3	8	0.5	610	8	0	0	0.16	0.03	2.2	20	1164
0	27	4.6	20	4.1	332	12	0	0	0.07	0.06	1.8	8	1165
0	27	2.4	7	0.4	515	5	0	0	0.14	0.03	2.0	18	1166
0	27	2.4	11	0.4	443	7	0	0	0.13	0.03	1.8	10	1167
0	31	2.8	12	0.5	512	8	0	0	0.15	0.03	2.0	12	1168
37	31	2.2	203	0.8	537	1,076	522	76	0.05	0.20	2.3	8	1169
56	28	4.4	292	1.6	970	1,061	647	93	0.16	0.28	2.4	24	1170
0	16	1.6	4	0.6	209	15	0	0	0.06	0.01	1.0	5	1171
0	8	0.6	4	0.4	126	10	0	0	0.03	0.01	0.7	2	1172
0	33	3.1	12	1.3	501	37	0	0	0.12	0.03	3.1	9	1173
29	32	4.8	103	0.5	489	697	378	44	0.23	0.11	1.4	20	1174
4	37	4.2	55	0.6	628	636	40	13	0.18	0.08	2.3	14	1175
4	35	4.2	55	0.5	607	620	355	42	0.18	0.08	2.3	13	1176
73	22	1.5	18	1.2	597	386	109	11	0.10	0.13	1.6	17	1177
0	24	2.5	24	1.2	300	589	13	2	0.15	0.06	1.7	5	1178
170	28	3.3	48	1.6	635	1,323	523	83	0.19	0.15	2.2	25	1179
27	31	2.7	88	0.9	497	835	363	51	0.05	0.14	2.5	8	1180
29	26	4.7	140	1.4	926	821	331	47	0.17	0.23	2.6	26	1181
0	12	2.7	37	1.4	564	2	2,651	265	0.08	0.19	1.0	12	1182
0	20	7.1	64	3.4	505	12	54,037	5,405	0.06	0.13	0.9	10	1183
0	TR	0.1	1	TR	10	1	TR	TR	TR	TR	TR	1	1184
0	15	3.1	82	0.9	554	34	954	95	0.14	0.07	1.2	32	1185
0	10	5.9	71	3.5	401	1,560	42	5	0.05	0.05	0.3	35	1186

Food No.	Food Description	Measure of edible portion	Weight (g)	Water (%)	Calories (kcal)	Protein (g)	Total fat (g)	Fatty acids Saturated (g)	Fatty acids Mono-unsaturated (g)	Fatty acids Poly-unsaturated (g)
VEGETABLES AND VEGETABLE PRODUCTS (CONTINUED)										
	SEAWEED									
1187	KELP, RAW	2 TBSP	10	82	4	TR	TR	TR	TR	TR
1188	SPIRULINA, DRIED	1 TBSP	1	5	3	1	TR	TR	TR	TR
1189	SHALLOTS, RAW, CHOPPED	1 TBSP	10	80	7	TR	TR	TR	TR	TR
1190	SOYBEANS, GREEN, COOKED, DRAINED	1 CUP	180	69	254	22	12	1.3	2.2	5.4
	SPINACH									
	RAW									
1191	CHOPPED	1 CUP	30	92	7	1	TR	TR	TR	TR
1192	LEAF	1 LEAF	10	92	2	TR	TR	TR	TR	TR
	COOKED, DRAINED									
1193	FROM RAW	1 CUP	180	91	41	5	TR	0.1	TR	0.2
1194	FROM FROZEN (CHOPPED OR LEAF)	1 CUP	190	90	53	6	TR	0.1	TR	0.2
1195	CANNED, DRAINED	1 CUP	214	92	49	6	1	0.2	TR	0.4
	SQUASH									
	SUMMER (ALL VARIETIES),SLICED									
1196	RAW	1 CUP	113	94	23	1	TR	TR	TR	0.1
1197	COOKED, DRAINED	1 CUP	180	94	36	2	1	0.1	TR	0.2
1198	WINTER (ALL VARIETIES), BAKED, CUBES	1 CUP	205	89	80	2	1	0.3	0.1	0.5
1199	WINTER, BUTTERNUT, FROZEN, COOKED, MASHED	1 CUP	240	88	94	3	TR	TR	TR	0.1
	SWEET POTATOES									
	COOKED (2" DIA, 5" LONG RAW)									
1200	BAKED, WITH SKIN	1 POTATO	146	73	150	3	TR	TR	TR	0.1
1201	BOILED, WITHOUT SKIN	1 POTATO	156	73	164	3	TR	0.1	TR	0.2
1202	CANDIED (2 1/2" × 2 PIECE)	1 PIECE	105	67	144	1	3	1.4	0.7	0.2
	CANNED									
1203	SYRUP PACK, DRAINED	1 CUP	196	72	212	3	1	0.1	TR	0.3
1204	VACUUM PACK, MASHED	1 CUP	255	76	232	4	1	0.1	TR	0.2
1205	TOMATILLOS, RAW	1 MEDIUM	34	92	11	TR	TR	TR	0.1	0.1
	TOMATOES									
	RAW, YEAR-ROUND AVERAGE									
1206	CHOPPED OR SLICED	1 CUP	180	94	38	2	1	0.1	0.1	0.2
1207	SLICE, MEDIUM, 1/4" THICK	1 SLICE	20	94	4	TR	TR	TR	TR	TR
	WHOLE									
1208	CHERRY	1 CHERRY	17	94	4	TR	TR	TR	TR	TR
1209	MEDIUM, 2 3/5" DIA	1 TOMATO	123	94	26	1	TR	0.1	0.1	0.2
1210	CANNED, SOLIDS AND LIQUID	1 CUP	240	94	46	2	TR	TR	TR	0.1
	SUN DRIED									
1211	PLAIN	1 PIECE	2	15	5	TR	TR	TR	TR	TR
1212	PACKED IN OIL, DRAINED	1 PIECE	3	54	6	TR	TR	0.1	0.3	0.1
1213	TOMATO JUICE, CANNED, WITH SALT ADDED	1 CUP	243	94	41	2	TR	TR	TR	0.1
	TOMATO PRODUCTS, CANNED									
1214	PASTE	1 CUP	262	74	215	10	1	0.2	0.2	0.6
1215	PUREE	1 CUP	250	87	100	4	TR	0.1	0.1	0.2
1216	SAUCE	1 CUP	245	89	74	3	TR	0.1	0.1	0.2
	SPAGHETTI/MARINARA/PASTA SAUCE. SEE SOUPS, SAUCES, AND GRAVIES.									
1217	STEWED	1 CUP	255	91	71	2	TR	TR	0.1	0.1

*For product with no salt added: If salt added, consult the nutrition label for sodium value.

Cholesterol (mg)	Carbo-hydrate (g)	Total dietary fiber (g)	Calcium (mg)	Iron (mg)	Potassium (mg)	Sodium (mg)	Vitamin A (IU)	Vitamin A (RE)	Thiamine (mg)	Ribo-flavin (mg)	Niacin (mg)	Ascorbic acid (mg)	Food No.
0	1	0.1	17	0.3	9	23	12	1	0.01	0.02	TR	TR	1187
0	TR	TR	1	0.3	14	10	6	1	0.02	0.04	0.1	TR	1188
0	2	0.2	4	0.1	33	1	119	12	0.01	TR	TR	1	1189
0	20	7.6	261	4.5	970	25	281	29	0.47	0.28	2.3	31	1190
0	1	0.8	30	0.8	167	24	2,015	202	0.02	0.06	0.2	8	1191
0	TR	0.3	10	0.3	56	8	672	67	0.01	0.02	0.1	3	1192
0	7	4.3	245	6.4	839	126	14,742	1,474	0.17	0.42	0.9	18	1193
0	10	5.7	277	2.9	566	163	14,790	1,478	0.11	0.32	0.8	23	1194
0	7	5.1	272	4.9	740	58	18,781	1,879	0.03	0.30	0.8	31	1195
0	5	2.1	23	0.5	220	2	221	23	0.07	0.04	0.6	17	1196
0	8	2.5	49	0.6	346	2	517	52	0.08	0.07	0.9	10	1197
0	18	5.7	29	0.7	896	2	7,292	730	0.17	0.05	1.4	20	1198
0	24	2.2	46	1.4	319	5	8,014	802	0.12	0.09	1.1	8	1199
0	35	4.4	41	0.7	508	15	31,860	3,186	0.11	0.19	0.9	36	1200
0	38	2.8	33	0.9	287	20	26,604	2,660	0.08	0.22	1.0	27	1201
8	29	2.5	27	1.2	198	74	4,398	440	0.02	0.04	0.4	7	1202
0	50	5.9	33	1.9	378	76	14,028	1,403	0.05	0.07	0.7	21	1203
0	54	4.6	56	2.3	796	135	20,357	2,035	0.09	0.15	1.9	67	1204
0	2	0.6	2	0.2	91	TR	39	4	0.01	0.01	0.6	4	1205
0	8	2.0	9	0.8	400	16	1,121	112	0.11	0.09	1.1	34	1206
0	1	0.2	1	0.1	44	2	125	12	0.01	0.01	0.1	4	1207
0	1	0.2	1	0.1	38	2	106	11	0.01	0.01	0.1	3	1208
0	6	1.4	6	0.6	273	11	766	76	0.07	0.06	0.8	23	1209
0	10	2.4	72	1.3	530	355	1,428	144	0.11	0.07	1.8	34	1210
0	1	0.2	2	0.2	69	42	17	2	0.01	0.01	0.2	1	1211
0	1	0.2	1	0.1	47	8	39	4	0.01	0.01	0.1	3	1212
0	10	1.0	22	1.4	535	877	1,351	136	0.11	0.08	1.6	44	1213
0	51	10.7	92	5.1	2,455	231	6,406	639	0.41	0.50	8.4	111	1214
0	24	5.0	43	3.1	1,065	85*	3,188	320	0.18	0.14	4.3	26	1215
0	18	3.4	34	1.9	909	1,482	2,399	240	0.16	0.14	2.8	32	1216
0	17	2.6	84	1.9	607	564	1,380	138	0.12	0.09	1.8	29	1217

Food No.	Food Description	Measure of edible portion	Weight (g)	Water (%)	Calories (kcal)	Protein (g)	Total fat (g)	Fatty acids Satu-rated (g)	Mono-unsatu-rated (g)	Poly-unsatu-rated (g)
VEGETABLES AND VEGETABLE PRODUCTS (CONTINUED)										
1218	TURNIPS, COOKED, CUBES	1 CUP	156	94	33	1	TR	TR	TR	0.1
	TURNIP GREENS, COOKED, DRAINED									
1219	FROM RAW (LEAVES AND STEMS)	1 CUP	144	93	29	2	TR	0.1	TR	0.1
1220	FROM FROZEN (CHOPPED)	1 CUP	164	90	49	5	1	0.2	TR	0.3
1221	VEGETABLE JUICE COCKTAIL, CANNED	1 CUP	242	94	46	2	TR	TR	TR	0.1
	VEGETABLES, MIXED									
1222	CANNED, DRAINED	1 CUP	163	87	77	4	TR	0.1	TR	0.2
1223	FROZEN, COOKED, DRAINED	1 CUP	182	83	107	5	TR	0.1	TR	0.1
1224	WATERCHESTNUTS, CANNED, SLICES, SOLIDS AND LIQUIDS	1 CUP	140	86	70	1	TR	TR	TR	TR
MISCELLANEOUS ITEMS										
1225	BACON BITS, MEATLESS	1 TBSP	7	8	31	2	2	0.3	0.4	0.9
	BAKING POWDERS FOR HOME USE DOUBLE ACTING									
1226	SODIUM ALUMINUM SULFATE	1 TSP	5	5	2	0	0	0.0	0.0	0.0
1227	STRAIGHT PHOSPHATE	1 TSP	5	4	2	TR	0	0.0	0.0	0.0
1228	LOW SODIUM	1 TSP	5	6	5	TR	TR	TR	TR	TR
1229	BAKING SODA	1 TSP	5	TR	0	0	0	0.0	0.0	0.0
1230	BEEF JERKY	1 LARGE PIECE	20	23	81	7	5	2.1	2.2	0.2
1231	CATSUP	1 CUP	240	67	250	4	1	0.1	0.1	0.4
1232		1 TBSP	15	67	16	TR	TR	TR	TR	TR
1233		1 PACKET	6	67	6	TR	TR	TR	TR	TR
1234	CELERY SEED	1 TSP	2	6	8	TR	1	TR	0.3	0.1
1235	CHILI POWDER	1 TSP	3	8	8	TR	TR	0.1	0.1	0.2
	CHOCOLATE, UNSWEETENED, BAKING									
1236	SOLID	1 SQUARE	28	1	148	3	16	9.2	5.2	0.5
1237	LIQUID	1 OZ	28	1	134	3	14	7.2	2.6	3.0
1238	CINNAMON	1 TSP	2	10	6	TR	TR	TR	TR	TR
1239	COCOA POWDER, UNSWEETENED	1 CUP	86	3	197	17	12	6.9	3.9	0.4
1240		1 TBSP	5	3	12	1	1	0.4	0.2	TR
1241	CREAM OF TARTAR	1 TSP	3	2	8	0	0	0.0	0.0	0.0
1242	CURRY POWDER	1 TSP	2	10	7	TR	TR	TR	0.1	0.1
1243	GARLIC POWDER	1 TSP	3	6	9	TR	TR	TR	TR	TR
1244	HORSERADISH, PREPARED	1 TSP	5	85	2	TR	TR	TR	TR	TR
1245	MUSTARD, PREPARED, YELLOW	1 TSP OR 1 PACKET	5	82	3	TR	TR	TR	0.1	TR
	OLIVES, CANNED									
1246	PICKLED, GREEN	5 MEDIUM	17	78	20	TR	2	0.3	1.6	0.2
1247	RIPE, BLACK	5 LARGE	22	80	25	TR	2	0.3	1.7	0.2
1248	ONION POWDER	1 TSP	2	5	7	TR	TR	TR	TR	TR
1249	OREGANO, GROUND	1 TSP	2	7	5	TR	TR	TR	TR	0.1
1250	PAPRIKA	1 TSP	2	10	6	TR	TR	TR	TR	0.2
1251	PARSLEY, DRIED	1 TBSP	1	9	4	TR	TR	TR	TR	TR
1252	PEPPER, BLACK	1 TSP	2	11	5	TR	TR	TR	TR	TR
	PICKLES, CUCUMBER									
1253	DILL, WHOLE, MEDIUM (3 3/4" LONG)	1 PICKLE	65	92	12	TR	TR	TR	TR	0.1
1254	FRESH (BREAD AND BUTTER PICKLES), SLICES 1 1/2" DIA, 1/4" THICK	3 SLICES	24	79	18	TR	TR	TR	TR	TR
1255	PICKLE RELISH, SWEET	1 TBSP	15	62	20	TR	TR	TR	TR	TR

Cholesterol (mg)	Carbo-hydrate (g)	Total dietary fiber (g)	Calcium (mg)	Iron (mg)	Potassium (mg)	Sodium (mg)	Vitamin A (IU)	Vitamin A (RE)	Thiamine (mg)	Ribo-flavin (mg)	Niacin (mg)	Ascorbic acid (mg)	Food No.
0	8	3.1	34	0.3	211	78	0	0	0.04	0.04	0.5	18	1218
0	6	5.0	197	1.2	292	42	7,917	792	0.06	0.10	0.6	39	1219
0	8	5.6	249	3.2	367	25	13,079	1,309	0.09	0.12	0.8	36	1220
0	11	1.9	27	1.0	467	653	2,831	283	0.10	0.07	1.8	67	1221
0	15	4.9	44	1.7	474	243	18,985	1,899	0.07	0.08	0.9	8	1222
0	24	8.0	46	1.5	308	64	7,784	779	0.13	0.22	1.5	6	1223
0	17	3.5	6	1.2	165	11	6	0	0.02	0.03	0.5	2	1224
0	2	0.7	7	0.1	10	124	0	0	0.04	TR	0.1	TR	1225
0	1	TR	270	0.5	1	488	0	0	0.00	0.00	0.0	0	1226
0	1	TR	339	0.5	TR	363	0	0	0.00	0.00	0.0	0	1227
0	2	0.1	217	0.4	505	5	0	0	0.00	0.00	0.0	0	1228
0	0	0.0	0	0.0	0	1,259	0	0	0.00	0.00	0.0	0	1229
10	2	0.4	4	1.1	118	438	0	0	0.03	0.03	0.3	0	1230
0	65	3.1	46	1.7	1,154	2,846	2,438	245	0.21	0.18	3.3	36	1231
0	4	0.2	3	0.1	72	178	152	15	0.01	0.01	0.2	2	1232
0	2	0.1	1	TR	29	71	61	6	0.01	TR	0.1	1	1233
0	1	0.2	35	0.9	28	3	1	TR	0.01	0.01	0.1	TR	1234
0	1	0.9	7	0.4	50	26	908	91	0.01	0.02	0.2	2	1235
0	8	4.4	21	1.8	236	4	28	3	0.02	0.05	0.3	0	1236
0	10	5.1	15	1.2	331	3	3	TR	0.01	0.08	0.6	0	1237
0	2	1.2	28	0.9	11	1	6	1	TR	TR	TR	1	1238
0	47	28.6	110	11.9	1,311	18	17	2	0.07	0.21	1.9	0	1239
0	3	1.8	7	0.7	82	1	1	TR	TR	0.01	0.1	0	1240
0	2	TR	TR	0.1	495	2	0	0	0.00	0.00	0.0	0	1241
0	1	0.7	10	0.6	31	1	20	2	0.01	0.01	0.1	TR	1242
0	2	0.3	2	0.1	31	1	0	0	0.01	TR	TR	1	1243
0	1	0.2	3	TR	12	16	TR	0	TR	TR	TR	1	1244
0	TR	0.2	4	0.1	8	56	7	1	TR	TR	TR	TR	1245
0	TR	0.2	10	0.3	9	408	51	5	0.00	0.00	TR	0	1246
0	1	0.7	19	0.7	2	192	89	9	TR	0.00	TR	TR	1247
0	2	0.1	8	0.1	20	1	0	0	0.01	TR	TR	TR	1248
0	1	0.6	24	0.7	25	TR	104	10	0.01	TR	0.1	1	1249
0	1	0.4	4	0.5	49	1	1,273	127	0.01	0.04	0.3	1	1250
0	1	0.4	19	1.3	49	6	303	30	TR	0.02	0.1	2	1251
0	1	0.6	9	0.6	26	1	4	TR	TR	0.01	TR	TR	1252
0	3	0.8	6	0.3	75	833	214	21	0.01	0.02	TR	1	1253
0	4	0.4	8	0.1	48	162	34	3	0.00	0.01	0.0	2	1254
0	5	0.2	TR	0.1	4	122	23	2	0.00	TR	TR	TR	1255

Food No.	Food Description	Measure of edible portion	Weight (g)	Water (%)	Calories (kcal)	Protein (g)	Total fat (g)	Fatty acids Satu-rated (g)	Fatty acids Mono-unsatu-rated (g)	Fatty acids Poly-unsatu-rated (g)
MISCELLANEOUS ITEMS (CONTINUED)										
1256	PORK SKINS/RINDS, PLAIN	1 OZ	28	2	155	17	9	3.2	4.2	1.0
	POTATO CHIPS									
	REGULAR									
	PLAIN									
1257	SALTED	1 OZ	28	2	152	2	10	3.1	2.8	3.5
1258	UNSALTED	1 OZ	28	2	152	2	10	3.1	2.8	3.5
1259	BARBECUE FLAVOR	1 OZ	28	2	139	2	9	2.3	1.9	4.6
1260	SOUR CREAM AND ONION FLAVOR	1 OZ	28	2	151	2	10	2.5	1.7	4.9
1261	REDUCED FAT	1 OZ	28	1	134	2	6	1.2	1.4	3.1
1262	FAT FREE, MADE WITH OLESTRA	1 OZ	28	2	75	2	TR	TR	0.1	0.1
	MADE FROM DRIED POTATOES									
1263	PLAIN	1 OZ	28	1	158	2	11	2.7	2.1	5.7
1264	SOUR CREAM AND ONION FLAVOR	1 OZ	28	2	155	2	10	2.7	2.0	5.3
1265	REDUCED FAT	1 OZ	28	1	142	2	7	1.5	1.7	3.8
1266	SALT	1 TSP	6	TR	0	0	0	0.0	0.0	0.0
	TRAIL MIX									
1267	REGULAR, WITH RAISINS, CHOCOLATE CHIPS, SALTED NUTS AND SEEDS	1 CUP	146	7	707	21	47	8.9	19.8	16.5
1268	TROPICAL	1 CUP	140	9	570	9	24	11.9	3.5	7.2
1269	VANILLA EXTRACT	1 TSP	4	53	12	TR	TR	TR	TR	TR
	VINEGAR									
1270	CIDER	1 TBSP	15	94	2	0	0	0.0	0.0	0.0
1271	DISTILLED	1 TBSP	17	95	2	0	0	0.0	0.0	0.0
	YEAST, BAKER'S									
1272	DRY, ACTIVE	1 PKG	7	8	21	3	TR	TR	0.2	TR
1273		1 TSP	4	8	12	2	TR	TR	0.1	TR
1274	COMPRESSED	1 CAKE	17	69	18	1	TR	TR	0.2	TR

Cholesterol (mg)	Carbo-hydrate (g)	Total dietary fiber (g)	Calcium (mg)	Iron (mg)	Potassium (mg)	Sodium (mg)	Vitamin A (IU)	Vitamin A (RE)	Thiamine (mg)	Ribo-flavin (mg)	Niacin (mg)	Ascorbic acid (mg)	Food No.
27	0	0.0	9	0.2	36	521	37	11	0.03	0.08	0.4	TR	1256
0	15	1.3	7	0.5	361	168	0	0	0.05	0.06	1.1	9	1257
0	15	1.4	7	0.5	361	2	0	0	0.05	0.06	1.1	9	1258
0	15	1.2	14	0.5	357	213	62	6	0.06	0.06	1.3	10	1259
2	15	1.5	20	0.5	377	177	48	6	0.05	0.06	1.1	11	1260
0	19	1.7	6	0.4	494	139	0	0	0.06	0.08	2.0	7	1261
0	17	1.1	10	0.4	366	185	1,469	441	0.10	0.02	1.3	8	1262
0	14	1.0	7	0.4	286	186	0	0	0.06	0.03	0.9	2	1263
1	15	0.3	18	0.4	141	204	214	28	0.05	0.03	0.7	3	1264
0	18	1.0	10	0.4	285	121	0	0	0.05	0.02	1.2	3	1265
0	0	0.0	1	TR	TR	2,325	0	0	0.00	0.00	0.0	0	1266
6	66	8.8	159	4.9	946	177	64	7	0.60	0.33	6.4	2	1267
0	92	10.6	80	3.7	993	14	69	7	0.63	0.16	2.1	11	1268
0	1	0.0	TR	TR	6	TR	0	0	TR	TR	TR	0	1269
0	1	0.0	1	0.1	15	TR	0	0	0.00	0.00	0.0	0	1270
0	1	0.0	0	0.0	2	TR	0	0	0.00	0.00	0.0	0	1271
0	3	1.5	4	1.2	140	4	TR	0	0.17	0.38	2.8	TR	1272
0	2	0.8	3	0.7	80	2	TR	0	0.09	0.22	1.6	TR	1273
0	3	1.4	3	0.6	102	5	0	0	0.32	0.19	2.1	TR	1274

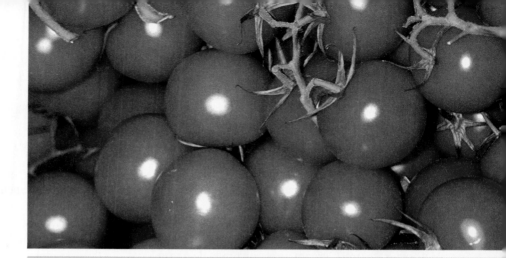

APPENDIX E

DRUG-FOOD INTERACTIONS

From *PDR Nurse's Drug Handbook 2007 Edition,* by G. R. Spratto and A. L. Woods, 2006. Clifton Park, NY: Thomson Delmar Learning and Medical Economics of Thomson Healthcare.

A. DRUGS THAT SHOULD BE TAKEN WHILE FASTING

Ampicillin
AzoGantanol/Gantrisin
Bacampicillin
Bethanechol (may experience nausea and vomiting)
Bisacodyl
Calcium carbonate
Captopril
Carbenicillin
Castor oil
Chloramphenicol
Cyclosporine gel caps only (do not take with fatty meals)
Demeclocycline (avoid high-calcium foods and dairy products)
Dicloxacillin
Digitalis preparations (not with high-fiber foods)
Disopyramide
Erythromycin base/estolate
Etidronate
Ferrous salts (not with tea, coffee, egg, cereals, fiber, or milk)
Flavoxate
Furosemide
Isoniazid

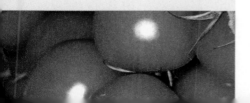

Isosorbide dinitrate

Ketoprofen (if GI distress occurs, may take with food)

Lansoprazole

Levodopa (not with high-protein foods; meals delay absorption and peak plasma concentration; avoid caffeine)

Lisinopril

Lomustil (empty stomach will reduce nausea)

Methotrexate (milk, cream, or yogurt may decrease absorption)

Methyldopa (not with high-protein foods; meals delay absorption and peak plasma concentration; avoid caffeine)

Nafcillin (inactivated by stomach acid; absorption variable with/without food)

Nalidixic acid

Naltrexone

Norfloxacin (milk, cream, or yogurt may decrease absorption)

Oxytetracycline (avoid dairy products and foods high in calcium)

Penicillamine (antacids, iron, and food decrease absorption)

Penicillin

Phenytoin (if GI distress occurs, may take with food; food effect depends on preparation)

Propantheline

Rifampicin

Sotalol

Sulfamethoxazole

Terbutaline sulfate

Tetracycline (avoid dairy products and foods high in calcium)

Theophylline (absorption of controlled release varies by preparation)

Thyroid hormone preparations (limit foods containing goitrogens)

Trientine (antacids, iron, and food reduce absorption)

Trimethoprim

B. DRUGS THAT SHOULD BE TAKEN WITH FOOD

Buspirone

Carbamazepine (erratic absorption)

Chlorothiazide

Clofazimine

Gemfibrozil

Grisefulvin (high-fat meals)

Isotretinoin

Labetatol

Lovastatin

Methenamine

Metoprolol

Nifedipine (grapefruit juice increases bioavailability)

Nitrofurantoin

Oxcarbazepine

Probucol (high-fat meals)

Propranolol

Spironolactone

Trazodone

Verapamil SR (absorption varies by manufacturer; too rapid absorption may cause heart block)

C. CONSTIPATING AGENTS

Antacids

Anticholinergic drugs

    Anticholinergics

    Antihistamines

    Phenothiazines

    Tricyclic antidepressants

Clonidine

Corticosteroids

Ganglionic blocking agents

Iron supplements

Laxatives (when abused)

Lithium

MAO inhibitors

Muscle relaxants

    NSAIDS

Octreotide

Opioids

Prostaglandin synthesis inhibitors

D. DIARRHEAL AGENTS

Adrenergic neuron blockers: reserpine, guanethidine

Antibiotics (especially broad-spectrum agents)

Cholinergic agonists and cholinesterase inhibitors

Erythromycin

Metoclopramide

Osmotic and stimulant laxatives

Quinidine

E. TYRAMINE-CONTAINING FOODS

Moderate amounts of tyramine:

    Banana peel

Broad beans

Cheese (all except cream cheese and cottage cheese)

Chianti, vermouth

Concentrated yeast extracts/brewer's yeast

Fermented cabbage products: sauerkraut, kimchee

Fermented soy products: fermented bean curd, soya bean paste, miso soup

Hydrolyzed protein extracts for sauces, soups, gravies

Imitation cheese

Liquid and powdered protein supplements

Meat extracts

Nonalcoholic beers

Prepared meats (sausage, chopped liver, pate, salami, mortadella)

Raspberries

Some non–United States brands of beer

Significant amounts of tyramine:

Avocado

Chocolate

Cream from fresh pasteurized milk

Distilled spirits

Peanuts

Red and white wines, port wines

Soy sauce

Yogurt

F. FOODS CONTAINING GOITROGENS

Asparagus

Brussels sprouts

Cabbage

Kale

Lettuce

Peas

Soy beans

Spinach

Turnip greens

Watercress

Other leafy green vegetables

G. COUMADIN ANTICOAGULANTS AND DIETARY EFFECTS

Consumption of vitamin K–enriched foods may counteract the effects of anticoagulants since the drugs act through antagonism of vitamin K. Advise the client on anticoagulants to maintain a steady, consistent intake of vitamin K–containing foods. The drug monograph for warfarin clearly lists these foods. Additionally, certain herbal teas (Woodruff, tonka beans, melitot) contain natural coumarins that can potentiate the effects of Coumadin and should be avoided. Large amounts of avocado also potentiate the drug's effects. Brussels sprouts and other cruciferous vegetables increase the catabolism of warfarin, thereby decreasing its anticoagulant activities.

H. GENERAL DRUG CLASS RECOMMENDATIONS

ACE inhibitors: Take captopril and moexipril 1 hr before or 2 hrs after meals; food decreases absorption. Avoid high-potassium foods as ACE increases K+.

Analgesic/Antipyretic: Take on an empty stomach as food may slow the absorption.

Antacids: Take 1 hr after or between meals. Avoid dairy foods as the protein in them can increase stomach acid.

Antianxiety agents: Caffeine may cause excitability, nervousness, and hyperactivity, lessening the antianxiety drug effects.

Antibiotics: Penicillin generally should be taken on an empty stomach; may take with food if GI upset occurs. Do not mix with acidic foods such as coffee, citrus fruits, and tomatoes as the acid interferes with absorption of penicillin, ampicillin, erythromycin, and cloxacillin.

Anticoagulants: High vitamin K produces blood-clotting substance and may reduce drug effectiveness. Vitamin E >400 IU may prolong clotting time and increase bleeding risk.

Antidepressant drugs: May be taken with or without food.

Antifungals: Avoid taking with dairy products; avoid alcohol.

Antihistamines: Take on an empty stomach to increase effectiveness.

Bronchodilators with theophylline: High-fat meals may increase bioavailability, while high-carbohydrate meals may decrease it. Food increases absorption of Theo-24 and Uniphyl, which may cause increased nausea and vomiting, headache, and irritability.

Cephalosporins: Take on an empty stomach 1 hr before or 2 hrs after meals. May take with food if GI upset occurs.

Corticosteroids: Take with food to decrease stomach upset.

Diuretics: Vary in interactions; some cause loss of potassium, calcium, and magnesium. Avoid salty food and natural black licorice as these increase K and Mg losses. Large doses of vitamin D can elevate blood pressure.

H_2 blockers: May take with or without regard to food.

HMG-CoA reductase inhibitors: Take lovastatin with the evening meal to enhance absorption.

Laxatives: Avoid dairy foods, as calcium can decrease absorption.

Macrolides: Take on an empty stomach 1 hr before or 2 hrs after meals. May take with food for GI upset.

MAO inhibitors: Have many dietary restrictions, so follow dietary guidelines as prescribed. Foods or alcoholic beverages containing tyramine may cause a fatal increase in blood pressure.

Nitroimadazole (metronidazole): Avoid alcohol or food prepared with alcohol for at least 3 days after finishing the medicine. Alcohol may cause nausea, abdominal cramps, vomiting, headaches, and flushing.

NSAIDS: Take with food or milk to prevent irritation of the stomach.

Quinolones: Take on an empty stomach 1 hr before or 2 hrs after meals. May take with food for GI upset but avoid calcium-containing foods such as milk, yogurt, and vitamins and minerals containing iron and antacids because they decrease drug concentrations. Caffeine-containing products may lead to excitability and nervousness.

Sulfonamides: Take on an empty stomach 1 hr before or 2 hrs after meals. May take with food if GI upset occurs.

Tetracyclines: Take on an empty stomach 1 hr before or 2 hrs after meals. May take with food but avoid dairy products, antacids, and vitamins containing iron.

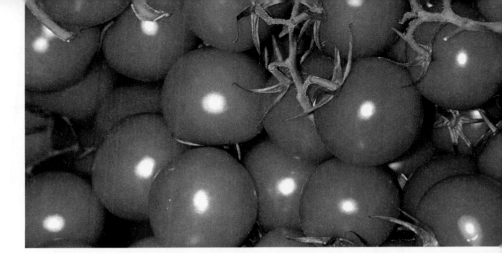

APPENDIX F

ENGLISH AND METRIC UNITS AND CONVERSIONS

Units of Measure in the English System

Unit	Abbreviation	Equivalent
dash		less than ⅛ teaspoon
few grains	f.g.	less than ⅛ teaspoon
drop		—
15 drops		—
1 teaspoon	tsp	⅓ tablespoon
1 tablespoon	Tbsp	3 teaspoons
1 fluid ounce	oz	2 tablespoons
1 cup	c	8 fluid ounces or 16 tablespoons
1 pint	pt	2 cups
1 quart	qt	2 pints or 4 cups
1 gallon	gal	4 quarts
1 peck	pk	2 gallons
1 bushel	bu	4 pecks
1 pound	lb	16 ounces

Units of Measure in the Metric System

Basic unit of *weight* is the *gram* (g)
Basic unit of *volume* is the *liter* (l)
Basic unit of *length* is the *meter* (m)
Temperature is measured in degrees *Celsius* (°C)

kilo: (*key*-low) = 1,000
deci: (*dess*-ee) = 0.1 (1/10)
centi: (*sent*-ee) = 0.01 (1/100)
milli: (*mill*-ee) = 0.001 (1/1000)

Unit Relationships within the Metric System

Weight				Volume		
1,000 grams	=	1 *kilo*gram		1000 liters	=	1 *kilo*liter*
100 grams	=	1 *hecto*gram*		100 liters	=	1 *hecto*liter*
10 grams	=	1 *deka*gram*		10 liters	=	1 *deka*liter*
		1 gram				1 liter
0.1 gram	=	1 *deci*gram*		0.1 liter	=	1 *deci*liter*
0.01 gram	=	1 *centi*gram*		0.01 liter	=	1 *centi*liter*
0.001 gram	=	1 *milli*gram		0.001 liter	=	1 *milli*liter
0.000001 gram	=	1 *micro*gram*		0.000001 liter	=	1 *micro*liter*

*Units not commonly used.

Converting from the English System to the Metric System

Convert to Metric	When You Know	Multiply By	To Find
Weight	ounces (oz)	28	grams (g)
	pounds (lb)	0.45	kilograms (kg)
	teaspoons (tsp)	5	milliliters (ml)
	tablespoons (Tbsp)	15	milliliters
	fluid ounces (fl oz)	30	milliliters
	cups (c)	0.24	liters (l)
Volume	pints (pt)	0.47	liters
	quarts (qt)	0.95	liters
	gallons (gal)	3.8	liters
	cubic feet (ft^3)	0.03	cubic meters (m^3)
	cubic yards (yd^3)	0.76	cubic meters
Temperature	Fahrenheit (°F) temperature	5/9 (after subtracting 32)	Celsius (°C) temperature

Source: Adapted from "Some References on Metric Information" by U.S. Department of Commerce, National Bureau of Standards.

Converting from the Metric System to the English System

Convert to Metric	When You Know	Multiply By	To Find
Weight	grams (g)	0.035	ounces (oz)
	kilograms (kg)	2.2	pounds (lb)
	metric tons (1,000 kg)	1.1	short tons
	milliliters (ml)	0.03	fluid ounces (fl oz)
	liters (l)	2.1	pints (pt)
	liters	1.06	quarts (qt)
Volume	liters	0.26	gallons (gal)
	cubic meters (m^3)	35	cubic feet (ft^3)
	cubic meters	1.3	cubic yards (yd^3)
Temperature	Celsius (°C) temperature	9/5 (then add 32)	Fahrenheit (°F) temperature

Source: Adapted from "Some References on Metric Information" by U.S. Department of Commerce, National Bureau of Standards.

Weight Equivalents

	Milligram	Gram	Kilogram	Grain	Ounce	Pound
1 microgram (mg)	0.001	0.000001				
1 milligram (mg)	1.0	0.001		0.0154		
1 gram (g)	1,000.0	1.0	0.001	15.4	0.035	0.0022
1 kilogram (kg)	1,000,000.0	1,000.0	1.0	15,400.0	35.2	2.2
1 grain (gr)	64.8	0.065		1.0		
1 ounce (oz)		28.3		437.5	1.0	0.063
1 pound (lb)		453.6	0.454		16.0	1.0

Volume Equivalents

	Cubic Millimeter	Cubic Centimeter	Liter	Fluid Ounce	Pint	Quart
1 cubic millimeter (mm^3)	1.0	0.001				
1 cubic centimeter (cm^3)	1,000.0	1.0	0.001			
1 liter (l)	1,000,000.0	1,000.0	1.0	33.8	2.1	1.06
1 fluid ounce (fl oz)		30.(29.57)	0.03	1.0		
1 pint (pt)		473.0	0.473	16.0	1.0	
1 quart (qt)		946.0	0.946	32.0	2.0	1.0

GLOSSARY

A

absorption—taking up of nutrients in the intestines

abstinence—avoidance

acid-base balance—the regulation of hydrogen ions in body fluids

acidosis—condition in which excess acids accumulate or there is a loss of base in the body

acne—pimples

acquired immune deficiency syndrome (AIDS)—caused by the human immunodeficiency virus (HIV) which weakens the body's immune system, leaving it susceptible to fatal infections

acute renal failure (ARF)—suddenly occurring failure of the kidneys

adipose tissue—fatty tissue

adolescent—person between the ages of 13 and 20

aerobic metabolism—Combining nutrients with oxygen within the cell; also called oxidation

albumin—protein that occurs in blood plasma

alcoholism—chronic and excessive use of alcohol

alkaline—base; capable of neutralizing acids

alkalosis—condition in which excess base accumulates in, or acids are lost from, the body

allergen—substance-causing an allergic reaction

allergic reaction—adverse physical reaction to specific substance(s)

allergy—sensitivity to specific substance(s)

amenorrhea—the stoppage of the monthly menstrual flow

amino acids—nitrogen-containing chemical compounds of which protein is composed

amniocentesis—a test to determine the status of the fetus in utero

amniotic fluid—fluid that surrounds fetus in the uterus

amphetamines—drugs intended to inhibit appetite

anabolism—the creation of new compounds during metabolism

anaerobic metabolism—reduces fats without the use of oxygen

anemia—condition caused by insufficient number of red blood cells, hemoglobin, or blood volume

anencephaly—absence of the brain

angina pectoris—pain in the heart muscle due to inadequate blood supply

anorexia nervosa—psychologically induced lack of appetite

anthropometric measurements—measurements of height, weight, head, skinfold

antibodies—substances produced by the body in reaction to foreign substance; neutralize toxins from foreign bodies

antioxidant—substance preventing damage from oxygen

anxiety—apprehension

appetite—learned psychological reaction to food caused by pleasant memories of eating

arteriosclerosis—generic term for thickened arteries

arthritis—chronic disease involving the joints

ascites—abnormal collection of fluid in the abdomen

ascorbic acid—vitamin C

aspartame—artificial sweetener made from two amino acids; does not require insulin for metabolism

aspirated—inhaled or suctioned

atherosclerosis—a form of arteriosclerosis affecting the intima (inner lining) of the artery walls

avitaminosis—without vitamins

B

balanced diet—one that includes all the essential nutrients in appropriate amounts

basal metabolism rate (BMR)—the rate at which energy is needed for body maintenance

beriberi—deficiency disease caused by a lack of vitamin B_1(thiamine)

bile—secretion of the liver, stored in the gallbladder, essential for the digestion of fats

bioavailable—ability of a nutrient to be readily absorbed and used by the body

biochemical tests—involving biology and chemistry

biotin—a B vitamin; necessary for metabolism

bolus—food in the mouth that is ready to be swallowed

bomb calorimeter—device used to scientifically determine the caloric value of foods

bonding—emotional attachment

botulism—deadliest of food poisonings; caused by the bacteria *Clostridium botulinum*

bran—outer covering of grain kernels

buffer systems—protective systems regulating amounts of hydrogen ions in body fluids

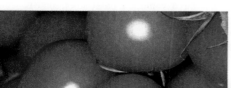

509

bulimia—condition in which patient alternately binges and purges

C

cachexia—severe malnutrition and body wasting caused by chronic disease

caliper—mechanical device used to measure percentage of body fat by skinfold measurement

calorie—also known as kcal or kilocalorie; represents the amount of heat needed to raise the temperature of one kilogram of water one degree Celsius (C)

calorie requirement—number of calories required daily to meet energy needs

capillaries—tiny blood vessels connecting veins and arteries

carbohydrate—the nutrient providing the major source of energy in the average diet

carboxypeptidase—pancreatic enzyme necessary for protein digestion

carcinogen—cancer-causing substance

cardiac sphincter—the muscle at the base of the esophagus that prevents gastric reflux from moving into the esophagus

cardiomyopathy—damage to the heart muscle caused by infection, alcohol, or drug abuse

cardiovascular—pertaining to the heart and entire circulatory system

cardiovascular disease (CVD)—disease affecting heart and blood vessels

carotenoids—plant pigments, some of which yield vitamin A

carrier—one who is capable of transmitting an infectious organism.

catabolism—the breakdown of compounds during metabolism

catalyst—a substance that causes another substance to react

cellular edema—swelling of body cells caused by inadequate amount of sodium in extracellular fluid

cellulose—indigestible carbohydrate; provides fiber in the diet

cerebrovascular accident (CVA)—either a blockage or bursting of blood vessel leading to the brain

chemical digestion—chemical changes in foods during digestion caused by hydrolysis

chemotherapy—treatment of diseased tissue with chemicals

cholecystectomy—removal of the gallbladder

cholecystitis—inflammation of the gallbladder

cholecystokinin—the hormone that triggers the gallbladder to release bile

cholelithiasis—gallstones

cholesterol—fatlike substance that is a constituent of body cells; is synthesized in the liver; also found in animal foods

chronic kidney disease—slow development of kidney failure

chylomicron—largest lipoprotein; transports lipids after digestion into the body

chyme—the food mass as it has been mixed with gastric juices

chymotrypsin—pancreatic enzyme necessary for the digestion of proteins

circulation—the body process whereby the blood is moved throughout the body

cirrhosis—generic term for liver disease characterized by cell loss

clinical examination—physical observation

coagulate—to thicken

cobalamin—organic compound known as vitamin B_{12}

coenzyme—an active part of an enzyme

collagen—protein substance that holds body cells together

colon—the large intestine

colostomy—opening from colon to abdomen surface

coma—state of unconsciousness

compensated heart disease—heart disease in which the heart is able to maintain circulation to all body parts

complementary proteins—incomplete proteins that when combined provide all nine essential amino acids

complete proteins—proteins that contain all nine essential amino acids

congestive heart failure (CHF)—a form of decompensated heart disease

coronary artery disease—severe narrowing of the arteries that supply blood to the heart

crash diets—fad-type diets intended to reduce weight very quickly; in fact they reduce water, not fat tissue

creatinine—an end (waste) product of protein metabolism

Crohn's disease—a chronic progressive disorder that causes inflammation, ulcers, and thickening of intestinal walls, sometimes causing obstruction

cumulative effects—results of something done repeatedly over many years

cystine—a nonessential amino acid

cysts—growths

D

daily values—represent percentage per serving of each nutritional item listed on new food labels based on daily intake of 2,000 calories

decompensated heart disease—heart disease in which the heart cannot maintain circulation to all body parts

deficiency disease—disease caused by the lack of a specific nutrient

dehydrated—having lost large amounts of water

dehydration—loss of water

demineralization—loss of mineral or minerals

dental caries—decayed areas on teeth; cavities

dentition—arrangement, type, and number of teeth

depression—an indentation; or feelings of extreme sadness

dermatitis—inflammation of the skin

descriptors—terms used to describe something

desensitize—to gradually reduce the body's sensitivity (allergic reaction) to specific items

diabetes mellitus—chronic disease in which the body lacks the normal ability to metabolize glucose

diabetic coma—unconsciousness caused by a state of acidosis due to too much sugar or too little insulin

dialysis—mechanical filtration of the blood; used when the kidneys are no longer able to perform normally

diaphragm—thin membrane or partition

dietary fiber—indigestible parts of plants; absorbs water in large intestine, helping to create soft, bulky stool; some is believed to bind cholesterol in the colon, helping to rid cholesterol from the body; some is believed to lower blood glucose levels

Dietary Guidelines for Americans—general goals for optimal nutrient intake

dietary laws—rules to be followed in meal planning in some religions

Dietary Reference Intakes (DRIs)—combines the Recommended Dietary Allowances, Adequate Intake, Estimated Average Requirements, and Tolerable Upper Intake Levels for individuals into one value representative of the average daily nutrient intake of individuals over time

dietary-social history—evaluations of food habits, including client's ability to buy and prepare foods

dietitian—a professional trained to assess nutrition status and recommend appropriate diet therapy

digestion—breakdown of food in the body in preparation for absorption

disaccharides—double sugars that are reduced by hydrolysis to monosaccharides; examples are sucrose, maltose, and lactose

diuretics—substances used to increase the amount of urine excreted

diverticulitis—inflammation of the diverticula

diverticulosis—intestinal disorder characterized by little pockets forming in the sides of the intestines; pockets are called diverticula

dumping syndrome—nausea and diarrhea caused by food moving too quickly from the stomach to the small intestine

duodenal ulcer—ulcer occurring in the duodenum

duodenum—first (and smallest) section of the small intestine

dysentery—disease caused by microorganism; characterized by diarrhea

dyslipidemia—increased lipids in the blood

dyspepsia—gastrointestinal discomfort of vague origin

dysphagia—difficulty swallowing

E

eclamptic stage—convulsive stage of toxemia

edema—the abnormal retention of fluid by the body

electrolyte—chemical compound that in water breaks up into electrically charged atoms called ions

elemental formulas—those formulas containing products of digestion of proteins, carbohydrates, and fats; also called hydrolyzed formulas

elimination—evacuation of wastes

elimination diet—limited diet in which only certain foods are allowed; intended to find the food allergen causing reaction

endocardium—lining of the heart

endogenous insulin—insulin produced within the body

endometrium—mucous membrane of the uterus

endosperm—the inner part of the kernel of grain; contains the carbohydrate

end-stage renal disease (ESRD)—the stage at which the kidneys have lost most or all of their ability to function

energy balance—occurs when the caloric value of food ingested equals the kcal expended

energy imbalance—eating either too much or too little for the amount of energy expended

energy requirement—number of calories required by the body each day

enriched foods—foods to which nutrients, usually B vitamins and iron, have been added to improve their nutritional value

enteral nutrition—feeding by tube directly into the client's digestive tract

enterotoxins—toxins affecting mucous membranes

enzyme—organic substance that causes changes in other substances

esophagitis—inflammation of mucosal lining of esophagus

esophagus—tube leading from the mouth to the stomach; part of the gastrointestinal system

essential hypertension—high blood pressure with unknown cause; also called primary hypertension

essential nutrients—nutrients found only in food

estrogen—hormone secreted by the ovaries

etiology—cause

exchange lists—lists of foods with interchangeable nutrient and kcal contents; used in specific forms of diet therapy

exogenous insulin—insulin produced outside the body

extracellular—outside the cell

extracellular fluid—water outside the cells; approximately 35% of total body fluid

F

fad diets—currently popular weight-reducing diets; usually nutritionally inadequate and not useful or permanent methods of weight reduction

fast foods—restaurant food that is ready to serve before orders are taken

fat cell theory—belief that fat cells have a natural drive to regain any weight lost

fats (lipids)—highest caloric-value nutrient

fat-soluble—can be dissolved in fat

fatty acids—a component of fats that determines the classification of the fat

feces—solid waste from the large intestine

fermentation—changing of sugars and starches to alcohol

fetal alcohol syndrome (FAS)—subnormal physical and mental development caused by mother's excessive use of alcohol during pregnancy

fetal malformations—physical abnormalities of the fetus

fetus—infant in utero

fibrosis—development of tough, stringy tissue

flatulence—gas in the intestinal tract

flavonoids—naturally occurring water-soluble plant pigments that act as antioxidants

folate/folic acid—a form of vitamin B, also called folacin; essential for metabolism

food customs—food habits

food diary—written record of all food and drink ingested in a specified period

food faddists—people who have certain beliefs about particular foods or diets

food poisoning—foodborne illness

free radical—atoms or groups of atoms with an odd (unpaired) number of electrons; can be formed when oxygen interacts with certain molecules

fructose—the simple sugar (monosaccharide) found in fruit and honey

fundus (of the stomach)—upper part of the stomach

G

galactose—the simple sugar (monosaccharide) to which lactose is broken down during digestion

galactosemia—inherited error in metabolism that prevents normal metabolism of galactose

galactosuria—galactose in the urine

gastric bypass—surgical reduction of the stomach

gastric juices—the digestive secretions of the stomach

gastric ulcer—ulcer in the stomach

gastrin—hormone released by the stomach

gastroesophageal reflux (GER)—backflow of stomach contents into the esophagus

gastrointestinal (GI) tract—pertaining to the stomach and intestines

gastrostomy—opening created by the surgeon directly into the stomach for enteral nutrition

genetic predisposition—inherited tendency

geriatrics—the branch of medicine involved with diseases of the elderly

germ—embryo or tiny life center of each kernel of grain

gerontology—the study of aging

gestational diabetes—diabetes occurring during pregnancy; usually disappears after delivery of the infant

glomerular filtration rate (GFR)—the rate at which the kidneys filter the blood

glomerulonephritis—inflammation of the glomeruli of the kidneys

glomerulus—filtering unit in the kidneys

glucagon—hormone from alpha cells of pancreas; helps cells release energy

glucose (dextrose)—the simple sugar to which carbohydrate must be broken down for absorption; also known as *dextrose*

gluten—protein found in grains

glycerol—a component of fat; derived form a water-soluble carbohydrate

glycogen—glucose as stored in the liver and muscles

glycogen loading—process in which the muscle store of glycogen is maximized; also called carboloading

glycosuria—excess sugar in the urine

goiter—enlarged tissue of the thyroid gland due to a deficiency of iodine

H

Heliobacter pylori—bacteria that can cause peptic ulcer

heme iron—part of hemoglobin molecule in animal foods

hemicellulose—dietary fiber found in whole grains

hemodialysis—cleansing the blood of wastes by circulating the blood through a machine that contains tubing of semipermeable membranes

hemolysis—the destruction of red blood cells

hemorrhage—unusually heavy bleeding

hepatitis—inflammation of the liver caused by viruses, drugs, and alcohol

HbgA1c—a blood test to determine how well blood glucose has been controlled for the last 3 months

hiatal hernia—condition wherein part of the stomach protrudes through the diaphragm into the chest cavity

high-density lipoproteins (HDLs)—lipoproteins that carry cholesterol from cells to the liver for eventual excretion

homeostasis—state of physical balance; stable condition

hormone—chemical messengers secreted by a variety of glands

human immunodeficiency virus (HIV)—a virus that weakens the body's immune system and ultimately leads to AIDS

hunger—physiological need for food

hydrogenation—the combining of fat with hydrogen, thereby making it a saturated fat and solid at room temperature

hydrolysis—the addition of water resulting in the breakdown of the molecule

hydrolyzed formulas—contain products of digestion of proteins, carbohydrates, and fats; also called elemental formulas; used for clients who have difficulty digesting food

hypercholesterolemia—unusually high levels of cholesterol in blood; also known as high serum cholesterol

hyperemesis gravidarum—nausea so severe as to be life-threatening

hyperglycemia—excessive amounts of sugar in the blood

hyperkalemia—excessive amounts of potassium in the blood

hyperlipidemia—excessive amounts of fats in the blood

hypermetabolic—higher than normal rate of metabolism

hypersensitivity—abnormally strong sensitivity to certain substance(s)

hypertension—higher than normal blood pressure

hyperthyroidism—condition in which the thyroid gland secretes too much thyroxine and T3; the body's rate of metabolism is unusually high

hypervitaminosis—condition caused by excessive ingestion of one or more vitamins

hypoalbuminemia—abnormally low amounts of protein in the blood

hypoglycemia—subnormal levels of blood sugar

hypokalemia—low level of potassium in the blood

hypothalamus—area at base of brain that regulates appetite and thirst

hypothyroidism—condition in which the thyroid gland secretes too little thyroxine and T$_3$; body metabolism is slower than normal

I

iatrogenic malnutrition—caused by treatment or diagnostic procedures

ileostomy—opening from ileum to abdomen surface

ileum—last part of the small intestine

immunity—ability to resist certain diseases

inborn errors of metabolism—congenital disabilities preventing normal metabolism

incomplete proteins—proteins that do not contain all of the nine essential amino acids

infarct—dead tissue resulting from blocked artery

inflammatory bowel disease (IBD)—chronic condition causing inflammation in the gastrointestinal tract

insecticide—agent that destroys insects

insulin—secretion of the islets of Langerhans in the pancreas gland; essential for the proper metabolism of glucose

insulin reaction—hypoglycemia leading to insulin coma caused by too much insulin or too little food

international units—units of measurement of some vitamins; $5 \mu g = 200$ international units

interstitial fluid—fluid between cells

intracellular—within the cell

intracellular fluid—water within cells; approximately 65% of total body fluid

intrinsic factor—secretion of stomach mucosa essential for B_{12} absorption

invisible fats—fats that are not immediately noticeable, such as those in egg yolk, cheese, cream, and salad dressings

iodized salt—salt that has had the mineral iodine added for the prevention of goiter

ions—electrically charged atoms resulting from chemical reactions

iron deficiency—intake of iron is adequate, but the body has no extra iron stored

iron-deficiency anemia—condition resulting from inadequate amount of iron in the diet, reducing the amount of oxygen carried by the blood to the cells

ischemia—reduced blood flow causing inadequate supply of nutrients and oxygen to, and wastes from, tissues

islets of Langerhans—part of the pancreas from which insulin is secreted

isoleucine—an amino acid

J

jaundice—yellow cast of the skin and eyes

jejunostomy—opening created by the surgeon in the intestine for enteral nutrition

jejunum—the middle section comprising about two-fifths of the small intestine

K

Kaposi's sarcoma—type of cancer common to individuals with AIDS

kcal—the unit used to measure the fuel value of foods

Keshan disease—condition causing abnormalities in the heart muscle

ketonemia—ketones collected in the blood

ketones—substances to which fatty acids are broken down in the liver

ketonuria—ketone bodies in the urine

ketoacidosis—condition in which ketones collect in the blood; caused by insufficient glucose available for energy

kilocalorie—*see* kcal

Krebs cycle—a series of enzymatic reactions that serve as the main source of cellular energy

kwashiorkor—deficiency disease caused by extreme lack of protein

L

lactase—enzyme secreted by the small intestine for the digestion of lactose

lactation—the period during which the mother is nursing the baby

lactation specialist—expert on breastfeeding

lacteals—lymphatic vessels in the small intestine that absorb fatty acids and glycerol

lacto-ovo vegetarian—vegetarians who will eat dairy products and eggs but no meat, poultry, or fish

lactose—the sugar in milk; a disaccharide

lactose intolerance—inability to digest lactose because of a lack of the enzyme lactase; causes abdominal cramps and diarrhea

lacto-vegetarians—vegetarians who eat dairy products

lean body mass—percentage of muscle tissue

lecithin—fatty substance found in plant and animal foods; a natural emulsifier that helps transport fats in the bloodstream; used commercially to make food products smooth

legumes—plant food that is grown in a pod; for example, beans or peas

leucine—an amino acid

lignins—dietary fiber found in the woody parts of vegetables

linoleic acid—fatty acid essential for humans; cannot be synthesized by the body

linolenic acid—one of three fatty acids needed by the body; cannot be synthesized by the body

lipid—fat

lipoproteins—carriers of fat in the blood

longevity—length of life

Lofenalac—commercial infant formula with 95% of phenylalanine removed

low-density lipoproteins (LDLs)—carry blood cholesterol to the cells

lumen—the hollow area in a tube

lymphatic system—transports fat-soluble substances from the small intestine to the vascular system

M

macrosomia—birthweight over 9 pounds

malignant—life-threatening

malnutrition—poor nutrition

maltase—enzyme secreted by the small intestine essential for the digestion of maltose

maltose—the double sugar (disaccharide) occurring as a result of the digestion of grain

maple syrup urine disease (MSUD)—disease caused by an inborn error of metabolism in which the body cannot metabolize certain amino acids

marasmus—severe wasting caused by lack of protein and all nutrients or faulty absorption; PEM

mechanical digestion—the part of digestion that requires certain mechanical movement such as chewing, swallowing, and peristalsis

megadose—extraordinarily large amount

megaloblastic anemia—anemia in which the red blood cells are unusually large and are not completely mature

mental retardation—below-normal intellectual capacity

metabolic—based on metabolism

metabolism—the use of food by the body after digestion which results in energy

metastasize—spread of cancer cells from one organ to another

milliequivalent—the concentration of electrolytes in a solution

mineral—one of many inorganic substances essential to life and classified generally as minerals

modular formulas—made by combining specific nutrients

mold—a type of fungus

monosaccharides—simplest carbohydrates; sugars that cannot be further reduced by hydrolysis; examples are glucose, fructose, and galactose

monosodium glutamate (MSG)—a form of flavor enhancer containing large amounts of sodium

monounsaturated fats—fats that are neither saturated nor polyunsaturated and are thought to play little part in atherosclerosis

morbid—damaging to health

morning sickness—early morning nausea common to some pregnancies

mucilage—gel-forming dietary fiber

mutations—changes in the genes

myelin—lipoprotein essential for the protection of nerves

myocardial infarction (MI)—heart attack; caused by the blockage of an artery leading to the heart

myocardium—heart muscle

myoglobin—protein compound in muscle that provides oxygen to cells

MyPyramid—outline for making selections based on *Dietary Guidelines for America, 2005*. From the U.S. Department of Agriculture

N

nasogastric (NG) tube—tube leading from the nose to the stomach for tube feeding

necrosis—tissue death due to lack of blood supply

negative nitrogen balance—more nitrogen lost than taken in

neoplasia—abnormal development of cells

neoplasm—abnormal growth of new tissue

nephritis—inflammatory disease of the kidneys

nephrolithiasis—kidney, or renal, stones

nephron—unit of the kidney containing a glomerulus

nephrosclerosis—hardening of renal arteries

neural tube defects (NTDs)—congenital malformation of brain and/or spinal column due to failure of neural tube to close during embryonic development

neuropathy—nerve damage

neurotoxins—toxins affecting the nervous system

niacin—B vitamin

niacin equivalent (NE)—unit for measuring niacin; 1 NE equals 1 mg niacin or 60 mg tryptophan

nitrogen—chemical element found in protein; essential to life

nitrogen balance—when nitrogen intake equals nitrogen excreted

nonheme iron—iron from animal foods that is not part of the hemoglobin molecule; and all iron from plant foods

nontropical sprue—a disorder of the gastrointestinal tract characterized by malabsorption; also called gluten sensitivity

normal weight—average weight for size and age

nourishing—foods or beverages that provide substantial amounts of essential nutrients

nutrient—chemical substance found in food that is necessary for good health

nutrient density—nutrient value of foods compared with number of calories

nutrient requirement—amount of specific nutrient needed by the body

nutrition—the result of those processes whereby the body takes in and uses food for growth, development, and the maintenance of health

nutritional status—one's physical condition as determined by diet

nutrition assessment—evaluation of nutritional status

nutritious—foods or beverages containing substantial amounts of essential nutrients

O

obesity—excessive body fat, 20% above average

obstetrician—doctor who cares for the mother during pregnancy and delivery

occlusions—blockages

oliguria—decreased output of urine to less than 500 ml a day

omega-3 fatty acids—polyunsaturated fatty acids found in fish oil; may contribute to reduction of coronary artery disease

oncologist—doctor specializing in the study of cancer

oncology—the study of cancer

on demand—feeding infants as they desire

opportunistic infections—caused by microorganisms that are present but that do not normally affect people with healthy immune systems

osmolality—number of particles per kilogram of solution; solutions with high osmolality exert more pressure than do those with fewer particles

osmosis—movement of a substance through a semipermeable membrane

osteomalacia—a condition in which bones become soft, usually in adult women, because of calcium loss

osteoporosis—condition in which bones become brittle because there have been insufficient mineral deposits, especially calcium

overweight—weight 10%–20% above average

oral diabetes medication—oral hypoglycemic agents; medications that may be given to type 2 diabetics to lower blood glucose

P

pancreas—gland that secretes enzymes essential for digestion and insulin, which is essential for glucose metabolism

pancreatic amylase—the enzyme secreted by the pancreas that is essential for the digestion of starch

pancreatic lipase—the enzyme secreted by the pancreas that is essential for the digestion of fat

pancreatic protease—the enzyme secreted by the pancreas that is essential for the digestion of protein

pancreatitis—inflammation of the pancreas

pantothenic acid—a B vitamin

parenteral nutrition—nutrition provided via a vein

pathogens—disease-causing agents

pectin—edible thickening agent

peer group—group of people approximately one's own age

peer pressure—pressure of one's friends and colleagues of the same age

pellagra—deficiency disease caused by a lack of niacin

pepsin—an enzyme secreted by the stomach that is essential for the digestion of proteins

peptic ulcer—ulcer of the stomach or duodenum

peptidases—enzymes secreted by the small intestine that are essential for the digestion of protein

pericardium—outer covering of the heart

periodontal disease—disease of the mouth and gums

peripheral vascular disease (PVD)—narrowed arteries some distance from the heart

peripheral vein—a vein that is near the surface of the skin

peristalsis—rhythmical movement of the intestinal tract; moves the chyme along

peritoneal dialysis—removal of waste products from the blood by injecting the flushing solution into the abdomen and using the client's peritoneum as the semipermeable membrane

pernicious anemia—severe, chronic anemia caused by a deficiency of vitamin B_{12}; usually due to the body's inability to absorb B_{12}

pH—symbol for the degree of acidity or alkalinity of a solution

phenylalanine—an amino acid

phenylalanine hydroxylase—liver enzyme necessary to metabolize the amino acid phenylalanine

phenylketonuria (PKU)—condition caused by an inborn error of metabolism in which the infant lacks an enzyme necessary to metabolize the amino acid phenylalanine

phenylpropanolamine—constituent of diet pills; can damage blood vessels

phlebitis—inflammation of a vein

physical trauma—extreme physical stress

physiological—relating to bodily functions

phytochemicals—substances occurring naturally in plant foods

pica—abnormal craving for nonfood substance

placenta—organ in the uterus that links blood supplies of mother and infant

plaque—fatty deposit on interior of artery walls

plateau period—period in which there is no change

polycystic kidney disease—rare, hereditary kidney disease causing cysts or growths on the kidneys that can ultimately cause kidney failure in middle age

polydipsia—abnormal thirst

polymeric formulas—commercially prepared formulas for tube feedings that contain intact proteins, carbo- hydrates, and fats that require digestion

polypeptides—10 or more amino acids bonded together

polyphagia—excess hunger

polysaccharides—complex carbohydrates containing combinations of monosaccharides; examples include starch, dextrin, cellulose, and glycogen

polyunsaturated fats—fats whose carbon atoms contain only limited amounts of hydrogen

polyuria—excessive urination

positive nitrogen balance—nitrogen intake exceeds outgo

precursor—something that comes before something else; in vitamins it is also called a provitamin, something from which the body can synthesize the specific vitamin

pregnancy-induced hypertension (PIH)—typically occurs during late pregnancy; characterized by high blood pressure, albumin in the urine, and edema

pressure ulcers—bedsores

primary hypertension—high blood pressure resulting from an unknown cause

prohormone—substance that precedes the hormone and from which the body can synthesize the hormone

protein energy malnutrition (PEM)—marasmus and kwashiorkor

proteins—the only one of six essential nutrients containing nitrogen

proteinuria—protein in the urine

provitamin—*see* precursor

psychosocial development—relating to both psychological and social development

purines—end products of nucleoprotein metabolism

pylorus—the end of the stomach nearest the intestine

R

resting energy expenditure (REE)—*see* basal metabolism rate

regurgitation—vomiting

renal stones—kidney stones

renal threshold—kidneys' capacity

resection—reduction

respiration—breathing

retardation—slowing

retinol—the preformed vitamin A

retinol equivalent (RE)—the equivalent of 3.33 IU of vitamin A

retinopathy—damage to small blood vessels in the eyes

riboflavin—the name for vitamin B_2

rickets—deficiency disease caused by the lack of vitamin D; causes malformed bones and pain in infants

S

saliva—secretion of the salivary glands

salivary amylase—also called ptyalin; the enzyme secreted by the salivary glands to act on starch

salmonella—an infection caused by the *Salmonella* bacteria

satiety—feeling of satisfaction; fullness

saturated fats—fats whose carbon atoms contain all of the hydrogen atoms they can; considered a contributory factor in atherosclerosis

scurvy—a deficiency disease caused by a lack of vitamin C

secondary hypertension—high blood pressure caused by another condition such as kidney disease

secretin—the hormone that causes the pancreas to release sodium bicarbonate to neutralize acidity of the chyme

self-esteem—feelings of self-worth

sepsis—infection of the blood

serum cholesterol—cholesterol in the blood

set-point theory—belief that everyone has a natural weight ("set point") at which the body is most comfortable

skeletal system—body's bone structure

skin tests—allergy tests using potential allergens on scratches on the skin

solute—the substance dissolved in a solution

solvent—liquid part of a solution

spina bifida—spinal cord or spinal fluid bulge through the back

spontaneous abortion—occurring naturally; miscarriage

Staphylococcus **(staph)**—genus of bacteria causing food poisoning called "staph" or "staphylococcal poisoning"

starch—polysaccharide found in grains and vegetables

stasis—stoppage or slowing

steatorrhea—abnormal amounts of fat in the feces

sterile—free of infectious organisms

stoma—surgically created opening in the abdominal wall

stomach banding—surgical reduction of stomach, but to lesser degree than bypass

sucralose—a sweetener made from molecule of sugar

sucrase—enzyme secreted by the small intestine to aid in digestion of sucrose

sucrose—a double sugar or disaccharide; examples are granulated, powdered, and brown sugar

T

tetany—involuntary muscle movement

thiamine—vitamin B_1

thrombosis—blockage, as a blood clot

thrombus—blood clot

tocopherols—vitamers of vitamin E

tocotrienols—a form of vitamin E

total parenteral nutrition—*see* TPN

toxicity—state of being poisonous

TPN—total parenteral nutrition; process of providing all nutrients intravenously

trans-fatty acids (TFAs)—produced by adding hydrogen atoms to a liquid fat, making it a solid

transferase—a liver enzyme necessary for the metabolism of galactose

trichinosis—disease caused by the parasitic roundworm *Trichinella spiralis*; can be transmitted through under-cooked pork

triglycerides—combinations of fatty acids and glycerol

trimester—3-month period; commonly used to denote periods of pregnancy

trypsin—pancreatic enzyme; helps digest proteins

tube feeding (TF)—feeding by tube directly into the stomach or intestine

24-hour recall—listing the types, amounts, and preparation of all foods eaten in the past 24 hours

type 1 diabetes—diabetes occurring suddenly between the ages of 1 and 40; clients secrete little, if any, insulin and require insulin injections and a carefully controlled diet

type 2 diabetes— diabetes occurring after age 40; onset is gradual, and production of insulin gradually diminishes; can usually be controlled by diet and exercise

U

ulcerative colitis—disease characterized by inflammation and ulceration of the colon, rectum, and sometimes entire large intestine

underweight—weight that is 10%–15% below average

urea—chief nitrogenous waste product of protein metabolism

uremia—condition in which protein wastes are circulating in the blood

ureters—tubes leading from the kidneys to the bladder

uric acid—one of the nitrogenous waste products of protein metabolism

urticaria—hives; common allergic reaction

V

valine—an amino acid

vascular disease—disease of the blood vessels

vascular osmotic pressure—high concentration of electrolytes in the blood; low blood volume or blood pressure

vascular system—circulatory system

vegans—vegetarians who avoid all animal foods

very-low-density lipoproteins (VLDLs)—lipoproteins made by the liver to transport lipids throughout the body

villi—the tiny, hairlike structures in the small intestines through which nutrients are absorbed

visible fats—fats in foods that are purchased and used as fats, such as butter or margarine

vitamins—organic substances necessary for life although they do not, independently, provide energy

vitamin supplements—concentrated forms of vitamins; may be in tablet or liquid form

W

water—major constituent of all living cells; composed of hydrogen and oxygen

water-soluble—can be dissolved in water

weaning—training an infant to drink from the cup instead of the nipple

wellness—a way of life that integrates body, mind, and spirit

whey—the liquid part of milk that separates from the curd (solid part) during the making of hard cheese

X

xerophthalmia—serious eye disease characterized by dry mucous membranes of the eye, caused by a deficiency of vitamin A

xerostomia—sore, dry mouth caused by a reduction of salivary secretions; may be caused by radiation for treatment of cancer

Y

yo-yo effect—refers to crash diets; the dieter's weight goes up and down over short periods because these diets do not change eating habits

American Academy of Pediatrics. (2003, June). *Pediatrics, 111*(6) Suppl. Retrieved January 19, 2005, from http://pediatrics.aapublications.org/content/vol1111/issue6/index/shtml#suppLS2.

American Cancer Society. (2003). *Resolve to reduce your risk of cancer.* Retrieved June 14, 2006, from http://www.cancer.org/docroot/NWS/content/NWS_2_1x_Resolve_to_Reduce_Your_Risk_of_Cancer.asp.

American Diabetes Association and the American Dietetic Association. (1995). *Exchange list for meal planning.* Alexandria, VA: American Diabetes Association.

Bitomsky, M. (2001, September 29). Yogurt, fermented drinks good for bowel disease. *Reuters Health.*

Brody, J. (2005, March). What's good for the heart is good for the head. *New York Times.*

California bans soda in public high schools. (n.d.). *MSNBC News.* Retrieved January 19, 2006, from http://www.msnbc.msn.com/id/9355436.

Chait, J. (2002, August). Siblings of African-Americans with diabetes often have kidney problems, too. *Diabetes Health Magazine—American Journal of Kidney Diseases.* Retrieved June 15, 2006, from http://www.diabeteshealth.com/read,1021,3083.html.

Farshchi, H., Taylor, M., & Macdonald, I. (2005, February). Deleterious effects of omitting breakfast on insulin sensitivity and fasting lipid profiles in healthy lean women. *American Journal of Clinical Nutrition, 81,* 388–396.

Food and Nutrition Board, Institute of Medicine, & National Academies of Science. (2002). *Dietary reference intakes for energy, carbohydrates, fiber, fat, fatty acids, cholesterol, protein, and amino acids.* Retrieved June 15, 2006, from http://www.iom.edu/?id=4340&redirect=0.

Food and Nutrition Board, National Academies of Science, & Institute of Medicine. (1997). Dietary *reference intakes for calcium, phosphorus, magnesium, vitamin D, and fluoride.* Retrieved June 15, 2006, from http://www.iom.edu/CMS/3788/4008/4253.aspx.

Food and Nutrition Board, National Academies of Sciences, & Institute of Medicine. (2001). *Dietary reference intakes for vitamin A, vitamin K, arsenic, boron, chromium, copper, iodine, iron, manganese, molybdenum, nickel, silicon, vanadium, and zinc.* Retrieved June 15, 2006, from http://www.iom.edu/CMS/3788/4574/8521.aspx.

Food and Nutrition Service, U.S. Department of Agriculture, Centers for Disease Control and Prevention, U.S. Department of Health and Human Services, & U.S. Department of Education. (2005, January). *Making it happen! School nutrition success stories.* Retrieved May 4, 2006, from http://www.cdc.gov/HealthyYouth/Nutrition/Making-It-Happen.

Food and Nutrition Service, U.S. Department of Agriculture. (2005, September). *MyPyramid for kids.* Retrieved January 19, 2006, from http://teamnutrition.usda.gov/Resources/mpk_poster2.pdf.

Food and Nutrition Service, U.S. Department of Agriculture. (2005, September). *Children's activity pyramid.* Retrieved January 19, 2006, from http://teamnutrition.usda.gov/Resources/moveit.pdf.

Food and Nutrition Service, U.S. Department of Agriculture. (1990). *Meal pattern requirements and offer versus serve manual.* Publication FNS-265.

Gebhardt, S. E., & Thomas, R. G. (2002). *Nutritive value of foods.* (Agricultural Research Home and Garden Bulletin, 72, 14–89.)

Hedley, A. A., Ogden, C. L., Johnson, C. L., Carroll, M. D., Curtin, L. R., & Flegal, K. M. (2004). Overweight and obesity among U.S. children, adolescents, and adults, 1999-2002. *Journal of the American Medical Association, 291,* 2847–50.

Hoyert, D. L., Kung, H. C., & Smith, B. L. (2005). Deaths: Preliminary data for 2003. *National Vital Statistics Reports, 53*(15). Hyattsville, MD: National Center for Health Statistics.

Human Nutrition Information Service, USDA. (1990, June). *Report of the Dietary Guidelines Committee on the Dietary Guidelines for Americans—1990.* Hyattsville, MD: U.S. Government Printing Office.

Human Nutrition Information Service, USDA. (2000). *Report of the Dietary Guidelines Advisory Committee on the*

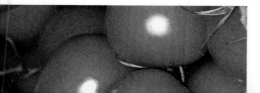

Dietary Guidelines for Americans—2000. Hyattsville, MD: U.S. Government Printing Office.

Lose an inch in a pinch. (2004, May). *Associated Press.* Retrieved from www.kmov.com.

Meisel, P. (2005). Hypertension, diabetes: Chocolate with a single remedy? *Hypertension, 46*(2), 398–405.

National Academy of Sciences. (1989). *Recommended dietary allowances* (10th ed.). Washington, DC: National Academy Press.

National Academy of Sciences. (1997). *Dietary reference intakes.* Washington, DC: National Academy Press.

National Academy of Sciences. (1998). *DRI report.* Retrieved from http://www.nap.edu.

National Academy of Sciences. (2001). *Adequate intakes for selected minerals.* Washington, DC: National Academy Press.

National Institutes of Health, Osteoporosis and Related Bone Diseases Resource Center. (2000, October). Osteoporosis overview. Retrieved June 15, 2006, from http://www.osteo.org/osteo.html.

National Institutes of Health. (2001, February). Study shows new link between salt sensitivity and risk of death [news release]. Retrieved June 15, 2006, from http://www.nih.gov/news/pr/feb2001/nhlbi-15.htm.

National Institutes of Health. (2005). Lifestyle changes especially effective at preventing type 2 diabetes in adults aged 60 and older. Data complied and retrieved December 2, 2005, from http://www.ndep.nih.gov/campaigns/tools.htm.

National Kidney Foundation. (2005, October 4). Canadian to help fight kidney disease. Retrieved from http://www.kidney.org/news/newsroom/newsitem.cFm?id=270.

Nelsonn, J. K., Moxness, K. E., Gastineau, C. F., & Jenson, M. D. (1994). *Mayo Clinic diet manual: A handbook of nutrition practices* (7th ed.). St. Louis, MO: Mosby.

Obesity. (2005). *Atlanta Journal-Constitution.* Retrieved June 15, 2006, from http://www.ajc.com/health/healthfd/shared/health/adam/ency/article/003101.html.

People eat more when they are served more. (2004, October). *Journal of Nutrition, 134,* 2546–2549.

Protein in human milk reduces risk of obesity. (2004, May). *Medical Study News.* Retrieved June 15, 2006, from http://www.news-medical.net/?id=1173

Rosenberg, K. D., Gelow, J. M., & Sandoval, A. P. (2004, May). Pregnancy intendedness and the use of periconceptual folic acid. *Pediatrics, 111*(5), 1142–1145.

Runners: Beware too much water. (2005, April 15). *CBS News.* Retrieved from http://www.cbsnews.com/stories/2005/04/12/earlyshow/contributors/emilysenay.

Spratto, G. R., & Woods, A. L. (2006). *PDR nurse's drug handbook.* Clifton Park, NY: Thomson Delmar Learning and Medical Economics of Thomson Healthcare.

Trecroci, D. (2005, November). Mark Consuelos encourages Type 2s and their loved ones to take "diabetes freedom" pledge. *Diabetes Health.* Retrieved June 15, 2006, from http://www.diabeteshealth.com/read,1038,4445.html.

Tufts University. (2005, June). Happiness and your heart. *Health and nutrition letter.*

Two-for-one portions are double trouble. (2003). *Discovery Health.* Retrieved June 15, 2006, from http://health.discovery.com/news/afp/20030630/portionsize.html.

U.S. Department of Agriculture. (1981). *Nutritive value of foods.* (Home and Garden Bulletin, 72.)

U.S. Department of Agriculture. (2002). *Nutritive value of foods (rev. ed.).* (Home and Garden Bulletin, 72.)

U.S. Department of Agriculture. (2005). *MyPyramid food intake patterns.* Retrieved December 2, 2005, from http://www.mypyramid.gov/professionals/pdf_food_intake.html.

U.S. Department of Agriculture, Agricultural Research Service. (2005). *USDA national nutrient database for standard reference, release 18.* Retrieved June 13, 2006, from http://www.ars.usda.gov/ba/bhnrc/ndl.

U.S. Department of Agriculture, Center for Nutrition Policy and Promotion. (2005, April). Publication CNPP-XX. Washington, DC: Author.

U.S. Department of Agriculture & U.S. Department of Health and Human Services. (1990). *Dietary guidelines for Americans* (3rd ed.). Retrieved May 5, 2005 from http://www.nal.usda.goc/fnic/dga/weight.htm.

U.S. Department of Agriculture & U.S. Department of Health and Human Services. (1990). Maintain healthy weight. In *Nutrition and your health: Dietary guidelines for Americans.* (Home and Garden Bulletin No. 232.) Retrieved May 5, 2005, from http://www.nal.usda.gov/fnic/dga/weight.htm.

U.S. Department of Agriculture & U.S. Department of Health and Human Services. (2005). *Dietary guidelines for Americans 2005* (6th ed.). Washington, DC: U.S. Government Printing Office.

U.S. Department of Agriculture & U.S. Department of Health and Human Services. (2005). *MyPyramid food guidance system.* Retrieved from http://www.mypyramid.gov.

U.S. Department of Agriculture & U.S. Department of Health and Human Services. (2005). *Nutrition and your health: Dietary guidelines for Americans* (6th ed.).

Walk slowly for weight loss. (2005, May). University of Colorado at Boulder [news release]. Retrieved June 15, 2006, from http://www.colorado.edu/news/releases/2005/252.html.

Wheat Foods Council. (2005). Twists and turns of fad diets. Retrieved from www.wheatfoods.org.

White, L. (2005). *Foundations of adult health nursing* (2nd ed.). Clifton Park, NY: Thomson Delmar Learning.

Yara, S. (2005, October). Best and worst vending machine snacks. *Forbes.com.* Retrieved June 15, 2006, from http://www.msnbc.msn.com/id/9620780.

BIBLIOGRAPHY

BOOKS

Cataldo, C. B. (2003). *Nutrition and diet therapy* (6th ed.). Belmont, CA: Wadsworth Publishing Company.

Dudek, S. G. (2006). *Nutrition essentials for nursing practice* (5th ed.). Philadelphia: Lippincott.

Grodner, M., Long, S., & DeYoung, S. (2004). *Foundations and clinical applications of nutrition: A nursing approach* (3rd ed.). St. Louis, MO: Mosby.

Lutz, C. A., & Rutherford, K. P. (2006). *Nutrition and diet therapy* (4th ed.). Philadelphia: Davis.

Mahan, L. K., & Escott-Stump, S. (2003). *Krause's food nutrition and diet therapy* (11th ed.). Philadelphia: Saunders.

Mitchell, M. K. (2002). *Nutrition across the life span* (2nd ed.). Philadelphia: Saunders.

National Kidney Foundation. (2005, October 4). Comedian to help fight kidney disease since having a transplant. Retrieved April 4, 2006, from www.kidney.org/news/newsroom/newsitem.cfm?id=270

Osteometer MediTech. (2004). *Risk factors.* Retrieved from www.osteometer.com/osteoporosis/facts.htm

Trahms, C. M., & Pipes P. (2001). *Nutrition in infancy and childhood* (7th ed.). New York: McGraw-Hill.

Wardlaw, G. M., & Insel, P. M. (2002). *Perspectives in nutrition* (6th ed.). New York: Mosby-Year Book.

Whitney, E. N., DeBruyne, L. K., Pinna, K., & Rolfes, S. R. (2007). *Nutrition for health & health care* (3rd ed.). Belmont, CA: Wadsworth Publishing Company.

Whitney, E. N., & Rolfes, S. R. (2005). *Understanding nutrition* (10th ed.). Belmont, CA: Wadsworth Publishing Company.

Williams, S. R. (2005). *Basic nutrition and diet therapy* (12th ed.). St. Louis, MO: Mosby.

Worthington-Roberts, B. S., & Williams, S. R. (Eds.). (2000). *Nutrition throughout the life cycle.* New York: McGraw-Hill.

PERIODICALS AND PUBLICATIONS

American Heart Association. (2005). AHA Scientific Statement. Dietary recommendations for children and adolescents. *Circulation, 112,* 1061–1075.

Amylin Pharmaceuticals. (n.d.). First-in-class, incretin mimetic. Retrieved from www.Byetta.com

Barclay, L. (2005). American Heart Association updates guidelines for children. Retrieved April 4, 2006, from www.medscape.com/viewarticle/513792

Browning, R., & Kram, R. (2005, May). Energetic cost and preferred speed of walking in obese vs. normal weight women. *Obesity Research, 13,* 891–899.

California wants to serve a warning with fries. (n.d.). *The New York Times.* Retrieved October 10, 2005, from www.nytimes.com

Calorie Control Council. (2005). Percentage of obese Americans increases in most states. Retrieved September 19, 2005, from www.caloriecontrol.org

Centers for Disease Control and Prevention. (2006). BMI—Body mass index: BMI for children and teens. Retrieved June 8, 2006, from www.cdc.gov/nccdphp/dnpa/bmi/childrens_BMI/about_childrens_BMI.htm

Centers for Disease Control and Prevention. (2005). Overweight and obesity: Home. Retrieved April, 12 2005 from www.cdc.gov

Centers for Disease Control and Prevention and National Center for Health Statistics. (n.d.). *Prevalence of overweight among children and adolescents: United States, 1999–2002.* Retrieved June 8, 2006, from www.cdc.gov/nchs/products/pubs/pubd/hestats/overwght99.htm

Collins, N. (2001, March/April). Tube feeding and pressure ulcers. *Advances in Skin and Wound Care.*

Diabetic-Lifestyle Online Magazine. (2004, December). Diabetes and osteoporosis. Retrieved from www.diabetic-lifestyle.com

Enger, S. M., Ross, R. K., Henderson, B., & Bernstein, L. (1997). Breastfeeding history, pregnancy experience and risk of breast cancer. *British Journal of Cancer, 76*(1), 118–123.

Food & Nutrition Board, Institute of Medicine. (1997). *Dietary reference intakes of calcium, phosphorus, magnesium, vitamin D, and fluoride.* Washington, DC: National Academy Press.

Food & Nutrition Board, Institute of Medicine. (2004). *Dietary reference intakes for water, potassium, sodium, chloride, and sulfate.* Washington, DC: National Academy Press.

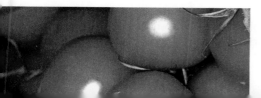

Food & Nutrition Board, Institute of Medicine. (1998). *Dietary reference intakes of thiamin, riboflavin, niacin, vitamin B₆, folate, vitamin B₁₂, pantothenic acid, biotin, and choline.* Washington, DC: National Academy Press.

Food & Nutrition Board, Institute of Medicine. (2000). *Dietary reference intakes for vitamin C, vitamin E, selenium and carotenoids.* Washington, DC: National Academy Press.

Food & Nutrition Board, Institute of Medicine. (2001). *Dietary reference intakes for vitamin A, vitamin K, arsenic, boron, chromium, copper, iodine, iron, manganese, molybdenum, nickel, silicon, vanadium and zinc.* Washington, DC: National Academy Press.

Food & Nutrition Board, Institute of Medicine. (2005). *Dietary reference intakes for energy, carbohydrate, fiber, fat, fatty acids, cholesterol, protein, and amino acids (macronutrients).* Washington, DC: National Academy Press.

Food Insight: Current topics in Food Safety and Nutrition. (2001, July/August). *IACP ON Tour: Exploring the Issues of Food Biotechnology,* 2–3.

Gutzin, S. J., et al. (2003). The safety of oral hypoglycemic agents in the first trimester of pregnancy: A meta analysis. *Canadian Journal of Pharmacology, 42*(4), 303–313.

Hamvas, J., Schwab, R., & Pap, A. (2001). Jejunal feeding in chronic pancreatitis with severe necrosis. *Journal of Pancreas* (Online), *2*(3), 112–116. [Full text] Available: www.jcplink.net/prev/200105/200105_5.pdf

Hedley, A. A., et al. (2004). Prevalence of overweight and obesity among US children, adolescents, and adults, 1999–2002. *Journal of the American Medical Association, 291*(23), 2847–2850.

Hu, F. B., Manson, J. E., Stampfer, M. J., Colditz, G., Liu, S., Solomon, C. G., & Willett, W. C. (2001). Diet, lifestyle, and the risk of type 2 diabetes mellitus in women. *The New England Journal of Medicine, 345,* 790–797.

Lakdawalla, D., Goldman, D., & Shang, B. (2005, September 26). The health and cost consequences of obesity among the elderly. *Health Affair.*

Lockyear, P. L. B. (2004). Childhood eating behaviors: Developmental and sociocultural consideration. *Medscape OB/GYN & Women's Health 9*(1). Retrieved April 4, 2005, from www.medscape.com/viewarticle/467523_print

Michels, K. B., Willett, W. C., Rosner, B. A., Manson, J. E., Hunter, D. J., Colditz, G. A., Hankinson, S. E., & Speizer, F. E. (1996). Prospective assessment of breastfeeding and breast cancer incidence among 89,887 women. *Lancet, 347,* 431–436.

MSNBC News. (n.d.). California bans soda in public high schools. Retrieved from www.msnbc.msn.com

Mukherjee, S., Anlonarakis, E., Asadvzzaman, S., Peters, J. (2005). Acute psychological stress-induced water intoxication. *International Journal of Psychiatry in Clinical Practice, 9*(2), 142–144.

National Geographic Society. (2005). Some couch potatoes born that way, fat study says. Retrieved June 10, 2005, from www.nationalgeographic.com/news/2005/01/0127_050127_couchpotato.html

Pearce, C. B., & Duncan, H. D. (2002). Enteral feeding, nasogastric, nasojejunal, percutaneous endoscopic, gastrostomy vs. jejunostomy; its indications and limitations. *Postgraduate Medical Journal 78,* 198–204.

Regions Hospital. Coming to the burn center. Retrieved December 2005, from www.regionshospital.com/Regions/Menu/0,11369,00.html

Stroud, M., Duncan, H., & Nightingale, J. (2003). Guidelines for enteral feeding in adult hospital patients. *Gut, 52,* vii1–vii12.

U.S. Department of Agriculture. (2005). *MyPyramid.* Retrieved from www.mypyramid.gov

U.S. Department of Health & Human Services. (2005). Citing "dangerous increase" in deaths, HHS launches new strategies against overweight epidemic. Retrieved June 12, 2005, from www.hhs.gov www.hhs/news/2004pres/20040309.html

U.S. National Library of Medicine. (2005). Gastric bypass (Medline). Retrieved September 19, 2005, from www.nlm.nih.gov/medlineplus/print/ency/article/009199.htm

University of Maryland Medical Center. (2005). How can gallstones and gallbladder disease be prevented? Retrieved September 19, 2006, from www.umm.edu/patiented/articles/how_can_gallstones_gallbladder_disease_be_prevented

INTERNET SITES

Agricultural Research Service, www.ars.usda.gov

AIDS.Org, www.aids.org

Alpha Nutrition, www.nutramed.com

American Cancer Society, www.cancer.org

American Heart Association, www.americanheart.com

American Obesity Association, www.obesity.org

American Society for Gastrointestinal Endoscopy, www.asge.org

American Society for Parenteral and Enteral Nutrition, www.clinnutr.org

Arthritis Foundation, www.arthritis.org

Cancer Supportive Care, www.cancersupportivecare.com

Cycling Performance Tips, www.cptips.com

Forbes.com, Inc., www.forbes.com

HeartInfo.Org, www.heartinfo.org

Indiana State University, www.web.indstate.edu

La Leche League International, www.lalecheleague.org

March of Dimes Birth Defects Foundation, www.marchofdimes.org

Mayo Foundation for Medical Education and Research, www.mayoclinic.com

McDonald's, www.mcdonalds.com

Medical College of Wisconsin, www.healthlink.mcw.edu

National Digestive Diseases Information Clearinghouse, www.digestive.niddk.nih.gov

National Geographic Society, www.nationalgeographic.com. Search nutrition.

National Kidney Foundation, www.kidney.org

National Heart, Lung, and Blood Institute, www.nhlbi.nib.gov

National Institute of Diabetes & Digestive & Kidney Diseases, www.niddk.nih.gov

National Institutes of Health, www.nih.gov

National Library of Medicine, www.nlm.nih.gov

National Osteoporosis Foundation, www.nof.org

New York Times, www.nytimes.com

Personal MD, www.personalmd.com

People Living with Cancer, www.plwc.org

Quest Health Library, www.questhealthlibrary.com

U.S. Centers for Disease Control and Prevention, www.cdc.gov

U.S. Department of Agriculture, www.usda.gov

U.S. Department of Health & Human Services. www.smallstep.gov

U.S. Food and Drug Administration, www.fda.gov

U.S. National Agricultural Library, www.nal.usda.gov

U.S. National Institute of Allergy and Infectious Disease, www.niaid.nih.gov

U.S. National Institutes of Health, www.nih.gov

U.S. National Library of Medicine, www.nlm.nih.gov

Wikipedia, www.wikipedia.org

WorldWide Anaesthetist, www.anaesthetist.com

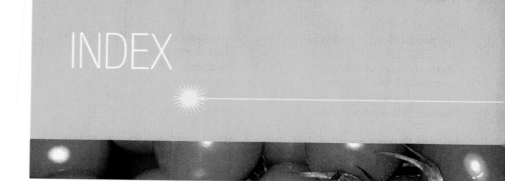

INDEX

STUDYWARE™ TO ACCOMPANY *NUTRITION & DIET THERAPY*, NINTH EDITION

Minimum System Requirements

Operating System: Microsoft Windows 98 SE, Windows 2000, or Windows XP

Processor: Pentium PC 500 MHz or higher (750 MHz recommended)

Memory: 64 MB of RAM (128 MB recommended)

Screen Resolution: 800 x 600 pixels

Color Depth: 16-bit color (thousands of colors)

Macromedia Flash Player V7.x. The Macromedia Flash Player is free, and can be downloaded from http://www.macromedia.com

Installation Instructions

1. Insert disc into CD-ROM drive. The StudyWare™ installation program should start automatically. If it does not, go to step 2.

2. From My Computer, double-click the icon for the CD drive.

3. Double-click the *setup.exe* file to start the program.

Technical Support

Telephone: 1-800-477-3692, 8:30 A.M.-5:30 P.M. Eastern Time

Fax: 1-518-881-1247

E-mail: *delmarhelp@thomson.com*

StudyWare™ is a trademark used herein under license.
Microsoft® and Windows® are registered trademarks of the Microsoft Corporation.
Pentium® is a registered trademark of the Intel Corporation.

IMPORTANT! READ CAREFULLY: This End User License Agreement ("Agreement") sets forth the conditions by which Thomson Delmar Learning, a division of Thomson Learning Inc. ("Thomson") will make electronic access to the Thomson Delmar Learning-owned licensed content and associated media, software, documentation, printed materials, and electronic documentation contained in this package and/or made available to you via this product (the "Licensed Content"), available to you (the "End User"). BY CLICKING THE "I ACCEPT" BUTTON AND/OR OPENING THIS PACKAGE, YOU ACKNOWLEDGE THAT YOU HAVE READ ALL OF THE TERMS AND CONDITIONS, AND THAT YOU AGREE TO BE BOUND BY ITS TERMS, CONDITIONS, AND ALL APPLICABLE LAWS AND REGULATIONS GOVERNING THE USE OF THE LICENSED CONTENT.

1.0 SCOPE OF LICENSE

1.1 <u>Licensed Content</u>. The Licensed Content may contain portions of modifiable content ("Modifiable Content") and content which may not be modified or otherwise altered by the End User ("Non-Modifiable Content"). For purposes of this Agreement, Modifiable Content and Non-Modifiable Content may be collectively referred to herein as the "Licensed Content." All Licensed Content shall be considered Non-Modifiable Content, unless such Licensed Content is presented to the End User in a modifiable format and it is clearly indicated that modification of the Licensed Content is permitted.

1.2 Subject to the End User's compliance with the terms and conditions of this Agreement, Thomson Delmar Learning hereby grants the End User, a nontransferable, nonexclusive, limited right to access and view a single copy of the Licensed Content on a single personal computer system for noncommercial, internal, personal use only. The End User shall not (i) reproduce, copy, modify (except in the case of Modifiable Content), distribute, display, transfer, sublicense, prepare derivative work(s) based on, sell, exchange, barter or transfer, rent, lease, loan, resell, or in any other manner exploit the Licensed Content; (ii) remove, obscure, or alter any notice of Thomson Delmar Learning's intellectual property rights present on or in the Licensed Content, including, but not limited to, copyright, trademark, and/or patent notices; or (iii) disassemble, decompile, translate, reverse engineer, or otherwise reduce the Licensed Content.

2.0 TERMINATION

2.1 Thomson Delmar Learning may at any time (without prejudice to its other rights or remedies) immediately terminate this Agreement and/or suspend access to some or all of the Licensed Content, in the event that the End User does not comply with any of the terms and conditions of this Agreement. In the event of such termination by Thomson Delmar Learning, the End User shall immediately return any and all copies of the Licensed Content to Thomson Delmar Learning.

3.0 PROPRIETARY RIGHTS

3.1 The End User acknowledges that Thomson Delmar Learning owns all rights, title and interest, including, but not limited to all copyright rights therein, in and to the Licensed Content, and that the End User shall not take any action inconsistent with such ownership. The Licensed Content is protected by U.S., Canadian and other applicable copyright laws and by international treaties, including the Berne Convention and the Universal Copyright Convention. Nothing contained in this Agreement shall be construed as granting the End User any ownership rights in or to the Licensed Content.

3.2 Thomson Delmar Learning reserves the right at any time to withdraw from the Licensed Content any item or part of an item for which it no longer retains the right to publish, or which it has reasonable grounds to believe infringes copyright or is defamatory, unlawful, or otherwise objectionable.

4.0 PROTECTION AND SECURITY

4.1 The End User shall use its best efforts and take all reasonable steps to safeguard its copy of the Licensed Content to ensure that no unauthorized reproduction, publication, disclosure, modification, or distribution of the Licensed Content, in whole or in part, is made. To the extent that the End User becomes aware of any such unauthorized use of the Licensed Content, the End User shall immediately notify Thomson Delmar Learning. Notification of such violations may be made by sending an e-mail to delmarhelp@thomson.com.

5.0 MISUSE OF THE LICENSED PRODUCT

5.1 In the event that the End User uses the Licensed Content in violation of this Agreement, Thomson Delmar Learning shall have the option of electing liquidated damages, which shall include all profits generated by the End User's use of the Licensed Content plus interest computed at the maximum rate permitted by law and all legal fees and other expenses incurred by Thomson Delmar Learning in enforcing its rights, plus penalties.

6.0 FEDERAL GOVERNMENT CLIENTS

6.1 Except as expressly authorized by Thomson Delmar Learning, Federal Government clients obtain only the rights specified in this Agreement and no other rights. The Government acknowledges that (i) all software and related documentation incorporated in the Licensed Content is existing commercial computer software within the meaning of FAR 27.405(b)(2); and (2) all other data delivered in whatever form, is limited rights data within the meaning of FAR 27.401. The restrictions in this section are acceptable as consistent with the Government's need for software and other data under this Agreement.

7.0 DISCLAIMER OF WARRANTIES AND LIABILITIES

7.1 Although Thomson Delmar Learning believes the Licensed Content to be reliable, Thomson Delmar Learning does not guarantee or warrant (i) any information or materials contained in or produced by the Licensed Content, (ii) the accuracy, completeness or reliability of the Licensed Content, or (iii) that the Licensed Content is free from errors or other material defects. THE LICENSED PRODUCT IS PROVIDED "AS IS," WITHOUT ANY WARRANTY OF ANY KIND AND THOMSON DELMAR LEARNING DISCLAIMS ANY AND ALL WARRANTIES, EXPRESSED OR IMPLIED, INCLUDING, WITHOUT LIMITATION, WARRANTIES OF MERCHANTABILITY OR FITNESS OR A PARTICULAR PURPOSE. IN NO EVENT SHALL THOMSON DELMAR LEARNING BE LIABLE FOR: INDIRECT, SPECIAL, PUNITIVE OR CONSEQUENTIAL DAMAGES INCLUDING FOR LOST PROFITS, LOST DATA, OR OTHERWISE. IN NO EVENT SHALL THOMSON DELMAR LEARNING'S AGGREGATE LIABILITY HEREUNDER, WHETHER ARISING IN CONTRACT, TORT, STRICT LIABILITY OR OTHERWISE, EXCEED THE AMOUNT OF FEES PAID BY THE END USER HEREUNDER FOR THE LICENSE OF THE LICENSED CONTENT.

8.0 GENERAL

8.1 Entire Agreement. This Agreement shall constitute the entire Agreement between the Parties and supercedes all prior Agreements and understandings oral or written relating to the subject matter hereof.

8.2 Enhancements/Modifications of Licensed Content. From time to time, and in Thomson Delmar Learning's sole discretion, Thomson Delmar Learning may advise the End User of updates, upgrades, enhancements and/or improvements to the Licensed Content, and may permit the End User to access and use, subject to the terms and conditions of this Agreement, such modifications, upon payment of prices as may be established by Thomson Delmar Learning.

8.3 No Export. The End User shall use the Licensed Content solely in the United States and shall not transfer or export, directly or indirectly, the Licensed Content outside the United States.

8.4 Severability. If any provision of this Agreement is invalid, illegal, or unenforceable under any applicable statute or rule of law, the provision shall be deemed omitted to the extent that it is invalid, illegal, or unenforceable. In such a case, the remainder of the Agreement shall be construed in a manner as to give greatest effect to the original intention of the parties hereto.

8.5 Waiver. The waiver of any right or failure of either party to exercise in any respect any right provided in this Agreement in any instance shall not be deemed to be a waiver of such right in the future or a waiver of any other right under this Agreement.

8.6 Choice of Law/Venue. This Agreement shall be interpreted, construed, and governed by and in accordance with the laws of the State of New York, applicable to contracts executed and to be wholly preformed therein, without regard to its principles governing conflicts of law. Each party agrees that any proceeding arising out of or relating to this Agreement or the breach or threatened breach of this Agreement may be commenced and prosecuted in a court in the State and County of New York. Each party consents and submits to the nonexclusive personal jurisdiction of any court in the State and County of New York in respect of any such proceeding.

8.7 Acknowledgment. By opening this package and/or by accessing the Licensed Content on this Web site, THE END USER ACKNOWLEDGES THAT IT HAS READ THIS AGREEMENT, UNDERSTANDS IT, AND AGREES TO BE BOUND BY ITS TERMS AND CONDITIONS. IF YOU DO NOT ACCEPT THESE TERMS AND CONDITIONS, YOU MUST NOT ACCESS THE LICENSED CONTENT AND RETURN THE LICENSED PRODUCT TO DELMAR LEARNING (WITHIN 30 CALENDAR DAYS OF THE END USER'S PURCHASE) WITH PROOF OF PAYMENT ACCEPTABLE TO THOMSON DELMAR LEARNING, FOR A CREDIT OR A REFUND. Should the End User have any questions/comments regarding this Agreement, please contact Thomson Delmar Learning at delmarhelp@thomson.com.